WORKBOOK

Edward B. Kuvlesky, NREMT-P, AAS
Craig N. Story, MPA

Prehospital Emergency Care

EIGHTH EDITION

Joseph J. Mistovich, MEd, NREMT-P
Chairperson and Professor
Department of Health Professions
Youngstown State University
Youngstown, Ohio

Keith J. Karren, PhD
Professor, Department of Health Sciences
Brigham Young University
Provo, Utah

Medical Editor
Howard A. Werman, MD

Legacy Author
Brent Q. Hafen, PhD

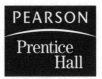

PEARSON

Prentice Hall

Upper Saddle River, New Jersey 07458

About the Writers

Edward B. Kuvlesky, NREMT-P, AAS, is Field Supervisor, Indian River County Fire Rescue, Indian River County, Florida.

Craig N. Story, MPA, is the former EMS program director at Polk Community College in Winter Haven, Florida. He is currently a full-time student completing a PhD in Education at the University of South Florida in Tampa, Florida.

Publisher: Julie Levin Alexander
Publisher's Assistant: Regina Bruno
Executive Editor: Marlene McHugh Pratt
Senior Managing Editor for Development: Lois Berlowitz
Development Editor: Triple SSS Press Media Development
Assistant Editor: Matthew Sirinides
Director of Marketing: Karen Allman
Executive Marketing Manager: Katrin Beacom
Marketing Specialist: Michael Sirinides
Managing Editor for Production: Patrick Walsh
Production Liaison: Faye Gemmellaro
Production Editor: Jessica Balch, Pine Tree Composition
Manufacturing Manager: Ilene Sanford
Manufacturing Buyer: Pat Brown
Cover Designer: Amanda Kavanagh
Cover Photography: Nathan Eldridge
Composition: Pine Tree Composition, Inc.
Printer/Binder: Bind-Rite Graphics
Cover Printer: Phoenix Color Corp.

Notice on Care Procedures

It is the intent of the authors and publisher that this workbook be used as part of a formal EMT education program taught by qualified instructors and supervised by a licensed physician. The procedures described in the textbook and this workbook are based on consultation with EMT and medical authorities. The authors and publisher have taken care to make certain that these procedures reflect currently accepted clinical practice; however, they cannot be considered absolute recommendations.

The material in this workbook contains the most current information available at the time of publication. However, federal, state, and local guidelines concerning clinical practices, including, without limitation, those governing infection control and universal precautions, change rapidly. The reader should note, therefore, that new regulations may require changes in some procedures.

It is the responsibility of the reader to familiarize himself or herself with the policies and procedures set by federal, state, and local agencies as well as the institution or agency where the reader is employed. The authors and the publisher of this workbook disclaim any liability, loss, or risk resulting directly or indirectly from the suggested procedures and theory, from any undetected errors, or from the reader's misunderstanding of the text. It is the reader's responsibility to stay informed of any new changes or recommendations made by any federal, state, and local agency as well as by his or her employing institution or agency.

Notice on Gender Usage

The English language has historically given preference to the male gender. Among many words, the pronouns "he" and "his" are commonly used to describe both genders. Society evolves faster than language, and the male pronouns still predominate in our speech. The authors have made great effort to treat the two genders equally, recognizing that a significant percentage of EMTs are female. However, in some instances, male pronouns may be used to describe both males and females solely for the purpose of brevity. This is not intended to offend any readers of the female gender.

Notice on "Case Studies"

The names used and situations depicted in the case studies throughout this workbook are fictitious.

Notice on Medications

The authors and the publisher of this workbook have taken care to make certain that the equipment, doses of drugs, and schedules of treatment are correct and compatible with the standards generally accepted at the time of publication. Nevertheless, as new information becomes available, changes in treatment and in the use of equipment and drugs become necessary. The reader is advised to carefully consult the instruction and information material included in the page insert of each drug or therapeutic agent, piece of equipment, or device before administration. This advice is especially important when using new or infrequently used drugs. Prehospital care providers are warned that use of any drugs or techniques must be authorized by their medical director, in accord with local laws and regulations. The publisher disclaims any liability, loss, injury, or damage incurred as a consequence, directly or indirectly, of the use and application of any of the contents of this workbook.

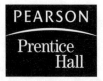

10 9 8 7 6 5 4 3 2 1
ISBN-13 978-0-13-174159-1
ISBN-10 0-13-174159-4

CONTENTS

INTRODUCTION

Welcome to the *Prehospital Emergency Care, Eighth Edition Workbook*. We have combined our writing skills and our knowledge as prehospital health care professionals and educators to produce a highly functional supplement for you. This is a self-instructional workbook, written to reinforce key concepts presented in the textbook. You can work on the chapters at your own pace and monitor your progress and understanding by checking the *Answer Key* and rereading text pages indicated in the key.

Every chapter includes five basic sections: Cognitive Objectives, Key Ideas, Terms and Concepts, Content Review, and Case Study. Three additional sections appear, as appropriate, in many of the chapters. These special sections are: Medical Terminology, Enrichment, and Documentation Exercise.

The content of the five basic sections is as follows: *Cognitive Objectives* lists knowledge objectives from the United States Department of Transportation's 1994 *Emergency Medical Technician-Basic: National Standard Curriculum*. The same objectives are listed at the beginning of the corresponding textbook chapter. *Key Ideas* summarizes the chapter's key concepts. *Terms and Concepts* reviews major terms that are introduced in bold type in the textbook chapter and are listed and defined at the end of the textbook chapter. *Content Review* presents questions to review your understanding of important information and concepts from the textbook chapter. *Case Study* presents one or more realistic scenarios—situations similar to those you may encounter on real emergency calls—and requires you to apply chapter information to solving patient management problems.

The content of the three special sections that appear in many chapters is as follows: *Medical Terminology* presents a chart of chapter-relevant medical terms that are frequently used in emergency care. For each term, the chart provides a pronunciation, breaks the term into a defined prefix, root, and suffix, and ends with a definition of the whole term. Questions following the chart reinforce the meanings and often highlight how the term might be used in an emergency situation. *Enrichment* provides questions about the Enrichment section of the corresponding textbook chapter. *Documentation Exercise* presents a real-life emergency-call scenario that is longer and more detailed than the Case Study scenarios, including detailed vital signs and other physical exam and patient history information that you would gather on such a call. A few questions to check understanding of the scenario follow. The final piece of the exercise is a blank prehospital care report form that you will fill out, using information from the scenario, as if you were the EMT who had responded to that call. Note that *no answers* are provided for the PCR form. There will be differences in the way each student completes the form, especially in the narrative segment. We recommend that after you fill out the document to the best of your ability, you discuss it with fellow students and your instructor to help you sharpen your documentation skills.

Great effort has been taken to provide high quality multiple-choice questions (with a few fill-ins here and there) because this is the accepted format of most standardized tests, such as a state or the National Registry exam. The *Course Review Self-Test* (160 items covering all chapters in the text) is entirely in multiple-choice format. The test items for the various chapters are in scrambled order, as they might be on a major standardized or national test. However, the chapter each item relates to and the text page on which the information was covered is, again, identifiable by consulting the Answer Key for the Self-Test.

We have provided detachable *Medication Cards* containing information about the six medications that the EMT can administer or assist the patient in administering, with on-line or off-line approval from medical direction.

The authors and the publisher have worked diligently to produce the finest study supplement possible. We welcome any comments you may have regarding this workbook and ask that you please address your suggestions to the publisher. We wish you much success in your studies and as an Emergency Medical Technician.

Ed Kuvlesky
Craig Story

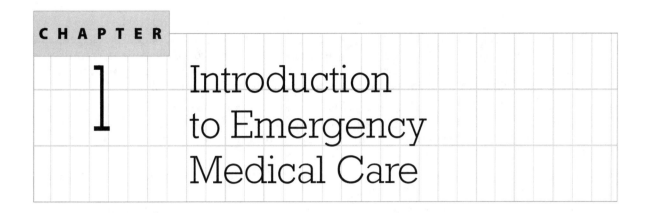

CHAPTER

1 Introduction to Emergency Medical Care

OBJECTIVES

Numbered objectives are from the United States Department of Transportation EMT-Basic National Standard Curriculum. Asterisked objectives, if any, pertain to material that is supplemental to the DOT curriculum.

The terminology used in these and subsequent objectives uses the titles First Responder, EMT-B (EMT-Basic), EMT-I (EMT-Intermediate), and EMT-P (EMT-Paramedic). These titles are in the process of being phased out and replaced with the terms Emergency Medical Responder (EMR), Emergency Medical Technician (EMT), Advanced Emergency Medical Technician (AEMT), and Paramedic. For consistency the updated terms will be used here. The job titles and the rationale for this transition are fully explained in the textbook.

Cognitive

1-1.1 Define Emergency Medical Services (EMS) systems.
1-1.2 Differentiate the roles and responsibilities of the EMT-Basic from other prehospital care providers.
1-1.3 Describe the roles and responsibilities related to personal safety.
1-1.4 Discuss the roles and responsibilities of the EMT-Basic toward the safety of the crew, the patient, and bystanders.
1-1.5 Define quality improvement and discuss the EMT-Basic's role in the process.
1-1.6 Define medical direction and discuss the EMT-Basic's role in the process.
1-1.7 State the specific statutes and regulations in your state regarding the EMS system.

KEY IDEAS

This chapter describes the EMS system and the roles and responsibilities of the EMT. Emphasis is placed on the personal safety of the EMT and the safety of other rescuers.

■ Prehospital care is provided by the EMS (Emergency Medical Services) system. Each state manages its EMS system in its own way, using federal guidelines.

■ EMS, fire, and law enforcement services may be accessed in many areas by the universal access number 9-1-1 and in other areas by non-9-1-1 numbers.

■ The four levels of emergency medical service practitioners identified in the *National EMS Scope of Practice Model* are Emergency Medical Responder (EMR), Emergency Medical Technician (EMT), Advanced Emergency Medical Technician (AEMT), and Paramedic.

■ The health-care system includes the EMS system, emergency departments, and specialized-care facilities such as trauma, burn, obstetrical, pediatric, poison, stroke, cardiac, spine injury, and hyperbaric centers.

- The responsibilities of the EMT include personal safety, the safety of others, patient assessment and emergency medical care, safe lifting and moving, transport and transfer of the patient, recordkeeping and data collection, and patient advocacy. Your first priority is your own safety, then the safety of other rescuers. Once the scene is safe, the patient's needs are your priority.

- The professional attributes required of the EMT are knowledge and skills, a professional appearance, good health, a calm and reassuring personality, leadership abilities, good judgment, moral character, stability and adaptability, resourcefulness, an ability to listen, and an ability to cooperate with others.

- Every EMS system must have a physician medical director who is legally responsible for the clinical and patient-care aspects of the system.

- The goal of quality improvement is to identify aspects of the system that can be improved and to implement programs to improve identified shortcomings.

TERMS AND CONCEPTS

1. Write the number of the correct term next to each definition.
   1. EMS system
   2. EMT
   3. Advanced Emergency Medical Technician (AEMT)
   4. Paramedic
   5. Emergency Medical Responder (EMR)
   6. Prehospital care

   ___4___ a. One who is trained in all aspects of prehospital care including intravenous lines, administering medications, decompressing chest injuries, reading electrocardiograms, and manual defibrillation.

   ___5___ b. The first person on the scene who has emergency-care training.

   ___1___ c. An organization that coordinates emergency care as part of the continuum of health care.

   ___6___ d. Care provided prior to transport to the hospital.

   ___3___ e. One who is certified to perform some (but not all) advanced prehospital emergency-care skills.

   ___2___ f. One who performs skills in three areas: controlling life-threatening situations, stabilizing nonlife threats, and nonmedical skills such as driving. Has completed a course based on the U.S. Department of Transportation curriculum.

CONTENT REVIEW

1. The roles and responsibilities of the EMT include
   a. insertion of intravenous lines.
   b. controlling life-threatening situations.
   c. decompressing the chest cavity.
   d. reading and interpreting electrocardiograms.

2. The EMT's responsibilities for scene safety include
   a. personal safety first, then other rescuers'/bystanders' safety, then patient safety.
   b. other rescuers'/bystanders' safety first, then personal safety, then patient safety.
   c. personal safety first; the EMT has no responsibility for the safety of others.
   d. patient safety first, then other rescuers'/bystanders' safety, then personal safety.

3. From the following list, select the items that are potential hazards that may be present at an emergency scene.
    1. A poorly lit, high-traffic area
    2. A car leaking gasoline
    3. A chemical spill
    4. A crime scene
    a. 2, 3
    b. 2, 4
    c. 1, 2, 3, 4
    d. 1, 2, 3

4. The risk of being struck by traffic at nighttime scenes is
    a. seldom a risk for the EMT or other emergency responders.
    b. reduced by wearing dark clothing and waving a flare from side to side.
    c. reduced by wearing reflective clothing and providing adequate scene lighting.
    d. an assumed risk that is "just a part of the job."

5. You are responding to the scene of a shooting. The dispatcher advises you that law enforcement is also responding. Upon arrival you observe a large crowd of people who appear to be fighting. The patient is lying next to the crowd. Law enforcement has not yet arrived. You should next
    a. be alert to any threat and approach the patient.
    b. retreat to a safe area and await law enforcement arrival.
    c. exit the vehicle and await law enforcement arrival.
    d. remain in the vehicle and await law enforcement arrival.

6. A process of internal and external reviews and audits of all aspects of an emergency medical system is called which of the following?
    a. Chart review
    b. Quality improvement
    c. Medical command
    d. Medical control

7. The EMT must wear protective equipment to decrease the risks of infectious-disease exposure. The protective clothing most commonly worn for this purpose includes
    a. leather gloves, hard hat, eye protection, boots.
    b. latex gloves, eye protection, mask, gown.
    c. turnout gear, helmet, boots, mask.
    d. leather gloves, helmet, boots, and self-contained breathing apparatus.

8. During a routine physical examination, your personal physician informs you that he is interested in becoming the medical director for the service that you work for. He asks you to describe the medical director's responsibilities. Which of the following are important responsibilities of the medical director?
    1. Is involved in EMS education programs and refresher courses
    2. Is only responsible for providing on-line medical direction
    3. Develops and establishes guidelines under which emergency service personnel function
    4. Is only responsible for providing off-line medical direction
    a. 1, 2
    b. 1, 3
    c. 2, 4
    d. 1, 2, 3

9. Which statement best describes the relationship between the EMT and the EMS system medical director?
   a. The prehospital care rendered by the EMT is not governed or controlled by the medical director.
   b. All care rendered by the EMT is considered an extension of the medical director's authority.
   c. The in-hospital care rendered by the EMT is considered an extension of the medical director's authority.
   d. The medical director advises the on-scene paramedic, who guides the EMT.

10. To be effective as an EMT, you must have the personality characteristics that are listed below. Using a 1–5 ranking system (5 is the highest), rate your own personality characteristics.

Personal rank

_____ Pleasant personality (ability to get along with others, reassuring and calming voice and manner)

_____ Leadership ability (takes control, sets priorities, able to give clear directions)

_____ Good judgment (able to make appropriate decisions quickly in unsafe or stressful conditions)

_____ Good moral character (high ethical standards)

_____ Stability (able to deal with feelings openly and honestly)

_____ Resourcefulness and improvisation (able to adapt to change quickly and use resources effectively)

_____ Ability to listen (able to be an effective listener)

_____ Cooperativeness (able to act as a leader while cooperating with others)

11. The EMT is responsible for the patient's privacy and valuables. The EMT should also honor patient requests, if possible. The term that best describes these responsibilities is
    a. EMS advocacy.
    b. patient's rights.
    c. EMS rights.
    d. patient advocacy.

12. 9-1-1 is frequently called the "Universal Number." What services can generally be accessed by calling 9-1-1?
    a. Law enforcement and fire services only
    b. Law enforcement and EMS only
    c. Law enforcement, EMS, and fire services
    d. Fire services and EMS only

CASE STUDY

It's 1:00 in the morning, and you have been dispatched to a single-vehicle auto crash. You wipe the sleep from your eyes and prepare to respond to the call. The dispatcher informs you that law enforcement is on-scene, and there is one patient who has a possible head injury. A fire/rescue truck is also responding to the call. The car has struck a power pole just over the top of a steep hill.

1. Which has the primary responsibility for traffic control at this scene?
   a. Fire/rescue department
   b. EMS/ambulance service
   c. Power company
   d. Law enforcement

2. Which has the primary responsibility for extrication/rescue at this scene?
   a. Fire/rescue department
   b. EMS/ambulance service
   c. Power company
   d. Law enforcement

3. Which has the primary responsibility for patient care and transport?
   a. Fire/rescue department
   b. EMS/ambulance service
   c. Power company
   d. Law enforcement

Law enforcement is on-scene controlling traffic as you arrive. The fire/rescue crew and power company have stabilized potential hazards. You evaluate the patient and determine that he has minor injuries and is in stable condition. While you are transporting the patient to the hospital, the patient asks you to please call his wife and let her know he is OK.

4. Which statement best describes the most appropriate action to take in response to the patient's request to call his wife and explain what has happened?
   a. Contact the police and let them call his wife.
   b. Contact your supervisor and let the supervisor call his wife.
   c. Explain that this is not a part of your responsibilities.
   d. Call the patient's wife and explain what has happened.

5. What information is most likely to be used by EMS system administration for quality improvement audits on this call?
   a. Prehospital care report of call
   b. Feedback from crews on scene
   c. Feedback from the patient involved
   d. Feedback from the patient's wife

6. Which of the following creates the greatest potential hazard at this scene?
   a. Highway traffic
   b. Gasoline leak
   c. Power lines
   d. Violent bystander

2 The Well-Being of the EMT

OBJECTIVES

Numbered objectives are from the United States Department of Transportation EMT-Basic National Standard Curriculum. Asterisked objectives, if any, pertain to material that is supplemental to the DOT curriculum.

Cognitive

1-2.1 List possible emotional reactions that the EMT-Basic may experience when faced with trauma, illness, death, and dying.

1-2.2 Discuss the possible reactions that a family member may exhibit when confronted with death and dying.

1-2.3 State the steps in the EMT-Basic's approach to the family confronted with death and dying.

1-2.4 State the possible reactions that the family of the EMT-Basic may exhibit due to their outside involvement in EMS.

1-2.5 Recognize the signs and symptoms of critical incident stress.

1-2.6 State possible steps that the EMT-Basic may take to help reduce/alleviate stress.

1-2.7 Explain the need to determine scene safety.

1-2.8 Discuss the importance of body substance isolation (BSI).

1-2.9 Describe the steps the EMT-Basic should take for personal protection from airborne and bloodborne pathogens.

1-2.10 List the personal protective equipment necessary for each of the following situations:
- Hazardous materials
- Rescue operations
- Violent scenes
- Crime scenes
- Exposure to bloodborne pathogens
- Exposure to airborne pathogens

KEY IDEAS

This chapter provides an overview of ways you can safeguard your emotional and physical well-being while providing emergency care.

■ Your ability to recognize and effectively deal with stressful situations is as essential for your well-being as it is for that of your patients and their family members.

■ The highly charged environment of emergency care requires that you recognize the warning signs of stress and remedy them before stress results in burnout.

■ Scene safety includes practicing body substance isolation to protect yourself from infectious disease and following proper rescue techniques to prevent accidental injury.

TERMS AND CONCEPTS

1. Write the number of the correct term next to each definition.
   1. Burnout
   2. Critical incident stress debriefing (CISD)
   3. Body substance isolation (BSI)
   4. Sterilization
   5. Personal protective equipment (PPE)

   ___1___ a. State of exhaustion and irritability

   ___3___ b. Strict infection control measures based on the presumption that all blood and body fluids are infectious

   ___2___ c. Session in which a team of counselors helps rescuers deal with an emotionally difficult experience

   ___5___ d. Items worn to guard against injury or disease transmission

   ___4___ e. Use of chemical or physical substances to kill all surface microorganisms

CONTENT REVIEW

1. Which of the following is one of the five emotional stages that dying patients will experience?
   a. Repression
   b. Denial
   c. Regression
   d. Confusion

2. Beside each of the following actions that you might take when dealing with a dying patient, family member, or bystander, write "A" for an appropriate action or "I" for an inappropriate action.

   ___A___ a. Talk to the unresponsive patient as if the patient is fully alert.

   ___I___ b. Always remove family members from the area or room during resuscitation efforts.

   ___I___ c. If a critically injured or ill patient asks you, "Am I going to die?", respond by saying, "Everything is going to be OK," or "You are going to be OK."

   ___A___ d. If a dying patient wants a message delivered to survivors, always listen carefully and deliver any message the patient conveys.

3. As an EMT, you should be alert to recognize warning signs of stress. Which of the following may signal stress?
   a. Irritability, loss of appetite, loss of interest in work
   b. Calm demeanor and renewed interest in work
   c. Planning long-term recreational events with family or friends
   d. Ability to get along well with coworkers and friends, able to make decisions

4. A session held prior to a critical incident stress debriefing (CISD) that helps to vent emotions and gather information is which of the following?
   a. Defusing
   b. Critical incident
   c. Peer support
   d. Follow-up service

5. Microorganisms that can spread disease by a person's contact with blood, inhalation of airborne droplets, or touching contaminated objects are generally referred to as
   a. pathogens.
   b. viruses.
   c. bacteria.
   d. contaminants.

6. Which of the following is considered the single most important way to prevent the spread of infection?
   a. Handwashing
   b. Sterilizing reusable equipment
   c. Bagging contaminated laundry
   d. Placing sharp objects in a container

7. Before attempting rescue or patient care in a situation such as a hazardous material or biological agent incident, a high-angle rescue, or a whitewater rescue, you, as an EMT, should usually
   a. contact your emergency-service supervisor for instructions.
   b. consult with law enforcement personnel prior to acting.
   c. call for specialized rescue teams or experts.
   d. quickly enter the emergency scene.

8. Number the steps below in the proper order from 1 to 5 for providing emergency care at a scene involving possible hazardous materials.

   _____5_____ a. Provide patient assessment and emergency care.

   _____2_____ b. Look for and compare placards or signs to the *DOT Hazardous Materials: The Emergency Response Guidebook*.

   _____3_____ c. Make sure the scene is controlled by a specialized hazardous materials team before you enter.

   _____1_____ d. Use binoculars to try to identify hazards before approaching the scene.

   _____4_____ e. Put on appropriate protective clothing, such as a self-contained breathing apparatus and a "hazmat" suit.

9. If you suspect potential violence at an emergency scene, you should
   a. request law enforcement assistance before entering the scene.
   b. enter cautiously and call for law enforcement assistance if needed.
   c. first remove patients from the scene and then call for police assistance.
   d. first secure the scene and then begin patient assessment and care.

10. If you are providing emergency care at a crime scene, you should take precautions to preserve the chain of evidence by
    a. waiting to start treatment until all evidence has been collected by police.
    b. avoiding disturbing the scene unless necessary to provide care.
    c. immediately removing the patient from the scene to begin care.
    d. contacting medical oversight for permission to enter the scene.

CASE STUDY

It's early afternoon, and you have just finished cleaning out the jump kit from a prior call when the alarm bell sounds. You are called to a scene at a railroad yard where one of the workers is trapped from the waist down between two rail cars. Specialty rescue teams are en route and the patient's wife, who has been called by his coworker, has just arrived at the scene. Your patient is responsive. He tells you that he knows that as soon as they separate the cars he will die. He asks that you leave him alone with his wife and that you do nothing heroic to try to intervene.

1. Of the five stages of emotional response to death and dying, which stage does your patient seem to be exhibiting regarding his imminent death?
    a. Denial
    b. Anger
    c. Depression
    d. Acceptance

2. The situation described above would be
    a. considered a high-stress incident.
    b. a routine part of the EMT's job.
    c. something the EMT must learn to live with.
    d. considered an average incident.

As predicted, as soon as the cars are separated, your patient rapidly loses responsiveness and becomes pulseless and apneic. He has sustained massive open crush injuries to his abdomen and pelvis. There is nothing that can be done to save his life, and he dies. In the days following this incident, you begin to have trouble sleeping and often have nightmares. You are having trouble concentrating, and your heart pounds every time you get dispatched on a call.

3. Your partner suggests that the EMS personnel who responded to this incident should attend a stress-management session. Who should *not* participate in the session?
    a. Police personnel
    b. Communications personnel
    c. Emergency department personnel
    d. Patient's family

4. Beside each of the following actions, write "A" for an appropriate action or "I" for an inappropriate action to be taken to mitigate the potential effects of stress.

    _____ a. Drink one or two beers each night when off duty to relieve stress.

    _____ b. Avoid any exercise for at least two months following a high-stress incident.

    _____ c. Avoid sharing details of stressful events with family, friends, or coworkers.

    _____ d. Request a rotation in duty to a busier station to put the stressful event into perspective.

1. Hepatitis B infection
   a. will always cause symptoms such as fever or headache.
   b. is only transmitted by direct contact such as shaking hands.
   c. is a minor medical ailment that resolves itself over a few days.
   d. may be prevented by obtaining a vaccination.

2. Which statement best describes the action to take if the EMT suspects exposure to the hepatitis B virus?
   a. Arrange for an immediate injection of HBIG (hepatitis B immunoglobulin).
   b. Arrange with your personal physician for an immediate hepatitis B vaccination.
   c. Report the incident to your supervisor and follow your local exposure-control policy.
   d. Contact the Centers for Disease Control for the latest treatment recommendations.

3. Tuberculosis
   a. is of little consequence due to its low rate of incidence in the United States.
   b. requires that self-contained breathing apparatus (SCBA) be worn by the EMT.
   c. spreads by droplets from the cough of a patient and from the patient's infected sputum.
   d. is a serious but not a highly infectious disease.

4. The OSHA respiratory protective standards for emergency response personnel includes the use of _____ when in contact with tuberculosis patients.
   a. Self-contained breathing apparatus (SCBA)
   b. Surgical mask
   c. HEPA or N-95 respirator
   d. J350 mask

5. Which of the following has been identified as a mode of transmission of the HIV virus, which causes acquired immune deficiency syndrome (AIDS)?
   a. Direct contact with an infected person, such as shaking hands
   b. Exposure to coughing or sneezing by an infected person
   c. Indirect contact, such as with eating utensils or bed linens used by an infected person
   d. Sexual contact with an infected person

6. Which statement is most correct regarding AIDS?
   a. It results from destruction of the body's hormonal balance.
   b. It is caused by a virus that destroys the body's ability to fight infections.
   c. It always presents with signs and symptoms.
   d. It is easier to contract via occupational exposure than is hepatitis B.

7. You are transferring a patient from one medical facility to another and notice on the patient's transfer orders that he has Hepatitis C. You know that Hepatitis C
   a. can be prevented by obtaining a vaccination.
   b. is the most common bloodborne infection in the United States.
   c. is easily transmitted via mucous membranes.
   d. causes no symptoms in about 10 percent of patients.

8. You and an EMT student intern are transporting a suspected severe acute respiratory syndrome (SARS) patient from a local hospital to a regional medical center for specialized treatment. The patient has a fever of 102 degrees F, is coughing heavily, and generally states that he "aches all over." You and the EMT student intern are wearing eye protection, a surgical mask, and a cover gown. What other action should you take to best protect yourself and your EMT intern?
   a. Remove the surgical mask from the patient to improve communication
   b. Look for signs of fever and respiratory symptoms for 48 hours
   c. Avoid touching your eyes, nose, or mouth with your gloved hands
   d. Avoid washing your hands after glove removal to limit droplet spread

9. You are at the station between calls watching TV with a coworker. A report comes on describing an outbreak of West Nile virus in your community. Your partner asks you what the signs and symptoms of West Nile virus are. Which response best describes severe signs and symptoms?
   a. Vision loss, headache, stiff neck, and muscle weakness
   b. Excessive thirst, yellow vision, and slurred speech
   c. Inability to urinate, nausea, and dizziness
   d. Dyspnea and difficulty in swallowing

10. Multidrug-resistant organisms
   a. are commonly encountered in patients at health spas, resorts, and pools.
   b. are considered to be of little threat or consequence to EMTs.
   c. are never transmitted by person-to-person contact.
   d. include MRSA, VRE, PRSP, and DRSP.

3 Medical, Legal, and Ethical Issues

OBJECTIVES

Numbered objectives are from the United States Department of Transportation EMT-Basic National Standard Curriculum. Asterisked objectives, if any, pertain to material that is supplemental to the DOT curriculum.

Cognitive

1-3.1 Define the EMT-Basic scope of practice.

1-3.2 Discuss the importance of Do Not Resuscitate (DNR) (advance directives) and local or state provisions regarding EMS application.

1-3.3 Define consent and discuss the methods of obtaining consent.

1-3.4 Differentiate between expressed and implied consent.

1-3.5 Explain the role of consent of minors in providing care.

1-3.6 Discuss the implications for the EMT-Basic in patient refusal of transport.

1-3.7 Discuss the issues of abandonment, negligence, and battery and their implications to the EMT-Basic.

1-3.8 State the conditions necessary for the EMT-Basic to have a duty to act.

1-3.9 Explain the importance, necessity, and legality of patient confidentiality.

1-3.10 Discuss the considerations of the EMT-Basic in issues of organ retrieval.

1-3.11 Differentiate the actions that an EMT-Basic should take to assist in the preservation of a crime scene.

1-3.12 State the conditions that require an EMT-Basic to notify local law enforcement.

KEY IDEAS

The EMT-Basic provides patient care in an increasingly complex legal and ethical environment. Important ethical and legal concepts are described in this chapter.

■ The EMT's scope of practice, or the actions and care that are legally allowed by the state in which the EMT is providing care, is determined by the National Highway and Traffic Administration's *National EMS Scope of Practice Model*, the National Standard Curriculum, state law, regulations, and policies.

■ The standard of care describes the care expected of a "reasonably prudent" EMT or how an EMT with similar training in a similar situation would perform. This encompasses what is often called "the reasonable person standard or test." The standard of care is established by EMT textbooks, the care expected by other EMTs in the community or region, local and state protocols, the National Standard Curriculum, and the EMS system's operating policies and procedures.

- Your legal obligation to provide service for a patient is called the "duty to act." Duties to your patient, yourself, your partner, and your equipment are also important concepts.

- Good Samaritan laws are generally designed to protect an individual from liability for acts performed in good faith unless those acts constitute gross negligence. The law provides limited protection for the EMT and vary from state to state.

- The EMT's legal right to function is contingent upon medical oversight.

- A conscious, competent, and rational adult has the right to refuse treatment or transportation.

- Informed consent is provided when the patient is informed of the care to be provided and understands the associated risks and potential consequences of refusing treatment or transportation.

- Permission to care for a patient is called consent. You must obtain consent from every patient prior to treatment. There are three forms of consent: expressed, implied, and minor.

- Three common types of advance directives are a living will, a Do Not Resuscitate (DNR) order, and a health-care durable power of attorney (health-care proxy). As a general rule, you should begin resuscitative efforts when you are unsure about the validity of advance directives.

- Document refusals of care completely and accurately. Make sure the patient is competent (an adult who is lucid and capable of making an informed decision) and not under the influence of drugs or alcohol, consult medical direction, and try again to persuade the patient to accept treatment prior to departing the scene.

- Four items must be demonstrated in a successful negligence action: (1) The EMT had a duty to act. (2) The EMT breached that duty to act. (3) The patient suffered an injury or harm that is recognized by the law as a compensable injury. (4) The injury was the result of the breach of the duty.

- Common intentional torts in EMS are abandonment, assault, battery, false imprisonment, and defamation (slander and libel).

- The Health Insurance Portability and Accountability Act (HIPAA) of 1996 protects the privacy of patient health-care information and provides the patient with control over how the information is used. Information obtained when treating a patient must be kept confidential.

- The Consolidated Omnibus Budget Reconciliation Act (COBRA) and the Emergency Medical Treatment and Active Labor Act (EMTALA) are federal regulations designed to ensure the public's access to emergency health care regardless of their ability to pay. Avoid potential liability by never making a decision to transport to a specific medical facility based on the patient's ability to pay.

- Appropriate crime scene actions include the following: touch or move only what is required to care for the patient, document anything unusual, do not cut through knots or bullet or stab holes in the patient's clothing, and preserve evidence in sexual assault cases.

- Law enforcement should be notified in cases of abuse, injuries related to a crime, and drug-related injuries. Follow your state laws.

- When dealing with difficult legal or ethical issues, always put the welfare of the patient first.

TERMS AND CONCEPTS

1. Write the number of the correct term next to each definition.

   1. advance directive
   2. duty to act
   3. expressed consent
   4. implied consent
   5. minor consent
   6. scope of practice
   7. battery
   8. Good Samaritan law
   9. informed consent
   10. slander
   11. tort

   _5_ a. Permission obtained from a parent or legal guardian for emergency treatment of a patient who is under legal age or who is a mentally incompetent adult.

   _4_ b. Assumes an unresponsive patient would agree to emergency treatment.

   _3_ c. Permission that must be obtained from every conscious, mentally competent adult before emergency treatment may be provided.

   _1_ d. Written instructions regarding future resuscitation and care, such as living wills, DNR orders, and health-care proxies.

   _2_ e. The obligation to care for a patient who requires it.

   _6_ f. The actions and care that are legally allowed to be provided by a health-care provider.

   _11_ g. A civil action.

   _7_ h. The act of touching a patient unlawfully.

   _8_ i. Generally protects a person from liability for acts performed in good faith unless those acts constitute gross negligence.

   _10_ j. Spoken defamation.

   _9_ k. The patient is provided information related to the care and consequences of care.

CONTENT REVIEW

1. Which of the following determines the EMT's scope of practice?
   a. The EMT's capability to perform medical procedures
   b. National EMS Act of 1999
   c. National Standard Curriculum
   d. Federal Medical Practice Act

2. On a call, you begin to dress the severely bleeding wound of an adult patient who has told you to go away and leave her alone. The patient appears competent. You can legally be charged with which of the following?
   a. Breech of duty
   b. Negligence
   c. Abandonment
   d. Battery

3. Which of the following provides some protection from liability for emergency care provided in good faith?
   a. Code of ethics
   b. Malpractice act
   c. Good Samaritan law
   d. Emergency-care statute

4. Emergency care that is expected of any EMT under similar circumstances is known as which of the following?
   a. Standard of care
   b. Code of care
   c. Patient-care guidelines
   d. Emergency-care guidelines

5. Under the law, to care for a patient, you must receive which of the following?
   a. Consent from the wife or husband of the patient
   b. The patient's expressed or implied consent
   c. Prior consent from medical oversight
   d. Consent that is written and witnessed

6. A 10-year-old is critically injured. The parents cannot be located. Treatment can be initiated under which of the following forms of consent?
   a. Implied consent
   b. Expressed consent
   c. Minor consent
   d. Incapacitated consent

7. Under the law, in order to refuse treatment, a *patient* must meet which of the following requirements?
   a. Be mentally competent
   b. Be free of any life-threatening injuries or conditions
   c. Sign a form releasing the EMT from liability
   d. Have a witness to the refusal of treatment

8. Which of the following is considered a valid indication of refusal of care from a competent adult?
   a. Nodding the head "yes" before treatment begins
   b. Pushing you away after treatment has begun
   c. Shrugging the shoulders
   d. Questioning the health-care provider

9. Stopping care without ensuring that another health-care professional with equivalent or better training will take over is called which of the following?
   a. Neglect
   b. Abandonment
   c. Refusal
   d. Battery

10. Confidential patient information may be released only under certain circumstances. Which of the following is one of these circumstances?
    a. While off-duty, another EMT asks you about patient care information.
    b. Your wife asks you what happened at a neighbor's house.
    c. A lawyer calls you and demands information related to the incident.
    d. A health-care provider needs to know in order to continue medical care.

11. Your legal obligation to provide service to a patient while you are on duty (and, in some states, even while you are off duty) is known as
    a. Good Samaritan law.
    b. duty to act.
    c. scope of practice.
    d. advance directive.

12. You are on the scene where a patient is refusing treatment and transport to the hospital. You are unsure whether the patient is able to make a rational decision. You should
    a. transport the patient against his wishes.
    b. have the patient sign a refusal-of-care form.
    c. contact medical oversight for a consultation.
    d. have a family member sign the refusal.

13. A willful threat to a patient that can occur without actual touching is called
    a. battery.
    b. false imprisonment.
    c. slander.
    d. assault.

14. The Health Insurance Portability and Accountability Act (HIPAA), as it relates to the EMT, includes which of the following general provisions?
    a. Limits on disclosure of patient information, training on specific policies, requirements for specific treatments provided, and timelines for reporting violations
    b. Limits on disclosure of patient information, training on specific policies, obtaining patient signatures, and the assignment of an EMS privacy officer
    c. Limits on patients' rights to information, patient training on specific policies, timelines for reporting violations, and the assignment of an EMS privacy officer
    d. Limits on patients' rights to information, training on specific policies, and requirements for specific treatments provided

15. The Consolidated Omnibus Budget and Reconciliation Act (COBRA) and the Emergency Medical Treatment and Active Labor Act (EMTALA) are both federal regulations designed to
    a. reduce potential errors associated with interfacility patient transfers.
    b. help patients pay for needed emergency medical care and rehabilitation.
    c. ensure public access to emergency care regardless of ability to pay.
    d. limit the legal liability exposure of EMS systems by providing limits of liability.

CASE STUDY 1

It's 4:00 in the morning, and you have been dispatched to care for a patient complaining of chest pain. Upon arrival you observe a male patient who appears to be in his mid-60s. He looks pale and sweaty. However, he appears to be alert and is able to give you his name, address, day of the week, and time of day. He describes his pain as severe but refuses to be treated or transported to the hospital. You describe the need for medical care to the patient. While you are explaining this information to him, he repeatedly cups his hand behind his ear and asks, "What? What are you telling me?" Unexpectedly, your partner asks the patient to sign a refusal-of-care release form. The patient signs the form quickly and hands it back. Your partner looks at you and says, "Let's go!"

1. What is the most important concern you should have relating to this patient's refusal of treatment?
   a. The patient's mental competence
   b. The patient's understanding of the possible consequences of refusal
   c. The patient's signing the release without reading it
   d. Lack of professional courtesy if you second-guess your partner's suggestion to go

2. Your next action in the situation described above should be to
   a. leave as soon as the refusal form has been signed.
   b. encourage the patient to seek help if additional symptoms develop.
   c. have a witness sign the refusal form along with the patient.
   d. try again to persuade the patient to accept treatment.

CASE STUDY 2

You are employed as an EMT for a public EMS agency. Your partner, Joe, and you are dispatched to a call for a child who is choking. You are dispatched at 3:00 P.M. You have about a 10-block response to the scene. En route, your unit runs out of gas. You look at Joe. Joe gives you a blank stare and says, "I guess I forgot to fill it up!" A secondary unit responds to the call and arrives in 10 minutes. You learn later that the secondary unit arrived on-scene and quickly removed a piece of hot dog from the child's airway. The child suffered permanent brain damage as a result of this incident.

1. Listed below are four items that must be demonstrated to be successful in a negligence action. Place a Y for yes or an N for no next to each item to determine if negligence occurred in this case.
   _____ a. The EMTs had a duty to act.
   _____ b. The EMTs breached the duty to act.
   _____ c. The patient suffered an injury.
   _____ d. The injury was the result of the negligence of the EMTs.

4 The Human Body

OBJECTIVES

Numbered objectives are from the United States Department of Transportation EMT-Basic National Standard Curriculum. Asterisked objectives, if any, pertain to material that is supplemental to the DOT curriculum.

Cognitive

1-4.1 Identify the following topographic terms: medial, lateral, proximal, distal, superior, inferior, anterior, posterior, midline, right and left, midclavicular, bilateral, and midaxillary.

1-4.2 Describe the anatomy and function of the following major body systems: respiratory, circulatory, musculoskeletal, nervous, and endocrine.
- Identify and define other common descriptive anatomical terms.
- Describe the anatomy and function of the skin.

KEY IDEAS

This chapter introduces basic terminology and concepts of the anatomy and physiology of the human body—information you will need to help you determine when the body is functioning normally and when it is not and to help you communicate with other health-care providers.

- The EMT must be able to identify the following positions: normal anatomical position, supine, prone, lateral recumbent, Fowler's, and Trendelenburg.

- The EMT must be able to define descriptive terms such as *midline, midclavicular line, midaxillary line, plantar,* and *palmar.*

- The EMT must be able to define the terms *anterior, superior, dorsal, lateral,* and *distal* and their opposites—*posterior, inferior, ventral, medial,* and *proximal.*

- The EMT must be able to understand and describe the anatomy and physiology of the following body systems: musculoskeletal, respiratory, circulatory, nervous, endocrine, and skin.

- The EMT must be able to identify and locate the central and peripheral pulse points.

MEDICAL TERMINOLOGY

Term	Prefix	Word Root Combining	Suffix	Definition
cerebrospinal (SAIR-uh-bro-SPI-nul)		cerebr/o (cerebrum, brain); spin (spine)	-al (pertaining to)	Referring to the brain and spinal cord. Example: *cerebrospinal fluid,* a cushion of fluid around the brain and spinal cord.
dermis (DER-mis)		derm/a/is (skin)		The middle layer of the skin. (The layers of the skin from outer- to innermost are the epidermis, the dermis, and the subcutaneous layer.)
epidermis (EP-uh-DER-mis)	epi- (upon, over, above)	derm/a/is (skin)		The outermost layer of the skin, above the dermis.
epiglottis (EP-uh-GLOT-is)	epi- (upon, over, above)	glottis (the sound-producing area of the larynx)		A small, leaf-shaped flap of tissue, located above the glottis, which covers the entrance of the larynx.
hypoperfusion (HY-po-per-FYU-zhun)	hypo- (below, under, deficient)	perfusion (delivery of oxygen and other nutrients to the cells)		The insufficient delivery of oxygen and other nutrients to the body's cells. Also called *shock.*
interpleural (in-ter-PLUR-ul)	inter- (between)	pleur (relating to the pleura, the membranes that line the lungs and thorax)	-al (pertaining to)	Pertaining to the area between the visceral and parietal pleura. Example: *interpleural space,* a tiny space with negative pressure, which allows the lungs to stay inflated.
intervertebral (in-ter-VER-tuh-brul)	inter- (between)	vertebra (segment of the spinal column)	-al (pertaining to)	Pertaining to the area between two vertebrae. Example: *intervertebral disc* is a fluid-filled pad between two vertebrae.
midaxillary (mid-AX-uh-lair-e)	mid- (center)	axil (armpit)	-ary (pertaining to)	Refers to the center of the armpit. Example: *midaxillary line,* an imaginary line extending downward from the center of either armpit.
midclavicular (mid-klav-IK-yu-ler)	mid- (center)	clavicle (collarbone)	-ular (pertaining to)	Refers to the center of the collarbone (clavicle). Example: *midclavicular line,* an imaginary line extending downward from the center of either collarbone.
myocardium (MY-o-KAR-de-um)		my/o (muscle); card/ium (heart)		The cardiac muscle that makes up the middle layer of the walls of the heart.
nasopharynx (NA-zo-FAIR-inks)		nas/o (nose); pharynx (throat)		Nasal portion of the pharynx, situated above the soft palate.
pericardium (PAIR-uh-KAR-de-um)	peri- (around)	card/ium (heart)		Doubled-walled sac that encloses and supports the heart.
physiology (FIZ-e-OL-uh-je)		physi/o (nature)	-logy (study of)	The study of the function of the living body and its parts.
subcutaneous (SUB-kyu-TAY-ne-us)	sub- (below, under, beneath)	cut (skin)	-aneous (pertaining to)	Pertaining to the layer of fatty tissue just below the dermis.

1. The word root *physi/o* in the medical term *physiology* means
   a. nature. *(circled)*
   b. study of.
   c. lung.
   d. spleen.

2. The prefix *inter-* in the medical term *intervertebral* translates to
   a. above.
   b. below.
   c. between. *(circled)*
   d. under.

3. The prefix *epi-* in the medical term *epiglottis* means
   a. leaf-shaped.
   b. over, above. *(circled)*
   c. two, double.
   d. separation.

4. A medical term that ends with the suffix *-logy*, as in *physiology*, indicates
   a. study of. *(circled)*
   b. tension.
   c. condition.
   d. pertaining to.

5. The medical term *subcutaneous* contains the word root *cut*. You know this to relate to the
   a. brain.
   b. finger.
   c. breast.
   d. skin. *(circled)*

6. In each space, write the prefix, word root, or suffix that matches the definition.

   axil   my/o
   card/ium   perfusion
   glottis   peri
   hypo   pleur
   inter   vertebra

perfusion	a.	Delivery of oxygen and other nutrients to the cells
my/o	b.	Relating to muscle
glottis	c.	The sound-producing area of the larynx
vertebra	d.	Segment of the spinal column
hypo	e.	Below, under deficient
card/ium	f.	Relating to the heart
per	g.	Around (an object)
axil	h.	Referring to the armpit
pleur	i.	Referring to the lining of the lung and thorax
inter	j.	Between (objects)

TERMS AND CONCEPTS

1. In each space, write the term described by the statement. Not all terms will be used.

anterior   midline

distal   normal anatomical position

inferior   posterior

lateral   prone

medial   superior

midaxillary   transverse line

midclavicular

transverse   a. An imaginary line drawn horizontally through the waist to divide the body into superior and inferior planes

posterior   b. The back or toward the back

prone   c. Lying on the stomach

superior   d. Above, toward the head

normal anatom e. Position in which the patient is standing erect, facing forward, with arms down at the sides and palms forward

mid axillary f. Refers to the center of the armpit

inferior   g. Below, toward the feet

lateral   h. Refers to the side, left or right of the midline, or away from the midline of the body

anterior   l. The front or toward the front

distal   j. Distant or far from the point of reference

midline   k. An imaginary line drawn vertically through the middle of the patient's body, dividing it into right and left planes

CONTENT REVIEW

1. When you are describing an injury to the right chest, _right_ refers to
   a. your right, while facing the patient.
   b. your right, while facing away from the patient.
   c. the patient's right, regardless of position.
   d. your right, while in a prone position.

2. Fill in each term of direction on the appropriate line.

anterior   midline
distal   palmar
inferior   plantar
lateral   posterior
medial   proximal
midaxillary   superior

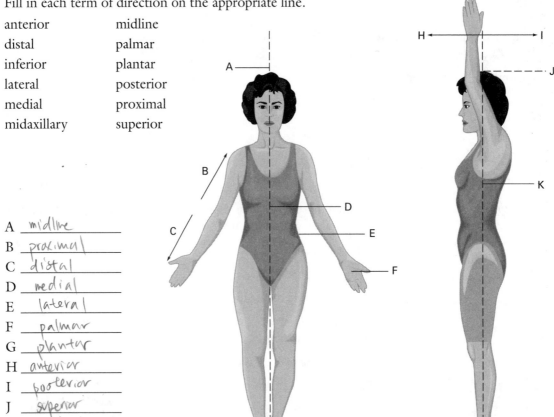

A   midline
B   proximal
C   distal
D   medial
E   lateral
F   palmar
G   plantar
H   anterior
I   posterior
J   superior
K   midaxillary
L   inferior

3. The emergency-department physician confirms that your patient has sustained *bilateral femur* fracture. This would indicate
   a. both right and left thigh bones are fractured.
   b. both right and left forearm bones are fractured.
   c. there are two fractures of one forearm bone.
   d. there are two fractures of one thigh bone.

4. Describing the location of your patient's burns as *posterior thigh* would indicate
   a. the back of the thigh.
   b. the front of the thigh.
   c. on the inner side of the thigh.
   d. on the outer side of the thigh.

5. You place a patient on his side so fluids can drain from his mouth. In what position have you placed him?
   a. Supine
   b. Prone
   c. Lateral recumbent or recovery position
   d. Fowler's position

29. For cells to function correctly, they require energy. The main source of energy comes from the cell's metabolizing

    a. glucose.

    b. carbon dioxide.

    c. amino acids.

    d. thiamine.

30. The hormone epinephrine contains all four properties (alpha 1, alpha 2, beta 1, and beta 2). Which of the following properties would cause the skin to become cool, pale, and diaphoretic from vasoconstriction in the skin?

    a. Alpha 1

    b. Alpha 2

    c. Beta 1

    d. Beta 2

CASE STUDY

You are a student EMT riding with an ambulance unit. At 1400 hours the unit is dispatched to a car-versus-tree crash. As you approach the scene, you notice a heavily damaged auto. The scene appears to be under control by police and rescue personnel. The experienced EMT reminds you to wear your body substance isolation (BSI) gear. You find the patient lying supine with a police officer supporting his neck.

1. Define the supine position.

The patient appears to be unresponsive. The senior EMT states he has conducted the initial assessment and will manage the airway while his partner retrieves the equipment to stabilize the spine. "You need to do a rapid trauma assessment (head-to-toe exam for obvious injuries)," he tells you. He supervises as you examine the head and neck. Then, as you cut away the patient's shirt, you note a large laceration to the center of the chest area above the nipple on the patient's right, your left as you face him. Further examination reveals a deformity to the upper arm (patient's left, your right) close to the shoulder.

2. How would you describe the lacerated chest?

    a. Large laceration to the right midclavicular line superior to the right nipple

    b. Large laceration to the right midaxillary line superior to the right nipple

    c. Large laceration to the right midclavicular line inferior to the right nipple

    d. Large laceration to the left midclavicular line superior to the left nipple

3. How would you describe the arm injury?

    a. Deformity to the proximal end of the left humerus

    b. Deformity to the proximal end of the right radius/ulna

    c. Deformity to the proximal end of the left calcaneus

    d. Deformity to the distal end of the left humerus

After exposing the lower body, you find that both right and left thighs are grossly deformed. A puncture wound is found on the left thigh away from the midline and close to the knee.

4. How would you describe the injuries?
   a. Right and left thigh area deformity with a puncture wound to the left medial thigh proximal to the patella
   b. Bilateral femoral region deformity with a puncture wound to the left lateral thigh proximal to the patella
   c. Bilateral femoral region deformity with a puncture wound to the left ventral area distal to the greater trochanter
   d. Bilateral femoral region deformity with a puncture wound to the left dorsal area distal to the patella

After the patient is secured to a spine immobilization device and loaded onto the wheeled stretcher, the senior EMT asks you to place the patient into a Trendelenburg position.

5. Describe the Trendelenburg position.

While transporting the patient to the hospital, the senior EMT commends you on your knowledge of anatomy and anatomical terms.

ENRICHMENT

1. Which organ contains the islets of Langerhans that are responsible for producing insulin?
   a. Pancreas
   b. Liver
   c. Kidney
   d. Appendix

2. Which solid organ is located in the left upper quadrant of the abdomen, helps with filtration of the blood, and serves as a reservoir of blood the body can use in an emergency?
   a. Small intestine
   b. Adrenal gland
   c. Spleen
   d. Gallbladder

3. Urine is carried from the kidneys to the bladder through which structure(s)?
   a. Ureters
   b. Urethra
   c. Duodenum
   d. Hepatic ducts

CHAPTER 5

Baseline Vital Signs and History Taking

OBJECTIVES

Numbered objectives are from the United States Department of Transportation EMT-Basic National Standard Curriculum. Asterisked objectives, if any, pertain to material that is supplemental to the DOT curriculum.

Cognitive

1-5.1 Identify the components of vital signs.
1-5.2 Describe the methods to obtain a breathing rate.
1-5.3 Identify the attributes that should be obtained when assessing breathing.
1-5.4 Differentiate between shallow, labored, and noisy breathing.
1-5.5 Describe the methods to obtain a pulse rate.
1-5.6 Identify the information obtained when assessing a patient's pulse.
1-5.7 Differentiate between a strong, weak, regular, and irregular pulse.
1-5.8 Describe the methods to assess the skin color, temperature, and condition (capillary refill in infants and children).
1-5.9 Identify the normal and abnormal skin colors.
1-5.10 Differentiate between pale, blue, red, and yellow skin color.
1-5.11 Identify the normal and abnormal skin temperature.
1-5.12 Differentiate between hot, cool, and cold skin temperature.
1-5.13 Identify normal and abnormal skin conditions.
1-5.14 Identify normal and abnormal capillary refill in infants and children.
1-5.15 Describe the methods to assess the pupils.
1-5.16 Identify normal and abnormal pupil size.
1-5.17 Differentiate between dilated (big) and constricted (small) pupil size.
1-5.18 Differentiate between reactive and nonreactive pupils and equal and unequal pupils.
1-5.19 Describe the methods to assess blood pressure.
1-5.20 Define systolic pressure.
1-5.21 Define diastolic pressure.
1-5.22 Explain the difference between auscultation and palpation for obtaining a blood pressure.
1-5.23 Identify the components of the SAMPLE history.
1-5.24 Differentiate between a sign and a symptom.
1-5.25 State the importance of accurately reporting and recording the baseline vital signs.
1-5.26 Discuss the need to search for additional medical information.

KEY IDEAS

This chapter focuses on the critical EMT skills of obtaining a patient history and taking vital signs. These skills are key elements of patient assessment, measuring the patient's response to prehospital emergency care, and providing essential information for hospital personnel.

- Baseline vital-sign measurements are your first assessments related to breathing; pulse; skin color, condition, and temperature; pupils; blood pressure; and pulse oximetry. All subsequent measurements of these "signs of life" will be compared to your initial baseline.

- Breathing assessments include rate, which is assessed by determining the number of breaths per minute, and quality. Breathing quality refers to how much air is moving in and out with each breath, as well as how well it is moving.

- Pulses are pressure waves generated by each heartbeat that can be felt in an artery that is near the skin surface. Pulses are assessed for rate (the number of heartbeats per minute) and quality (strength and regularity). In the adult patient, a rapid pulse (greater than 100 bpm) is called tachycardia, while a slow pulse (less than 60 bpm) is called bradycardia.

- Skin provides many important clues about the patient's status. When assessing the patient's skin, you should note its color, condition, and temperature.

- Capillary refill is considered a more reliable sign of circulatory status in infants and children who are less than 6 years of age than in older children or adults.

- The size, equality, and reactivity of the patient's pupils can provide helpful information and clues about what might be wrong with your patient.

- Blood pressure is assessed by using a sphygmomanometer to measure the amount of pressure exerted against the arterial walls when the left ventricle of the heart contracts (systolic pressure) and when the left ventricle of the heart is at rest (diastolic pressure). Blood pressure is measured in millimeters of mercury (mmHg). The pulse pressure is the difference between the systolic and diastolic blood pressures.

- Comparing the pulse and blood pressure in a patient who is supine and then standing is called testing orthostatic vital signs (tilt test). An increase in the pulse by 10–20 bpm and a decrease in the blood pressure by 10–20 mmHg may indicate significant blood or fluid loss.

- The pulse oximeter is used to detect hypoxia and to monitor airway management and oxygen therapy. An SpO_2 reading of 97 percent is normal, while in a compromised patient a reading of less than 95 percent may indicate hypoxia and require oxygen and ventilation. Inaccurate readings may be produced by hypoperfusion states (shock), hypothermia, excessive patient movement, the patient's use of nail polish, carbon monoxide, or anemia; during some seizures; or in cigarette smokers.

- Vital signs should be taken and recorded as often as necessary to provide proper care. Generally, reassessing vital signs every 15 minutes is reasonable for a stable patient, but an unstable patient requires vital signs taken every 5 minutes.

- Obtaining a medical history for your patient can be done easily using the SAMPLE history. SAMPLE is an acronym to remind you to ask about and record information about signs and symptoms (OPQRST), allergies, medications, pertinent past history, last oral intake, and events leading to the injury or illness.

- Assessment activities may embarrass your patients or make them anxious, so it is important that you reassure them and make every effort to maintain their dignity.

MEDICAL TERMINOLOGY

Term	Prefix	Word Root Combining Form	Suffix	Definition
auscultation (OS-kul-TAY-shun)		auscultat (to listen to)	-ion (process)	Listening with a stethoscope
bradycardia (brad-uh-KAR-de-uh)	brady- (slow)	card (heart)	-ia (condition of)	A slow heart rate, less than 60 beats per minute
cyanosis (si-uh-NO-sis)		cyan (dark blue)	-osis (condition of)	A bluish color of the skin and mucous membranes that indicates poor oxygenation of tissues
diastolic (dye-us-TOL-ik)		diastol (expansion)	-ic (pertaining to)	The blood pressure that occurs during the relaxation phase of the heart cycle; the bottom number of the blood pressure reading
sphygmomanometer (sfig-mo-mah-NOM-uh-ter)		sphygm/o (pulse); meter (measuring instrument)		Instrument used to measure blood pressure
systolic (sis-TOL-ik)		systol (contraction)	-ic (pertaining to)	The blood pressure that occurs during the contraction phase of the heart cycle; the top number of the blood pressure reading
tachycardia (tak-uh-KAR-de-uh)	tachy- (fast)	card (heart)	-ia (condition of)	A rapid heart rate, more than 100 beats per minute

1. In each space, write the prefix, word root, or suffix that matches the definition.

auscultat   ic
brady   osis
card   sphygm/o
cyan   systol
diastol   tachy

_____ a. Contraction

_____ b. Pulse

_____ c. Expansion

_____ d. Fast

_____ e. To listen to

_____ f. Pertaining to

_____ g. Slow

_____ h. Heart

_____ i. Dark blue

_____ j. Condition of

TERMS AND CONCEPTS

1. Write the number of the correct term next to each definition.

   1. auscultation
   2. diastolic blood pressure
   3. palpation
   4. signs
   5. stridor
   6. symptoms
   7. systolic blood pressure
   8. pulse pressure
   9. tachycardia
   10. bradycardia

   _____ a. A harsh, high-pitched airway sound

   _____ b. Assessment by listening with a stethoscope

   _____ c. Assessment by feeling

   _____ d. Conditions that you can observe

   _____ e. Pressure in the arteries when the heart's left ventricle contracts

   _____ f. Pressure in the arteries when the heart's left ventricle rests

   _____ g. Conditions that must be described by the patient

   _____ h. In the adult, a pulse rate less than 60 beats per minute

   _____ i. The difference between the systolic and diastolic blood pressures

   _____ j. In the adult, a pulse rate greater than 100 beats per minute

CONTENT REVIEW

1. There are six vital signs that are commonly assessed by the EMT. Which vital sign is missing from the following list?

   Breathing

   Pulse

   Pupils

   Blood pressure

   Pulse oximeter

   a. Neurological check
   b. Core temperature
   c. Skin
   d. ECG

2. Breathing is usually assessed by counting the number of respirations
   a. in a 15-second period and multiplying by 4.
   b. in a 20-second period and multiplying by 3.
   c. in a 30-second period and multiplying by 2.
   d. in a 60-second period.

3. Chest wall motion of about a one-inch expansion, no use of accessory muscles of breathing, and an inhalation and exhalation of about equal length. This describes which breathing pattern or type?
   a. Normal
   b. Shallow
   c. Labored
   d. Noisy

4. Assessing the quality of a patient's breathing provides the EMT what critical information?
   a. How much air is moving and how well it is moving
   b. Only how much air the patient is moving
   c. Only how well the air is moving in and out of the patient
   d. An indication of the patient's perfusion status

5. Fill in the name of each pulse on the appropriate line.
   Brachial
   Carotid
   Dorsalis pedis
   Femoral
   Posterior tibial
   Radial

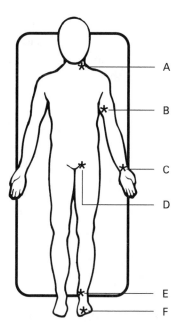

   A _____
   B _____
   C _____
   D _____
   E _____
   F _____

6. In most cases, to assess your patient's pulse, palpate the artery and count the number of beats
   a. for 15 seconds and multiply by 4.
   b. for 20 seconds and multiply by 3.
   c. for 30 seconds and multiply by 2.
   d. for 60 seconds.

7. To assess the pulse of your 6-month-old patient, you should initially check the _____ pulse.
   a. carotid
   b. brachial
   c. radial
   d. femoral

8. For the 6-month-old patient, what would be considered a normal pulse rate?
   a. 60 beats per minute
   b. 80 beats per minute
   c. 100 beats per minute
   d. 120 beats per minute

9. In terms of pulse quality, which of the following would be considered normal for an adult?
   a. Weak and irregular at 60 beats per minute
   b. Strong and regular at 60 beats per minute
   c. Bounding and irregular at 60 beats per minute
   d. Thready and regular at 60 beats per minute

10. Which of the following may be a sign of extreme vasoconstriction or blood loss?
   a. Pale conjunctiva
   b. Red nail beds
   c. Blue-gray oral mucosa
   d. Yellow skin

11. When assessing skin color in infants, children, and dark-skinned people, the EMT should additionally check the
   a. posterior portion of both forearms.
   b. tops of both feet.
   c. palms of hands and soles of feet.
   d. base of the neck.

12. How would you assess the relative skin temperature of your patient?
   a. Assess by placing the palm of your hand on the patient.
   b. Assess by using your forearm.
   c. Assess by placing the back of your hand on the patient.
   d. Assess by using the fingertips of your right hand.

13. Which of the following is a sign of normal skin condition?
   a. Clammy
   b. Wet
   c. Cool
   d. Dry

14. Which of the following is a correct upper limit for capillary-refill time assessed at normal room temperature?
   a. 3 seconds for infants and children
   b. 2 seconds for female patients
   c. 5 seconds in the elderly
   d. 2 seconds for male patients

15. When assessing the patient's pupils with a light, which of the following is commonly assessed in the baseline vitals?
   a. Halo effect
   b. Corneal status
   c. Sensitivity to light
   d. Reactivity

16. Blood pressure is a reflection of the pressure in which of the following?
   a. Ventricles
   b. Arteries
   c. Veins
   d. Capillaries

17. When evaluating a patient's blood pressure, it is important to understand that
    a. the systolic blood pressure is determined by auscultation of the last sound.
    b. the diastolic blood pressure is determined by auscultation of the first sound.
    c. the blood pressure when using a sphygmomanometer is always reported as an odd number.
    d. a pulse pressure less than 25 percent of the systolic blood pressure is considered to be a narrow pulse pressure.

18. You are auscultating the blood pressure of a 34-year-old female. To estimate the systolic pressure in the adult female patient at rest who is less than 40 years of age, which of the following blood-pressure readings is considered normal for this patient?
    a. 124/82
    b. 134/82
    c. 124/94
    d. 134/94

19. When measuring a patient's blood pressure by auscultation, you need
    a. a sphygmomanometer and your fingertips.
    b. a sphygmomanometer and a penlight.
    c. a sphygmomanometer and a stethoscope.
    d. only a sphygmomanometer.

20. Number the steps below in the proper order—from 1 to 6—for measuring a patient's blood pressure once you have selected and applied the proper-size sphygmomanometer.

    _____ a. Note the systolic and diastolic sounds.

    _____ b. Deflate cuff at 2 mmHg per second.

    _____ c. Palpate the radial pulse, inflate to 70 mmHg, and increase by 10 mmHg until the radial pulse is no longer palpable. Note the number and deflate the cuff.

    _____ d. Inflate the cuff 30 mmHg above the noted number.

    _____ e. Place the stethoscope in your ears.

    _____ f. Position the patient's arm.

21. In a stable patient, vital signs should be taken every _____ minutes.
    a. 5
    b. 10
    c. 15
    d. 20

22. Identify which element of the SAMPLE history applies to each statement below by writing S, A, M, P, L, or E, according to the key.

S   Sign or symptom
A   Allergies
M   Medications
P   Pertinent past history
L   Last oral intake
E   Events leading to the illness or injury

_____ a.   Medic Alert tag notes "reacts to penicillin."

_____ b.   Ate large meal 2 hours ago.

_____ c.   Patient complains of nausea.

_____ d.   Requires insulin daily to control diabetes.

_____ e.   Diagnosed with emphysema 10 years ago.

_____ f.   Patient has chest pain that radiates down the left arm.

_____ g.   Mother reports that patient gets rashes from poison ivy.

_____ h.   Patient was outside shoveling snow.

_____ i.   Obvious deformity noted in right lower leg.

_____ j.   Has taken only small amounts of liquids since early morning.

_____ k.   Takes aspirin two to three times each day for arthritis pain.

_____ l.   Husband says patient has had epilepsy since head injury last year.

23. A paramedic asks you to help him test orthostatic vital signs on a patient you are both treating. This test is conducted to help determine if
    a.   the patient has experienced a neurological emergency.
    b.   the patient has a cardiac problem.
    c.   significant blood or fluid loss has occurred.
    d.   the patient has significant hypoxia.

24. Pulse oximetry
    a.   is a method of detecting hypoxia in patients.
    b.   reading of 97 percent eliminates the potential of hypoxemia in a patient.
    c.   provides an accurate reading in shock and hypothermia patients.
    d.   readings are always accurate if the patient is wearing fingernail polish.

CASE STUDY

As you read the following scenario, remember that baseline vital signs and the SAMPLE history are key elements of patient assessment and provide essential information for hospital personnel.

It is about 10:00 PM on a Thursday night, and you are talking to your shift supervisor about conducting a training program at next month's shift meeting. The alarm sounds. "Rescue One, respond to a difficulty breathing at 1600 Osban Street, cross street New Jersey Avenue." You find your 60-year-old male patient sitting up in bed with his wife at his bedside. Mr. Baker is in obvious distress and reports that he can't breathe. He is breathing at a rate of 26 breaths per minute. He is using accessory muscles, and you hear wheezing and gurgling with each breath. You find that his radial pulse is weak and irregular at a rate of 50 beats per minute. His skin is slightly cyanotic, cool, and moist. Using your penlight, you assess his pupils and find them to be equal, reactive, and of normal size. You auscultate his blood pressure at 80/50 mmHg and his SpO_2 reading is 90 percent.

1. How would you describe this patient's respiratory status?
   a. Normal respiratory status
   b. Minor respiratory distress
   c. Moderate respiratory distress
   d. Severe respiratory distress

2. What might Mr. Baker's skin color, temperature, and condition indicate in this situation?
   a. Hyperperfusion
   b. Normal perfusion
   c. Hypoperfusion and liver failure
   d. Hypoperfusion and inadequate oxygenation

3. What is the relationship between Mr. Baker's pulse and his blood pressure?
   a. The pulse rate is bradycardic and may be responsible for the lowered blood pressure.
   b. The pulse rate is tachycardic and may be responsible for the lowered blood pressure.
   c. The relationship is normal, given Mr. Baker's age.
   d. The relationship is normal, given Mr. Baker's respiratory status.

While your partner starts Mr. Baker on high-flow oxygen therapy, you begin to get his history from his wife. Mrs. Baker is upset and very worried about her husband. She tells you that he had a heart attack 5 years ago and takes Digoxin (a medication to strengthen his heart's contractions) and Lasix (a water pill) daily. Mr. Baker also occasionally takes nitroglycerin for episodes of chest pain, but she says he denied having chest pain today. Although she told him that he shouldn't, he shoveled snow this morning and since then has been increasingly short of breath. He did not eat supper and only ate a bowl of soup at lunch. Mrs. Baker says that her husband has no allergies.

4. Identify the elements of the SAMPLE history found in this scenario.

5. Based on his current status, how frequently should you reassess Mr. Baker's vital signs?
   a. Every 5 minutes
   b. Every 10 minutes
   c. Every 15 minutes
   d. Every 20 minutes

6 Preparing to Lift and Move Patients

OBJECTIVES

Numbered objectives are from the United States Department of Transportation EMT-Basic National Standard Curriculum. Asterisked objectives, if any, pertain to material that is supplemental to the DOT curriculum.

Cognitive

1-6.1 Define body mechanics.

1-6.2 Discuss the guidelines and safety precautions that need to be followed when lifting a patient.

1-6.4 Describe the guidelines and safety precautions for carrying patients and/or equipment.

1-6.5 Discuss one-handed carrying techniques.

1-6.6 Describe correct and safe carrying procedures on stairs.

1-6.7 State the guidelines for reaching and their applications.

1-6.8 Describe correct reaching for log rolls.

1-6.9 State the guidelines for pushing and pulling.

KEY IDEAS

This chapter presents proper methods of lifting and moving patients and equipment. It is not enough to know this material. You need to continuously use the information every day and on every response.

■ Proper use of body mechanics can greatly decrease injuries. The four basic principles of body mechanics are (1) Keep the weight of the object close to the body. (2) To lift a heavy object, use leg, hip, and gluteal muscles plus contracted abdominal muscles. (3) "Stack" shoulders over hips, hips over feet. (4) Reduce the height or distance an object must be lifted.

■ Poor posture can fatigue your back and promote injury.

■ Communication and teamwork are essential to safe lifting and moving.

■ It is important to be able to perform the following techniques: power lift, squat lift, one-handed carrying technique, stair-chair technique, reaching techniques, and pushing and pulling techniques.

TERMS AND CONCEPTS

1. Define each of the following terms.
   a. Body mechanics

   b. Power grip

   c. Power lift

CONTENT REVIEW

1. You are much more likely to injure your back when performing which task?
   a. Reaching a great distance to lift a light object
   b. Reaching a short distance to lift a heavy object
   c. Reaching up to shoulder height to lift a light object
   d. Lifting a light object while keeping it close to you

2. You are preparing to move a heavy object; which muscles will provide the most power with the greatest degree of safety?
   a. Leg, hip, and gluteal muscles
   b. Back and shoulder muscles
   c. Chest and arm muscles
   d. Abdominal and intercostal muscles

3. The body mechanics principle called "stacking" means
   a. stacking objects to be lifted one on top of the other.
   b. keeping your shoulders, hips, and feet in vertical alignment.
   c. eliminating curvature from your spine.
   d. staying under an object being lifted overhead.

4. To help prevent injury and manage stress, you should follow a physical fitness program that includes what four ingredients?

5. When performing a power lift, which of the following is correct?
   a. Stand to the side of object and lift hips before upper body
   b. Turn feet inward, lock knees, and lift hips before upper body
   c. Lock the back and lift upper body before hips
   d. Bend forward at the waist and lift upper body before hips

6. When performing the squat lift with a weak leg or ankle, you should
   a. place the weaker leg slightly behind your good leg.
   b. place the weaker leg slightly forward of the good leg.
   c. place the weaker leg beside and parallel to the good leg.
   d. not use the squat lift with a weak leg.

7. You are preparing to carry a heavy tool using the one-handed carrying technique. You know you should avoid
   a. leaning to the opposite side.
   b. bending your knees.
   c. locking your back.
   d. bending at the hips.

8. You and your partner are preparing to navigate stairs using a stair chair. You should
   a. tilt the stair chair forward.
   b. position the patient facing the stairs.
   c. keep one hand on the railing.
   d. use a spotter to direct and navigate.

9. If you have to reach for an object that is greater than _____ from your body, you should reposition yourself closer to the object.
   a. 5 inches
   b. 10 inches
   c. 20 inches
   d. 3 feet

10. When you need to push or pull an object, which of the following is correct?
   a. Push rather than pull, and keep the load at knee level.
   b. Push rather than pull, and keep the load between hips and shoulders.
   c. Pull rather than push, and keep the load at shoulder level.
   d. Pull rather than push, and keep the load at hip level.

11. In which of the following situations would use of the rapid extrication technique be inappropriate?
   a. The patient presents with loss of sensation and motor response to the lower extremities.
   b. The patient is bleeding severely; the vehicle appears unstable and may slide down a ravine.
   c. The patient seems uninjured, but there is what appears to be an electric line across the vehicle.
   d. The patient has stopped breathing, and a weak central pulse is palpated on the neck.

CASE STUDY

You and your partner Kyle work in an East Coast community and are dispatched to a guarded beach for an injured surfer. As you and Kyle approach the scene, you are met by lifeguard captain Vicky. She explains that the patient has deeply lacerated his leg and will need to be carried across the beach and over the dune line to the parking lot. Fortunately, there is a ramp that leads to a boardwalk, and a set of stairs connects the boardwalk with the parking lot. Vicky says she has three lifeguards who can assist with moving the patient. Kyle suggests a four-corner carry with the wheeled stretcher in the up position (legs fully extended), thus reducing the chance of dropping the patient. If the carriers need a break, this position will allow the stretcher to rest on the extended wheels without lowering the patient to ground level, thus reducing the chance of injury. You commend Kyle for his foresight and planning.

1. After the patient has been loaded and you are ready to move him, you instruct the rescuers on the corners of the stretcher to
   a. keep their backs leaning to the opposite side of the patient to compensate the weight.
   b. keep their backs locked and stay as close to the stretcher as possible, avoiding leaning.
   c. relax their back muscles and bend at the waist to keep the stretcher moving forward.
   d. grip the stretcher handles with only their fingers, avoiding contact between palms and handles.

2. As you and the team reach the boardwalk, you instruct them to
   a. continue to carry the stretcher because once you are in motion stopping will result in fatigue.
   b. continue to carry the stretcher because it is important that the patient receive a smooth ride.
   c. lower the stretcher onto its wheels so the stretcher does part of the work, with the rescuers at the back pushing it along the boardwalk.
   d. lower the stretcher onto its wheels so the stretcher does part of the work, with the rescuers at the front pulling it along the boardwalk.

3. As you reach the stairs, your team takes a brief break. You instruct your team to lower the stretcher (legs retracted) so the wheels won't catch on the stairs. You should also instruct them to
   a. have a spotter at the bottom to help guide them.
   b. flex the body at the hips and not the waist.
   c. keep the weight and arms close to the body.
   d. all of these.

4. You and Kyle will use the power-lift technique to lift the stretcher into the up position. Regarding the power lift, which of the following is *not* correct?
   a. This technique is not recommended for use with heavy patients.
   b. This technique offers you the best defense against injury.
   c. This technique protects the patient with a safe and stable move.
   d. This technique is useful for rescuers with weak knees or thighs.

PREPARATORY: CHAPTERS 1–6

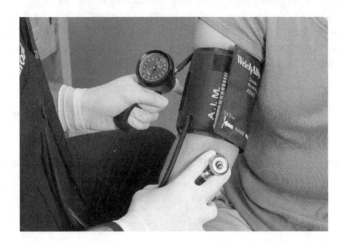

The U.S. Department of Transportation Emergency Medical Technician: National Standard Curriculum is divided into eight modules. The Prehospital Emergency Care textbook is divided into modules that correspond to the DOT curriculum modules.

The first module, "Preparatory," is an introduction to the EMS system and some basic concerns, including your safety and well-being as an EMT, certain legal and ethical issues, fundamental anatomy and physiology, and essential skills of measuring vital signs and taking a patient history.

Q   The opening chapters made it clear that an EMT can come in contact with an infectious disease, sustain injury, and be affected by severe stress. How worried should I be about these hazards?

A   There certainly are a number of factors that should be taken very seriously. You will be doing a lot of lifting and moving, you will be working at hazardous accident scenes, you will be treating patients who may have infectious diseases, and your job may sometimes be quite stressful. However, by using appropriate protective clothing and equipment, exercising good health and hygiene practices, using the principles of body mechanics, and knowing how to manage stress, you can have a long, safe, and rewarding career in EMS.

Q   What about consent, abandonment, falsification—all those legal issues? Should I be afraid of getting sued?

A   You may be the subject of a lawsuit at some time during your career. However, you have some protection under the Good Samaritan laws, and you are not likely to be *successfully* sued if you do your job to the best of your ability according to the training you have received and if you carefully document every call.

Q   A lot of terminology was taught in Chapter 4. How much medical terminology do I have to know?

A   The EMT must have enough understanding of the human body to be able to perform adequate assessment and emergency care and enough command of terminology to be able to communicate clearly with other health-care providers. Obviously, the higher the level of training one attains the greater the command of terminology that is and will be required. However, standard medical vocabulary is based on the medical prefixes, suffixes, and root words that are contained in the exercises in this workbook. A commitment to memorization of and use of the various combining terms will allow the committed student to understand terms that may appear, at first sight, to be complicated.

How much terminology you need to know depends upon how far you plan to advance in a health-care career. If you have plans to attain paramedic or some other level of health-care certification, it would be to your advantage to commit yourself to memorization and use of the root words, prefixes, and suffixes contained in various chapters of this workbook.

Q   **It's hard to remember all those vital-signs measurements and history-taking questions that were taught in Chapter 5. Are there any shortcuts?**

A   Many EMTs carry basic vital-signs ranges and the SAMPLE-history questions on quick-reference cards. However, taking vital-signs measurements and patient histories are among the most basic functions of your profession as an EMT, and it is best to know this information "cold." Remembering them will get much easier as you practice your skills and gain experience.

7 Airway Management, Ventilation, and Oxygen Therapy

OBJECTIVES

Numbered objectives are from the United States Department of Transportation EMT-Basic National Standard Curriculum. Asterisked objectives, if any, pertain to material that is supplemental to the DOT curriculum.

Cognitive

2-1.1 Name and label the major structures of the respiratory system on a diagram.

2-1.2 List the signs of adequate breathing.

2-1.3 List the signs of inadequate breathing.

2-1.4 Describe the steps in performing the head-tilt/chin-lift.

2-1.5 Relate the mechanism of injury to opening the airway.

2-1.6 Describe the steps in performing the jaw thrust.

2-1.7 State the importance of having a suction unit ready for immediate use when providing emergency care.

2-1.8 Describe the techniques of suctioning.

2-1.9 Describe how to artificially ventilate a patient with a pocket mask.

2-1.10 Describe the steps in performing the skill of artificially ventilating a patient with a bag-valve mask while using the jaw thrust.

2-1.11 List the parts of the bag-valve mask system.

2-1.12 Describe the steps in performing the skill of artificially ventilating a patient with a bag-valve mask for one and two rescuers.

2-1.13 Describe the signs of adequate artificial ventilation using the bag-valve mask.

2-1.14 Describe the signs of inadequate artificial ventilation using the bag-valve mask.

2-1.15 Describe the steps in artificially ventilating a patient with a flow restricted, oxygen-powered ventilation device.

2-1.16 List the steps in performing the actions taken when providing mouth-to-mouth and mouth-to-stoma artificial ventilation.

2-1.17 Describe how to measure and insert an oropharyngeal (oral) airway.

2-1.18 Describe how to measure and insert a nasopharyngeal (nasal) airway.

2-1.19 Define the components of an oxygen delivery system.

2-1.20 Identify a nonrebreather face mask and state the oxygen flow requirements needed for its use.

2-1.21 Describe the indications for using a nasal cannula versus a nonrebreather face mask.

2-1.22 Identify a nasal cannula and state the flow requirements needed for its use.

KEY IDEAS

In this chapter, your knowledge of the respiratory system and airway management will be put to use. After completion of this chapter, you should be able to establish and maintain an airway, as well as ensure effective ventilation and oxygen administration. It is important to do the following:

- Review the anatomy and physiology of the respiratory system in both adults and infants/children.

- Understand the two manual methods of opening an airway, and explain the circumstances in which each should be used.

- Understand that the EMT may insert an oropharyngeal or nasopharyngeal airway adjunct to assist in establishing and maintaining an open airway, and understand the circumstances in which each should be used.

- Understand how to assess for adequate or inadequate breathing.

- Know the methods that the EMT can use to artificially ventilate the patient, and understand the advantages and disadvantages of each.

- Know the techniques for ventilating patients with and without suspected spinal injury.

- Know the signs that indicate the patient is being ventilated adequately.

- Describe the appropriate procedure for initiating oxygen therapy, including preparing the equipment, and the steps for discontinuing oxygen administration.

MEDICAL TERMINOLOGY

Term	Prefix	Word Root Combining Form	Suffix	Definition
bilateral (bi-LAT-uh-rul)	bi- (two, double)	later (side)	-al (pertaining to)	On both sides
bradypnea (brad-ip-NEE-uh)	brady- (slow)	pnea (to breathe or breathing)		A breathing rate slower than the normal rate
cyanosis (si-uh-NO-sis)		cyan (dark blue)	-osis (condition of)	A bluish color of the skin and mucous membranes that indicates poor oxygenation of tissues
deoxygenated (de-OK-suh-jun-ate-id)	de- (down, away from)	oxy (oxygen); gen (formation, produce)	-ate (use, action); -ed (indicates adjective formed from verb)	Containing low amounts of oxygen, as with venous blood
hemoglobin (HEE-muh-glo-bin)		hem/o (blood); globin (globule)		A complex protein molecule found on the surface of the red blood cell that is responsible for carrying a majority of the oxygen in the blood
hypoxia (hi-POX-ee-uh)	hyp/o- (below, deficient)	oxy (oxygen)	-ia (condition of)	A reduction of oxygen delivery to the tissues
laryngectomy (lair-in-JEK-tuh-me)		laryng (larynx)	-ectomy (surgical excision)	A surgical procedure in which a patient's larynx is removed

Term	Prefix	Word Root Combining Form	Suffix	Definition
nasopharynx (NAY-zo-FAIR-inks)		nas/o (nose); pharynx (pharynx, throat)		Nasal portion of the pharynx, situated above the soft palate
oropharynx (OR-o-FAIR-inks)		or/o (mouth); pharynx (pharynx, throat)		Portion of the pharynx that extends from the mouth to the oral cavity at the base of the tongue
tachypnea (tak-ip-NEE-uh)	tachy- (fast)	pnea (to breathe or breathing)		A breathing rate faster than the normal rate
tracheostomy (tray-kee-OS-tuh-me)		trache/o (trachea)	-stomy (new opening)	A surgical opening in the trachea into which a tube is inserted for the patient to breathe through

1. The prefix *bi-* in the medical term *bilateral* means
   a. two, double.
   b. before.
   c. slow.
   d. half.

2. *Cyan,* the word root in *cyanosis,* indicates
   a. to suck in.
   b. hollow air sac.
   c. dark blue.
   d. to the right.

3. The suffix *-ectomy* in the medical term *laryngectomy* indicates
   a. pertaining to the epiglottis.
   b. surgical excision.
   c. inflammation or infection.
   d. sound production.

4. The word root *trache/o* in the medical term *tracheostomy* means
   a. traction.
   b. trachea.
   c. tract.
   d. transition.

5. The suffix *-stomy* when used in the term *tracheostomy* relates to a/an
   a. structure.
   b. tube.
   c. contraction.
   d. opening.

TERMS AND CONCEPTS

1. In each space, write the number of the term described by the statement. Not all terms will be used.

   1. Agonal respirations
   2. Alveoli
   3. Bradypnea
   4. Cricoid cartilage
   5. Cyanosis
   6. Epiglottis
   7. Esophagus
   8. Hemoglobin
   9. Hypopnea
   10. Hypoxia
   11. Mucous membrane
   12. Nasal cannula
   13. Nasopharynx
   14. Nonrebreather mask
   15. Oropharyngeal airway
   16. Oropharynx
   17. Oxygenated
   18. Pleura
   19. Retractions
   20. Tachypnea
   21. Tidal volume
   22. Tracheostomy

   _____ a. A breathing rate slower than the normal rate

   _____ b. Gasping respirations that have no pattern and occur infrequently

   _____ c. Two layers of connective tissue that surround the lungs

   _____ d. Air sacs in the lungs; point of gas exchange with the pulmonary capillaries

   _____ e. Bluish color of skin and mucous membranes that indicates poor oxygenation

   _____ f. Depressions seen in the neck, above the clavicles, between the ribs, or below the rib cage from excessive muscle use during breathing

   _____ g. A surgical procedure that creates a stoma in the neck for the patient to breathe through

   _____ h. Volume of air inhaled and exhaled in one respiration

   _____ i. A breathing rate faster than the normal rate

   _____ j. Molecule that carries oxygen in the blood

   _____ k. Portion of the pharynx that extends from the mouth to the base of the tongue

   _____ l. A reduction of oxygen delivery to the tissues

   _____ m. Portion of the pharynx that extends from the nostrils to the soft palate

   _____ n. Passage for foods and liquids to enter the stomach

   _____ o. Flap of tissue that closes over the trachea during swallowing

   _____ p. Oxygen delivery device that includes a one-way valve and reservoir and can deliver up to 100 percent oxygen

   _____ q. Semicircular hard plastic device that is inserted into the mouth and holds the tongue away from the back of the pharynx

   _____ r. Inadequate tidal volume in a breathing patient

CONTENT REVIEW

1. Which anatomical feature may cause more frequent airway obstruction in infants and children than in adults?
   a. Nose and mouth are proportionately larger.
   b. Cricoid cartilage is wider and more rigid.
   c. Tongue takes up relatively more space.
   d. Diaphragm and intercostal muscles are less developed.

2. Fill in each term naming a structure of the upper airway on the appropriate line.

   Cricoid cartilage
   Epiglottis
   Esophagus
   Larynx
   Mandible
   Nasal cavity
   Nasopharynx
   Oropharynx
   Soft palate
   Thyroid cartilage
   Tongue
   Trachea
   Vocal cords

   A _____
   B _____
   C _____
   D _____
   E _____
   F _____
   G _____
   H _____
   I _____
   J _____
   K _____
   L _____
   M _____

3. A major muscle of breathing that separates the chest cavity from the abdominal cavity is which of the following?
   a. Diaphragm
   b. Alveolus
   c. Visceral pleura
   d. Bronchiole

4. The point at which the trachea bifurcates (splits) into the right and left mainstem bronchi is termed the
   a. larynx.
   b. carina.
   c. pleura.
   d. bronchiole.

5. While inspecting an injured patient's mouth, you find broken teeth in the oropharynx, and suctioning equipment is not immediately available. You should
   a. perform five quick abdominal thrusts.
   b. perform five back blows with your hand.
   c. sweep the mouth with your index finger.
   d. sit the patient up to help secure the airway.

6. Describe the steps to perform the head-tilt/chin-lift maneuver.

7. When treating a patient with a suspected spinal injury, which method of opening the airway should be used?
   a. Jaw-thrust maneuver
   b. Head-tilt/chin-lift maneuver
   c. Lateral-flexion maneuver
   d. Hyperextension maneuver

8. To help prevent obstruction of the trachea when performing the head-tilt/chin-lift maneuver on infants or children, the head should be placed in which position?
   a. Flexed
   b. Tilted
   c. Extended
   d. Neutral

9. When suctioning, you should use what type of body substance isolation protection?
   a. Gloves
   b. Mask
   c. Protective eyewear
   d. All of these

10. Your patient is unresponsive and has a large amount of vomitus in the oropharynx. Which suction catheter should be used?
   a. English catheter
   b. French catheter
   c. Hard catheter
   d. Soft catheter

11. Suction should only be applied for _____ seconds in the adult patient and _____ seconds for infants and children.
    a. 20, 10
    b. 20, 5
    c. 15, 5
    d. 10, 5

12. You are preparing to suction the patient with inadequate breathing who is producing large amounts of frothy secretions that are continuous and require constant suctioning. You should
    a. suction for 15 seconds, provide oxygen by nonrebreather mask for 15 seconds, repeat.
    b. suction for 15 seconds, provide oxygen by nonrebreather mask for 5 minutes, repeat.
    c. suction for 15 seconds, provide positive-pressure ventilation for 2 minutes, repeat.
    d. Suction for 15 seconds, provide positive-pressure ventilation for 10 minutes, repeat.

13. You have decided to use an oropharyngeal airway on a deeply unresponsive patient. How would you measure for the proper size?
    a. Measure the airway from the tip of the patient's nose to the tip of the earlobe.
    b. Measure the airway from the patient's earlobe to the bottom of the angle of the jaw.
    c. Measure the airway from the level of the front teeth to the angle of the jaw.
    d. Oropharyngeal airways should not be used if the patient is deeply unresponsive.

14. After selecting the correct-size nasopharyngeal airway and lubricating the airway with a water-soluble lubricant, the airway should be inserted into the larger nostril until
    a. the patient gags, and then pull back slightly.
    b. resistance is met or bleeding occurs.
    c. the flange rests on the flare of the nostril.
    d. the bevel comes in contact with the septum.

15. Cells that are not receiving an adequate amount of oxygen are suffering from
    a. hypoxia.
    b. hypoventilation.
    c. hyperperfusion.
    d. hemoglobin.

16. You must assess your patient for adequate or inadequate breathing. Briefly describe what you would observe about the following four factors in a patient who is breathing adequately.
    a. Rate

    b. Rhythm

    c. Quality

    d. Depth

17. Which of the following is a late and significant sign of hypoxia?
    a. Headache
    b. Hypertension
    c. Cyanosis
    d. Restlessness

18. What are the normal respiratory rate limits for the following patients?
    Adult: _____ to _____ respirations a minute
    Child: _____ to _____ respirations a minute
    Infant: _____ to _____ respirations a minute

19. From the answers below, choose the one that best indicates that your patient is breathing adequately.
    a. Bilateral chest rise
    b. Tachypnea
    c. Bradypnea
    d. Agonal breathing

20. You are treating a medical patient who is responding to painful stimuli with moaning. His breathing is adequate. The best method to protect this patient from aspirating is to
    a. place the patient on a nonrebreather mask at 15 lpm.
    b. place the patient in a modified lateral (recovery) position.
    c. insert an oropharyngeal airway.
    d. apply cricoid pressure while he is in a supine position.

21. After auscultating the chest of an elderly patient who has fallen out of bed, you note that the breath sounds on both sides are dramatically decreased. You should
    a. place the patient back into bed.
    b. administer oxygen by nonrebreather mask.
    c. provide positive-pressure ventilation.
    d. help the patient to a sitting position.

22. Which of the following statements regarding the use of cricoid pressure (Sellick's maneuver) is correct?
    a. It cannot be used in the deeply unresponsive apneic patient.
    b. It collapses the trachea against the cervical vertebrae.
    c. It helps to protect the airway from regurgitated stomach contents.
    d. It can be used in the patient with an altered mental status.

23. You know that exhaled breath contains about
    a. 21 percent oxygen.
    b. 16 percent oxygen.
    c. 5 percent oxygen.
    d. 0.05 percent oxygen.

24. You are preparing to ventilate your patient with the pocket mask. Which of the following is an advantage of performing mouth-to-mask ventilations with the pocket mask?
    a. The mask eliminates direct contact with the patient.
    b. There is no need for the use of an oral airway.
    c. Nearly 100 percent oxygen concentrations can be reached.
    d. The device eliminates the need to watch for chest rise.

25. When ventilating the apneic patient with a pulse using the bag-valve mask (BVM), the adult patient should be ventilated every _____ seconds, and the infant and child should be ventilated every _____ seconds.
   a. 5 to 6, 3 to 5
   b. 2 to 3, 3 to 5
   c. 8 to 10, 5 to 6
   d. 3 to 5, 5 to 6

26. Fill in the parts of the bag-valve mask unit on the appropriate lines.

   Bag
   Face mask
   Intake valve/oxygen-reservoir valve
   Nonrebreathing patient valve
   Oxygen reservoir
   Oxygen-supply connecting tube
   A_____
   B_____
   C_____
   D_____
   E_____
   F_____

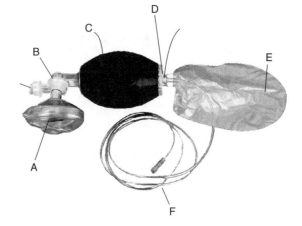

27. The bag-valve mask with a reservoir, when attached to an oxygen source, can deliver nearly 100 percent oxygen. What percentage of oxygen is delivered to the patient by bag-valve mask without an oxygen source?
   a. 61 percent
   b. 41 percent
   c. 21 percent
   d. 11 percent

28. Which of the following is a desirable feature of the bag-valve mask?
   a. It allows a single operator to easily maintain a tight mask seal.
   b. It allows delivery of ventilations enriched from an oxygen source.
   c. It can be easily taught to the emergency medical responder (EMR) and layperson.
   d. It protects the airway from regurgitation of vomitus.

29. Your patient is experiencing agonal breathing, and you suspect a spinal injury. You should
   a. perform a head-tilt/chin-lift to open the airway, then ventilate.
   b. pull on the head to align the airway, then ventilate.
   c. establish in-line stabilization and perform a jaw-thrust maneuver, then ventilate.
   d. establish in-line stabilization, but do not ventilate because the patient is breathing.

30. From the following, choose the correct statement pertaining to use of the flow-restricted, oxygen-powered ventilation device (FROPVD).
   a. It is unnecessary to use an airway adjunct while in use.
   b. It is the ventilation of choice for children and infants.
   c. Gastric distention is a rare side effect.
   d. Improper use may rupture the lungs.

31. When ventilating with the flow-restricted, oxygen-powered ventilation device, the trigger or button on the valve should be released
    a. as soon as the chest begins to rise.
    b. after the chest has risen fully.
    c. after the audible alarm sounds.
    d. after 5 to 7 seconds of activation.

32. While ventilating a patient with the FROPVD, the chest does not rise adequately. You should *first*
    a. depress the trigger or button up to twice as long.
    b. follow foreign body airway obstruction maneuvers.
    c. reevaluate the position of the head, chin, and mask seal.
    d. use an alternative means to ventilate the patient.

33. To determine the correct tidal volume and rate for the automatic transport ventilator (ATV), you should
    a. watch the stomach rise and fall.
    b. consult with medical oversight.
    c. set the inspiration time for 10 seconds.
    d. estimate the tidal volume by observing the pulse oximeter.

34. Although there are different sizes of oxygen tanks, when full, all contain the same pressure, which is
    a. approximately 1,000 pounds per square inch.
    b. approximately 2,000 pounds per square inch.
    c. approximately 3,000 pounds per square inch.
    d. approximately 4,000 pounds per square inch.

35. Which of the following, when it comes into contact with oxygen under pressure, may cause an explosion to occur?
    a. Ambient air
    b. Petroleum jelly
    c. All adhesive tapes
    d. Sterile water

36. Which type of pressure regulator has only one gauge, which registers the content of the oxygen tank?
    a. Therapy regulator
    b. Treatment regulator
    c. High-pressure regulator
    d. Continuous-flow regulator

37. You are preparing to change the oxygen tank to a full one. To remove any dust or debris, before placing the yoke of the pressure regulator onto the oxygen cylinder, you should
    a. tap the valve with the yolk of the regulator.
    b. wipe the valve stem with a clean, damp cloth.
    c. quickly open and shut the valve on the cylinder.
    d. gently rinse the valve under running water.

38. You have transferred your patient over to the receiving-facility staff. When discontinuing the oxygen administration to the patient, you should
    a. turn off the oxygen, then remove the mask from the patient's face.
    b. remove the mask from the patient's face, then turn off the oxygen.
    c. hyperoxygenate the patient for 5 minutes, then remove the mask.
    d. turn off the oxygen, then ask the patient to breathe for 2 minutes.

39. While preparing to administer oxygen to your patient, you know the liter flow typically needed to keep the reservoir bag filled on the nonrebreather mask is
    a. 2 liters per minute.
    b. 5 liters per minute.
    c. 10 liters per minute.
    d. 15 liters per minute.

40. You are attempting to treat a child with a nonrebreather mask, but the child will not tolerate the mask and pushes it away from his face. What is the recommended way to continue the treatment?
    a. Hold the mask on the face, while diverting the child's attention.
    b. Ask the parent to hold the mask on the face until the child accepts the mask.
    c. Have someone familiar with the child hold the mask close to the child's face.
    d. Administer the oxygen by using the flow-restricted, oxygen-powered ventilation device.

41. The nasal cannula is not a preferred method of administering oxygen in the prehospital setting and is mainly indicated
    a. when the patient will not tolerate a nonrebreather mask.
    b. as an adjunct to the nonrebreather mask.
    c. when the patient requests its use.
    d. for transports lasting longer than 30 minutes.

42. The proper liter-flow range for the nasal cannula is commonly set at _____ liters per minute.
    a. 1–6
    b. 8–10
    c. 15
    d. 22–44

43. The only mask recommended for oxygen delivery in the prehospital setting is which one of the following?
    a. Simple face mask
    b. Partial rebreather mask
    c. Nonrebreather mask
    d. Venturi mask

44. If your patient's dentures are securely in place, before ventilating, you should
    a. remove them to achieve a better mask seal.
    b. remove them to avoid the danger of breaking them in the mouth.
    c. leave them in the mouth so they will not be misplaced.
    d. leave them in the mouth to achieve a better mask seal.

45. You arrive on the scene and find a 62-year-old male lying on the garage floor. The police indicate that this is an attempted suicide. They indicate the patient had the car running in the garage with all the doors shut. As you assess the patient, you note that he is breathing at 24

times per minute with adequate volume. Your partner attaches the pulse oximeter prior to your placing the patient on oxygen. You would anticipate the SpO_2 reading to be

a. less than 70 percent.
b. approximately 90 percent.
c. 93 to 95 percent.
d. close to 100 percent.

46. In the healthy patient chemoreceptors in the brain sense changes in _____ levels and send impulses to the respiratory muscles to increase or decrease the rate and depth of respirations, thus controlling the respiratory effort.

a. hydrogen
b. carbon dioxide
c. oxygen
d. nitrogen

47. The patient suffering from a condition known as chronic obstructive pulmonary disease (COPD) typically has chronically high carbon dioxide levels; thus the chemoreceptors must rely on which of the following to regulate breathing?

a. Carbon monoxide
b. Oxygen
c. Nitrogen
d. Hydrogen

48. You are assessing a patient that displays signs of hypoxia; you immediately assess the airway for adequacy of breathing. The patient presents with poor tidal volume and tachypnea. You should next

a. apply oxygen by nasal cannula.
b. apply oxygen via nonrebreather mask.
c. provide positive-pressure ventilations.
d. provide blow-by oxygen at 100 percent.

49. Which of the following positions may lead to inadequate ventilations and severe hypoxia by pushing the abdominal contents upward against the diaphragm, limiting its movement?

a. Supine
b. Recovery
c. Semi-Fowler
d. Prone

50. You are preparing to suction your patient using a rigid (Yankauer) catheter. You know the tip of the catheter may stimulate the vagus nerve, causing the patient to become

a. bradycardic.
b. apneic.
c. tachypneic.
d. hypovolemic.

51. You are assessing the adequacy of your patient's breathing. What two variables must you know before you can accurately assess the breathing?

a. Respiratory rate and tidal volume
b. Respiratory volume and minute rate
c. Spirometer volume and respiratory effort
d. Oximeter reading and minute volume

52. You have assessed your patient and determined he is breathing 12 times a minute with an inadequate tidal volume. You should immediately increase the tidal volume by
    a. instructing the patient to increase his breaths per minute by breathing faster.
    b. delivering a ventilation with the BVM when the patient begins to breath in.
    c. placing the patient in the tripod position and instructing him to use accessory muscles.
    d. delivering smaller-volume breaths at an increased minute rate using the BVM.

53. You are providing ventilations to a pulseless adult patient using the laryngeal-mask airway (LMA). What ventilation rate should this patient receive?
    a. 3 to 5 ventilations per minute
    b. 5 to 7 ventilations per minute
    c. 8 to 10 ventilations per minute
    d. 12 to 14 ventilations per minute

54. You are preparing to provide ventilations to your apneic newborn patient with a pulse. At what rate should you ventilate this patient?
    a. 10 to 12 ventilations per minute
    b. 12 to 20 ventilations per minute
    c. 20 to 30 ventilations per minute
    d. 40 to 60 ventilations per minute

55. You are attempting to ventilate your pulseless and apneic trauma patient; the jaw thrust is ineffective in opening the airway. You should
    a. continue to apply the jaw thrust until the airway is maintained.
    b. perform the head-tilt/chin-lift maneuver to ventilate the patient.
    c. call for ALS backup and wait for their arrival to perform an emergency airway.
    d. place the patient in the coma or left lateral recumbent position and transport immediately.

56. You are preparing to ventilate your adult patient that is breathing at a rate of 40 breaths per minute (tachypnea), which leads to an inadequate tidal volume (hypopnea). You should
    a. ventilate at the patient's rate, then slowly adjust the rate to one breath every 5 to 6 seconds.
    b. continue to ventilate at the patient's rate until the respiratory effort spontaneously decreases.
    c. ventilate at a lower than normal rate—every 8 to 12 seconds—until the patient's rate decreases.
    d. provide ventilations of one breath every 5 to 6 seconds, then increase the rate to every 3 to 4 seconds.

57. You are preparing to ventilate your adult stoma patient with the bag-valve mask. Which of the following is an acceptable practice when ventilating the adult stoma patient?
    a. When suctioning, insert a soft suction catheter approximately 6 to 8 inches.
    b. Perform a head-tilt/chin-lift or jaw-thrust maneuver to manage the airway.
    c. Select a mask—usually the child or infant mask—to fit securely over the stoma.
    d. Administer the ventilation over a 3- to 4-second period, watching for abdominal rise.

58. You have responded to a report of a child choking on a toy. You find the responsive child choking but moving air when inhaling and exhaling, You should
    a. perform a head-tilt/chin-lift maneuver to clear the airway.
    b. instruct the patient to cough to try to dislodge the object.
    c. administer abdominal thrusts to expel the object from the airway.
    d. instruct the mother to perform a blind finger sweep of the mouth.

CASE STUDY 1

You and your partner, Ashley, are dispatched to a local church for an elderly woman suffering from shortness of breath. As you walk in, a member of the clergy directs you to the back of the church, where you find a woman sitting bolt upright in a tripod position, obviously very anxious. You introduce yourselves to the patient, and she replies with gasping breaths, "I'm Mary. Help me. I can't breathe." You reassure her and, anticipating possible respiratory arrest, call for paramedic backup from another station.

1. From your brief interaction with Mary, what indications lead you to believe she is experiencing serious respiratory distress? (Name at least three.)

2. At this time, which of the following would be the most appropriate for Mary?
   a. Nasal cannula at 6 liters per minute
   b. Venturi mask at 10 liters per minute
   c. Simple face mask at 10 liters per minute
   d. Nonrebreather mask at 15 liters per minute

A friend of Mary's tells you that Mary has emphysema (chronic obstructive pulmonary disease) and sometimes has to be on oxygen at home. As you assess Mary's breathing sounds, you detect a gurgling noise and then notice a pink frothy secretion coming from her mouth. Ashley advises you that Mary's respiratory rate is 36 per minute.

3. Which suction catheter and technique would be most appropriate for Mary in this situation?
   a. Use a rigid catheter, insert the catheter without suction, apply suction for 15 seconds.
   b. Use a rigid catheter, insert the catheter with suction, suction for 20 seconds.
   c. Use a French catheter, insert into the mouth without suction, apply for 15 seconds.
   d. Use a soft catheter, insert into the mouth without suction, apply for 20 seconds.

It becomes apparent that Mary's breathing is inadequate and that positive-pressure ventilation is needed. You decide to use the bag-valve mask, with you and Ashley delivering the ventilations. Before using the mask and the associated airway adjuncts, Ashley explains the procedure to Mary.

4. Keeping in mind that Mary is still slightly responsive, which of the following adjuncts and techniques is most appropriate for Mary at this time?
   a. Oropharyngeal airway inserted by using the 180-degree-turn advancing technique
   b. Oropharyngeal airway inserted by using a tongue-depressor technique
   c. Nasopharyngeal airway inserted bevel first until the flange rests on the nostril
   d. Nasopharyngeal airway inserted flange first until the bevel rests on the nostril

Despite your best team efforts, Mary becomes unresponsive and is no longer breathing on her own. Her pulse can be felt and is bounding. Dispatch advises you that the estimated time of arrival for the paramedic backup unit is less than one minute.

5. What should you and Ashley do, now that Mary is not breathing on her own?
   a. Start cardiopulmonary resuscitation (CPR) until the paramedic unit arrives.
   b. Continue to ventilate and suction the patient as you did when she was responsive.
   c. Continue to ventilate the patient but, because she is unresponsive, suction is not needed.
   d. Roll the patient to clear the airway, and start CPR immediately.

CASE STUDY 2

You and your partner, Joshua, are dispatched to a construction site where there is a report of a young female worker who fell from the third floor. Dispatch advises you that Engine Company 4 and a paramedic backup unit from your system are both responding. Your unit arrives on-scene. As you approach the patient, a coworker states that the patient fell head first from the third floor onto the dirt where she lies now. Another worker tells you the patient was unconscious when he rolled her from her stomach to her back. As you visually examine the patient, you notice that she is breathing with agonal respirations and is bleeding freely from the mouth.

1. In the above situation, how would you open the mouth and airway?
    a. In-line stabilization with the hyperextension/head-lift maneuver
    b. In-line stabilization with the head-tilt/chin-lift maneuver
    c. In-line stabilization with the jaw-thrust maneuver
    d. In-line stabilization with the crossed-finger technique

2. After opening the mouth and airway, you find a copious amount of blood with teeth in the oropharynx. How should you remove the foreign material?
    a. Turn the patient's head to the side to permit drainage.
    b. Roll the patient to a prone position and finger sweep.
    c. Suction, using the soft or French catheter.
    d. Suction, using the rigid or hard catheter.

The patient's agonal respirations are clearly inadequate. With the oral airway in place, Joshua will stabilize the patient's head and hold the bag-valve mask in place while you squeeze the bag to ventilate the patient. You squeeze the bag, but the patient's chest does not rise.

3. Which of the following may cause the chest not to rise with ventilations?
    a. Incorrect position of the head and chin
    b. Air escaping from around the mask
    c. Airway obstruction
    d. Any or all of the above may cause a failure.

After reevaluating and adjusting your patient and airway technique, the patient's chest is rising and falling normally with every squeeze of the bag. The backup paramedic unit arrives, with the engine company following. The paramedic lieutenant states, "This type of airway problem can be very difficult to control. You did a good job." You and Joshua assist the paramedics with spinal immobilization and give them your report. Joshua assists the paramedics further on the way to the hospital.

AIRWAY: CHAPTER 7

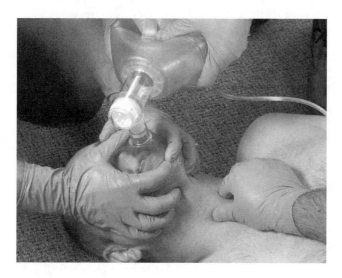

The module on airway management concerns basic techniques for establishing and maintaining an open airway and providing artificial ventilation and oxygen therapy.

Q   Why is Chapter 7 an entire module all by itself?

A   Airway care is of critical importance. Without a patent airway, no patient will survive, no matter what else is done for him or her.

Q   How important is it to learn the head-tilt/chin-lift and jaw-thrust maneuvers, suctioning procedures, and how to insert an airway adjunct?

A   These are essential. When a patient's mental status declines, perhaps to the point of unresponsiveness (unconsciousness), the muscles of the airway relax, and the tongue may fall back into the airway. The patient's head may flex forward or extend backward, causing poor alignment or closing off of airway passages. The patient may lose the gag reflex or the ability to cough and clear his or her own airway so that fluids and foreign particles must be suctioned to keep the airway clear. An airway adjunct may be required to help keep the airway open once you have opened it. These are the basic airway-management techniques every EMT must master and be ready to use.

Q   Why is it important to know both child and adult airway anatomy?

A   The airway anatomy of infants and children differs from that of adults in several significant ways. The head is larger and thus more likely to tip forward when the child is supine. The mouth and nose are smaller, but the tongue is relatively larger in the mouth. The trachea is narrower and thus more likely to become blocked. The chest wall is softer and should respond more obviously to artificial ventilations. These differences must be kept in mind when performing airway and ventilation procedures, and appropriate sizes of equipment, such as airway adjuncts, must be chosen.

Q **Why does breathing have to be assessed? Isn't it easy to tell if a person is breathing or not breathing? What does "inadequate breathing" mean?**

A It's easy to tell if a person is breathing or not breathing. It is not so easy to tell if a person is breathing inadequately, that is, not taking in enough oxygen to sustain life. A person is breathing inadequately when the rate is outside normal ranges, either too fast or too slow; when the breathing pattern is irregular; or when there is a poor quality of breathing (breath sounds are decreased or absent when you listen to the chest with a stethoscope; the chest wall is not rising and falling adequately with each breath or the two sides of the chest rise and fall unequally; the breathing is shallow and you cannot feel an adequate amount of air coming from the person's mouth or nose with exhalation). When a person is breathing inadequately (or not breathing at all), positive-pressure ventilation with supplemental oxygen must be provided.

Q **What is "positive-pressure ventilation"?**

A "Positive-pressure ventilation" is another term for artificial ventilation or artificial respiration. It is any of several means of forcing air into a patient's lungs (by exerting positive pressure) when the patient cannot breathe or breathe adequately on his or her own. Mouth-to-mask ventilation is preferred because it protects the rescuer from the patient's secretions, delivers a greater tidal volume of air than the bag-valve mask, and requires only a single rescuer. Bag-valve mask ventilation performed by two rescuers is the next preferred method, followed by the flow-restricted, oxygen-powered ventilation device. One-rescuer bag-valve-mask ventilation is the least preferred method because of the difficulties of one person holding a mask seal and providing adequate tidal volumes of air.

Q **What about providing oxygen by nonrebreather mask? Is this another form of positive-pressure ventilation?**

A When the patient can benefit from additional oxygen but is able to breathe adequately on his or her own, oxygen may be provided (at a flow rate of 15 liters per minute) by nonrebreather mask. This is not the same as positive-pressure ventilation because no pressure is exerted to force the oxygen into the lungs. The oxygen supplied through the nonrebreather mask is breathed in by the patient. Oxygen may be supplied by nasal cannula, which provides oxygen at a maximum flow rate of 6 liters per minute, only if the patient will not tolerate a nonrebreather mask.

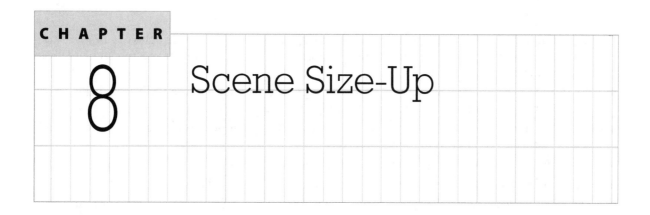

OBJECTIVES

Numbered objectives are from the United States Department of Transportation EMT-Basic National Standard Curriculum. Asterisked objectives, if any, pertain to material that is supplemental to the DOT curriculum.

Cognitive

3-1.1 Recognize hazards/potential hazards.
3-1.2 Describe common hazards found at the scene of a trauma and medical patient.
3-1.3 Determine if the scene is safe to enter.
3-1.4 Discuss common mechanisms of injury/nature of illness.
3-1.5 Discuss the reason for identifying the total number of patients at the scene.
3-1.6 Explain the reason for identifying the need for additional help or assistance.
   * Explain how to gain scene control.
   * Explain how to establish rapport with the patient.

KEY IDEAS

This chapter covers the importance of proper scene size-up. Because the prehospital environment can be hostile and uncontrolled, it is extremely important to follow basic guidelines and use good sense when working as an EMT. It is imperative that the EMT pay close attention to the scene size-up on every call. By doing so, you may save your life as well as that of your partner and patient.

- The EMT must ensure the safety of the EMS crew first, then that of the patient and bystanders.

- Note scene characteristics such as blood and other hazards that may require the use of personal protective equipment (PPE) and body substance isolation (BSI) measures.

- Survey the total scene before entering, looking for hazards that make the scene unstable, and do not enter if you are not trained to stabilize the hazards.

- The scene size-up consists of evaluating the five components in a stepwise manner: taking necessary BSI and other personal protection precautions; evaluating the scene for safety hazards; determining the mechanism of injury (MOI) or the nature of illness (NOI); determining the number of patients; and determining the need for additional resources.

- Beware of low-oxygen, toxic-substance, and confined-space areas, such as sewers, caverns, wells, manholes, silos, and closed storage areas. Never enter unless you are certain it is safe.

- Never enter a known crime scene unless it has been secured by the police. Be cautious and ready to retreat.

- At a crime scene, take steps to help preserve evidence. However, remember that your primary concern is treating the patient. Limit potential exposure to hazards by practicing recommendations suggested in the text.
- While on the scene of vehicle crashes, prevent emergency personnel and the EMT from being struck by traffic by practicing scene-safety recommendations suggested in the text.
- The EMT must be prepared to call upon additional specialized rescue resources to ensure not only his own well-being but also the successful rescue of the patient.
- Note whether the patient's problem is traumatic or medical in nature.
- The trauma-scene size-up includes determining the mechanism of injury.
- The medical-scene size-up requires collecting evidence that may help identify the nature of the illness.
- Determine the number of patients, and call for additional resources, if needed, prior to making contact with the patient.
- Reduce the patient's anxiety by bringing order to the environment, introducing yourself, gaining consent, positioning yourself, using good communication skills, being courteous, and using touch when appropriate.
- The scene size-up is a dynamic process that requires the EMT to continuously assess and reassess the emergency scene for potential hazards.

TERMS AND CONCEPTS

1. For each patient-care situation described below, indicate if it is a traumatic (T) or a medical (M) condition.

    _____ a. Six-inch laceration to the right anterior forearm

    _____ b. Gunshot wound to the right chest at nipple level on the midaxillary line

    _____ c. Shortness of breath with audible wheezing on expiration

    _____ d. Burn to the right anterior aspect of the thigh

    _____ e. Ingestion of 20 to 30 capsules of an unknown medication

    _____ f. Hot, dry, flushed skin

2. Write the number of the correct term next to each definition.
    1. Index of suspicion
    2. Mechanism of injury (MOI)
    3. Nature of illness (NOI)
    4. Scene safety
    5. Scene size-up

    _____ a. An overall assessment of the scene to which an EMT has been called

    _____ b. An anticipation that certain types of accidents and mechanisms will produce specific types of injuries

    _____ c. Factor involved in producing an injury to a patient, including the strength, direction, and nature of the force that caused the injury

    _____ d. Steps taken to ensure the safety and well-being of the EMT, coworkers, patients, and bystanders

    _____ e. The type of medical condition or complaint from which a patient is suffering

CONTENT REVIEW

1. One of the first goals of an EMT responding to a scene is scene safety. With this goal in mind, the EMT is concerned with the well-being of which of the following?
   a. The EMTs, patients, and bystanders
   b. The EMTs and patients only
   c. The EMTs only
   d. The patients only

2. Ensuring scene safety begins
   a. after patient contact is made.
   b. after arrival at the scene.
   c. while approaching the scene.
   d. while receiving dispatch information.

3. The EMT must use different levels of body substance isolation protection. Which BSI protection device should be used with every patient contact?
   a. Protective gown
   b. Eye protection
   c. Protective gloves
   d. HEPA or N-95 respirator

4. To help protect the patient's privacy from onlookers and to control bystanders, it is most effective to
   a. ask some of the bystanders to turn their backs to the patient while holding an unfolded bed sheet at shoulder height.
   b. advise the bystanders to immediately leave the scene or you will be forced to notify the police.
   c. request that the police immediately remove the bystanders from the scene.
   d. request that the police arrest curious bystanders for interfering with the patient's confidentiality.

5. As you arrive on the perimeter of a motor vehicle accident scene, you notice that there appear to be more patients than your unit can effectively handle. You should *first*
   a. proceed to the scene and evaluate the patients' needs.
   b. proceed to the patients and begin treatment.
   c. stage off the scene until law enforcement arrives.
   d. call for additional resources.

6. You are on a motor vehicle accident scene where power lines are lying across the vehicle. Which statement is correct?
   a. Consider all power lines to be energized until a power-company representative advises you they are not.
   b. If the power lines are not arcing or smoking, you may assume the lines are safe and not energized.
   c. You should approach the vehicle and remove the wires by using a wooden or fiberglass pole.
   d. If a local firefighter states, "The power was cut by the fire department," you can assume that it is safe.

You introduce your partner and yourself to the patient, and your partner radios dispatch to inform them that patient contact has been made and that you are OK. You explain to the patient that the mask you are wearing is a precaution you take when a patient is coughing a lot. When you ask the patient to tell you why she had her husband call the ambulance, the patient replies, "I've been coughing uncontrollably for the past week. I need relief." The patient says she has not seen a doctor about her condition and doesn't know what may be causing it. She denies having any other symptoms, but you make a note of some clues in the environment that you will report to the hospital staff: a thermometer on the nightstand and pink-tinged tissues in a wastebasket by the bed, indications that the patient may be running a fever and coughing up blood-tinged sputum. You gather a couple of bottles of over-the-counter cough medications the patient has been taking in an effort to control her cough and bring them to the hospital.

3. While you are transporting this patient to the hospital, which of the following would be appropriate?
   a. Because the patient and the scene present signs of TB, you continue to wear the respirator and advise the hospital of the precaution.
   b. The patient and the scene present signs of TB, but because TB is not contagious, you take off the N-95 or HEPA respirator.
   c. Because the patient has not received a doctor's diagnosis of TB, you take off the N-95 or HEPA respirator.
   d. Because you are in the ambulance and not in the patient's house, the N-95 or HEPA respirator is not needed and you take it off.

9 Patient Assessment

OBJECTIVES

Numbered objectives are from the United States Department of Transportation EMT-Basic National Standard Curriculum. Asterisked objectives, if any, pertain to material that is supplemental to the DOT curriculum.

Cognitive

PART 1: Scene Size-Up

3-1.4 Discuss common mechanisms of injury/nature of illness.
3-1.5 Discuss the reason for identifying the total number of patients at the scene.
3-1.6 Explain the reason for identifying the need for additional help or assistance.
    * Explain how to gain scene control.
    * Explain how to establish rapport with the patient.

PART 2: Initial Assessment

3-2.1 Summarize the reasons for forming a general impression of the patient.
3-2.2 Discuss methods of assessing altered mental status.
3-2.3 Differentiate between assessing the altered mental status in the adult, child, and infant patient.
3-2.4 Discuss methods of assessing the airway in the adult, child, and infant patient.
3-2.5 State reasons for management of the cervical spine once the patient has been determined to be a trauma patient.
3-2.6 Describe the methods used for assessing if a patient is breathing.
3-2.7 State what care should be provided to the adult, child, and infant patient with adequate breathing.
3-2.8 State what care should be provided to the adult, child, and infant patient without adequate breathing.
3-2.9 Differentiate between a patient with adequate and inadequate breathing.
3-2.10 Distinguish between methods of assessing breathing in the adult, child, and infant patient.
3-2.11 Compare the methods of providing airway care to the adult, child, and infant patient.
3-2.12 Describe the methods used to obtain a pulse.
3-2.13 Differentiate between obtaining a pulse in the adult, child, and infant patient.
3-2.14 Discuss the need for assessing the patient for external bleeding.
3-2.15 Describe normal and abnormal findings when assessing skin color.
3-2.16 Describe normal and abnormal findings when assessing skin temperature.
3-2.17 Describe normal and abnormal findings when assessing skin condition.
3-2.18 Describe normal and abnormal findings when assessing capillary refill in the infant and child patient.
3-2.19 Explain the reason for prioritizing a patient for care and transport.

PART 3: Focused History and Physical Exam

For a Trauma Patient

3-3.1 Discuss the reasons for reconsideration concerning the mechanism of injury.

3-3.2 State the reasons for performing a rapid trauma assessment.

3-3.3 Recite examples and explain why patients should receive a rapid trauma assessment.

3-3.4 Describe the areas included in the rapid trauma assessment and discuss what should be evaluated.

3-3.5 Differentiate when the rapid assessment may be altered in order to provide patient care.

3-3.6 Discuss the reason for performing a focused history and physical exam.

For a Medical Patient

3-4.1 Describe the unique needs for assessing an individual with a specific chief complaint with no known prior history.

3-4.2 Differentiate between the history and physical exam that are performed for responsive patients with no known prior history and responsive patients with a known prior history.

3-4.3 Describe the needs for assessing an individual who is unresponsive.

3-4.4 Differentiate between the assessment that is performed on a patient who is unresponsive or has an altered mental status and other medical patients requiring assessment.

PART 4: Detailed Physical Exam

3-5.1 Discuss the components of the detailed physical exam.

3-5.2 State the areas of the body that are evaluated during the detailed physical exam.

3-5.3 Explain what additional care should be provided while performing the detailed physical exam.

3-5.4 Distinguish between the detailed physical exam that is performed on a trauma patient and that of the medical patient.

PART 5: Ongoing Assessment

3-6.1 Discuss the reasons for repeating the initial assessment as part of the ongoing assessment.

3-6.2 Describe the components of the ongoing assessment.

3-6.3 Describe trending of assessment components.

KEY IDEAS

Performing an accurate and reliable assessment is your most important function as an EMT. All treatment and transport decisions will be based on the information gathered during the assessment. It is important to develop a consistent routine for assessing all patients. This chapter introduces basic assessment skills.

- The purposes of assessing patients include the following: determining if the incident is a medical or traumatic emergency, to identify and manage life threats; determining the transport priority; examining the patient; providing care based on the findings; monitoring the patient; communicating information to the medical staff; and documenting the call.

- Patient assessment includes the scene size-up, initial assessment, focused history and physical exam (conducted somewhat differently for a trauma patient and a medical patient), detailed physical exam, and ongoing assessment. Communication and documentation are also key elements of patient assessment.

- The scene size-up includes taking body substance isolation (BSI) precautions, evaluating scene hazards, determining the mechanism of injury or the nature of the illness, establishing the number of patients, and identifying the need for additional resources that may be required.

- The initial assessment is conducted on *all patients*. The primary purpose of the initial assessment is to identify and manage immediately life-threatening conditions to the airway, breathing, and circulation. The six steps conducted in this sequence are (1) forming a general impression of the patient, (2) assessing mental status, (3) assessing the airway, (4) assessing breathing, (5) assessing circulation, and (6) establishing patient priorities for transport and further assessment and care.

- The focused history and physical exam has three parts. For a trauma patient or an unresponsive medical patient, it is conducted in this sequence: (1) physical exam, (2) baseline vital-sign assessment, (3) history taking (using the acronym SAMPLE to represent categories of information to obtain during the history). For a responsive medical patient, the steps of the focused history and physical exam are generally conducted in this sequence: (1) SAMPLE history, (2) physical exam, (3) baseline vital-sign assessment. For a patient who is unresponsive or who has a significant mechanism of injury, altered mental status, suspected multiple injuries, or critical findings in the initial assessment, the physical exam is a rapid head-to-toe trauma or medical assessment. For a responsive patient who has a specific, localized injury or medical complaint and no significant mechanism of injury, no multiple injuries, and is alert and oriented, the physical exam will focus on the area of the injury or complaint.

- The detailed physical exam is a more thorough version of the rapid trauma or rapid medical assessment. It is a detailed head-to-toe examination typically conducted in the ambulance en route to the hospital, if time and the patient's condition permit, to discover any additional injuries or conditions that may previously have been overlooked.

- The ongoing assessment is conducted at frequent intervals, beginning immediately after the focused history and physical exam, or immediately after the detailed physical exam if one is conducted. The purposes of the ongoing assessment are to determine any changes in the patient's condition, to assess the effectiveness of your emergency care, and to intervene as necessary.

MEDICAL TERMINOLOGY

Term	Prefix	Word Root Combining Form	Suffix	Definition
apnea (AP-nee-uh)	a- (no, not, without, lack of)	pnea (breathing)		The absence of breathing
dyspnea (DISP-nee-uh)	dys- (bad, difficult)	pnea (breathing)		Difficult or labored breathing
hemiplegia (hem-uh-PLEE-ja)	hemi- (half)	plegia (paralysis)		Paralysis of an arm and leg on one side of the body
icteric, icterus (ik-TAIR-ik, IK-ter-us)		icter (jaundice)	-ic (pertaining to) -us (condition of)	Yellow skin or sclera
paraplegia (pair-uh-PLEE-ja)	para- (beside)	plegia (paralysis)		Paralysis of both legs
quadriplegia (kwad-ruh-PLEE-ja)	quadri- (four)	plegia (paralysis)		Paralysis of both arms and both legs

1. In each space, write the prefix, word root, or suffix that matches the definition.

a   ic   plegia

dys   icter   pnea

hemi   para   quadri

_____ a. Breathing   _____ f. Four

_____ b. Difficult   _____ g. Beside

_____ c. No, not, without, lack of   _____ h. Half

_____ d. Jaundice   _____ i. Paralysis

_____ e. Pertaining to

TERMS AND CONCEPTS

1. Write the number of the correct term next to each definition.

   1. Apnea
   2. Aspiration
   3. AVPU
   4. Battle's sign
   5. Cerebrospinal fluid
   6. Chief complaint
   7. Flail segment

   8. Focused medical assessment
   9. Focused trauma assessment
   10. Initial assessment
   11. Paradoxical motion
   12. Rapid medical assessment
   13. Rapid trauma assessment

   _____ a. Head-to-toe physical exam that is swiftly conducted on a patient with a significant mechanism of injury

   _____ b. Breathing a substance into the lungs

   _____ c. Two or more adjacent ribs that are fractured in two or more places

   _____ d. The patient's answer to the question, "Why did you call the ambulance?"

   _____ e. Black-and-blue discoloration to the mastoid area behind the ear, a late sign of skull or head injury

   _____ f. The movement of a section of the chest in the opposite direction from the rest of the chest during respiration

   _____ g. A head-to-toe physical exam that is swiftly conducted on an unresponsive medical patient or a medical patient who is suspected to also have injuries

   _____ h. Exam that is focused on a specific injury site, performed on a patient with no significant mechanism of injury

   _____ i. The portion of the assessment conducted immediately following scene size-up for the purpose of discovering immediately life-threatening conditions

   _____ j. Exam that is focused on the parts of the body indicated by the ill patient's chief complaint, signs, or symptoms

   _____ k. The absence of breathing

   _____ l. Fluid that surrounds and cushions the brain and spinal cord

   _____ m. A mnemonic for alert, responds to verbal stimulus, responds to painful stimulus, unresponsive—to characterize levels of responsiveness

CONTENT REVIEW

1. The primary rationale for conducting a patient assessment is to
   a. completely manage all injuries and medical conditions.
   b. gather a comprehensive and complete patient medical history.
   c. perform a careful and complete physical exam of the patient.
   d. determine the illness or injury and establish transport priorities.

2. The _____ and the _____ are the first two stages of performing a patient assessment.
   a. scene size-up, focused history and physical exam
   b. initial assessment, focused history and physical exam
   c. scene size-up, initial assessment
   d. initial assessment, detailed physical exam

SCENE SIZE-UP

3. You have been dispatched to a scene where the patient's family is extremely hostile. A family member has made physical threats to you and your partner. Which of the following is the best action to take in this situation?
   a. Use scene-control techniques to regain control.
   b. Move as rapidly as possible to leave the scene.
   c. Request immediate law-enforcement backup.
   d. Work back-to-back with your partner for protection.

INITIAL ASSESSMENT

4. You have arrived on the scene of a 25-year-old male who was struck by a car. The distraught driver of the car states that he was traveling about 30 miles per hour and his car struck the patient on his left side. The patient's head is turned to the side, his eyes are open, and he responds appropriately to your questions. He appears to be in moderate distress. A laceration to his forehead with minor bleeding is also observed. The next best action to take given this information is to
   a. open the patient's airway using the head-tilt/chin-lift maneuver.
   b. bring the head to a neutral in-line position while maintaining in-line stabilization of the head and neck.
   c. call for paramedic backup, and then open the patient's airway using the head-tilt/chin-lift maneuver.
   d. maintain the position of the head and provide in-line stabilization of the head and neck.

5. Once in-line stabilization of the head and neck is established, it must be maintained until
   a. a cervical-spine immobilization device is applied.
   b. the rapid trauma assessment has been completed.
   c. the patient is fully immobilized to a backboard.
   d. the patient is transferred to the care of hospital personnel.

6. An initial assessment
   a. must be completed prior to treatment of any life threats that may be discovered.
   b. does not necessarily need to be completed in a specific sequence to be effective.
   c. is performed on all patients, regardless of the mechanism of injury or nature of illness.
   d. is only performed on those patients who are critically injured or are critically ill.

7. Which of the following is the correct sequence for performing the initial assessment?
   1. Form a general impression
   2. Assess circulation
   3. Assess mental status
   4. Assess airway
   5. Assess breathing
   6. Establish patient priorities
   a. 6, 4, 5, 2, 3, 1
   b. 1, 4, 5, 2, 3, 6
   c. 1, 3, 4, 5, 2, 6
   d. 3, 4, 5, 1, 2, 6

8. The patient's general age, sex, whether the patient seems ill or injured, and items you notice in the patient's immediate environment can be obtained during which of the following steps of the initial assessment?
   a. General impression
   b. Assessment of breathing
   c. Assessment of mental status
   d. Establishment of patient priorities

9. Which question will best help you to establish a patient's chief complaint?
   a. "Where do you hurt?"
   b. "Can you take one finger and point to the pain?"
   c. "Does anything make the pain worse?"
   d. "Why did you call EMS today?"

10. On approach to a patient, you note that his eyes are closed. The sound of your voice causes the patient to open his eyes. This patient would be considered
    a. alert and oriented.
    b. alert and disoriented.
    c. alert and responsive to verbal stimuli.
    d. responsive to verbal stimuli.

11. Which patient has the "highest" or best level of consciousness?
    a. A patient who grabs your hand when you elicit a pain response
    b. A patient who displays flexion posturing when you elicit a pain response
    c. A patient who mumbles incoherent words when you speak to her
    d. A patient who displays no action when you elicit a pain response

12. Which of the following is an appropriate method of eliciting a pain response in an unresponsive patient?
    a. Gracilis squeeze
    b. Trapezius pinch
    c. Needle stick
    d. Hair twist

13. Assessment of the airway in the responsive patient
    a. is accomplished by talking with the patient.
    b. is performed prior to the evaluation of mental status.
    c. is not necessary if the patient is looking at you.
    d. is performed as part of the scene size-up.

14. Unresponsive patients or patients with a severely altered mental status, such as those only responding to painful stimuli with flexion or extension, have a high incidence of airway occlusion due to
    a. uncontrolled coughing resulting in bronchoconstriction.
    b. relaxation of the muscles in the upper airway.
    c. spasm of the muscles in the upper airway.
    d. esophageal rupture resulting in epiglottic spasm.

15. Which partial airway obstruction sound is correctly paired with the appropriate management technique for resolving the obstruction?
    a. Gurgling respirations—quickly provide positive-pressure ventilation
    b. Snoring respirations—use a head-tilt/chin-lift or jaw-thrust maneuver
    c. Crowing respirations—provide deep suction of the airway
    d. Stridor—use a tongue blade to visualize for an airway obstruction

16. Which of the following most likely indicates inadequate breathing in an adult patient?
    a. Pink nail beds, conjunctiva, and oral mucosa
    b. Cyanosis and deteriorating mental status
    c. Adequate chest-wall movement with breathing
    d. Respirations at a rate of 20 per minute

17. Positive-pressure ventilation may be delivered by a
    a. nasal cannula.
    b. partial rebreathing face mask.
    c. bag-valve mask device.
    d. nonrebreather face mask.

18. Which statement is most correct regarding concepts related to evaluation of the patient's skin:
    a. In a cold environment the vessels in the skin dilate to increase the blood flow to the skin.
    b. In a hot environment the vessels in the skin constrict, causing the blood to be shunted to the core of the body.
    c. The alpha properties of circulating epinephrine cause the vessels in the skin to constrict, shunting blood away from the skin.
    d. Anemic, hypoxic patients will become cyanotic more rapidly than patients without anemia.

19. When assessing the pulse in the initial assessment, determine
    a. the pulse rate in one minute.
    b. if the pulse is present or not.
    c. only the regularity of the pulse.
    d. only the strength of the pulse.

20. In order for a pulse to be palpable, the systolic blood pressure must be at least
    a. 40 mmHg.
    b. 50 mmHg.
    c. 60 mmHg.
    d. 70 mmHg.

21. Where is the least reliable place to check for skin color?
    a. Mucous membranes of the mouth
    b. Nail beds
    c. Mucous membranes that line the eyelids
    d. Under the tongue

22. Select the skin color that is correctly paired with a potential cause.
    a. Cyanotic: reduced tissue oxygenation
    b. Red: blood loss from internal or external causes
    c. Yellow: kidney failure
    d. Pale or mottled: hypertension or increased perfusion

23. Which of the following skin-temperature and skin-condition combinations is most commonly a sign of shock?
    a. Hot, dry skin
    b. Cool, dry skin
    c. Cold, dry skin
    d. Cool, clammy skin

24. If capillary refill is _____ in the infant, child, or adult male, tissue perfusion is inadequate. (Select the shortest time period that indicates inadequate perfusion.)
    a. greater than 1 second
    b. greater than 2 seconds
    c. greater than 3 seconds
    d. greater than 4 seconds

25. Your supervisor has asked you to assist with quality improvement (QI) by reviewing records of patient care. The supervisor wants you to determine if the following patients required rapid assessment and transport. Next to each patient description, write Y (yes) if rapid assessment and transport is required or N (no) if rapid assessment and transport is not required.

    _____ 1. An unresponsive diabetic who does not respond to painful stimuli

    _____ 2. A patient complaining of severe right lower abdominal pain

    _____ 3. A responsive patient complaining of minor chest discomfort with a BP of 120/80

    _____ 4. A responsive patient with cool, clammy skin who collapsed at work

    _____ 5. A responsive patient with a minor cut on her leg

    _____ 6. A patient who was stung by a bee and looks ill

    _____ 7. A patient who is complaining of a headache and is unable to obey commands

    _____ 8. A patient complaining of shortness of breath

FOCUSED HISTORY AND PHYSICAL EXAM—TRAUMA PATIENT

26. You have determined that a trauma patient requires rapid assessment and transport after completion of the initial assessment. You should next
    a. move the patient to the stretcher, then perform a rapid trauma assessment.
    b. perform a rapid trauma assessment, then move the patient to the stretcher.
    c. perform a focused trauma assessment (focused on specific injuries), then move the patient to the stretcher.
    d. move the patient to the stretcher, then perform a focused trauma assessment.

27. You did such a good job reviewing patient-care reports for your supervisor that she has returned and asked you to perform additional quality-improvement reviews. The supervisor asks you to review reports to see if significant mechanisms of injury are present to justify a rapid trauma assessment. Next to each description, write Y (yes) if there is significant mechanism of injury present or N (no) if there is not.

    _____ 1. A patient involved in a rollover collision

    _____ 2. A patient who fell from 6 feet

    _____ 3. A patient who was struck by a car

    _____ 4. A patient with a gunshot wound to the hand

    _____ 5. A patient whose impact causes deformity to a steering wheel

    _____ 6. A patient who was in the passenger seat of a vehicle in which the driver died

28. A significant mechanism of injury for an infant or child is a
    a. fall from a standing position.
    b. fall from 4 feet.
    c. vehicle collision at a medium speed.
    d. low-speed vehicle collision where child was restrained.

29. Which of the following is the proper order for performing the focused history and physical exam in the trauma patient with a significant mechanism of injury, altered mental status, suspected multiple injuries, or critical findings in the initial assessment?
    1. Rapid trauma assessment
    2. Focused trauma assessment
    3. Baseline vital signs
    4. SAMPLE history
    a. 2, 3, 4
    b. 1, 3, 4
    c. 3, 4, 1
    d. 3, 4, 2

30. Which of the following is the proper order for performing the focused history and physical exam in the trauma patient with no significant mechanism of injury and no multiple injuries and who is alert and oriented?
    1. Rapid trauma assessment
    2. Focused trauma assessment
    3. Baseline vital signs
    4. SAMPLE history
    a. 3, 2, 4
    b. 4, 2, 3
    c. 1, 3, 4
    d. 2, 3, 4

31. You have responded to a traffic accident in which the patient sustained an injury to his head. He fails to open his eyes to pain, he is unresponsive to verbal stimuli, and displays a flexor response to pain. What is the patient's Glasgow Coma Scale, and what is the appropriate management for this patient?
    a. 5; Immediately establish an airway and administer oxygen by nonrebreather mask.
    b. 5; Immediately establish an airway and hyperventilate, using positive-pressure ventilation.
    c. 4; Complete the rapid trauma exam and then administer oxygen by nonrebreather mask.
    d. 3; Apply direct pressure to the head injury and then administer oxygen by nonrebreather mask.

32. Which statement is most correct regarding patients with a head injury?
    a. A patient with a Glasgow Coma Score of less than 8 has a severe alteration in brain function.
    b. A normal response, which does not require immediate reporting in a patient with a head injury, occurs when the patient is unresponsive, then regains responsiveness for a short time, and then begins to exhibit a deteriorating mental status.
    c. Place is the first orientation to be lost in an altered mental status.
    d. Person is the first orientation to be lost in an altered mental status.

33. During the rapid trauma assessment, it is necessary to examine the patient for DCAP-BTLS. Write what each letter in DCAP-BTLS stands for.

D _____

C _____

A _____

P _____

B _____

T _____

L _____

S _____

34. There are five general techniques used during patient assessment. Which assessment technique is missing from this list?

   Inspect

   Palpate

   Auscultate

   Listen

   a. Pelvic push
   b. Sensory check
   c. Neurological check
   d. Smell

35. When assessing the neck during the rapid trauma assessment, the EMT should inspect for
   a. tracheal articulation.
   b. carotid artery disease.
   c. jugular vein distention.
   d. laryngeal distortion.

36. Regarding assessing the chest for breath sounds during the rapid trauma assessment, which statement is correct?
   a. Auscultation of the chest is not performed in the rapid trauma assessment.
   b. The EMT should auscultate the right and left chest at the base of the lungs only.
   c. The EMT should auscultate the right and left chest at the apex and base of the lungs.
   d. The EMT should auscultate the right and left chest at the apex of the lungs only.

37. When assessing the abdomen during the rapid trauma assessment, the EMT should palpate for
   a. tenderness.
   b. aortic compromise.
   c. crepitus.
   d. an unstable bowel.

38. During the rapid trauma assessment, when should the EMT *not* palpate the pelvis?
   a. When the patient complains of pain in the pelvic region
   b. When the patient has a history of cardiovascular disease
   c. When the patient is under 12 or over 65 years of age
   d. When the patient complains of lower abdominal cramps

39. Following inspection and palpation of the extremities in the rapid trauma assessment, the EMT should check for PMS. "PMS" refers to
    a. pulses, motor function, and sensation.
    b. pulses, motor function, and severity.
    c. pain, motor function, and sensation.
    d. pain, motor function, and severity.

40. In order to inspect the posterior body during the rapid trauma assessment, the EMT should
    a. log roll the patient while maintaining in-line stabilization.
    b. reach under the patient's body to palpate the spine.
    c. have the patient sit up so the back can be examined.
    d. not attempt to examine the posterior body.

41. When spinal injury is suspected, the cervical-spine immobilization collar (CSIC) should be applied
    a. before the rapid trauma assessment is begun.
    b. after the head is assessed.
    c. after the neck is assessed.
    d. after the rapid trauma assessment is completed.

42. The vital signs should be reassessed and recorded every _____ minutes in the unstable trauma or medical patient.
    a. 15
    b. 10
    c. 8
    d. 5

43. During the focused history and physical exam, the EMT should obtain a SAMPLE history. Write the type of information that each letter in SAMPLE stands for.

    S _____

    A _____

    M _____

    P _____

    L _____

    E _____

44. You are treating a responsive trauma patient who complains of a minor injury. There is no significant mechanism of injury or critical finding. During the focused history and physical exam, however, you develop a suspicion that more injuries may exist. Your next action should be to
    a. secure the patient to the stretcher and transport immediately.
    b. secure the patient to the stretcher and perform a rapid trauma assessment en route to the hospital.
    c. immediately perform a rapid trauma assessment.
    d. immediately perform a detailed physical exam.

45. Which of the following is the proper order for performing the focused history and physical exam in the responsive medical patient?
 1. Perform a focused medical assessment
 2. Obtain baseline vital signs
 3. Perform a rapid medical assessment
 4. Obtain the SAMPLE history

 a. 2, 3, 4
 b. 2, 4, 1
 c. 4, 2, 1
 d. 4, 1, 2

46. Which of the following is the proper order for performing the focused history and physical exam in the unresponsive medical patient?
 1. Perform a focused medical assessment
 2. Obtain baseline vital signs
 3. Perform a rapid medical assessment
 4. Obtain the SAMPLE history

 a. 2, 1, 4
 b. 3, 2, 4
 c. 1, 2, 4
 d. 4, 3, 2

47. During the rapid medical assessment, the abdomen should be inspected for scars, discoloration, or distention. Palpate for which of the following?
 a. Tenderness, bowel obstruction, distention, and rigidity
 b. Deformity, tenderness, penetrations, and pulsating masses
 c. Rigidity, abdominal pain, distention, and lacerations
 d. Tenderness, rigidity, distention, and pulsating masses

48. When assessing the extremities during the rapid medical assessment, be sure to check around the hands, feet, and ankles for
 a. peripheral edema.
 b. alterations in nail-bed formation.
 c. jaundice.
 d. hepatic spots ("liver" spots).

49. Which baseline vital sign is missing from the list below?
 Respiration
 Pulse
 Skin
 Blood pressure
 Pulse oximetry

 a. Pupils
 b. Capillary refill
 c. Glasgow Coma Scale
 d. Chest auscultation

50. During the SAMPLE history for a responsive medical patient, the OPQRST questions are asked to elicit more information about the patient's symptoms, especially pain. Write the type of information that each of the letters OPQRST stands for.

O _____

P _____

Q _____

R _____

S _____

T _____

51. The unresponsive medical patient should be transported in which position?
   a. Supine
   b. Prone
   c. Recovery
   d. Fowler's

52. Which statement is most correct regarding patient medications?
   a. Gather prescription medications only.
   b. Gather prescription and over-the-counter medications.
   c. Gather over-the-counter medications only.
   d. It is not important to gather medications.

53. You have responded to a call for a medical patient who just "doesn't feel well." You should
   a. perform a focused medical assessment of the head and neck.
   b. perform a detailed physical exam.
   c. perform a rapid medical assessment.
   d. transport rapidly without additional interventions.

DETAILED PHYSICAL EXAM AND ONGOING ASSESSMENT

54. A complete detailed physical exam most often is performed
   a. just prior to transport in all patients.
   b. on a patient who required a head-to-toe rapid medical or trauma assessment.
   c. when requested by medical direction.
   d. on all patients who request EMS services.

55. Which statement is most correct regarding assessment or management of the medical patient?
   a. It is not important to determine the last oral intake when testing a patient's blood glucose level.
   b. A fasting blood glucose in the diabetic patient may be 12 to 14 mg/Dl.
   c. If an unresponsive medical patient requires ventilation, put him in a lateral recumbent position.
   d. Pain is typically produced by ischemia, inflammation, infection, and obstruction.

CASE STUDY 1

It is a Friday night, and you have just completed a stand-by assignment at a local high school football game when you are dispatched to a motor vehicle crash. You determine that the scene is safe. You observe a car that has rolled over and has significant damage. The only patient was ejected from the vehicle. As you approach, you can see that the patient is about 45 years old and looks severely injured. His eyes are closed and he looks pale. You direct your partner to provide in-line stabilization of the head and neck. The patient does not respond to your voice. He responds to a painful stimulus by arching his back and extending his arms and legs. His airway is open and clear; his breathing is shallow at 6 per minute. Your partner slides his finger up to palpate the carotid pulse and tells you it is strong and regular.

1. What are the most appropriate actions to take, given the above description?
   a. Provide oxygen via nonrebreather mask at 15 lpm, then check for pulses.
   b. Place a cervical-spine immobilization collar and complete the initial assessment.
   c. Provide hyperventilation while maintaining in-line stabilization.
   d. Complete the initial assessment, and then provide oxygen via nonrebreather mask at 15 lpm.

2. This patient will require
   a. a rapid trauma assessment on-scene and a detailed physical exam—if time and the patient's condition permit—while en route to the hospital.
   b. a rapid trauma assessment and components of the detailed physical exam while en route to the hospital.
   c. a focused trauma assessment and a detailed physical exam—if time and the patient's condition permit—while en route to the hospital.
   d. a focused trauma assessment and components of the detailed physical exam while en route to the hospital.

3. You know that the patient's blood pressure is at least
   a. 80 mmHg.
   b. 70 mmHg.
   c. 60 mmHg.
   d. 50 mmHg.

CASE STUDY 2

You have just finished filling up the unit with gas when you are dispatched to a house for an unknown medical emergency. You have your disposable gloves and eye protection on. The scene appears safe as you approach the older home. An elderly woman meets you at the door and says frantically, "George won't wake up! He takes a nap every afternoon, and I can't wake him up." In response to additional questioning, she tells you there is no trauma involved and her husband is the only patient. As you enter the room, you observe the patient (an approximately 70-year-old male) lying face up on his bed. You hear a snoring sound on inhalation and exhalation of each breath. He has a pillow behind his head, and his skin looks blue. There are no signs of trauma. His eyes remain closed in spite of your attempts to arouse him with your voice. The patient also fails to respond to a painful stimulus. You tell your partner to remove the pillow from behind the patient's head and open the airway. Your partner opens the airway and assesses the patient's breathing. You assess the patient's circulatory status.

1. For each item in the following list, write Y (yes) or N (no) to indicate if it is a potential clue to an airway problem in this patient.

_____ a. The patient's wife was unable to wake the patient.

_____ b. The patient's skin color is cyanotic.

_____ c. The patient is unresponsive to painful stimulus.

_____ d. A snoring sound is evident on inspiration and expiration.

_____ e. A pillow is positioned under the patient's head.

2. What is the preferred method your partner should use to open the airway?
   a. Jaw-thrust maneuver
   b. Head-tilt/neck-lift maneuver
   c. Head-tilt/chin-lift maneuver
   d. Head-tilt maneuver

3. In this patient, which of the following would most likely require the EMT to provide positive-pressure ventilation?
   a. Inadequate respiratory rate or inadequate tidal volume
   b. History of asthma or slow capillary refill
   c. Impaired lung capacity or high blood pressure
   d. Rapid heart rate or flushed skin color

4. Management of this patient should include
   a. a focused medical assessment.
   b. a focused trauma assessment.
   c. a rapid medical assessment.
   d. a rapid trauma assessment.

5. This patient's Glasgow Coma Score is:
   a. 3
   b. 4
   c. 5
   d. 6

CASE STUDY 3

You are in the middle of studying for a promotional exam for your agency when you get a call for a man who cut his hand. You have your disposable gloves and eye protection on as you leave the vehicle. Two young men greet you on the street before you can exit the vehicle. They yell, "Hurry up, man! Fred is gonna die!" The scene appears safe as you approach the residence located in a run-down neighborhood. As you are walking to the back of the house, you ask, "Why did you call EMS today?" One of the two replies, "Fred got mad at his girlfriend and put his fist through the window." You ask him if Fred is the only patient injured. He nods.

As you enter the backyard, you see the patient sitting on the back steps holding his arm. His girlfriend is yelling at him, then starts yelling at you: "He's not hurt! He doesn't need an ambulance!" "Knock it off!" the patient snaps at her. The patient, who appears to be about 25 years old, has a towel wrapped around his lower arm. He looks up in disgust as you approach. Obviously, his girlfriend is upsetting him, and he is upsetting her. His color is pink. He appears to be in minor distress. His shirt is covered with blood. He responds to your questions appropriately and relates the same story his friend told you. You ask your partner to get the baseline vitals. The patient's respirations are adequate, and you place him on oxygen by nonrebreather mask. You check the patient's radial pulse, and it feels strong and regular at about 90 per minute. The SpO$_2$ is 96 percent. His skin is warm and dry. On examination, you discover a large laceration on the anterior surface of the patient's wrist, which is bleeding moderately.

1. To maintain scene control, you should
    a. transport the patient rapidly from the scene.
    b. suggest a task for the girlfriend that will remove her from the area.
    c. actively listen to the patient's description of the injury that occurred.
    d. order the girlfriend to leave the area at once.

2. The best method to control this patient's bleeding would be
    a. elevation.
    b. tourniquet.
    c. direct pressure.
    d. pressure points.

3. This patient would most likely require which of the following?
    a. Rapid trauma assessment followed by SAMPLE history, then vitals
    b. Rapid trauma assessment followed by vitals, then SAMPLE history
    c. Focused trauma assessment followed by vitals, then SAMPLE history
    d. Focused trauma assessment followed by SAMPLE history, then vitals

CASE STUDY 4

You have just left your main station after replacing some supplies when you are dispatched to a downtown office for a patient complaining of chest pain. You have disposable gloves and eye protection on. The scene appears safe as you arrive in front of a local insurance company. Several employees are awaiting your arrival. You ask them, "Why did you call EMS today?" A young worker replies, "It's my boss. He says he is OK, but he doesn't look well at all. He told me his chest hurts." The worker tells you there is no trauma involved in this incident and the boss is the only patient.

As you enter a plush office, you observe the patient, who appears to be approximately 55 years old, leaning back in a large desk chair. He is pale, and your general impression is that he looks ill. There is no sign of trauma. You introduce yourself and ask the patient, "What seems to be the problem?" The patient replies, "Nothing, really. A little indigestion, maybe. I don't know why they called you, but I guess as long as you're here you may as well check me out. My chest hurts. But I'm sure it must be something I ate." His breathing appears adequate. His radial pulse is weak and slow. His skin is cool and clammy. While you are obtaining a history, your partner obtains the baseline vital signs. He reports the following: respirations normal at 20 per minute; pulse weak and regular at 50 per minute; skin pale, cool, and moist; pupils equal and reactive; blood pressure 90/60. The SpO$_2$ is 97 percent.

1. What history-taking method should you use on this patient?
    a. OPQRST questions only
    b. SAMPLE history, including OPQRST questions
    c. SAMPLE history only
    d. DCAP-BTLS and SAMPLE history

2. Which of the following is the best question to ask to evaluate the quality of this patient's pain?
    a. Is the pain dull and squeezing?
    b. Where do you feel the pain?
    c. Can you take one finger and point to where the pain is located?
    d. How would you describe the pain?

3. The physical exam on this patient should be
   a. a medical assessment focused on the neck, chest, abdomen, and extremities.
   b. a head-to-toe rapid medical assessment.
   c. a head-to-toe rapid trauma assessment.
   d. a detailed physical exam.

4. Appropriate management for this patient should include
   a. cardiopulmonary resuscitation.
   b. oxygen by nonrebreather mask and immediate transport.
   c. positive-pressure ventilation and immediate transport.
   d. departing the scene, as the patient has refused treatment.

CASE STUDY 5

You are reviewing policies and treatment protocols with an EMT intern when a call comes in for a "sick child." You, your partner, and the EMT intern quickly respond to the call and arrive on the scene in less than 4 minutes. You are wearing disposable gloves and eye protection. The scene appears safe as you arrive in front of a neatly kept home in a working-class neighborhood. As you enter the home, you observe the patient on a couch. The patient's mother tells you the patient is 5 years old. He is lying on his back. He does not look at you as you enter the room. He looks pale, and your general impression is that he looks ill. His eyes appear to be sunken into the sockets. There is no sign of trauma, and the mother reports no traumatic event. You introduce yourself, gain consent, and ask the mother, "Why did you call EMS today?" The mother replies, "Ryan has been sick for the last week. He's been throwing up constantly." The patient does not respond to your voice, but he responds appropriately to pain. His breathing appears adequate at 20 per minute. The SpO_2 is 96 percent. His radial pulse is weak and rapid. His skin is cool and clammy.

1. You should next
   a. check for bleeding only.
   b. check the capillary refill, and check for bleeding.
   c. check for pulse, motor, and sensory function in the extremities.
   d. check for a carotid pulse.

2. This patient should be given
   a. a medical assessment focused on his abdomen.
   b. a head-to-toe rapid medical assessment.
   c. a trauma assessment focused on his chest and abdomen.
   d. a head-to-toe rapid trauma assessment.

3. Regarding a transport decision, this patient should be considered
   a. a medium-priority patient.
   b. a high-priority patient.
   c. stable and would not be assigned to a category.
   d. a low-priority patient.

4. Your treatment for this patient should include
   a. oxygen by nasal cannula.
   b. oxygen by nonrebreather mask.
   c. insertion of an oropharyngeal airway.
   d. positive-pressure ventilation by bag-valve mask.

10 Communication

OBJECTIVES

Numbered objectives are from the United States Department of Transportation EMT-Basic National Standard Curriculum. Asterisked objectives, if any, pertain to material that is supplemental to the DOT curriculum.

Cognitive

3-7.1 List the proper methods of initiating and terminating a radio call.
3-7.2 State the proper sequence for delivery of patient information.
3-7.3 Explain the importance of effective communication of patient information in the verbal report.
3-7.4 Identify the essential components of the verbal report.
3-7.5 Describe the attributes for increasing effectiveness and efficiency of verbal communications.
3-7.6 State legal aspects to consider in verbal communication.
3-7.7 Discuss the communication skills that should be used to interact with the patient.
3-7.8 Discuss the communication skills that should be used to interact with the family, bystanders, and individuals from other agencies while providing patient care and the difference between skills used to interact with the patient and those used to interact with others.
3-7.9 List the correct radio procedures in the following phases of a typical call:
To the scene
At the scene
To the facility
At the facility
To the station
At the station

KEY IDEAS

This chapter focuses on the role of communications in the delivery of emergency medical services. A good understanding of EMS communications skills and equipment is essential to your success as an EMT. Reliable communications systems are critical to all aspects of an EMS call. Key concepts include:

■ Standard components of an emergency communications system include a base station and mobile or portable transmitters/receivers. Additional components, such as repeaters and digitalized encoders and decoders, are used to enhance communication capabilities within an EMS system.

■ The Federal Communications Commission (FCC) has jurisdiction over all radio operations in the country, including those used by EMS systems.

- Communications within an EMS system are dependent on adhering to basic rules of radio communication at all times.
- Effective interpersonal communications depend on the three "Cs": competence, confidence, and compassion.
- Digital data terminals receive dispatch information and transmit critical information back to dispatch.
- Patients with special needs, such as the hearing impaired, children, and the elderly, require special consideration to ensure effective communication at the scene of an emergency.

TERMS AND CONCEPTS

1. Write the number of the correct term next to each definition.
   1. Base station
   2. Decoder
   3. Encoder
   4. Repeater
   5. Mobile (digital) data terminal

   _____ a. Device that converts sound waves into digital codes for transmission

   _____ b. The central dispatch and coordination area of an EMS communications system

   _____ c. Devices that receive transmissions from one source and rebroadcast them at a higher power on another frequency

   _____ d. Device that recognizes and responds to only certain codes imposed on a radio broadcast

   _____ e. Receives and transmits digital dispatch information

CONTENT REVIEW

1. An EMS base station
   a. generally uses a low output of between 50 and 75 watts of transmission power.
   b. should be located in a low-lying area, free from potential damaging high winds.
   c. does not require close proximity to the hospital that serves as the medical command center.
   d. serves as a dispatch and coordination area and is in contact with other system elements.

2. Repeaters are used within an EMS communications system to allow
   a. communications over a wide geographic area.
   b. all personnel the opportunity to monitor all statewide radio transmissions.
   c. communications between EMS agencies in adjoining jurisdictions.
   d. communications to be transmitted through the air via cells.

3. Cellular telephones within an EMS system
   a. usually have poor sound quality.
   b. seldom become overwhelmed during disaster situations.
   c. are usually difficult to maintain and are cost prohibitive.
   d. often improve communication privacy.

4. One role of the FCC in EMS communications systems is to
   a. purchase base-station radio equipment.
   b. license base stations.
   c. serve as a repeater for base-station operations.
   d. conduct radio-operations training for EMS personnel.

5. Which of the following is a "ground rule" for radio operations?
   a. Use the radio just as if you were talking on a telephone.
   b. Keep transmissions brief, organized, and to the point.
   c. Never listen for other radio traffic before transmitting.
   d. Don't waste valuable airtime by repeating back orders or information.

6. The role of dispatch in an EMS communications system is to obtain information about the nature of the emergency, direct the appropriate emergency service(s) to the scene, and
   a. notify the medical command center of the request for service.
   b. alert the local news media to provide essential information.
   c. provide the caller with instructions about what to do until help arrives.
   d. contact the medical director to provide a link for medical direction.

7. In addition to communicating with dispatch to acknowledge the dispatch information and again while en route to report your estimated time of arrival at the scene, number the list below in the proper order from 1 to 5 to show the other times you should communicate with dispatch.
   _____ To announce your arrival back at base
   _____ To announce your arrival on-scene and request further assistance
   _____ To announce you are "clear" and available for another call
   _____ To announce your arrival at the hospital
   _____ To announce your departure from the scene and your estimated hospital arrival time

8. When communicating with medical direction, you should use a standard format that includes your unit identification and service level; the patient's age, sex, and chief complaint; a brief, pertinent history of the present illness, including scene assessment and mechanism of injury; past major illnesses; and
   a. the name of the patient's insurance provider.
   b. a detailed description of the patient's past illnesses.
   c. a comprehensive description of the findings of the physical exam.
   d. the patient's mental status.

9. After receiving an order or instructions from medical direction, you should
   a. always say thank you before you "sign off."
   b. repeat the instructions word for word.
   c. click your "press to talk" button twice to signal your understanding.
   d. acknowledge the instructions by saying "10–4."

10. If you receive orders from medical direction that do not appear to be appropriate, you should always
   a. question the order to clarify if there has been a misunderstanding.
   b. follow the orders as given by medical direction.
   c. double-check with your partner before following the orders.
   d. request to speak with someone else.

11. When interacting with bystanders or other EMRs when you arrive on the scene, you should
   a. obtain permission from police and fire personnel before beginning patient care.
   b. obtain complete information from on-scene emergency providers before making patient contact.
   c. ask for information about what happened and what care has been given.
   d. quickly and loudly point out any errors in treatment provided by on-scene emergency providers.

12. Your patient is a non-English-speaking traveler in your community. Which of the following is an appropriate action in this situation?
   a. See if a companion or a bystander can interpret.
   b. Talk loudly and slowly to make yourself understood.
   c. No action is necessary—nothing can be done in this circumstance.
   d. Draw pictures to communicate with the non-English speaker.

CASE STUDY

You were dispatched to the carousel on the playground at 1031 Bruce Road for an injured child. Your partner notifies dispatch of your arrival. You note no signs of danger as you park the ambulance and then put on your gloves and protective eyewear. As you approach the group gathered near a picnic table, you can hear the sound of a child crying. You introduce yourself to the woman holding the crying child on her lap and ask what happened and what you can to do to help. The mother of your patient, Mrs. Smith, thanks you for coming so quickly and tells you that her son, Mikey, tripped while running and cut his chin. She says he did not lose consciousness. Mikey's crying has quieted, and he's watching you closely. You ask him if you can look at his chin. He nods his permission. His mother removes the washcloth that she had been using to control the bleeding. You observe an approximately one-inch laceration. You explain what you are going to do, and then, as you gently apply a sterile dressing and bandage to Mikey's injury, you reassure him quietly. He tells you that he is 3 years old and has a dog and three big sisters. He also says he never rode in an "ambliance." You see no other signs of injury.

Your partner obtains a set of baseline vitals. Mikey's blood pressure is 80/68 mmHg. His heart rate is strong at 80 beats per minute. His respirations are 28 per minute, full and adequate. His skin is slightly flushed, warm, and moist. His capillary refill is less than 2 seconds. His pupils are normal and equal in size and reactivity, and the SpO_2 is 96 percent on room air. You obtain a SAMPLE history. When asked, Mikey says his chin "hurts bad." His mother reports that he is a healthy child who takes no medications and has no known allergies. Mikey tells you that he had a Popsicle in the car on his way to the park. Mrs. Smith says that they arrived about an hour ago and that Mikey was fine before he fell as he ran to get on the carousel. You secure Mikey in the child restraint seat on the stretcher in the back of the ambulance and then help Mrs. Smith get settled and secured to the jump seat. You perform the ongoing assessment on Mikey, finding him still completely alert and oriented. His dressing remains dry. His vital signs are essentially unchanged. You radio the hospital with your report.

In the space below, write the report you would give orally at the following times:

1. Arrival on scene (to dispatch):

2. En route to the hospital (to the receiving hospital):

3. At the hospital when you transfer care:

ENRICHMENT

1. You are working in an EMS system that utilizes radio codes. Which statement best describes an advantage of radio codes?
   a. They provide clear, concise information.
   b. They lengthen radio airtime.
   c. They are generally understood by the patient.
   d. They are regulated by the Federal Communications Commission.

2. Which of the following statements is accurate regarding Ten-Codes?
   a. They are the primary code system used by EMS systems.
   b. They are published by the FCC.
   c. They are generally understood by the patient.
   d. They are less favored than the use of standard English.

3. To ensure accuracy and synchronicity, most EMS systems use military time rather than standard AM and PM designations. Choose the military time that correctly represents 8:32 PM standard time.
   a. 0832 hours
   b. 1832 hours
   c. 2032 hours
   d. 2232 hours

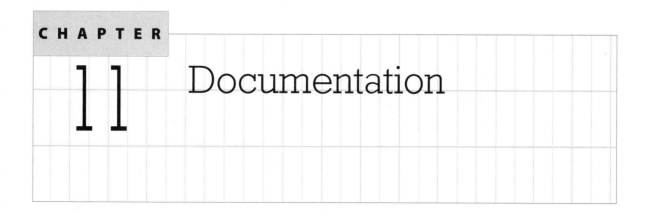

CHAPTER 11 Documentation

OBJECTIVES

Numbered objectives are from the United States Department of Transportation EMT-Basic National Standard Curriculum. Asterisked objectives, if any, pertain to material that is supplemental to the DOT curriculum.

Cognitive

3-8.1 Explain the components of the written report and list the information that should be included in the written report.

3-8.2 Identify the various sections of the written report

3-8.3 Describe what information is required in each section of the prehospital care report and how it should be entered.

3-8.4 Define the special considerations concerning patient refusal.

3-8.5 Describe the legal implications associated with the written report.

3-8.6 Discuss all state and/or local record and reporting requirements.

KEY IDEAS

The focus of this chapter is the written documentation of patient care. As an EMT, the documentation of all of your encounters with patients is an essential part of doing your job. Key ideas and concepts include:

- Documentation serves many functions. Among them are medical uses, such as ensuring continuity of care and establishing a baseline of patient status; administrative uses, such as billing and insurance information; and as a legal record of assessment, care given, and patient response. Documentation may also be used for educational, research, and quality improvement purposes.

- The traditional format for the patient-care report is the written prehospital-care report (PCR), which is designed to provide a complete and accurate picture of your contact with the patient.

- Documentation is governed by two basic rules: "If it wasn't written down, it wasn't done," and "If it wasn't done, don't write it down."

TERMS AND CONCEPTS

1. Write the number of the correct term next to each definition.

   1. Minimum data set
   2. Pertinent negatives
   3. Prehospital-care report (PCR)
   4. Triage tag

   _____ a. Document containing only key patient information, used during a multiple-casualty incident

   _____ b. Signs and symptoms that might be expected in certain situations but that the patient denies

   _____ c. Information that the U.S. Department of Transportation recommends all patient-care reports include

   _____ d. Documentation of an EMT's contact with a patient

CONTENT REVIEW

1. The *primary* purpose of high-quality documentation is
   a. as a resource for quality-improvement review.
   b. to assist in the preparation of patient bills.
   c. to ensure the continuity of patient care.
   d. as a resource in malpractice suits.

2. The documentation provided in the PCR
   a. typically becomes a part of the patient's permanent medical record.
   b. is of little use in a lawsuit brought against the EMT.
   c. is seldom created in an electronic form.
   d. may not be used for preparing bills or for submission to insurance.

3. The use of accurate and synchronous clocks
   a. is seldom important in EMS documentation.
   b. is critical for proper EMS documentation.
   c. is only important for dispatch purposes.
   d. is only important for medical information.

4. The narrative section of the patient-care report should include the patient's chief complaint, the SAMPLE history, and
   a. your diagnosis of the patient's problem.
   b. pertinent information about the scene.
   c. all remarks made by bystanders.
   d. your conclusions about the incident.

5. Which of the following would be considered a pertinent negative for a patient who was the unrestrained driver of a car involved in a serious motor vehicle accident?
   a. The patient complains of abdominal pain.
   b. The patient reports that it hurts to take a deep breath.
   c. The patient denies back and neck pain.
   d. The patient denies any allergies to food or drugs.

6. At least _____ set(s) of vital signs should be taken and recorded on all patient transports.
   a. one
   b. two
   c. three
   d. four

7. Under most state laws, you may *not* provide confidential information about a patient in which of the following situations?
   a. reporting to another health-care provider when transferring care.
   b. in response to questions from friends of the patient.
   c. when providing information to the police as part of a criminal investigation.
   d. if you are subpoenaed to appear in court and provide information in a legal case.

8. When dealing with a patient that has refused treatment
   a. document your explanation of possible consequences of failing to accept care, and have the patient sign the form acknowledging refusal of treatment.
   b. only discuss the situation with the patient, as required by patient-privacy provisions.
   c. documentation of the call is generally less involved and easier to document.
   d. issues of patient competency are rarely a concern of the EMT.

9. Objective information is
   a. a sign.
   b. a symptom.
   c. based on an individual's perception.
   d. symptoms the patient denies having.

10. Which of the following best describes the appropriate way to correct an error on the written patient-care report?
    a. Use correction fluid to cover the incorrect entry.
    b. Use multiple heavy lines to block out the incorrect entry.
    c. Draw a single line through the incorrect entry and initial it.
    d. Report the error verbally but do not alter the report.

11. Which of the following are commonly used for patient-care reports in a multiple-casualty incident?
    a. Triage tags
    b. Casualty codes
    c. Regularly used patient-care reports
    d. Multiple-casualty forms

12. Which of the following situations may require additional, special documentation by the EMT?
    a. Suspected abuse of a child or an elderly patient
    b. Patient care provided to a patient complaining of chest pain
    c. Patient care given to victims of motor vehicle accidents
    d. Patient care provided to a patient with difficulty breathing

13. The Department of Transportation has designated certain information on the PCR to be the minimum data set (MDS). Select the item that is *not* part of the minimum data set and that you would *not* be likely to see on a PCR form.
    a. Crew member names
    b. Chief complaint
    c. Next of kin
    d. Pulse rate

14. When writing the PCR, you may use approved abbreviations to help document your findings. In each space, write the abbreviation that stands for the given term.

a	Pt	Rx	TID
c	q	s	Tx
PO	QID	STAT	x

_____ a. Four times a day

_____ b. Times

_____ c. Before

_____ d. Patient

_____ e. Prescription

_____ f. Every

_____ g. Treatment

_____ h. With

_____ i. Immediately

_____ j. Without

_____ k. Orally, by mouth

_____ l. Three times a day

CASE STUDY

You get dispatched to the local high school on a report of a fall. Upon arrival at the school, you report to the office, where you find that your patient slipped on a wet floor and "twisted his ankle." Your 50-year-old patient is Mr. Henderson, the school principal. He says, "I'm sorry you were sent out for nothing. I'm more embarrassed than hurt." You introduce yourself and ask if you can check him over anyway, as long as you're here. He agrees.

On your initial assessment, you find him to be alert and oriented, having no apparent difficulty breathing and in no apparent distress. You see no signs of bleeding. Mr. Henderson lets your partner check his pulse, which is strong and regular. His skin is pink, warm, and dry.

During your focused physical exam, you find that Mr. Henderson's right ankle, which he reports is "a little sore," is markedly swollen, discolored, and very tender to gentle palpation. His foot is slightly pale but warm to the touch. His pedal pulse is present, and he has good sensation and motion. Vital signs: blood pressure 138/78 mmHg, pulse 68 beats per minute, and respirations 18 per minute and adequate; PaO_2 is 96 percent on room air. Skin is still normal, as are pupils. You complete your SAMPLE history and find that Mr. Henderson has no allergies and takes no medications. He denies any medical problems or any other injuries. He had soup and a sandwich for lunch about a half hour ago. He says that he has felt fine all day but slipped on some water on the floor as he was leaving the cafeteria.

You urge Mr. Henderson to allow you to splint his ankle and transport him to the hospital so that he can get X-rays to see if his ankle is broken. He refuses, saying, "Thanks for checking me out, but you guys have to be available for real emergencies. I've already called my wife, and she's on her way to take me to the doctor. She ought to be here in 10 minutes or so. Bad enough that I fell down in front of half the school. There's no way I'm going out of here on that stretcher." You agree that he's stable enough to be transported by car but remind him that he shouldn't bear any weight on his ankle until he's been seen by the doctor. You also remind him that if any problems arise or if he changes his mind, he should call 9-1-1.

1. In the space below, write the narrative section of the patient-care report for this call.

2. Before leaving the scene, what else should you do?
    a. Have the patient read the patient-care report and sign the refusal form.
    b. Call medical control and have the patient speak to the physician.
    c. Direct the patient to contact his own physician for advice.
    d. Contact the patient's wife in an attempt to have her convince him to be transported.

3. While walking toward your ambulance, a coworker of Mr. Henderson approaches you. The coworker is visibly upset. He explains he is the safety officer for the school; he asks you what happened to Mr. Henderson and if he is injured. How should you respond to the safety officer?
    a. Explain that, legally, you cannot discuss the call because of patient confidentiality rights.
    b. Discreetly discuss the call only in general terms, not disclosing anything specific about the injuries.
    c. Do not discuss the call, but allow him to read the PCR, because it is public information.
    d. Because he is the safety officer, you may disclose all of the information you have about the patient.

ENRICHMENT

1. The mnemonics SOAP, CHART, and CHEATED are often used by EMS personnel to
    a. determine the level of responsiveness or mental status.
    b. describe the patient's mechanism of injury.
    c. convey the pertinent negatives as described by the patient.
    d. organize the information on the PCR.

2. When using any of the following mnemonics—SOAP, CHART, or CHEATED—you know that the "A" refers to
    a. arrival on-scene.
    b. actions on-scene.
    c. absent physical findings.
    d. assessment.

PATIENT ASSESSMENT: CHAPTERS 8–11

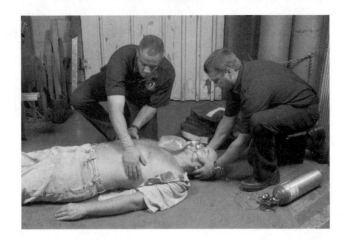

As an EMT, your most important functions will be assessing the patient and providing emergency care and transport to the hospital. Of these, performing an accurate and reliable patient assessment will be the most important because all of your decisions about care and transport will be based on it.

Q   **Why is the patient assessment procedure broken down into separate steps?**

A   It is very important to follow an assessment routine that is systematic. This will ensure that you assess every patient consistently and appropriately, based on that patient's illness or injury, and that you will not overlook any important parts of the assessment.

Q   **Why is scene size-up considered part of patient assessment?**

A   In addition to the scene-safety considerations involved in sizing up the scene, important clues to the patient's condition can also be observed. The most important of these observations is whether or not there is a mechanism of injury that would indicate that this is a trauma patient, as well as clues to the nature of a medical patient's illness, such as medications or an unusually warm or cold environmental temperature.

Q   **Why is the initial assessment so important?**

A   The purpose of the initial assessment is to identify any immediate life threats and treat them at once, as they are found. Once life threats have been controlled, a more thorough assessment and additional care can be provided.

Q   **Why is there a different sequence to the focused history and physical exam for a trauma patient and for a medical patient?**

A   For a trauma patient, the physical exam and baseline vital-signs measurements are performed first and the SAMPLE history last. This is because the greatest amount of information about a traumatic injury can be gathered from physical assessments and because life-threatening injuries not discovered during the initial assessment must be quickly found and managed. For a medical patient, on the other hand, the greatest amount of information is usually gained from the SAMPLE history—the patient's symptoms, for example, what medical conditions the patient has been suffering from, what medications the patient has been taking, and what brought on the current emergency. Because the patient who is responsive and able to provide this information may become unresponsive or have a deteriorating mental status, it is important to gain this information first for a medical patient.

Q **For whom, and when, should the detailed physical exam be performed?**

A If a patient required a head-to-toe physical exam (rapid trauma assessment or rapid medical assessment) during the focused history and physical exam, that patient is a candidate for a detailed physical exam en route to the hospital. The purpose of the detailed physical exam is to discover any conditions previously overlooked. However, if the patient is critical or unstable, there may not be time to perform a detailed exam. Perform a detailed physical exam only when time and the patient's condition permit.

Q **Why must an ongoing assessment be performed on every patient?**

A A patient's condition may change, and treatments or interventions may become ineffective. To monitor the patient's condition and interventions, an ongoing assessment must be performed at least every 5 minutes on an unstable patient, and every 15 minutes on a stable patient.

12 General Pharmacology

OBJECTIVES

Numbered objectives are from the United States Department of Transportation EMT-Basic National Standard Curriculum. Asterisked objectives, if any, pertain to material that is supplemental to the DOT curriculum.

Cognitive

4-1.1 Identify which medications will be carried on the unit.
4-1.2 State the medications carried on the EMS unit by the generic name.
4-1.3 Identify the medications with which the EMT may assist the patient with administering.
4-1.4 State the medications the EMT can assist the patient with by the generic name.
4-1.5 Discuss the forms in which the medications may be found.
   * List and explain the various routes of drug administration used by the EMT.
   * List and describe the essential medication information that should be understood by the EMT.
   * List and describe the key steps in administering medications to a patient.
   * Describe the reassessment strategies used following medication administration.
   * List sources that can be used to gather medication information.

KEY IDEAS

As an EMT, you will have the responsibility of administering certain medications carried on the EMS unit. You also may assist with the administration of certain prescribed medications that may be taken by the patient. Improper administration of these medications can result in dangerous or fatal consequences. It is vital that you be completely familiar with the medications and the proper procedures for administration. This chapter reviews these important concepts:

■ You may *not* administer or assist with administration of any medication other than the medications covered in this chapter and that are also identified in local protocol.

■ The medications carried on the EMS unit that may be administered under the approval of medical direction are oxygen, oral glucose, aspirin, and activated charcoal.

■ The medications prescribed for the patient that may be administered under the approval of medical direction are prescribed metered-dose inhaler (MDI), nitroglycerin, and epinephrine.

■ Medications can have up to four different names: chemical, generic, trade, and official. The EMT must be familiar with the generic and trade names.

■ Drugs can be administered by the following common routes: sublingual, oral, inhalation, and injection (intramuscular).

- There are six essential terms associated with medication administration: indications, contraindications, dose, administration, actions, and side effects.

- There are seven key steps to administering medications: obtain an order from medical direction; select the proper medication; verify the patient's prescription; check the expiration date; check for discoloration or impurities; verify the form, route, and dose; and provide documentation.

- The five "rights" of medication administration—right patient, right medication, right route, right dose, and right date—provide an important reminder of the critical elements of administering medications to patients.

TERMS AND CONCEPTS

1. Write the number of the correct term next to each definition.

1. Medication	7. Epinephrine
2. Drug	8. Metered-dose inhaler
3. Pharmacology	9. Nitroglycerin
4. Activated charcoal	10. Oral glucose
5. Aspirin	11. Side effects
6. Contraindications	

_____ a. A chemical substance that is used to treat or prevent a disease or condition

_____ b. Treatment with a substance that is used as a remedy for illness

_____ c. The study of drugs

_____ d. Dilates arterioles and veins and reduces the cardiac workload

_____ e. Situations when a drug should not be administered

_____ f. Administered to a patient with a history of diabetes with a low blood glucose level

_____ g. Commonly prescribed to patients with a history of asthma, emphysema, and chronic bronchitis

_____ h. Used to treat patients suffering from a severe allergic reaction

_____ i. Reduces platelets from forming clots

_____ j. Designed to absorb or bind to some ingested poisons

_____ k. Actions that are not desired and that occur in addition to the desired effects

CONTENT REVIEW

1. The EMT may not administer or assist in the administration of any medication other than the medications listed in this chapter. In addition, these drugs must be
   a. clearly identified by the official name on all prescriptions.
   b. clearly identified by the official or chemical name on all prescriptions.
   c. identified in local protocols as acceptable for the EMT to administer.
   d. only administered by oral or sublingual route.

2. Medications administered by the EMT are
   a. administered without medical direction.
   b. carried on the unit or prescribed for the patient.
   c. only given by the oral or sublingual route.
   d. only those medications that are prescribed for the patient.

3. Which of the following is a medication that can be administered by the EMT?
   a. Epinephrine
   b. Diazepam
   c. Lasix
   d. Lidocaine

4. You have responded to a patient complaining of chest pain. The patient states that his medication is upstairs on his dresser. Select the best response to this situation.
   a. Leave the patient momentarily to retrieve the patient's medication.
   b. Ask the patient to walk upstairs and retrieve the medication.
   c. Ask a family member to retrieve the medication.
   d. Help the patient up the stairs to retrieve the medication.

5. Which of the following is also known as the brand name of a drug?
   a. Trade name
   b. Generic name
   c. Chemical name
   d. Official name

6. Which of the following generic and trade names are *incorrectly* paired?
   a. Metaproterenol—Alupent®, Metaprel®
   b. Isoetharine—Serevent®
   c. Epinephrine—Adrenalin®
   d. Albuterol—Proventil®

7. Which of the following generic and trade names are *incorrectly* paired?
   a. Nitroglycerin—Nitrostat®
   b. Salmeterol—Ventolin®
   c. Ipratropin—Atrovent®
   d. Nitroglycerin spray—Nitrolingual Spray®

8. Medication that is placed under the tongue is an example of medication given by which of the following?
   a. The inhalation route
   b. The intramuscular route
   c. The oral route
   d. The sublingual route

9. A suspension must be
   a. shaken before it is administered.
   b. given sublingually.
   c. inhaled.
   d. injected.

10. Situations when a drug should not be given are known as which of the following?
    a. Actions
    b. Contraindications
    c. Side effects
    d. Negative markers

11. What are the six essential items of medication information that the EMT should understand to ensure safe, proper, and effective medication administration?
    a. Indications, contraindications, dose, administration, actions, and side effects
    b. Indications, negative markers, dose, administration, actions, and side effects
    c. Indications, negative markers, dose, forms, prescriptions, and side effects
    d. Indications, negative markers, dose, administration, actions, and adverse actions

12. Which of the following is an example of a drug given by the injection or intramuscular route?
    a. Alupent®
    b. Epinephrine
    c. Glutose®
    d. Isoetharine

13. Number the key steps below, for administration of a medication, in the proper order from 1 to 7.
    _____ a. Document medication administration.
    _____ b. Obtain an order from medical direction.
    _____ c. Ensure selection of the proper medication.
    _____ d. Check the expiration date.
    _____ e. Verify the form, route, and dose.
    _____ f. Verify the patient's prescription.
    _____ g. Check for discoloration or impurities.

14. Which of the following is a source of information about a patient's prescription medication?
    a. Package inserts
    b. Wilson's Formulary Service
    c. Doctors' Reference System
    d. National Drug Guide

Complete the following chart.

Generic Name	Trade Name	Used for
Oxygen	15.	Wide range of emergencies
16.	Glutose®, Insta-glucose®	17.
Activated charcoal	SuperChar®, InstaChar®, Actidose®, LiquiChar®	18.
Nitroglycerin	Nitrostat®	19.
20.	Nitrolingual Spray®	21.
Epinephrine	22.	Allergic reactions
Albuterol	23.	Breathing difficulty associated with respiratory conditions
Metaproterenol	24.	25.
26.	Bronkosol®, Bronkometer®	27.
Salmeterol Xinafoate	28.	Breathing difficulty associated with respiratory conditions
29.	Tornalate	30.
Levalbuterol	31.	Breathing difficulty associated with respiratory conditions
Pirbuterol	32.	33.
Terbutaline	34.	Breathing difficulty associated with respiratory conditions
Aspirin	35.	36.

CASE STUDY

You are helping an EMT intern study for an upcoming final exam when the alarm bell sounds. You respond to a call for a patient complaining of chest pain. You have completed the scene size-up and the initial assessment. The patient is a 56-year-old male who responds to painful stimuli only. The patient's wife tells you that he has been complaining of chest pain for the past 2 hours. He stopped talking just a few minutes before your arrival. A neighbor of the patient suggests that you give the patient her nitroglycerin. She takes it for a heart problem.

1. What is your best reaction to the neighbor's suggestion?
    a. Give the patient the neighbor's nitroglycerin.
    b. Contact the patient's personal physician for orders to administer the medication to the patient.
    c. Never administer medication to a patient unless it is prescribed and/or you are ordered to do so by medical direction.
    d. Take the medication with you and administer while en route to the hospital after checking the patient's vital signs.

2. Suppose that nitroglycerin prescribed to this patient is discovered on his person. *The nitroglycerin can and should be placed into the mouth of this patient.* Select the best response to this statement.
    a. The statement is true; you should administer the medication while holding the mouth closed with one hand.
    b. The statement is false; the medication should not be administered to a patient with an altered level of consciousness.
    c. The statement is true if the medication is administered by the oral route instead of the sublingual route.
    d. The statement is false; the patient must be unresponsive to pain before the medication can be administered.

3. Nitroglycerin is used for which of the following?
    a. Altered mental status
    b. Poisoning and overdose
    c. Chest pain
    d. Difficulty breathing

Note: *Medication Reference Cards appear at the back of this workbook. There is a card for each of the following medications that EMTs are permitted to administer or assist with administering, with approval from medical direction:* **activated charcoal, aspirin, epinephrine auto-injector, metered-dose inhaler, nitroglycerin,** *and* **oral glucose.** *Each card includes information on medication names, indications, contraindications, form, dosage, administration, actions, side effects, and reassessment. You will be able to carry these cards with you for ready reference.*

13 Respiratory Emergencies

OBJECTIVES

Numbered objectives are from the United States Department of Transportation EMT-Basic National Standard Curriculum. Asterisked objectives, if any, pertain to material that is supplemental to the DOT curriculum.

Cognitive

4-2.1 List the structure and function of the respiratory system.

4-2.2 State the signs and symptoms of a patient with breathing difficulty.

4-2.3 Describe the emergency medical care of the patient with breathing difficulty.

4-2.4 Recognize the need for medical direction to assist in the emergency medical care of the patient with breathing difficulty.

4-2.5 Describe the emergency medical care of the patient with breathing distress.

4-2.6 Establish the relationship between airway management and the patient with breathing difficulty.

4-2.7 List signs of adequate air exchange.

4-2.8 State the generic name, medication forms, dose, administration, action, indications, and contraindications for the prescribed inhaler.

4-2.9 Distinguish between the emergency medical care of the infant, child, and adult patient with breathing difficulty.

4-2.10 Differentiate between upper airway obstruction and lower airway disease in the infant and child.

KEY IDEAS

This chapter describes respiratory distress and respiratory failure. Emphasis is placed on ensuring an open airway and providing high-flow oxygen or positive-pressure ventilation, as needed, and not on trying to diagnose a specific underlying disease.

■ There is a wide variety of signs and symptoms of breathing difficulty. They may include any of these: shortness of breath; restlessness; increased pulse rate or breathing rate; decreased breathing rate; skin color changes; noisy breathing; inability to speak; retractions; shallow, slow, or irregular breathing; abdominal breathing; coughing; patient in a tripod position; unusual anatomy (barrel chest); altered mental status; nasal flaring; tracheal tugging or deviations; paradoxical motion; and/or pursed-lip breathing.

■ Time is critical to the patient who is breathing inadequately. If signs of inadequate breathing are exhibited by the patient, you should immediately begin positive-pressure ventilation with supplemental oxygen. If the breathing is adequate, but the patient is complaining of breathing difficulty or showing signs of respiratory distress, oxygen must be administered by a nonrebreather mask at 15 lpm.

- Metered-dose inhalers (MDI) are used by some patients with chronic or recurring breathing problems. If the patient has a prescribed MDI, contact medical direction for an order to assist the patient with administering the medication. It may be necessary to coach the patient during the procedure to be sure the medication is taken in by the patient in an effective manner.

- An increased work of breathing in the infant and child is an indication that he or she is compensating for inadequate oxygen and carbon dioxide exchange and may deteriorate into respiratory failure. You must recognize the wide range of symptoms and immediately provide oxygen if the infant or child is breathing adequately or provide positive-pressure ventilation with supplemental oxygen if there are signs of inadequate breathing.

MEDICAL TERMINOLOGY

Term	Prefix	Word Root Combining Form	Suffix	Definition
apnea (AP-nee-ah)	a- (no, not, without, lack of)	pnea (to breathe or breathing)		Absence of breathing; respiratory arrest
bronchoconstriction (BRONG-koh-kun-STRIK-shun)		bronch/o (bronchi); constriction (narrowing an opening)		Constriction of the smooth muscles of the bronchi and bronchioles, causing a narrowing of the air passageways
bronchospasm (brong-koh-SPAZ-um)		bronch/o- (bronchi); spasm (constriction)		Spasm or constriction of the smooth muscles of the bronchi and bronchioles
dyspnea (DISP-nee-ah)	dys- (bad, difficult, painful)	pnea (to breathe or breathing)		Shortness of breath or perceived difficulty in breathing
diaphoresis (DYE-ah-for-EE-sis)	dia- (through, between)	phoresis (migration of ions)		Profuse sweating
hypotension (high-poh-TEN-shun)	hypo- (below, under, deficient)	tens (tension)	-ion (process)	Blood pressure lower than normal
tachycardia (tak-i-KAR-dee-ah)	tachy- (fast)	card (heart)	-ia (condition of)	Heart rate faster than normal
tachypnea normal (tak-ip-NEE-ah)	tachy- (fast)	pnea (to breathe or breathing)		Breathing rate faster than
syncope (SIN-koh-pee)	syn- (together, with)		-cope (strike, cut)	Fainting; transient loss of consciousness

1. The medical term *apnea* contains the word root *pnea*. You know this refers to
   a. heart.
   b. breathing.
   c. pain.
   d. lungs.

2. The prefix *tachy-* used in the medical term *tachypnea* means
   a. slow.
   b. irregular.
   c. regular.
   d. fast.

3. The prefix *a-* in the medical term *apnea* refers to
   a. no, not, without, lack of.
   b. bad, difficult, painful.
   c. out, away from.
   d. through, between.

4. The medical term *dyspnea* contains the prefix *dys-*. You know this means
   a. upon, over, above.
   b. below, under, deficient.
   c. out, away from.
   d. bad, difficult, painful.

5. You know that combining the prefix *a-* and the word root *pnea* creates a medical term that means
   a. inflammation of the cornea.
   b. absence of breathing; respiratory arrest.
   c. constriction of the bronchi.
   d. faster than the normal breathing rate.

TERMS AND CONCEPTS

1. Write the number of the correct term next to each definition.

    1. Apnea
    2. Bronchodilator
    3. Bronchospasm
    4. Dyspnea
    5. Grunting
    6. Metered-dose inhaler (MDI)
    7. Respiratory arrest
    8. Respiratory failure
    9. Spacer
    10. Tripod position

    _____ a. A drug that relaxes the smooth muscle of the bronchi and bronchioles

    _____ b. When breathing stops completely

    _____ c. Constriction of the smooth muscle of the bronchi and bronchioles

    _____ d. Device consisting of a plastic container and a canister used to inhale an aerosolized medication

    _____ e. A chamber that is connected to a MDI to collect medication until it is inhaled

    _____ f. A period with absence of breathing

    _____ g. A sound heard during exhalation in infants suffering from severe respiratory distress

    _____ h. Inadequate oxygenation of the blood and elimination of carbon dioxide

    _____ i. Shortness of breath or difficulty in breathing

    _____ j. Patient sits upright, leans slightly forward, and supports the body with arms in front and elbows locked

2. Which two of the terms listed in item 1 above have essentially the same meaning?

    _____ and _____

CONTENT REVIEW

1. Your patient is experiencing difficulty breathing but has adequate tidal volume and respiratory rate. This patient is said to be _____ and your treatment should include _____.
    a. in respiratory failure; initiating immediate ventilation with BVM
    b. apneic; beginning aggressive ventilation at once
    c. experiencing dyspnea; administering oxygen at 6 liters per minute (lpm) via nasal cannula
    d. in respiratory distress; administering oxygen via nonrebreather mask

2. You are treating your patient that complains of shortness of breath. The patient appears to be quite agitated and aggressive. You know this is likely due to
    a. hypercarbia.
    b. hyperventilation.
    c. hypoxia.
    d. hypotension.

3. While treating your patient that is experiencing difficulty breathing, you find the skin to be pale, cool, and clammy (diaphoretic). You know this sign likely indicates
   a. late sign of hypoxia.
   b. early sign of hypoxia.
   c. late sign of hyperventilation.
   d. early sign of hyperventilation.

4. The tripod position is commonly indicative of which of the following?
   a. Severe respiratory distress
   b. Moderate respiratory distress
   c. Mild respiratory distress
   d. Apnea/respiratory arrest

5. Which of the following is a sign of severe respiratory distress?
   a. Speaking a couple of words between breaths
   b. Pink, warm skin
   c. Pulse oximeter reading of 97 percent
   d. Respiratory rate of 50 in infants

6. You are treating a patient complaining of breathing difficulty. You know that a patient in a state of hypercarbia (high CO_2 levels) will present with which of the following?
   a. Patient will speak with stuttering speech.
   b. Lung sounds will become diminished.
   c. Pupils will become fixed and dilated.
   d. Patient will be confused and disoriented.

7. You are assessing your patient that complains of difficulty breathing. You hear crowing sounds with each breath; you suspect
   a. a partial airway obstruction.
   b. fluid in the lower lungs.
   c. injured or ruptured diaphragm.
   d. inadequate blood flow to the lungs.

8. Your elderly patient is experiencing an acute onset of breathing difficulty. The patient is obviously very agitated and aggressive toward your attempts to treat him. You suspect the patient
   a. has had a reaction to medication.
   b. may be in an acute state of hypoxia.
   c. is hearing impaired and confused about your intentions.
   d. is an upset elderly person who is difficult to assess.

9. You are treating an unresponsive 3-year-old who is exhibiting signs of breathing difficulty with decreased tidal volume. The respiratory rate is 14 per minute. Which of the following is correct?
   a. Immediately begin positive-pressure ventilation.
   b. Begin positive-pressure ventilation after the physical exam.
   c. Immediately apply oxygen by nonrebreather mask at 15 lpm.
   d. Apply oxygen by nasal cannula at 6 lpm after the physical exam.

10. You are treating an elderly man who complains of breathing difficulty. He is breathing 18 times a minute with good chest rise and fall, and you feel a good volume of air at his nose and mouth upon exhalation. Which of the following is correct?
    a. Begin positive-pressure ventilation.
    b. Apply oxygen by nasal cannula at 6 lpm.
    c. Apply oxygen by nonrebreather mask at 15 lpm.
    d. No ventilation or oxygen therapy is required.

11. Upon arrival on the scene, you make contact with a patient who is experiencing difficulty breathing. You observe that the patient's eyelids are beginning to droop and his head bobs with each respiration. Your immediate action should be to
    a. place the patient on a nonrebreather mask.
    b. interview the patient to determine the specific complaint.
    c. place the patient in the Trendelenburg position.
    d. administer positive-pressure ventilations with the BVM.

12. The adult with breathing difficulty and increased pulse rate and the infant or child with breathing difficulty and slow pulse rate should both be transported immediately following the
    a. initial assessment.
    b. focused history.
    c. physical exam.
    d. ongoing assessment.

13. Which of the following adult patients complaining of difficulty breathing should be placed on a nonrebreather mask at 15 liters per minute?
    a. Respiratory rate of 20 with good air movement
    b. Respiratory rate of 18 with poor tidal volume
    c. Respiratory rate of 28 with adequate tidal volume
    d. Respiratory rate of 8 with little air movement

14. Suprasternal-notch retractions indicate that the patient
    a. has a history of heart surgery.
    b. is experiencing substernal chest pain.
    c. is making an extreme effort to breathe.
    d. has a history that includes asthma.

15. Bradycardia in the adult, child, or infant is a sign of which of the following?
    a. Severe hypoglycemia
    b. Impending respiratory failure
    c. Possible myocardial infarction
    d. Imminent shock

16. When an area of the chest moves inward during inhalation and outward during exhalation, it is a common sign of chest injury leading to breathing difficulty known as which of the following?
    a. Diaphragm breathing
    b. Accessory muscle use
    c. Paradoxical motion
    d. Intercostal retractions

17. If you are in doubt whether to ventilate with positive pressure or not, you should
    a. use a nonrebreather mask.
    b. contact medical direction for orders.
    c. provide positive-pressure ventilation.
    d. wait for paramedic backup.

18. You have placed the pulse oximeter on your patient complaining of breathing difficulty. The pulse oximeter reading is 88 percent while the patient is breathing room air. Which of the following statements best describes your findings?
    a. This is a normal reading for a patient breathing room air.
    b. This reading is an indication of severe hypoxia.
    c. This reading indicates a mild case of hypoxia.
    d. Reading below 90 percent is impossible; check the oximeter.

19. Number the list below in the proper order from 1 to 5 to provide emergency care for the patient with adequate breathing who is complaining of breathing difficulty.
    _____ Complete the focused history and physical exam.
    _____ Place the patient in a position of comfort and then transport.
    _____ Assess the vital signs.
    _____ Administer oxygen at 15 lpm by nonrebreather mask.
    _____ Determine if the patient has a prescribed MDI and contact medical direction for permission to administer it.

20. Your patient complains of shortness of breath. Following auscultation of the chest you find decreased breath sounds on the right side; there is no evidence of trauma. You suspect
    a. spontaneous pneumothorax.
    b. bilateral hemothorax.
    c. pneumonia.
    d. flail segment.

21. To determine if your emergency medical care has decreased the patient's breathing difficulty or if further intervention is necessary, you should
    a. perform an ongoing assessment prior to transporting the patient.
    b. perform an ongoing assessment while en route to the hospital.
    c. perform the focused history and physical exam while transporting.
    d. perform the focused history and physical exam before transporting.

22. For administering an MDI, which of the following procedures is correct?
    a. Coach the patient to breathe through the nose.
    b. Coach the patient to hold his or her breath as long as possible after inhalation of the medication.
    c. Depress the canister as the patient begins to exhale.
    d. Shake the canister for 10 seconds before removing the cap.

23. Which of the following is a sign of respiratory difficulty in children?
    a. Use of accessory muscles
    b. Hypertension and urticaria
    c. Sore or hoarse throat
    d. Respiratory rate of 15 to 30 breaths each minute

24. Which of the following is a sign of respiratory failure in infants and children?
    a. Seesaw or rocky breathing
    b. Increased muscle tone
    c. Bilateral breath sounds
    d. Rigid and painful abdomen

25. Your 4-year-old patient displays head bobbing and irregular breathing. You should
    a. administer oxygen; transport after completing the assessment.
    b. hold the nonrebreather mask next to the child's face; transport at once.
    c. immediately begin positive-pressure ventilation; transport at once.
    d. immediately administer oxygen by nonrebreather mask; transport after completing the assessment.

26. A child experiencing respiratory difficulty should be placed in which position?
    a. Supine position
    b. Prone position
    c. Position of comfort
    d. Tripod position

27. Regarding epiglottitis in the infant or child, which of the following is true?
    a. Epiglottitis is usually self-rectifying and is seldom an emergency.
    b. The child usually sits straight up, juts the neck out, and drools.
    c. You should inspect the throat and mouth with a tongue depressor.
    d. You should perform foreign body airway obstruction maneuvers if respiratory distress is evident.

28. A cough that produces a sound like a barking seal is the hallmark sign of which of the following?
    a. Complete airway obstruction
    b. Partial airway obstruction
    c. Epiglottitis, swollen epiglottis
    d. Croup, swelling of the larynx

29. Which of the following conditions can lead to faster muscle fatigue and early respiratory failure in the patient complaining of difficulty breathing?
    a. Difficulty breathing out (exhaling)
    b. Eupnea, relaxed breathing
    c. Increased lung sounds
    d. Increased tidal volume

30. You notice while assessing your patient who is having trouble breathing that his jugular veins are distended during inhalation and then return to normal during exhalation. You recognize this as
    a. paradoxical movement from a flail segment.
    b. an ominous sign of a traumatic brain injury with herniation.
    c. tachycardia, an increase in the heart rate above normal.
    d. kussmaul's sign, a severely increased pressure in the chest or around the heart.

31. You are treating your patient that has an extremely fast respiratory rate (tachypnea). You know that this fast respiratory rate will likely result in
    a. adequate tissue perfusion due to the increased breathing rate.
    b. inadequate tidal volume due to inadequate filling of the lungs.
    c. inadequate blood pressure due to increased oxygenation of the cells.
    d. overinflation of the lungs leading to increased oxygenation of the tissue.

32. Your patient has signs of subcutaneous emphysema. Which of the following is correct pertaining to this condition?
    a. Subcutaneous emphysema is easily seen by visual inspection of the chest.
    b. Due to gravity the air will settle to the lower chest in the seated patient.
    c. Subcutaneous emphysema is an indication of an air leak in the chest or neck.
    d. Subcutaneous emphysema cannot be felt; it must be auscultated with the stethoscope.

33. You are treating your patient that is breathing 36 times per minute with shallow tidal volume. The SpO$_2$ reading is 86 percent on room air. You should immediately
    a. ventilate with a BVM at 10 to 12 times per minute, imposing the ventilations over the patient's breathing rate.
    b. ventilate with a bag-valve mask at the patient's spontaneous respiratory rate.
    c. administer oxygen at 15 lpm due to the patient's ample spontaneous respiratory rate.
    d. place the patient on a nasal cannula at a low concentration due to the hyperventilation rate of the patient.

34. You are treating your patient suffering from bronchoconstriction with a Beta 2 metered-dose inhaler (MDI). You note an increase in the heart rate following the administration of the MDI. What is likely the reason for this increase in heart rate?
    a. Decreasing of the workload of the lungs increases the heart rate.
    b. Tachycardia is caused by the dilation of the smooth muscles.
    c. Beta 4 properties are a side effect to this type of MDI.
    d. Beta 2 MDI inhalers also have trace amounts of Beta 1 properties.

CASE STUDY

It's 8:15 in the morning. You and your partner, Angie, have just received the report from the previous shift. With a cup of coffee in hand, you walk to the ambulance to inventory the supplies and equipment. The alerting system sounds: "Unit 105 respond to 155 Wick Avenue for an elderly patient complaining of difficulty breathing. Alert time 0816 hours." You and Angie get underway at once. En route, dispatch advises that they are on the phone with the son of the patient and that he is very apprehensive. You arrive at the scene and are met at the ambulance by the son. "Hurry! My mother is having trouble breathing." You quickly reassure him as he leads you to the patient. You find an elderly woman, Mrs. Frederick, sitting on the side of the bed, with slight use of accessory muscles. A quick survey of the house and room doesn't reveal indications of trauma. The patient's chest is rising and falling adequately. There is good air volume exchange. Auscultation of the lungs reveals breath sounds bilateral with a slight wheezy sound. The respiratory rate is 20 per minute. The patient responds appropriately and states, "I've been—(breath)—short of breath—(breath)—over an hour—(breath)—Hope—(breath)—you can—(breath)—help me."

1. From the information provided, what should your assessment and first emergency-care step be?
    a. The patient is critical. Immediately begin positive-pressure ventilation.
    b. Breathing is adequate. Apply oxygen via nonrebreather mask at 15 lpm.
    c. Patient is hyperventilating. Apply a nasal cannula at 6 lpm.
    d. Patient is hyperventilating. Place a paper bag over the nose and mouth.

2. Using the OPQRST questions to evaluate the history of the present illness, the question, "Does lying flat make the breathing difficulty worse?" relates to which of the following?
   a. Provocation
   b. Quality
   c. Radiation
   d. Severity

During the focused history and physical exam, you learn that Mrs. Frederick has a history of asthma and has no known allergies. She does take Albuterol when her breathing is difficult, but she has not taken any today. You inspect around the lips and mouth for cyanosis; none is found. Angie advises that the vitals are blood pressure 160/76, breathing rate 22 per minute, pulse of 100 and regular.

3. Which of the following might cause the rapid breathing in this patient?
   a. Most asthmatics have rapid breathing continuously.
   b. The body attempts to make up for inadequate oxygenation.
   c. The patient's age (the elderly have higher respiratory rates.)
   d. This is a common side effect of Albuterol.

4. Which of the following is correct regarding Albuterol?
   a. Alpha agonist bronchoconstrictor, constricts the smooth muscles, dilates the airway
   b. Alpha agonist bronchodilator, relaxes the smooth muscles, dilates the airway
   c. Beta agonist bronchodilator, relaxes the smooth muscles, dilates the airway
   d. Beta pacifist bronchoconstrictor, contracts the smooth muscles, constricts the airway

5. Before you and Angie assist in the administration of the patient's MDI, what three criteria must first be met (indications)?

6. After you administer an MDI, if there is little or no effect, you should
   a. check the expiration date, then readminister the dose.
   b. consult medical direction to consider readministering.
   c. shake the MDI for 15 seconds, then readminister the dose.
   d. have the patient begin deep breathing to increase the effect of the medication.

After administering the MDI, you perform an ongoing assessment. Mrs. Frederick advises that her breathing difficulty has decreased dramatically. The vitals are blood pressure 140/62, respiratory rate 14 per minute, and pulse 74 and regular. After auscultating the lungs, you hear bilateral breath sounds without wheezes. Angie records and documents all the findings and readies the patient for transport.

7. In what position should you place this patient on the stretcher?
   a. Trendelenburg
   b. Lateral recumbent
   c. Supine
   d. Fowlers or semi-Fowlers

1. Which of the following medical conditions is caused by an obstruction of blood flow in the pulmonary arteries due to an occlusion?
   a. Spontaneous pneumothorax
   b. Pulmonary embolism
   c. Pulmonary edema
   d. Emphysema

2. Choose the medical condition that describes a sudden rupture of a portion of the visceral lining of the lung, causing the lung to partially collapse.
   a. Spontaneous pneumothorax
   b. Pulmonary embolism
   c. Pulmonary edema
   d. Chronic emphysema

3. Your partner has just finished auscultation of the lungs on an elderly patient complaining of respiratory difficulty. She described the lung sounds as a high-pitched whistling sound heard on both inspiration and exhalation. You recognize this to be
   a. wheezing.
   b. crackles.
   c. rhonchi.
   d. rales.

4. Choose the medical condition that is characterized by the destruction of the alveolar walls and distention of the alveolar sacs. It is more common in male patients, who may have a thin, barrel-chest appearance.
   a. Chronic bronchitis
   b. Emphysema
   c. Asthma
   d. Pulmonary embolism

5. You are treating a patient who is complaining of difficulty breathing. The patient has a history of congestive heart failure (CHF), and you suspect the patient is suffering from acute cardiogenic pulmonary edema. Which of the following treatments is considered dangerous and may exacerbate the condition, causing the patient to become worse?
   a. If breathing is adequate, place the patient on a nonrebreather mask at 15 lpm.
   b. If breathing is inadequate, begin positive-pressure ventilations immediately.
   c. Place the pulse oximeter probe on the patient's finger to obtain a SpO_2 value.
   d. Place the patient in the Trendelenburg or supine position to decrease fluid buildup.

SCENARIO 1: DOCUMENTATION EXERCISE

Read the following scenario and think about how you would document this call if you were the EMT who responded to the scene. Then answer the multiple-choice questions and fill in the sample prehospital-care report, basing your documentation on information from the scenario.

It's 1800 hours in the evening; you and your partner Captain Walls have just sat down for a well-deserved dinner break. Suddenly, the alerting system sounds: "Unit 1, respond to grid 534, 55 Seaman Way for a 62-year-old female, short of breath." As you exit the dining area, Captain Walls acknowledges the call with dispatch. After a short emergency response, you arrive on the scene of a well-kept single-family residence. You apply gloves and eye protection as you exit the ambulance. You both quickly scan the scene, looking for any safety hazards. Not suspecting any potential hazards, you approach the house and ring the doorbell. There is no response, so you carefully open the front door and announce your presence. You hear a muffled voice state, "I—(breath)—am—(breath)—in—(breath)—the—(breath)—bed—(breath)—room." You cautiously proceed to the back bedroom, very carefully assessing the scene.

As you and Captain Walls enter the bedroom, you find a patient who appears to be in her early 60s sitting on the edge of the bed in a tripod position. Captain Walls asks, "What seems to be the problem today?" She looks as if she is gasping for air, so Captain Walls quickly asks her if she is having trouble breathing. She nods her head indicating yes. You ask her name. She states very quickly with a gasp, "Mrs. Springer." Mrs. Springer seems very agitated, restless, and even somewhat confused by your presence. There are no stridorous or crowing sounds with inhalation or exhalation. Captain Walls indicates that the rate of Mrs. Springer's breathing is rapid at approximately 30 per minute. He also notes that her chest appears to be rising and falling, but little air is felt flowing from her mouth and nose, and she is using accessory muscles to breathe. You quickly place a nonrebreather on Mrs. Springer and set the liter flow to 15 lpm. You assess the radial pulse and find a strong, regular pulse. The skin is pale, cool, and clammy. A quick look at the patient's nail beds reveals a bluish-gray color. You quickly apply the pulse oximeter, which provides an SpO$_2$ reading of 86 percent on room air.

Captain Walls gives you a look that you recognize as meaning this is a priority call. He then calls for ALS backup. You reassess Mrs. Springer's mental status. She is now only responding to your verbal command to open her eyes with incomprehensible mumbling. Captain Walls proceeds to set up the cot

as you proceed with the rapid medical exam. Her pupils are sluggish to respond to light and are slightly dilated. The area around her nose and mouth is cyanotic along with her oral mucosa. You find no jugular venous distention, tracheal tugging, or subcutaneous emphysema to the neck. You quickly inspect and palpate the chest and find no evidence of trauma or scars. Auscultation reveals a bubbly sound produced during inhalation in the lower lobes of the lungs with decreased breath sounds bilaterally. Her abdomen is soft and not tender. Her lower extremities do not show any edema. Her distal pulses are present in all four extremities. She does not obey your commands to wiggle her toes or grasp your fingers. You pinch each extremity, which causes Mrs. Springer to moan slightly. You do not note any edema to the small of the back in the lower lumbar area.

As Captain Walls is positioning the cot, you obtain a set of baseline vital signs. The blood pressure is 190/86; the heart rate is 124 beats per minute and irregular; the respiratory rate is 30 per minute and labored; the skin is pale, cool, and clammy; and the pupils remain dilated and sluggish to respond to light. The SpO$_2$ reading is now at 87 percent. As you are positioning Mrs. Springer, you note that her chest is barely rising and falling. You quickly assess her breathing and find very little air movement. You immediately begin to ventilate her with a bag-valve-mask device. You ask Captain Walls to connect the BVM device to oxygen at 15 lpm. You quickly position the stretcher next to the bed and place the patient on the cot in a supine position as you continue to ventilate at 12 times per minute. With the patient continuously receiving positive-pressure ventilation, you enlist the help of a First Responder at the scene to load the patient into the ambulance. As Captain Walls prepares for immediate transport to the medical facility, the ALS crew arrives. The paramedic climbs into the back of the unit and begins to provide ALS care.

A family member drives up to the scene and tells Captain Walls that she is Mrs. Springer's daughter. The daughter is placed in the front seat of the ambulance, and Captain Walls begins to collect a history from her. The daughter indicates that the patient is not under the care of a physician and takes no medications. She states her mother has no known allergies. She notes her mother called her earlier and stated she was cleaning the bathroom with a strong disinfectant cleaner. She said she didn't feel good and was going to lie down in bed. She called a little later and said that she was having trouble breathing while lying flat and said that sitting upright on the edge of the bed made her breathing easier. The daughter denies that her mother complained of any other symptoms.

You conduct an ongoing assessment and note the heart rate is 122 beats per minute and irregular. The breathing is 26 times a minute with better volume. The patient seems more relaxed and less aggravated. She opens her eyes to your command. The pulse oximeter now indicates 98 percent SpO_2 with positive-pressure ventilations. The blood pressure is 188/90, and the skin is warm and dry without the bluish-gray color.

The paramedic in the back of the ambulance indicates that she is ready for transport. Captain Walls pulls from the scene and heads toward the medical facility, which is 3 minutes away. You are beginning to perform another ongoing assessment as Captain Walls indicates you are at the emergency department.

1. Which of the following signs or symptoms did *not* contribute to the decision as to whether or not to provide positive-pressure ventilation?
   a. SpO_2 of 86 percent
   b. Patient's age
   c. Agitation and restlessness
   d. Bluish-gray color

2. The medical term used to describe the bluish-gray color of the nailbeds, which indicates severe hypoxia, is known as
   a. cyanosis.
   b. jaundice.
   c. flushed.
   d. urticaria.

3. The bubbly sound heard in the lower-lung lobes with each inhalation while auscultating Mrs. Springer's chest is known as
   a. wheezes or stridor.
   b. rhonchi or sonorous.
   c. stridor or crowing.
   d. crackles or rales.

4. Captain Walls used the acronym OPQRST when questioning the patient's daughter. Mrs. Springer's daughter indicated that her mother's breathing became worse while lying flat. This is reported as which of the following?
   a. O—onset
   b. P—provocation
   c. Q—quality
   d. S—severity

EMERGENCY TRIP SHEET

TRIP #
MEDIC #
BEGIN MILES
END MILES
CODE___/___ PAGE___/___
UNITS ON SCENE

NAME   SEX   M   F   DOB ___/___/___
ADDRESS   RACE
CITY   STATE   ZIP
PHONE (   )   -   PCP DR.
RESPONDED FROM   CITY
TAKEN FROM   ZIP
DESTINATION   REASON
SSN   -   -   MEDICARE #   MEDICAID #
INSURANCE CO   INSURANCE #   GROUP #
RESPONSIBLE PARTY   ADDRESS
CITY   STATE   ZIP   PHONE (   )   -
EMPLOYER

TIME	ON SCENE (1)	ON SCENE (2)	ON SCENE (3)	EN-ROUTE (1)	EN-ROUTE (2)	AT DESTINATION
BP						
PULSE						
RESP						
EKG						

MEDICAL HISTORY

MEDICATIONS

ALLERGIES

C/C

EVENTS LEADING TO C/C

ASSESSMENT

TREATMENT

EMS SIGNATURE

BILLING USE ONLY

DAY

DATE

RECEIVED				
DISPATCHED				
EN-ROUTE				
ON SCENE				
TO HOSPITAL				
AT HOSPITAL				
IN-SERVICE				

CREW	CERT	STATE #

IV THERAPY
SUCCESSFUL   Y   N   # OF ATTEMPTS _____
ANGIO SIZE _____ga.
SITE _____
TOTAL FLUID INFUSED _____ cc
BLOOD DRAW   Y   N   INITIALS

INTUBATION INFORMATION
SUCCESSFUL   Y   N   # OF ATTEMPTS _____
TUBE SIZE _____ mm
TIME _____ INITIALS _____

CONDITION CODES				

TREATMENTS

TIME	TREATMENT	DOSE	ROUTE	INIT

GCS E___ V___ M___ TOTAL =
GCS E___ V___ M___ TOTAL =

HOSPITAL CONTACTED

CPR BEGUN BY   B   P   TIME BEGUN

AED USED   Y   N   BY:

RESUSCITATION TERMINATED - TIME

(   ) OSHA REGULATIONS FOLLOWED

CHAPTER

14 Cardiac Emergencies

OBJECTIVES

Numbered objectives are from the United States Department of Transportation EMT-Basic National Standard Curriculum. Asterisked objectives, if any, pertain to material that is supplemental to the DOT curriculum.

Cognitive

4-3.1   Describe the structure and function of the cardiovascular system.

4-3.2   Describe the emergency medical care of the patient experiencing chest pain/discomfort.

4-3.3   List the indications for automated external defibrillation (AED).

4-3.4   List the contraindications for automated external defibrillation.

4-3.5   Define the role of the EMT-Basic in the emergency cardiac-care system.

4-3.6   Explain the impact of age and weight on defibrillation.

4-3.7   Discuss the position of comfort for patients with various cardiac emergencies.

4-3.8   Establish the relationship between airway management and the patient with cardiovascular compromise.

4-3.9   Predict the relationship between the patient experiencing cardiovascular compromise and basic cardiac life support.

4-3.10 Discuss the fundamentals of early defibrillation.

4-3.11 Explain the rationale for early defibrillation.

4-3.12 Explain that not all chest pain patients result in cardiac arrest and do not need to be attached to an automated external defibrillator.

4-3.13 Explain the importance of prehospital ACLS intervention if it is available.

4-3.14 Explain the importance of urgent transport to a facility with Advanced Cardiac Life Support if it is not available in the prehospital setting.

4-3.15 Discuss the various types of automated external defibrillators.

4-3.16 Differentiate between the fully automated and the semi-automated defibrillator.

4-3.17 Discuss the procedures that must be taken into consideration for standard operations of the various types of automated external defibrillators.

4-3.18 State the reasons for assuring that the patient is pulseless and apneic when using the automated external defibrillator.

4-3.19 Discuss the circumstances that may result in inappropriate shocks.

4-3.20 Explain the considerations for interruption of CPR when using the automated external defibrillator.

4-3.21 Discuss the advantages and disadvantages of automated external defibrillators.

4-3.22 Summarize the speed of operation of automated external defibrillation.

4-3.23 Discuss the use of remote defibrillation through adhesive pads.

4-3.24 Discuss the special considerations for rhythm monitoring.

4-3.25 List the steps in the operation of the automated external defibrillator.

4-3.26 Discuss the standard of care that should be used to provide care to a patient with persistent ventricular fibrillation and no available ACLS.

4-3.27 Discuss the standard of care that should be used to provide care to a patient with recurrent ventricular fibrillation and no available ACLS.

4-3.28 Differentiate between the single rescuer and multirescuer care with an automated external defibrillator.

4-3.29 Explain the reasons for pulses not being checked between shocks with an automated external defibrillator.

4-3.30 Discuss the importance of coordinating ACLS-trained providers with personnel using automated external defibrillators.

4-3.31 Discuss the importance of post-resuscitation care.

4-3.32 List the components of post-resuscitation care.

4-3.33 Explain the importance of frequent practice with the automated external defibrillator.

4-3.34 Discuss the need to complete the Automated Defibrillator: Operator's Shift Checklist.

4-3.35 Discuss the role of the American Heart Association in the use of automated external defibrillation.

4-3.36 Explain the role medical direction plays in the use of automated external defibrillation.

4-3.37 State the reasons why a case review should be completed following the use of the automated external defibrillator.

4-3.38 Discuss the components that should be included in a case review.

4-3.39 Discuss the goal of quality improvement in automated external defibrillation.

4-3.40 Recognize the need for medical direction of protocols to assist in the emergency medical care of the patient with chest pain.

4-3.41 List the indications for the use of nitroglycerin.

4-3.42 State the contraindications and side effects for the use of nitroglycerin.

4-3.43 Define the function of all controls on an automated external defibrillator, and describe event documentation and battery defibrillator maintenance.

KEY IDEAS

In this chapter the assessment and emergency care of a patient suffering cardiovascular emergencies such as chest discomfort or pain and cardiac arrest are described.

- Signs and symptoms of cardiac compromise and acute coronary syndromes may vary widely from patient to patient. However, chest discomfort or pain is the most common chief complaint and most important signal of patients suffering from an acute coronary syndrome.

- All adult patients complaining of chest discomfort or pain should be treated as a cardiac emergency until proven otherwise.

- Prehospital treatment by the EMT of the responsive patient suffering chest discomfort or pain should focus on assessment, early interventions such as administration of high-flow oxygen, and transport—not on diagnosing the specific type of cardiac emergency the patient is experiencing.

- Not all patients experiencing chest discomfort or pain will go into cardiac arrest. If the patient does go into cardiac arrest, the EMT must be prepared to rapidly apply the automated external defibrillator (AED) and perform CPR.

- The EMT can assist in fibrinolytic-therapy decision making by attaining answers to important questions that will determine if fibrinolytics are appropriate for the patient or not and promptly presenting the results to emergency-department staff.

- The female may present with different signs and symptoms from those of a male when experiencing a cardiac event.

- Successfully resuscitating a cardiac-arrest patient is dependent upon the "chain of survival." This chain has four links: (1) early access, (2) early CPR, (3) early defibrillation, and (4) early Advanced Cardiac Life Support (ACLS). The provision of **high-quality chest compressions** and **early defibrillation** are two of the most critical factors.

- There are two basic types of external defibrillators: manual and automated. The automated external defibrillator (AED) is either fully automated or semiautomated.

- The rhythms for which automated external defibrillation is appropriate are ventricular fibrillation and pulseless ventricular tachycardia.

- The AED is indicated for use on nontrauma cardiac arrest patients older than 1 year of age who are unresponsive, with no breathing and no pulse. For patients from 1 to 8 years of age, an adult AED with a dose-attenuator system is preferred.

- CPR or AED priority:
  - Less than 1 year of age—do not apply; perform CPR only and transport rapidly
  - One to 8 years of age—adult AED with dose-attenuator system preferred
    - If arrest witnessed—AED, then CPR
    - If arrest unwitnessed—CPR, then AED
  - Older than 8 years of age
    - If arrest witnessed (or response time is less than 4 minutes)—AED, then CPR
    - If arrest unwitnessed (or response time is more than 4–5 minutes)—CPR, then AED

- Basic semiautomated AED sequence for two rescuers:
  - Take BSI precautions.
  - If CPR is in progress, stop CPR and check for airway, breathing, and pulse or begin CPR while your partner prepares the AED.
  - Attach defibrillation cables to the pads, attach pads to the patient's unclothed chest.
  - Turn the AED power on, and if required, begin event narrative (biphasic AEDs require the power to be turned on before pad placement).
  - When analysis begins, clear the patient.
  - Initiate analysis of the rhythm.
  - If a shock is advised, clear everyone from the patient and quickly deliver the shock.
  - Resume CPR (beginning with chest compressions) for 2 minutes (5 sets of 30:2 compressions to ventilations).
  - Recheck the pulse.

- Transport if two (or three) shocks are delivered or a total of two (or three) "No Shock" messages are received. Hypothermic patients should receive only one shock before immediate transport.

- The two- (or three-) shock rule begins again if the patient regains a pulse, then deteriorates back into cardiac arrest.

- The AED must be checked on a daily basis using the Automated Defibrillator: Operator's Shift Checklist to prevent device failure.

- AED operators should practice with the device every 90 days to refresh skills.

MEDICAL TERMINOLOGY

Term	Prefix	Word Root Combining Form	Suffix	Definition
angina pectoris (an-JYE-nah PEC-toris)		angina (to choke); pector (chest)		A symptom commonly associated with coronary artery disease.
asystole (a-sis-TOL-le)	a (no, not, without)	systole (contraction)		The absence of electrical activity and pumping action in the heart
atherosclerosis (ath-ER-oh skleh roh sis)		athero (fatty substance); sclera (hardening)	-osis (condition of)	Narrowing of arteries from fatty substances being deposited on the inner surface of the artery
atria (AY-tre-uh)		atri (atrium, entrance room)		The two upper chambers of the heart
arteriole (ar-TEER-e-ol)		arter (artery, road, channel)	-ole (small)	Smallest artery, leading to a capillary
arteriosclerosis (ar-TEER-e-oh-skleh-roh-sis)		arter (artery, road, channel); sclera (hardening)	-osis (condition of)	A condition that causes the arteries to become stiff and less elastic
artery (AR-tuh-re)		arter (artery, road, channel)		Blood vessel that carries blood away from the heart
capillary (KAP-uh-lair-e)		capillaries (hairlike)		Tiny blood vessel connecting to venules; site for gas and nutrient exchange
dysrhythmia (dis-RYTH-me-ah)	dys (bad, difficult, painful)	rhyth (rhythm)		An abnormal rhythm of the heart
myocardial infarction (my-OH-car-dee-al in-FARC-shun)		myo (muscle); card (heart); infarct (necrosis of an area)	ia (condition of) -ion (process)	Occurs when a portion of the heart muscle dies because of the lack of an adequate supply of oxygenated blood
perfusion (per-FU-zhun)	per- (through)	fus (pour)	-ion (process)	Delivery of oxygen and nutrients to the body cells and removal of wastes by blood flowing through the capillaries
pulmonary artery (PUL-mun-air-e AR-tuh-re)		pulmo (lung) artery	-ary (pertaining to)	Vessel carrying oxygen-depleted blood from the heart's right ventricle to the lungs
pulmonary vein (PUL-mun-air-e vane)		pulmo (lung) vein	-ary (pertaining to)	Vessel carrying oxygen-rich blood from the lungs to the left atrium of the heart
vein (vane)		ven (vein)		Vessel that carries blood toward the heart
ventricles (VEN-trik-ulz)		ventriculus (little belly, small cavity)		The two lower chambers of the heart

1. In each space, write the word form that matches the given definition. Not all terms will be used.

arter	card	ion	pulmo
ary	fus	myo	ven
atri	infarct	per	ventriculus

_____ a. Through

_____ b. Atrium

_____ c. Pour

_____ d. Artery

_____ e. Process

_____ f. Pertaining to

_____ g. Vein

_____ h. Small cavity

_____ i. Necrosis of an area

_____ j. Muscle

_____ k. Heart

TERMS AND CONCEPTS

1. Write the number of the correct term next to each definition. Not all terms will be used.

1. Arteriole
2. Atria
3. Capillary
4. Cardiac conduction system
5. Coronary arteries
6. Pulmonary vein
7. Valves
8. Venae cavae
9. Ventricles
10. Venule

_____ a. The two upper chambers of the heart

_____ b. Membranes located within the heart to prevent backflow of blood

_____ c. Two lower chambers of the heart

_____ d. Vessel carrying oxygen-rich blood from the lungs to the left atrium of the heart

_____ e. The smallest vein

_____ f. The two major veins that carry oxygen-depleted blood back to the heart

_____ g. Specialized contractile and conductive tissue of the heart that generates electrical impulses and causes the heart to beat

_____ h. Network of arteries that supply the heart with blood

_____ i. The smallest artery

2. The four terms below name heart rhythms that are detected by an AED. Write the number of each term next to its appropriate definition.

1. Asystole
2. Pulseless electrical activity (PEA)
3. Ventricular fibrillation (VF or V-Fib)
4. Ventricular tachycardia (V-Tach)

_____ a. A condition in which the heart generates a relatively normal electrical rhythm, but there is decreased or absent cardiac output as a result of cardiac muscle failure or blood loss

_____ b. A very rapid heart rhythm that is generally too fast to perfuse the body's organs adequately

_____ c. A continuous, uncoordinated trembling of the heart muscle that does not produce any cardiac output or perfusion of the body's organs

_____ d. A heart rhythm indicating absence of electrical activity in the heart; also known as "flatline"

CONTENT REVIEW

1. On the appropriate line, identify each structure of the circulatory system.

Alveoli   Lung capillaries
Arteries   Pulmonary artery
Arterioles   Pulmonary vein
Body capillaries   Veins
Bronchi   Venules

A _____
B _____
C _____
D _____
E _____
F _____
G _____
H _____
I _____
J _____

AIR (OXYGEN)

A
B
C
D
E

F
G
H
I
J

Heart (blood)

2. The three components of the circulatory system include the
   a. liver, kidneys, and the blood.
   b. heart, blood vessels, and the blood.
   c. heart, lungs, and the blood.
   d. liver, lungs, and the heart.

3. Hypoperfusion resulting from nervous-system interference
   a. creates a vascular system that is too small for the amount of available blood.
   b. is only a theoretical consideration and never occurs in a clinical situation.
   c. creates a vascular system that is too large for the amount of available blood.
   d. directly affects the normal pumping action of the heart.

4. Which is the proper sequence for the initial assessment of the responsive cardiac patient who is suffering chest discomfort or pain?
   a. Assess circulation, breathing, airway, skin
   b. Assess airway, breathing, circulation, skin
   c. Assess breathing, circulation, airway, skin
   d. Assess skin, airway, breathing, circulation

5. Which is the *first* emergency-care step for the responsive patient who is suffering chest discomfort or pain?
   a. Administer nitroglycerin.
   b. Perform positive-pressure ventilation with supplemental oxygen.
   c. Administer oxygen at 15 lpm by nonrebreather mask.
   d. Perform cardiopulmonary resuscitation (CPR).

6. Using the OPQRST questions to evaluate the history of the present illness, the question, "On a scale of 1 to 10, how would you rate your discomfort or pain?" is an example of which of the following?
   a. Onset
   b. Quality
   c. Severity
   d. Provocation

7. Some acute-coronary-syndrome patients, such as those suffering a heart attack, may not follow a typical pattern of signs and symptoms. This atypical pattern is widely known as
   a. a suspicious heart attack.
   b. an unconfirmed heart attack.
   c. a quiet heart attack.
   d. a silent heart attack.

8. Nitroglycerin in a spray or tablet form is administered by what route?
   a. Sublingual
   b. Topical
   c. Intravenous
   d. Intramuscular

9. Which statement is a contraindication for the administration of nitroglycerin?
   a. The patient has signs and symptoms of chest discomfort.
   b. The patient's systolic blood pressure is below 100 mmHg.
   c. The patient's systolic blood pressure is 10 mmHg lower than the baseline reading.
   d. The patient has a suspected head injury.

10. Which is correct regarding managing a patient with chest discomfort or pain?
    a. The EMT must be able to diagnose what condition is causing the chest discomfort.
    b. The EMT's assessment and care will be the same regardless of the cause of the patient's chest discomfort or pain.
    c. The EMT will administer nitroglycerin only to patients known to be suffering from angina pectoris.
    d. The EMT needs to know which condition is likely to deteriorate into cardiac arrest.

11. While preparing to administer nitroglycerin spray to your patient experiencing chest pain, he states that he takes Viagra. What should you do?
    a. Do not administer nitroglycerin, and contact medical direction for orders.
    b. Administer the first nitroglycerin spray, and reevaluate the patient.
    c. Double the dose of nitroglycerin, then contact medical direction.
    d. Reduce the nitroglycerin dose by half, and reevaluate the patient.

12. Which of the following is a candidate for automated external defibrillation?
    a. An adult medical patient who is in cardiac arrest
    b. An unresponsive adult with a pulse
    c. An adult trauma patient who is in cardiac arrest
    d. A responsive adult who is having severe chest pain or discomfort

13. According to the American Heart Association, which of the following is a primary cause of death in infants and children?
    a. Myocardial infarction
    b. Blunt trauma
    c. Seizures
    d. Respiratory compromise

14. The American Heart Association describes a sequence of events called the Chain of Survival. Choose two items that are components of the chain that are *most critical* to patient survival of cardiac arrest.
    a. High-quality cardiac compressions and early defibrillation
    b. Access and Advanced Cardiac Life Support (ACLS)
    c. Defibrillation and ACLS
    d. CPR and ACLS

15. The application of an electric shock to help the heart reorganize its electrical activity and restore its normal rhythm is known as which of the following?
    a. Vagal stimulation
    b. Shock therapy
    c. Defibrillation
    d. Cardiovascular therapy

16. The most frequent initial rhythm in sudden cardiac arrest is
    a. asystole.
    b. pulseless electrical activity.
    c. ventricular fibrillation.
    d. ventricular tachycardia.

17. Which of the following is a characteristic of the fully automated external defibrillator but is *not* a characteristic of the semiautomated external defibrillator?
    a. It can deliver a first shock quickly, usually within the first minute.
    b. It allows for "hands-free" defibrillation by use of adhesive pads.
    c. The machine, not the operator, administers the defibrillation.
    c. The machine may be able to provide a record of its operation.

18. Survival from ventricular fibrillation, sudden cardiac arrest decreases by _____ to _____ percent for each 1-minute delay to patient defibrillation.
    a. 2, 3
    b. 3, 4
    c. 5, 6
    d. 7, 10

19. The AED is contraindicated in patients less than
    a. 8 years of age.
    b. 4 years of age.
    c. 2 years of age.
    d. 1 year of age.

20. Select the proper description for the anterior-lateral placement of the defibrillator electrodes.
    a. $(-)$(sternum) on left upper-chest wall, $(+)$(apex) on right lower ribs at the anterior axillary line to the right of the nipple
    b. $(+)$(apex) on left upper-chest wall, $(-)$(sternum) on right lower ribs at the anterior axillary line to the right of the nipple
    c. $(-)$(sternum) right upper border of the sternum, $(+)$ (apex) on left anterior axillary line below and to the left of the nipple
    d. $(-)$(sternum) left upper border of the sternum, $(+)$(apex) on right anterior axillary line to the right of the nipple

21. Place the following steps for using a semiautomated (biphasic) AED in the proper sequence.
    1. Turn on power button.
    2. Attach pad to cables and apply pad to the patient's chest.
    3. Begin or resume CPR, and prepare the AED.
    4. Stop CPR, say "Clear," and press the button to begin analysis.
    5. Begin narrative (if equipped with recorder).
    6. BSI, and perform an initial assessment.
    7. Clear patient, and press button to deliver shock if "Deliver shock" message is given.
    a. 6, 3, 1, 2, 5, 4, 7
    b. 6, 3, 1, 4, 2, 5, 7
    c. 5, 6, 1, 3, 4, 7, 2
    d. 3, 6, 1, 5, 4, 2, 7

22. You are transporting an unresponsive patient who has been successfully defibrillated. The patient suddenly becomes pulseless and has no respirations. Select the best action to take.
    a. Stop the vehicle, deliver one shock, resume transport.
    b. Stop the vehicle, turn off the motor, deliver two (or three) shocks, resume transport.
    c. Stop the vehicle, deliver two (or three) shocks, resume transport.
    d. Initiate CPR only, and continue en route to the hospital.

23. AED failure is most commonly attributed to which of the following?
    a. Operator error
    b. Cable failure
    c. Internal electronics failure
    d. Battery failure

24. It is recommended that all AED operators refresh or practice operational skills with the device every
    a. month.
    b. 3 months.
    c. 6 months.
    d. year.

25. Which of the following best describes an acceptable and safe use of an AED?
    a. Application of an AED on a patient who is lying in rainwater
    b. AED use on a patient who is on a metal catwalk
    c. Placement of an AED pad on top of a nitroglycerin patch
    d. AED use on a patient who is on the floor of a business

CASE STUDY 1

You and your partner, Manny, are dispatched to a residence where there is a report of an elderly man having a heart attack. You are met at the door by the patient's wife, and she thanks you for your prompt response. She leads you to the back porch where you find her husband sitting, clutching his chest. You introduce yourselves, and the patient says his name is Fred Hansen. A quick visual assessment reveals that the patient is pale and slightly short of breath and seems very anxious.

1. You instruct Manny to place Mr. Hansen on oxygen. Which is the most appropriate means of delivering the oxygen?
    a. The patient's own home-oxygen apparatus
    b. Nasal cannula at 6 lpm
    c. Nonrebreather mask at 15 lpm
    d. Positive-pressure ventilation with supplemental oxygen

As you perform the initial assessment, you note that Mr. Hansen's radial pulse is very weak and irregular. You compare his radial pulse with the carotid pulse and find that the carotid is strong, but both are irregular.

2. On the basis of the information you gathered on arrival plus this additional information, you determine that
    a. Mr. Hansen is experiencing cardiac compromise; however, early transport is not necessary.
    b. Mr. Hansen is experiencing cardiac compromise and early transport is necessary.
    c. Mr. Hansen is not experiencing cardiac compromise; however, early transport is necessary.
    d. Mr. Hansen is not experiencing cardiac compromise, and early transport is not necessary.

Mr. Hansen states the only medicine that his physician prescribes for him is an aspirin a day and nitroglycerin for chest pain. You ask Mr. Hansen if he took any nitroglycerin with this episode of chest discomfort. He states, "One about 5 minutes before you arrived, but the pain is getting worse." You reassure Mr. Hansen as you quickly obtain the vital signs: pulse 70 per minute, weak and irregular; respirations 24 per minute; BP 152/74; SpO_2 of 94 percent. Skin is slightly pale and sweaty. Pupils are normal. Then you call medical direction for permission to administer additional nitroglycerin. Permission is granted by Dr. Smith for a total of three doses, including the dose Mr. Hansen has already taken, as long as the patient's blood pressure is stable.

3. Shortly after you administer sublingual nitroglycerin spray, Mr. Hansen complains of a headache. You should
   a. reassure him that this is a common side effect and the pain should pass.
   b. immediately remove the tablet; the headache indicates an allergic response.
   c. have him swallow the tablet; this will speed its absorption.
   d. reestablish contact with medical direction to ask for direction.

4. Mr. Hansen's chest discomfort has improved dramatically. You should
   a. relax, since the crisis is over, and complete the medical report.
   b. continue to evaluate him en route and update the receiving emergency department of any changes
   c. administer the third nitroglycerin tablet to increase the therapeutic level
   d. contact medical direction for permission to administer an aspirin to reduce the chest discomfort

CASE STUDY 2

You have been dispatched to the scene of a cardiac arrest. Dispatch advises that an ALS vehicle is also responding to the incident. You arrive and observe a male patient who appears to be in his mid-60 supine on the floor. A family member is performing adequate CPR on the patient. You calculate the total downtime as 3 minutes. You hear the siren of the approaching ALS vehicle.

1. Your next best action is to
   a. take over CPR, then stop and verify absence of pulse/breathing; do nothing further until ALS arrives.
   b. stop CPR, perform an initial assessment, and verify the absence of pulse/breathing.
   c. obtain a detailed history of the event as the family member continues CPR, then stop and verify the absence of pulse/breathing.
   d. have the family member continue CPR and radio dispatch to determine the exact ETA of the ALS vehicle, then verify the absence of pulse/breathing.

2. The patient is pulseless and not breathing. Your next best action is to
   a. prepare the AED for operation by turning the power button on.
   b. resume CPR and prepare the AED for operation.
   c. resume CPR and do nothing further until ALS arrives.
   d. place the adhesive monitoring-defibrillation pads on the patient's chest.

3. The patient's rhythm is analyzed, and the AED shows that applying a shock will not benefit the patient ("no shock"). What is your next best action?
   a. Resume CPR and transport the patient rapidly.
   b. Reanalyze the rhythm, wait 30 seconds, then reanalyze the rhythm again.
   c. Contact medical direction for additional orders.
   d. Recheck the pulse; if no pulse, resume CPR for 2 minutes, then reanalyze the rhythm.

CASE STUDY 3

You are working alone at a large convention complex as an EMT providing emergency medical coverage. You have been assigned to cover a concert for the evening. At the completion of the concert, you receive a call for a man down. You respond quickly to the site of the emergency. When you arrive, you observe a 50-year-old male who is supine on the floor of the restroom. You estimate the downtime at less than 2 minutes. You perform an initial assessment on the patient and determine that he is unresponsive, is not breathing, and is pulseless.

1. What is your next best action?
   a. Begin CPR.
   b. Call EMS for assistance.
   c. Attach the AED's external adhesive pads, turn the unit on, and initiate rhythm analysis.
   d. Use a pocket mask and attempt to give one ventilation to confirm an open airway.

2. You have delivered two shocks and rechecked the pulse. The patient is still pulseless. What is the next best action to take?
   a. Perform CPR for 2 minutes, then call for help from EMS dispatch.
   b. Reanalyze the rhythm and repeat two (or three) more shocks.
   c. Do nothing; resuscitation efforts are futile.
   d. Leave the patient briefly to call for help from EMS dispatch.

3. Let us assume that instead of the patient being pulseless, you recheck the pulse and find that the patient has a palpable carotid pulse. What is your next best action?
   a. Check the blood pressure.
   b. Check the breathing.
   c. Check the pupils.
   d. Check skin color and temperature.

CASE STUDY 4

You are on-scene treating a 70-year-old cardiac-arrest patient. A neighbor tells you that he saw the patient collapse while mowing his yard. The neighbor's wife called EMS while the neighbor quickly started CPR. You have been working on the patient for what seems like a long time. The ALS unit has not yet arrived. You have administered a total of three shocks according to your local protocol.

1. What is your next best action?
   a. Recheck the pulse, continue CPR (if required), and reanalyze for additional shocks.
   b. Recheck the pulse, and continue CPR (if required) until the arrival of the ALS unit.
   c. Recheck the pulse, continue CPR (if required), and transport the patient.
   d. Continue CPR for 2 minutes, and reanalyze for additional shocks.

ENRICHMENT

1. The primary contributing factor to coronary artery disease is
   a. arteriosclerosis
   b. lactic-acid formation
   c. peripheral vasodilation
   d. atherosclerosis

2. Which of the following most accurately states the factors that affect the signs and symptoms and the severity of acute coronary syndrome?
   a. The patient's resting pulse rate, the artery occluded, how much blood the coronary artery supplies to the heart, and the size or portion of the heart muscle not being supplied with oxygenated blood
   b. The site of the occlusion, the artery occluded, how much blood the occluded coronary artery supplies to the heart, the size or portion of the heart muscle not being supplied with oxygenated blood, and the length of time the artery has been occluded
   c. The patient's resting pulse rate, the patient's resting blood pressure, the artery occluded, how much blood the coronary artery supplies to the heart, and the size or portion of the heart muscle not being supplied with oxygenated blood
   d. The patient's resting pulse rate, the patient's resting blood pressure, the size or portion of the heart muscle not being supplied with oxygenated blood, and the length of time the artery has been occluded

3. Small coronary arteries that widen and supply oxygenated blood to an area of the heart where the larger coronary artery is narrowed from plaque deposits are called
   a. circumferential circulation.
   b. collateral circulation.
   c. Pott's circulation.
   d. sudoriferous circulation.

4. Angina pectoris
   a. is infrequently associated with coronary artery disease.
   b. typically occurs when a decreased workload is placed on the heart.
   c. most commonly will last from 2 to 5 minutes.
   d. is a symptom of inadequate blood supply to the heart muscle.

5. The signs and symptoms of angina pectoris may include
   a. steady discomfort in the lower abdomen.
   b. chest pain or discomfort that lasts longer than 20 minutes.
   c. nausea and or vomiting.
   d. numbness or tingling of the lips.

6. Appropriate emergency medical care for angina pectoris includes
   a. administering a patient's prescribed nitroglycerin.
   b. establishing an open airway and providing oxygen at 8 lpm.
   c. applying the pulse oximeter when en route to the hospital.
   d. administering a patient's prescribed metered-dose inhaler.

7. An acute myocardial infarction
   a. most frequently is the result of coronary artery spasm.
   b. occurs when a portion of the heart muscle dies.
   c. is commonly known as Graves' disease.
   d. will cause heart-muscle death within 2–5 minutes.

8. In the patient suffering from acute myocardial infarction,
   a. ventricular fibrillation infrequently results in cardiac arrest.
   b. ventricular fibrillation usually occurs within the first 4 hours.
   c. thrombolytic drugs will reverse heart-muscle damage.
   d. ischemic heart tissue can cause dysrhythmias.

9. Complete the chart by indicating if the sign or symptom is most likely associated with angina pectoris, acute myocardial infarction, or heart failure. Indicate with a check mark if the item is a common sign or symptom. One, two, or three check marks may be used for each sign or symptom.

Signs/Symptoms	Angina Pectoris	Acute Myocardial Infarction	Heart Failure
Steady discomfort usually located in the center of the chest but may be more diffuse throughout the front of the chest			
Chest discomfort radiating to the jaw, arms, shoulders, or back			
Nausea or vomiting			
Severe dyspnea			
Cyanosis			
Anxiety			
Dyspnea			
Signs and symptoms of pulmonary edema			
Complaint of indigestion pain			
Distended neck veins—JVD (late sign)			
Sense of impending doom			
Distended and soft, spongy abdomen			
Tachypnea			
Diaphoresis			
Discomfort usually described as pressure; tightness; or an aching, crushing, or heavy feeling			
Edema in the ankles, feet, and hands			
Lightheadedness or dizziness			
Fatigue on any exertion			
Crackles and possibly wheezes on auscultation of the chest			
Tachycardia			
Weakness			
Upright position with legs, feet, arms, and hands dangling			
Decreased SpO$_2$ (oxygen saturation) reading			

10. Heart failure
    a. can be categorized as upper-chamber or lower-chamber failure.
    b. may be caused by hypoperfusion, kidney failure, or liver failure.
    c. seldom results in peripheral edema, or swelling of the extremities.
    d. results when blood is not adequately ejected from the ventricle.

11. The management of the heart-failure patient with pulmonary edema
    a. is vastly different from treatment of the patient with an acute myocardial infarction.
    b. commonly results in a pneumothorax from positive-pressure ventilation treatment.
    c. becomes more complicated if the patient is taking a "water pill."
    d. can result in drastic improvement following positive-pressure ventilation.

12. The stage in which electrical charges of the heart muscle change from positive to negative and cause the heart muscle to contract is known as
    a. repolarization.
    b. depolarization.
    c. automaticity.
    d. conduction.

13. A normal ECG has stages that represent different activities in the normal heart cycle. Which of the following represents the second waveform, which signifies depolarization (contraction) of the ventricles of the heart?
    a. P wave
    b. PR interval
    c. QRS complex
    d. T wave

14. The T wave in a normal ECG represents which of the following?
    a. Repolarization, or relaxation, of the ventricles
    b. Depolarization, or contraction, of the atria
    c. Depolarization, or contraction, of the ventricles
    d. Repolarization, or relaxation, of the atria

15. From below, choose the ECG interval that represents the time it takes the heart's electrical impulses to travel from the atria to the ventricles.
    a. RR interval
    b. PR interval
    c. PP interval
    d. PS interval

SCENARIO 2: DOCUMENTATION EXERCISE

Read the following scenario, and think about how you would document this call if you were the EMT who responded to the scene. Then answer the multiple-choice questions and fill in the sample prehospital-care report (p. 132), basing your documentation on information from the scenario.

It is 6:00 PM on a Saturday afternoon. You and your partner, John, are on the way to a local grocery store to pick up some items for supper when dispatch calls: "Squad 104, respond to 635 South Florida Avenue, cross street Hallam Drive, for a 65-year-old male patient with chest discomfort." You advise dispatch that you are responding to the call.

In about 5 minutes you arrive on the scene. It is a residential area of small apartments and mobile homes. You ring the doorbell of a small but tidy mobile home and wait for an answer. A woman who appears to be in her mid-60s answers the door. With BSI precautions on, you and your partner enter. You introduce yourself and your partner and ask, "What's the problem today?" As you are walking toward a back bedroom, she tells you that her husband, Mr. Chambless, has been complaining of severe indigestion.

You enter the room and observe Mr. Chambless sitting up in bed, holding the center part of his chest with a balled fist. His opposite hand clasps his fist. His eyes are open as you enter the room. His skin looks blue, and you notice copious amounts of sweat on his forehead. He seems to be restless as he rocks back and forth in bed. He is breathing adequately with no audible, abnormal respiratory sounds.

You begin your assessment by saying, "Hello, Mr. Chambless. My name is Jill, and this is John. We're EMTs and we're here to help you. What's the problem today?" Mr. Chambless replies, "My chest hurts!" You place the AED next to the patient. You have a nonrebreather oxygen mask and oxygen prepared, and you place it on Mr. Chambless. You adjust the flow rate to 15 lpm. You assess the radial pulse. It appears to be rapid at a rate of approximately 120 beats per minute, and Mr. Chambless's skin is cool and clammy.

John quickly begins to take the vital signs as you begin a focused history and physical exam. You ask, "When did the pain start? What were you doing when it started? Did it start all of a sudden?" Mr. Chambless replies, "I was sitting here reading the newspaper, and it started all of a sudden. It was about an hour ago when it started. You guys gotta help me. It really hurts!" You quickly say, "We're doing everything we can for you, and to help you we need to ask you some additional questions." John finishes taking Mr. Chambless's pulse. He tells you it is 120, regular and strong. His skin is cool, clammy, and cyanotic. John places the pulse oximeter, and you note his SpO_2 is 96 percent.

Given the information that you have gained, you believe that ALS backup is required, and you quickly advise dispatch of the need. John continues with the vital signs while you continue with the focused history and physical exam. You ask Mr. Chambless, "Does anything make the discomfort better or worse?" He says, "No, it just hurts. I can't make it go away! Nothing seems to help it!" You ask him, "Can you describe the discomfort you are having? Is it sharp or dull, pressing or squeezing? What does it feel like?" He says, "It feels like someone is sitting on my chest. I don't really know how else to describe it." John states that the patient's respirations are 18 per minute, full and regular, and that the breath sounds are clear and equal bilaterally. You continue your assessment by inquiring, "Does this discomfort you are experiencing move or radiate to any other part of your body?" He replies, "You know . . . now that you said that, it does. It hurts in my shoulder and left arm—the inside part of my left arm." "Mr. Chambless, I really appreciate your cooperation. Is the oxygen helping you?" "Well, yes, it does seem to be helping me," he replies.

Mrs. Chambless is standing in the corner and appears to be disturbed by the activities taking place in her bedroom. You place your hand on her shoulder and speak to her softly. "Mrs. Chambless, we are doing everything we can right now. Could you please help us by getting any medications together that Mr. Chambless is currently taking and bring them to me?" She says, "Yes, yes. I am so worried about him. You know he is all I have. I'll get the medications together for you." Mrs. Chambless heads toward the bathroom.

John tells you the blood pressure is 180/90, and the pupils are equal and reactive. You quickly look at Mr. Chambless's neck veins, and they appear flat. His abdomen is distended and nontender, and you note no palpable masses. You don't see any swelling in his lower extremities or back region. John finishes the vital signs. You ask him to bring the cot into the house as you continue your focused history and physical exam. "Mr. Chambless, have you ever had any discomfort like this before?" You wait for his response. "No, I don't think I have," he states. "On a scale of 1–10, with 10 being the worst discomfort you have ever had, how would you rate your current discomfort?" you ask. He replies, "It's at least a 9 or a 10, it really hurts." "Mr. Chambless, when did this start? I know you told me about an hour ago. It's 6:05 PM now so it started about 5:00 PM, right?" you ask. He responds by saying, "No, it really started about 4:30 this afternoon."

Mrs. Chambless returns to the room with her husband's medications. The only medication he is taking is an over-the-counter medication for arthritis. You ask Mr. Chambless if he is allergic to any medications, and he shakes his head no. You ask Mr. Chambless if he is allergic to aspirin. He shakes his head no again. You ask him to chew a baby aspirin and then swallow a second 160 mg tablet.

A knock on the door is followed by the voice of Paramedic Robin Riki. She enters the room. You introduce Mr. Chambless to Robin and provide a brief report to Robin. You help Robin and her partner move Mr. Chambless to the front of the mobile home and into the ALS vehicle.

1. Mr. Chambless is most likely suffering from
   a. angina pectoris.
   b. acute myocardial infarction.
   c. congestive heart failure.
   d. acute hypertension.

2. What physical findings or information suggests that Mr. Chambless's condition is critical and requires ALS assistance?
   a. His abdominal distention
   b. His respiratory rate of 18 per minute
   c. The timing of his chest discomfort
   d. His mental status

EMERGENCY TRIP SHEET

TRIP #	
MEDIC #	
BEGIN MILES	
END MILES	
CODE___/___ PAGE___/___	
UNITS ON SCENE	

BILLING USE ONLY			
DAY			
DATE			
RECEIVED			
DISPATCHED			
EN-ROUTE			
ON SCENE			
TO HOSPITAL			
AT HOSPITAL			
IN-SERVICE			

NAME	SEX M F DOB ___/___/___
ADDRESS	RACE
CITY STATE	ZIP
PHONE ( ) -	PCP DR.
RESPONDED FROM	CITY
TAKEN FROM	ZIP
DESTINATION	REASON
SSN - - MEDICARE #	MEDICAID #
INSURANCE CO INSURANCE #	GROUP #
RESPONSIBLE PARTY ADDRESS	
CITY STATE ZIP PHONE ( ) -	
EMPLOYER	

CREW	CERT	STATE #

TIME	ON SCENE (1)	ON SCENE (2)	ON SCENE (3)	EN-ROUTE (1)	EN-ROUTE (2)	AT DESTINATION
BP						
PULSE						
RESP						
EKG						

IV THERAPY
SUCCESSFUL Y N # OF ATTEMPTS ___
ANGIO SIZE _____ga.
SITE _____
TOTAL FLUID INFUSED _____ c
BLOOD DRAW Y N INITIALS

INTUBATION INFORMATION
SUCCESSFUL Y N # OF ATTEMPTS ___
TUBE SIZE _____ mm
TIME _____ INITIALS ___

MEDICAL HISTORY

CONDITION CODES	▓		▓

TREATMENTS

MEDICATIONS

TIME	TREATMENT	DOSE	ROUTE	IN

ALLERGIES

C/C

EVENTS LEADING TO C/C

ASSESSMENT

TREATMENT

GCS E___ V___ M___ TOTAL =

GCS E___ V___ M___ TOTAL =

HOSPITAL CONTACTED

CPR BEGUN BY   B   P   TIME BEGUN

EMS SIGNATURE

AED USED Y N BY:

RESUSCITATION TERMINATED - TIME

( ) OSHA REGULATIONS FOLLOW

3. Mr. Chambless's clenched fist positioned over the center of his chest is called _____ sign.
   a. Wilson's
   b. Orchid
   c. Levine's
   d. Cardiac

4. The use of the AED on Mr. Chambless is
   a. appropriate and should have been placed during the initial assessment.
   b. appropriate and should have been placed following obtaining the vital signs.
   c. inappropriate unless he becomes pulseless and breathless.
   d. inappropriate; the AED should not have been taken from the vehicle.

5. The method used for assessing the patient's chest discomfort is referred to as the _____ method.
   a. cardiac history
   b. referral
   c. OPQRST
   d. summary

SCENARIO 3: DOCUMENTATION EXERCISE

Read the following scenario, and think about how you would document this call if you were the EMT who responded to the scene. Then answer the multiple-choice questions and fill in the sample prehospital-care report (p. 135), basing your documentation on information from the scenario.

It's a beautiful autumn day, and you and your partner, Tara, are the crew responsible for providing emergency medical care at a local football game. It's halftime, and the local team is winning 28 to 3. Both teams have left the field and are in the locker room. Suddenly, the portable radio squawks: "Unit 2, respond to the visitor's locker room for an elderly patient down; CPR is being administered; ALS Medic One is your backup." You mark or advise dispatch that you are en route to the locker room.

You and Tara quickly apply gloves and eye protection as you respond to the visiting team's locker room a short distance away. As you tell dispatch you are at the locker room, Tara pulls the stretcher from the rear of the ambulance. You both place the necessary equipment, including the AED, on the stretcher and walk briskly toward the locker room. As you enter the locker room you quickly scan the area, looking for any hazards. You notice that the room is filled to capacity with upset, screaming players and others. Tara solicits the help of a distressed but in-control adult standing in the room. She asks him to please help by moving all nonessential people out of the room.

As you approach the vicinity of the patient, you radio to dispatch that you have made patient contact and that this is a priority call. You recognize the patient as the coach from the visiting team. He is lying supine with a moribund look about him. Bystanders are administering CPR. An assistant coach states, "He was really giving it to the team, then his face turned red, and he fell to the floor. We immediately felt for a pulse and started CPR." Tara asks the bystanders to stop CPR while you perform an assessment of the airway, breathing, and circulation. You find that the patient is pulseless and apneic. Further observation reveals cyanosis around his lips and neck. You ask the bystanders to resume CPR and reassure them by saying what a good job they are doing.

Tara states she will ready the AED. As she exposes the patient's chest, you notice a large midchest scar extending from the suprasternal notch to the area just above the umbilicus. The assistant coach says, "The coach had a heart bypass 2 years ago." Tara attaches the defibrillation pads to the cables and then attaches them to the patient's bared chest. After the pads are attached, she states in a loud, clear voice, "Stop CPR and clear the patient." Tara looks at the AED screen and recognizes the following rhythm.

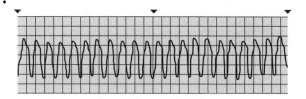

The AED indicates a "Deliver shock" message. Tara makes sure everyone is clear of the patient by looking from the patient's head to the feet. In a loud voice she says, "I'm clear, you're clear, everyone is clear." She presses the shock button to deliver the shock. The patient's body convulses with a quick jerk and then relaxes. Tara and you quickly begin CPR and continue for 2 minutes completing 5 sets of 30:2 compressions to ventilations. You feel for a carotid pulse and notice a bounding strong pulse. The patient remains apneic. Tara quickly starts positive-pressure ventilations with the BVM and supplemental oxygen. You hear on your portable radio that ALS Medic One has arrived on the scene.

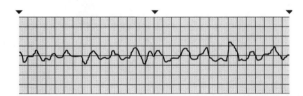

Medic One's crew, Lieutenant Wilson and Paramedic Springer, approach you for a report on the patient's status. You report that the patient was a witnessed cardiac arrest and prior to this event the coach was visibly upset. You mention that you found him on the floor with effective CPR being performed. An estimated time of 2 minutes passed from the time the patient went into cardiac arrest until you arrived on-scene. You relay that you immediately applied the AED and quickly explain the rhythm you found. You tell him that one shock was administered and that the patient just now has regained a pulse but remains apneic.

Tara continues to ventilate the patient with positive-pressure ventilations. As paramedic Springer positions the cot, you obtain a set of vital signs. The blood pressure is 138/64; the heart rate is 106 beats per minute, bounding but irregular. The skin is cool, pale, and clammy, but the color is improving. The SpO_2 is 94 percent. The pupils are dilated and very sluggish to respond to light. Lieutenant Wilson thanks you for a job well done. The patient is positioned on the cot and immediately loaded into Medic One and transported to the hospital 8 minutes away.

The next morning you and Tara receive a phone call at the station from the coach's wife, stating her gratitude for helping to save his life. You explain that you and Tara are but one link in the Chain of Survival and that there are others who deserve credit as well. You politely thank her for her comments and wish her and her husband well.

1. After Tara applied the AED, she found the patient in the following rhythm. You recognize this rhythm to be
   a. ventricular fibrillation.
   b. ventricular tachycardia.
   c. asystole.
   d. pulseless electrical activity (PEA).

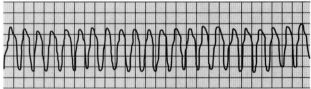

2. Tara asked everyone to stay clear of the patient when the AED entered the analyzing phase. Which of the following is a reason why it is important to ensure everyone stays clear of the patient during this time?
   a. The AED may sense the bystander's heart rate and shut off.
   b. The AED defibrillation pads may become ineffective.
   c. The patient's body may deliver a residual (leftover) shock.
   d. The AED may sense movement and report inaccurately.

3. You explained to the coach's wife that your efforts were one of several in the Chain of Survival that helped save her husband's life. You know that the links in the Chain of Survival, according to the American Heart Association, are
   a. early access, early CPR, early defibrillation, early ALS.
   b. early notification, early CPR, early diagnosis, early treatment.
   c. early diagnosis, early CPR, early hospitalization, early rehabilitation.
   d. early CPR, early ALS, early defibrillation, early hospitalization.

EMERGENCY TRIP SHEET

RIP #	
MEDIC #	
BEGIN MILES	
END MILES	
CODE ___/___	PAGE ___/___
UNITS ON SCENE	

BILLING USE ONLY				
DAY				
DATE				
RECEIVED				
DISPATCHED				
EN-ROUTE				
ON SCENE				
TO HOSPITAL				
AT HOSPITAL				
IN-SERVICE				

NAME _____ SEX M F DOB ___/___/___

ADDRESS _____ RACE

CITY _____ STATE _____ ZIP

PHONE (   )   -   _____ PCP DR.

RESPONDED FROM _____ CITY

TAKEN FROM _____ ZIP

DESTINATION _____ REASON

SSN ___ - ___ - ___ MEDICARE # _____ MEDICAID #

INSURANCE CO _____ INSURANCE # _____ GROUP #

RESPONSIBLE PARTY _____ ADDRESS

CITY _____ STATE ___ ZIP ___ PHONE (   )   -

EMPLOYER

CREW	CERT	STATE #

TIME	ON SCENE (1)	ON SCENE (2)	ON SCENE (3)	EN-ROUTE (1)	EN-ROUTE (2)	AT DESTINATION
BP						
PULSE						
RESP						
EKG						

IV THERAPY
SUCCESSFUL Y N # OF ATTEMPTS _____
ANGIO SIZE _____ ga.
SITE _____
TOTAL FLUID INFUSED _____ cc
BLOOD DRAW Y N INITIALS

INTUBATION INFORMATION
SUCCESSFUL Y N # OF ATTEMPTS _____
TUBE SIZE _____ mm
TIME _____ INITIALS _____

MEDICAL HISTORY

CONDITION CODES | | | | |

MEDICATIONS

TREATMENTS

TIME	TREATMENT	DOSE	ROUTE	INIT

ALLERGIES

C/C

EVENTS LEADING TO C/C

ASSESSMENT

TREATMENT

GCS E___ V___ M___ TOTAL =

GCS E___ V___ M___ TOTAL =

HOSPITAL CONTACTED

CPR BEGUN BY B P TIME BEGUN

EMS SIGNATURE

AED USED Y N BY:

RESUSCITATION TERMINATED - TIME

(   ) OSHA REGULATIONS FOLLOWED

15 Altered Mental Status and Diabetic Emergencies

OBJECTIVES

Numbered objectives are from the United States Department of Transportation EMT-Basic National Standard Curriculum. Asterisked objectives, if any, pertain to material that is supplemental to the DOT curriculum.

Cognitive

4-4.1 Identify the patient taking diabetic medications with altered mental status and the implications of a diabetes history.

4-4.2 State the steps in the emergency medical care of the patient taking diabetic medicine with an altered mental status and a history of diabetes.

4-4.3 Establish the relationship between airway management and the patient with altered mental status.

4-4.4 State the generic and trade names, medication forms, dose, administration, action, and contraindications for oral glucose.

4-4.5 Evaluate the need for medical direction in the emergency medical care of the diabetic patient.

* State the steps in the emergency care of the patient with an altered mental status and an unknown history.

KEY IDEAS

This chapter focuses on the patient with an altered mental status caused by a condition associated with diabetes. Emphasis is placed on assessing the patient's mental status, determining if the patient has a history of diabetes controlled by medication, and determining if the patient is alert enough to swallow before administering oral glucose with permission from medical direction.

■ It is important to distinguish between the patient with an altered mental status who has a history of diabetes controlled by medication and the patient with an altered mental status who does not have a known history of diabetes.

■ Airway management is a major concern in the patient with an altered mental status.

■ With on-line or off-line approval from medical direction, oral glucose may be administered to the patient with an altered mental status and a history of diabetes controlled by medication who is alert enough to swallow.

MEDICAL TERMINOLOGY

Term	Prefix	Word Root Combining Form	Suffix	Definition
hypoglycemia (HY-po-gly-SEE-mee-uh)	hypo- (below, under, deficient)	glyc (glucose, sweet, sugar)	-emia (blood condition)	Low blood sugar
hyperglycemia (HY-per-gly-SEE-mee-uh)	hyper- (above, beyond, excessive)	glyc (glucose, sweet, sugar)	-emia (blood condition)	High blood sugar
polyuria (POL-ee-YOO-ree-uh)	poly- (many, much, excessive)	ur (urine)	-ia (condition of)	Excessive urination
polyphagia (POL-ee-FAY-juh)	poly- (many, much, excessive)	phag (to eat, engulf)	-ia (condition of)	Excessive hunger
polydipsia (POL-ee-DIP-see-uh)	poly- (many, much, excessive)	dips (thirst, to drink)	-ia (condition of)	Excessive thirst

1. The medical term *hypoglycemia* contains the word root *glyc*. You know this refers to
   a. protein.
   b. globe.
   c. glomerulus.
   d. sugar.

2. The suffix *-emia* in such medical terms as *hyperglycemia* means
   a. blood condition.
   b. pertaining to.
   c. surgical repair.
   d. diabetic condition.

3. The prefix *poly-* in such medical terms as *polyuria* means
   a. many, much, excessive.
   b. similar, same, likeness.
   c. cut, away, from.
   d. below, under, deficient.

4. The medical term *polyuria* contains the word root *ur*, which you know to mean
   a. uterus.
   b. urine.
   c. uvea.
   d. ureter.

5. The medical term *polyphagia* contains the word root *phag*, which refers to
   a. sweating, perspiration.
   b. thirst, to drink.
   c. to eat, engulf.
   d. drum membrane.

TERMS AND CONCEPTS

1. Write the number of the correct term next to each definition.

   1. Altered mental status
   2. Diabetes mellitus
   3. Glucose
   4. Hyperglycemia
   5. Hypoglycemia
   6. Insulin

   _____ a. High blood glucose

   _____ b. Hormone secreted by the pancreas that promotes the movement of glucose into the sugar-storing cells

   _____ c. Disease characterized by the body's inability to produce insulin

   _____ d. Condition in which the patient displays a change ranging from disorientation to complete unresponsiveness

   _____ e. Low blood glucose

   _____ f. Form of sugar that is the body's basic source of energy

CONTENT REVIEW

1. You are treating your diabetic patient with an altered mental status. You know the altered mental status indicates
   a. the plantar nervous system has been affected.
   b. the brachial nervous system has been affected.
   c. the peripheral nervous system has been affected.
   d. the central nervous system has been affected.

2. Which of the following can be considered a frequent medical cause of altered mental status?
   a. Hypertension
   b. Pancreatitis
   c. Stroke
   d. Hypothermia

3. Your EMS medical director has approved orders to obtain patient blood-glucose levels through the use of a blood-glucose meter (glucometer). Which statement is true pertaining to the use of glucometers?
   a. The glucometer analyzes glucose in the blood by obtaining a drop of arterial blood.
   b. Glucometers measure blood-glucose levels in grams per liter (g/l).
   c. Glucometers are complex diagnostic equipment that require extensive special training.
   d. The glucometer analyzes glucose in the blood by obtaining a drop of capillary blood.

4. Your altered-mental-status patient is lying in bed, and no mechanism of injury is evident. You would suspect that the altered mental status is a result of which of the following?
   a. Head trauma
   b. Environmental exposure
   c. A medical illness
   d. An insect sting

5. Glucometers measure the glucose in the blood in milligrams per deciliter (mg/dl). Which of the following blood-glucose levels would indicate hyperglycemia?
   a. 50 mg/dl
   b. 80 mg/dl
   c. 120 mg/dl
   d. 150 mg/dl

6. You are assessing a patient with an altered mental status. Which of the following signs would cause you to suspect that the decreased mental status is due to trauma rather than a medical illness?
   a. Pupils that are pinpoint, or dilated
   b. Flexion or extension posturing
   c. Lacerations to the tongue, indicating seizure
   d. Loss of bowel control

7. Your patient has experienced a rapid onset of altered mental status and has cool, moist skin, an elevated heart rate, and other signs that indicate he is experiencing a diabetic emergency. He has no medical ID tag or medications on his person, and you are unable to confirm that he has a history of diabetes controlled by medication. However, he is clearly still able to swallow. Which of the following emergency-care measures should you provide?
   a. Ensure an open airway.
   b. Provide oxygen by nasal cannula at 4 lpm
   c. Administer oral glucose.
   d. Position the patient in a Trendelenburg position.

8. Which of the following best describes diabetes Type II?
   a. The blood-glucose level is usually controlled by diet.
   b. No insulin is produced by the body.
   c. It is commonly acquired during the childhood years.
   d. Insulin must be injected daily.

9. You are assessing a patient that has a history of diabetes mellitus. The patient presents with tachycardia, diaphoresis, and pale, cool skin typically seen in the hypoglycemic patient. Which of the following is responsible for these signs?
   a. Release of epinephrine (adrenalin)
   b. Increasing blood pressure (hypertension)
   c. Narrowing of blood vessels (vasoconstriction)
   d. Inflammation of the renal glomeruli (glomerulitis)

10. You are assessing your patient who has a history of diabetes. Which of the following questions will not aid you in your assessment of this patient?
    a. Did you take your medication today?
    b. Have you eaten (or skipped any) regular meals today?
    c. Did you do any unusual exercise or physical activity today?
    d. Does a history of cancer run in your family's medical history?

11. Signs and symptoms that mimic a stroke, such as weakness or paralysis on one side of the body, may occur more frequently in the diabetic patient who is
    a. young.
    b. hyperglycemic.
    c. elderly.
    d. on cardiac medications.

12. Which of the following indicates that a patient has a history of diabetes that is controlled by medication?
    a. Medical identification device (Medic Alert bracelet or tag)
    b. Unequal pupils
    c. Pale, cool, diaphoretic skin
    d. 1-cc syringes are found

13. You are treating a patient with an altered mental status who has diabetes that is controlled by medication. After establishing and maintaining the airway, you should next
    a. administer oral glucose per protocol.
    b. determine if the patient can swallow.
    c. reassess airway, breathing, and circulation.
    d. perform an ongoing assessment.

14. Select the correct statement regarding reassessment following administration of oral glucose.
    a. Reassess the patient's mental status, expecting an improvement in 3 minutes or less.
    b. Reassess the patient's mental status, understanding that improvement may not be apparent for 20 minutes or more.
    c. Assume that the patient's mental status will not deteriorate once oral glucose has been administered.
    d. If the patient loses responsiveness or seizes, insert a tongue depressor to prevent the patient from biting his or her tongue.

15. While attending a continuing education class on diabetes mellitus, you are asked which of the following best describes glucagon. You know that glucagon
    a. contains sugars to control the blood levels.
    b. is a hormone that stimulates the breakdown of glycogen.
    c. transports simple sugars into the cells from the bloodstream.
    d. prevents the free movement of glucose across the blood–brain barrier.

16. You are assessing a 42-year-old patient that presents with a furrowed tongue, sunken eyes, and poor skin turgor (tenting). You suspect the patient is dehydrated; you should
    a. place the patient in a Trendelenburg position.
    b. apply cold packs to the external neck great veins.
    c. immediately palpate the abdomen for abnormalities.
    d. check the patient's blood-glucose level (BGL).

17. You are treating a patient that you suspect is suffering from diabetic ketoacidosis (DKA). You know that the diabetic ketoacidosis patient's altered mental status is caused by
    a. dehydration and acidosis affecting the brain.
    b. a lack of glucose affecting the brain.
    c. rapid onset of hypoglycemia affecting the brain.
    d. decrease in blood from hypotension affecting the brain.

CASE STUDY

You and your partner, Emil, are dispatched to a local park, where there is a report of a young female acting strangely. You approach the scene and find an approximately 30-year-old female in a jogging outfit sitting on a bench. It appears that she is anxious and speaking with inappropriate words. You notice a medical identification bracelet that informs you she is an insulin-dependent diabetic. The patient's airway is patent, and her breathing appears adequate. You place her on oxygen. The patient does not answer any of your questions appropriately, and none of the bystanders who have gathered know her. Her vital signs include heart rate 104 per minute, blood pressure 100/64, respirations 20 per minute. The skin is cool and moist. You and Emil both suspect a diabetic emergency and decide that she is alert enough to swallow. You ask Emil to prepare to administer oral glucose following the protocol established off-line by your medical direction.

1. From the above information, list the signs that support your suspicion that the patient is suffering from a diabetic emergency.

2. You place the patient on oxygen. Which of the following is most appropriate for this patient?
   a. Nasal cannula at 6 lpm
   b. Nonrebreather mask at 15 lpm
   c. Simple face mask at 15 lpm
   d. Positive-pressure ventilation

3. You and your partner determine that the patient has met the three criteria for administration of oral glucose. Which of the following criteria would *not* aid you in your decision?
   a. The patient's blood pressure.
   b. The patient must have an altered mental status.
   c. The patient must have a history of diabetes controlled by medication.
   d. The patient must be able to swallow.

4. Approval to administer oral glucose was given off-line in the above scenario. In some jurisdictions, approval to administer oral glucose must be given on-line. Which of the following best describes "on-line" medical direction?
   a. Approval given by radio or phone
   b. Approval given by standing orders
   c. Approval given by prearranged written protocol
   d. Approval given by the EMS supervisor

After you administer the oral glucose, the patient begins feeling much better. En route to the hospital, she is able to converse normally. She informs you her name is Pat, that she lives on Third Avenue, and she knows it's Tuesday. She took her insulin this morning but went for a jog and forgot to eat lunch. You continue to assess her during transport to the hospital.

ENRICHMENT

1. Insulin is secreted when the blood-glucose level is elevated. Insulin has three main functions. Which of the following is a function of the hormone glucagon rather than insulin?
   a. Increases the movement of glucose out of the blood and into the cells
   b. Converts noncarbohydrate substances into glucose
   c. Causes the liver to take up glucose out of the blood and convert it to glycogen
   d. Decreases blood-glucose levels

2. The hormone glucagon is secreted by the pancreas. Its major role in the body is to
   a. raise and maintain the blood-glucose level.
   b. facilitate the movement of glucose out of the blood.
   c. increase insulin levels in the blood and brain.
   d. slow the secretion of glycogen, which lowers glucose levels.

3. Diabetes mellitus (DM) patients suffering from the lack of insulin will typically complain of frequent thirst (polydipsia), frequent urination (polyuria), and hunger (polyphagia). This is referred to as the "three Ps." Which best describes the reason these patients often complain of the three Ps?
   a. The liver collects the hormone insulin, which helps to regulate water absorption.
   b. The kidneys spill glucose into the urine; the large molecule of glucose draws water.
   c. The glycogen molecule is very small, which draws water from the kidneys into the cells.
   d. The pancreas overproduces the hormone insulin, which draws water from the cells.

4. Type I and Type II DM each have specific characteristics. Which characteristic best describes Type I diabetes mellitus?
   a. Most often, the pancreas will not produce and secrete any insulin.
   b. Typically it is diagnosed in patients older than 50 years of age.
   c. It is characteristically found in the heavy or obese patient.
   d. Rarely will these patients suffer from DKA or hypoglycemia.

5. Which of the following is typical of the patient suffering from DKA?
   a. Blood glucose levels are drastically low, usually below 40 mg/dl.
   b. Signs and symptoms of DKA occur immediately following the onset of hypoglycemia.
   c. The electrolytes in the body become balanced to form a homeostatic state.
   d. The cells begin to burn fat for energy as glucose collects in the blood.

6. Most often the signs and symptoms of DKA are produced by dehydration and acid buildup. Which of the following is a very late sign of DKA?
   a. Acetone breath
   b. Polyuria
   c. Coma
   d. Kussmaul's respirations

7. In the absence of glucose, some cells of the body are able to use fats and proteins as an energy source. Which of the following organ cells can use only glucose as a source of fuel and will dysfunction, shut down, and eventually begin to die without it?
   a. Cardiac muscle cells
   b. Skeletal muscle cells
   c. Brain tissue cells
   d. Liver cells

SCENARIO 4: DOCUMENTATION EXERCISE

Read the following scenario and think about how you would document this call if you were the EMT who responded to the scene. Then answer the multiple-choice questions and fill in the sample prehospital-care report, basing your documentation on information from the scenario.

You and your partner, Lieutenant Graves, are returning to the station from the hospital after completing a call. The radio sounds with an emergency tone: "Squad 11 respond to 1729 17th Avenue for an elderly male that is confused. Time out 1634 hours." Lieutenant Graves acknowledges the call, "Squad 11 en route." After a short emergency response, your unit arrives at the scene of a older, run-down single-family residence. You both put on gloves and eye protection as you scan the area for possible safety hazards. Seeing no obvious or potential hazards, you approach the house and knock on the front door.

A well-dressed, middle-aged woman answers. She introduces herself and says she is the patient's younger sister who lives across town. She states she tried to call her brother on the phone for the past few hours and then became worried so she drove over to check on him. As you enter the house you quickly scan, looking for any hazards or obstacles that may inhibit moving the patient. She leads you to the living room, where you find a man you estimate to be about 60 years old sitting on the couch rocking back and forth while repeating words that don't make sense. The patient seems agitated, perhaps even aggressive. He speaks in loud shouts but without slurred speech.

Lieutenant Graves begins the initial assessment. He touches the patient gently on the shoulder and asks him, "What seems to be the problem today?" The patient responds with an inappropriate statement but follows you with his eyes. His sister says, "He has diabetes and sometimes will have episodes like this. We've had the ambulance out here before." Your general impression is that the patient is weak, pale, and sweating profusely. Lieutenant Graves asks the patient his name, and he responds with a sluggish, mumbled "Dale." "Did you eat lunch today?" Lieutenant Graves asks. Dale responds with a delayed "No." You ask him if he took his insulin today. He responds "Yes." You observe that the patient has an adequate airway with respirations approximately 20 per minute. You place a nonrebreather mask on the patient at 15 lpm. You then assess the radial pulse and find it to be around 80 beats per minute and regular. The skin is very diaphoretic and cool. There is no noted cyanosis. Lieutenant Graves calls for ALS backup and positions the cot next to the patient.

You begin a rapid medical exam. Dale's pupils respond normally to light. You do not notice any acetone smell from the mouth; however, the patient is drooling copious amounts of saliva. There is no noted unilateral facial droop. You find no jugular-vein distention or tracheal tugging. You quickly inspect and palpate the chest and find no evidence of trauma or scars. Auscultation of the lungs reveals that they are clear in all fields with a normal tidal volume. His abdomen is soft and not tender. The lower extremities do not show any edema. The upper extremities are unremarkable and good distal pulses are found in all extremities. Dale does not respond to your request to wiggle his fingers and toes but responds with a loud "Ouch" when you pinch each extremity. There is no edema to the lower lumbar area of the back.

Lieutenant Graves asks Dale's sister if she can provide answers to some medical questions. She responds, "I hope I can remember everything." He reassures her. She states that Dale has no known allergies; he takes an injection of insulin in the morning and one right before dinner every day; he takes no other medications except for over-the-counter vitamins. She adds, "He always eats a good breakfast every morning, but he must have missed his lunch today."

Lieutenant Graves obtains a set of baseline vital signs. The blood pressure is 162/84; the heart rate is 86 beats per minute and regular; the respiratory rate is 18 per minute and nonlabored; the skin is pale, cool, and very diaphoretic; the pupils respond appropriately to light; the SpO_2 reading on the pulse oximeter is 99 percent with the oxygen. You prepare to obtain a blood glucose level per your off-line protocol. You let Dale's arm and hand dangle from the edge of the couch and briefly warm the fingers by placing them in your hands. Lieutenant Graves prepares the glucometer and test strip for the application of capillary blood. You grasp a finger close to the distal end and clean it with alcohol prep. The finger is pricked, and you gently squeeze a drop of blood onto the test strip. Lieutenant Graves takes the glucometer while you place a bandage on the pricked site, and Lieutenant Graves remarks, "The BGL is 42 mg/dl."

You determine that Dale is alert enough to swallow and prepare for the administration of oral glucose. You administer small amounts of oral glucose between his cheek and gum, making sure not to compromise his airway. You and Lieutenant Graves position Dale on the cot and prepare him for transport. As you move him to the ambulance, the ALS backup, Medic Six, arrives on the scene. You perform an ongoing assessment and find that Dale is becoming more alert and aware of his surroundings. His vital signs are blood pressure 158/80, heart rate 80 beats per minute and regular, respiratory rate 20 per minute and nonlabored. His skin is less diaphoretic but still pale. The SpO$_2$ reading on the pulse oximeter remains 99 percent with the oxygen. Dale remarks, "Oh, I must have been out for awhile. I should have eaten lunch." You assist the crew of Medic Six and transport Dale to the emergency department located approximately 10 minutes away.

1. Why is it significant for Lieutenant Graves to ask if the patient has eaten or taken his insulin today?
   a. If the patient ate without taking insulin, this is a critical mistake, which could lead to death.
   b. Administering insulin and then not eating signifies the patient is a danger to himself.
   c. Taking insulin injections and then not eating will likely lead to a high blood-glucose level.
   d. If the patient took his insulin but did not eat, you would suspect hypoglycemia.

2. How would the smell of acetone on the patient's breath be of value in your assessment of the diabetic patient?
   a. Acetone breath may indicate a buildup of ketones, a sign of DKA.
   b. This smell is evidence that the patient has consumed alcohol and may be intoxicated.
   c. Acetone breath indicates the need for immediate administration of ipecac syrup.
   d. The fruity acetone breath is an indication of impending unresponsiveness.

3. Why is it important to let the patient's hand dangle and to warm the patient's fingertips when obtaining a blood-glucose level?
   a. Bleeding is better controlled when the hand is lowered and warmed.
   b. Lowering the hand lessens the likelihood of developing complications like thrombus.
   c. This allows better blood flow to the fingers and provides a better sample.
   d. Lowering the hand will keep the blood from coagulating and ruining the sample.

4. This patient's blood-glucose level (BGL) was 42 mg/dl. Which of the following statements best describes this finding?
   a. The BGL is above the normal range. This patient shows signs of hyperglycemia.
   b. The BGL is within the normal range. However, the patient exhibits abnormal behavior.
   c. The BGL is below normal, but the patient is responsive. This is a normal response.
   d. The BGL is below normal with signs and symptoms. This patient is hypoglycemic.

5. What criteria did this patient have to meet before you were able to treat him with oral glucose? The patient must
   a. be over 30 years of age, have a history of diabetes controlled by diet, and have an intact gag reflex.
   b. have an altered mental status, have a history of diabetes controlled by medication, and have the ability to swallow.
   c. be responsive to tactile stimulation, have a history of diabetes controlled by diet, and have an intact gag reflex.
   d. have an altered mental status, have a history of diabetes controlled by diet or medication, and be able to respond to commands.

EMERGENCY TRIP SHEET

BILLING USE ONLY				
DAY				
DATE				
RECEIVED				
DISPATCHED				
EN-ROUTE				
ON SCENE				
TO HOSPITAL				
AT HOSPITAL				
IN-SERVICE				

TRIP #

MEDIC #

BEGIN MILES

END MILES

CODE___/___ | PAGE___/___

UNITS ON SCENE

NAME   SEX M F DOB ___/___/___

ADDRESS   RACE

CITY   STATE   ZIP

PHONE (   )   -   PCP DR.

RESPONDED FROM   CITY

TAKEN FROM   ZIP

DESTINATION   REASON

SSN   -   -   MEDICARE #   MEDICAID #

INSURANCE CO   INSURANCE #   GROUP #

RESPONSIBLE PARTY   ADDRESS

CITY   STATE   ZIP   PHONE (   )   -

EMPLOYER

CREW	CERT	STATE #

	ON SCENE (1)	ON SCENE (2)	ON SCENE (3)	EN-ROUTE (1)	EN-ROUTE (2)	AT DESTINATION
TIME						
BP						
PULSE						
RESP						
EKG						

IV THERAPY
SUCCESSFUL Y N # OF ATTEMPTS _____
ANGIO SIZE _____ga.
SITE _____
TOTAL FLUID INFUSED _____ cc
BLOOD DRAW Y N INITIALS _____

INTUBATION INFORMATION
SUCCESSFUL Y N # OF ATTEMPTS _____
TUBE SIZE _____ mm
TIME _____ INITIALS _____

MEDICAL HISTORY

MEDICATIONS

ALLERGIES

C/C

EVENTS LEADING TO C/C

ASSESSMENT

TREATMENT

EMS SIGNATURE

CONDITION CODES				

TREATMENTS				
TIME	TREATMENT	DOSE	ROUTE	INIT

GCS | E___ V___ M___ TOTAL =

GCS | E___ V___ M___ TOTAL =

HOSPITAL CONTACTED

CPR BEGUN BY   B   P   TIME BEGUN

AED USED Y N BY:

RESUSCITATION TERMINATED - TIME

(   ) OSHA REGULATIONS FOLLOWED

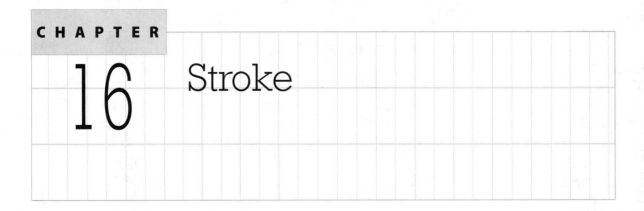

CHAPTER

16 Stroke

OBJECTIVES

Numbered objectives are from the United States Department of Transportation EMT-Basic National Standard Curriculum. Asterisked objectives, if any, pertain to material that is supplemental to the DOT curriculum.

Cognitive

* Describe the assessment of the patient with an altered mental status and a loss of speech, sensory, or motor function.
* List the common signs and symptoms of a nontraumatic brain injury.
* Describe the emergency care for a patient with an altered mental status and a loss of speech, sensory, or motor function.
* Describe the conditions most likely to cause altered mental status with a loss of speech, sensory, or motor function.

KEY IDEAS

An altered mental status may sometimes be accompanied by a loss of speech, sensory, or motor function. This chapter focuses on the assessment and management of patients with these signs.

■ Altered mental status with loss of function may be caused by external trauma or by a nontraumatic brain injury, such as that caused by stroke.

■ It is important to closely monitor and manage the airway and breathing of the patient who is suffering an altered mental status with loss of speech, sensory, and motor function.

MEDICAL TERMINOLOGY

Term	Prefix	Word Root Combining Form	Suffix	Definition
aphagia (ah-FAY-juh)	a- (lack of)	phag (to eat, engulf)	-ia (condition of)	Lack of the ability to eat or swallow
aphasia (ah-FAY-zhuh)	a- (no, not, without, lack of)	phas (to speak)	-ia (condition of)	Lack of the ability to speak
atherosclerosis (ath-uh-roh-skluh-RO-sis)		ather/o (fatty substance, porridge); scler (hardening)	-osis (condition of)	Condition of hardening of the arteries caused by fatty deposits that progress to calcified plaque
dysphagia (dis-FAY-juh)	dys- (bad, difficult, painful)	phag (to eat, engulf)	-ia (condition of)	Difficulty in eating or swallowing
dysphasia (dis-FAY-zhuh)	dys- (bad, difficult, painful)	phas (to speak)	-ia (condition of)	Difficulty in speaking
embolism (EM-boh-lizm)		embol (to cast, to throw)	-ism (condition of)	Condition in which a blood clot obstructs a blood vessel
hemiparesis (hem-ee-puh-REE-sis)	hemi- (half)		-paresis (weakness)	Slight paralysis or weakness that affects one side of the body
hemiplegia (hem-ee-PLEE-juh)	hemi- (half)		-plegia (paralysis, stroke)	Paralysis that affects one-half of the body
monoplegia (mon-oh-PLEE-juh)	mono- (one)		-plegia (paralysis, stroke)	Paralysis that affects only one extremity
paraplegia (pair-uh-PLEE-juh)	para- (beside, alongside, abnormal)		-plegia (paralysis, stroke)	Paralysis of both legs or the lower portion of the body
quadriplegia (kwahd-ruh-PLEE-juh)	quadri- (four)		-plegia (paralysis, stroke)	Paralysis in all four extremities
subarachnoid (sub-ah-RAK-noyd)	sub- (below, under, beneath)	arachn/e (spider)	-oid (resemble, form)	Below the arachnoid membrane; between the arachnoid membrane and the pia mater
thrombosis (throm-BOH-sis)		thromb (clot of blood)	-osis (condition of)	Condition in which there is a blood clot within the vascular system

©2008 by Pearson Education, Inc.   **CHAPTER 16** Stroke   **147**

1. The medical term *aphasia* contains the word root *phas.* You know this means
   a. without.
   b. paralysis.
   c. to eat, hunger.
   d. to speak.

2. *Dysphagia,* a medical term, contains the prefix *dys-,* which means
   a. down, away from.
   b. bad, difficult, painful.
   c. through, between.
   d. apart, separate.

3. The medical term *atherosclerosis* includes the word root *scler,* which means
   a. spine.
   b. narrowing.
   c. shoulder.
   d. hardening.

4. Your patient has a history of hemiparesis. You know that the prefix *hemi-* means
   a. half.
   b. water.
   c. different.
   d. below, under.

5. The medical term *quadriplegia* includes the suffix *-plegia,* which refers to
   a. weakness.
   b. paralysis, stroke.
   c. surgical repair.
   d. formation.

TERMS AND CONCEPTS

1. Write the number of the correct term next to each definition.
   1. Neurological deficit
   2. Nontraumatic brain injury
   3. Stroke
   4. Transient ischemic attacks (TIAs)

   _____ a. Brief, intermittent episodes with strokelike symptoms that disappear typically within 10 to 15 minutes and resolve within 24 hours

   _____ b. A medical injury to the brain, such as a stroke, that is not caused by an external injury

   _____ c. Any deficiency in the brain's functioning

   _____ d. A sudden disruption in blood flow to the brain that results in brain-cell damage

CONTENT REVIEW

1. Which of the following is a sign or symptom of neurological deficit?
   a. Slurred speech
   b. Substernal chest pain
   c. Hypoglycemia
   d. Hypotension

2. One kind of nontraumatic (medical) brain injury is a stroke. Using the illustrations as your guide, choose possible causes of a stroke from the list below.

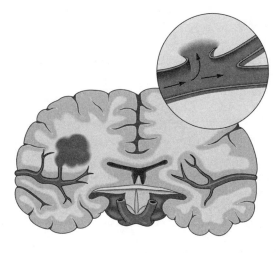 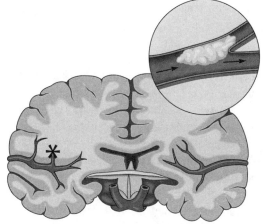

   1. Rupture of a blood vessel in the brain
   2. Blockage of a blood vessel in the brain
   3. Laceration of the carotid artery
   4. Dilation of the blood vessels in the brain
   a. 1 and 2
   b. 3 and 4
   c. 2 and 3
   d. 1 and 4

3. Which of the following is a common risk factor of hemorrhagic strokes?
   a. Hypoglycemia
   b. Chronic hypertension
   c. Alcoholism
   d. Chronic asthma

4. An ischemic stroke is one in which an inadequate amount of blood is being delivered to a portion of the brain due to a blood clot. The ischemic stroke is also known as a
   a. brain bleed.
   b. brain attack.
   c. brain accident.
   d. brain incident.

5. Which of the following signs and symptoms is a rare finding in the stroke patient?
   a. Hypertension
   b. Hemiplegia
   c. Hypotension
   d. Hemiparesis

6. A stroke that results from a piece of plaque or other substance that breaks off from inside a vessel or the heart and travels into the brain, becoming lodged in a cerebral vessel and cutting off circulation to the brain tissue, is known as
   a. acute stroke.
   b. embolic stroke.
   c. hemorrhagic stroke.
   d. systemic stroke.

7. Which of the following is a likely sign or symptom of stroke?
   a. Hemiparesis of the right arm and foot
   b. Paralysis to both right and left legs
   c. Bilateral paralysis of right and left arms
   d. Substernal nonradiating chest pain

8. You are treating a patient that you suspect suffered a stroke. The patient's breathing has become faster than normal with a decreased tidal volume. You should
   a. administer positive-pressure ventilation with supplemental oxygen.
   b. administer oxygen via nonrebreather mask.
   c. administer oxygen via nasal cannula.
   d. administer oxygen via Venturi mask.

9. You are treating a patient with signs and symptoms of a stroke who is unresponsive. In which position is it most appropriate to place this patient?
   a. Supine position, legs elevated
   b. Supine position, head and chest elevated
   c. Lateral recumbent position
   d. Prone position with knees to the side

10. When using the Cincinnati Prehospital Stroke Scale to evaluate your patient, you know that an abnormal arm drift is defined as when, after the patient extends both arms with eyes closed,
    a. both arms drift downward together.
    b. both arms drift upward together.
    c. one arm drifts upward.
    d. one arm drifts downward.

11. Because the patient with a nontraumatic brain injury may deteriorate rapidly, you should frequently perform which of the following?
    a. A rapid trauma assessment
    b. A focused trauma assessment
    c. A detailed physical exam
    d. An ongoing assessment

12. Strokes most often affect elderly patients with certain kinds of medical history. Which of the following contributes to strokes?
    a. A history of heart disease
    b. A history of osteoporosis
    c. A history of diabetes
    d. A history of emphysema

13. Your patient has experienced the signs and symptoms of a transient ischemic attack (TIA). However, he is feeling better and is refusing treatment. You must encourage the patient to be treated because
    a. approximately one-third of those who suffer a TIA will have a stroke.
    b. approximately one-half of those who suffer a TIA will have a heart attack.
    c. nearly all of the patients who suffer a TIA sustain permanent neurological deficit.
    d. nearly all of the patients who suffer TIA experience electrolyte imbalances.

14. It is extremely important to recognize the signs and symptoms of a stroke early. Which of the following strongly suggests that your patient may be suffering from a stroke?
    a. The patient has dilated pupils that constrict equally when a light source is applied.
    b. The patient uses wrong words when repeating, "You can't teach an old dog new tricks."
    c. The patient presents with an elevated blood-glucose level with pale, cool, diaphoretic skin.
    d. The patient experiences sudden and complete paralysis to the lower extremities.

15. You are assessing an elderly patient who appears to have suffered a stroke. Why is it important to determine if there is a history of diabetes?
    a. An elderly diabetic patient should not be given oxygen.
    b. An elderly stroke patient is likely to develop diabetes.
    c. Elderly hyperglycemic diabetics suffer more strokes than elderly nondiabetics.
    d. An elderly diabetic patient who is hypoglycemic may present with signs and symptoms similar to a stroke.

16. You suspect your patient is suffering from a stroke. What information is crucial to obtain from family or bystanders that will aid in proper treatment?
    a. When was the last meal consumed?
    b. Has the patient experienced a loss of time?
    c. Does the patient seem more agitated than normal?
    d. What was the time of onset of the symptoms?

17. Rapid transport of the stroke patient is critical because
    a. hyperventilation with a bag-valve mask may be necessary.
    b. increased secretions may compromise the airway.
    c. the emergency department may be able to administer clot-dissolving drugs.
    d. the patient will likely become unresponsive to voice commands.

CASE STUDY

You and your partner, Lynn, are dispatched to an unknown medical problem in a high-rise apartment. You are met in the parking lot by a security guard, who directs you to the elevator. He says, "José, the other guard, is with the patient, Mrs. Peters, and he will meet you up there." José directs you to the bedroom, where you find an elderly female lying in bed. As you introduce yourself, the patient looks at you with a terrified glare. You reassure her and ask if she can understand you. She nods her head to indicate yes. The patient tries to communicate, but her speech is incomprehensible. Her feelings of frustration are obvious. You explain that you will ask yes-or-no questions, and she can reply by shaking or nodding her head.

1. Mrs. Peters's breathing is approximately 14 per minute with good tidal volume. Which is most appropriate?
   a. Place her on oxygen at 15 lpm via nonrebreather mask.
   b. Mrs. Peters's breathing is adequate, so there is no need for oxygen.
   c. Place her on oxygen at 6 lpm via nasal cannula.
   d. Administer positive-pressure ventilation with supplemental oxygen.

Further interviewing reveals that Mrs. Peters's only medical history is hypertension. You notice significant facial drooping and paralysis to the right side of her body. Lynn suggests that the portable suction unit be set up and ready for immediate use. You agree. You prepare Mrs. Peters for transport, carefully protecting her paralyzed extremities so as not to injure them.

2. Briefly explain why the suction unit may be needed even though Mrs. Peters's airway is adequate.

As you and Lynn are transporting Mrs. Peters in the elevator, the patient grabs her head with her left hand. You ask her if she has a terrible headache. She nods yes, then becomes unresponsive, and her breathing becomes inadequate at 8 breaths per minute.

3. With this change in the patient's status, which of the following is now most appropriate?
   a. Administer oxygen at 15 lpm via nonrebreather mask.
   b. Administer positive-pressure ventilation at 10 to 12 ventilations per minute with supplemental oxygen.
   c. Administer positive-pressure ventilation at 20 ventilations per minute with supplemental oxygen.
   d. Administer positive-pressure ventilation at greater than 24 ventilations per minute with supplemental oxygen.

ENRICHMENT

1. The type of stroke that occurs when the cerebral artery is blocked by a clot or other foreign matter is known as a/an
   a. hemorrhagic stroke.
   b. ischemic stroke.
   c. hyperglycemic stroke.
   d. compression stroke.

2. The type of stroke that occurs from bleeding within the brain from a ruptured cerebral artery is known as a/an
   a. hemorrhagic stroke.
   b. ischemic stroke.
   c. hyperglycemic stroke.
   d. compression stroke.

3. Which sign or symptom would you associate with the patient suffering from a hemorrhagic stroke?
   a. Gradual onset
   b. Rapidly improving mental status
   c. History of low blood pressure
   d. Severe headache

SCENARIO 5: DOCUMENTATION EXERCISE

Read the following scenario, and think about how you would document this call if you were the EMT who responded to the scene. Then answer the multiple-choice questions and fill in the sample prehospital-care report, basing your documentation on information from the scenario.

You and your partner, Cory, are attending an on-duty continuing education class when your portable radio sounds: "Unit 3 respond to 428 45th Street for a man in his 50s acting inappropriately." You and Cory walk briskly toward the ambulance. You both check the map book to confirm the location, then mark en route. After a short emergency response, you arrive on the scene of a modest single-family residence. You both put on protective gloves and eyewear and scan the area for any obvious hazards. As you are placing the equipment on your cot, a frantic woman meets you at the rear of the ambulance. She cries, "Hurry! It's my husband, Brian. I think he's had a stroke." As you approach and enter the home, you again scan the area for possible hazards and note the best access and egress of the house.

As you and Cory enter the living room, you find an approximately 50-year-old man sitting on the floor leaning against the sofa. Cory asks, "What seems to be the problem today?" The patient responds in a muffled voice, "I don't know." You ask him his name and if he hurts anywhere. He responds with slurred speech, "My name is Brian, and I have a headache." You notice the airway is intact with good air exchange at a rate of approximately 14 breaths per minute. Brian's face seems drawn down on the right side. His chest is rising and falling, with adequate air moving in and out of the mouth and nose and no use of accessory muscles. Cory quickly assesses the radial pulse and finds the pulse strong and regular. The skin is warm and dry with no cyanosis noted. The pulse oximeter reveals a reading of 98 percent on room air just before Cory applies oxygen via a nonrebreather mask at 15 lpm.

You notify dispatch that this is a priority call and to send ALS backup immediately and notify the hospital emergency department of a possible stroke alert.

You look to the patient and his wife and explain that you suspect a possible stroke. As you and Cory lift the patient from the floor and place him on the stretcher, you notice the patient is supporting his right arm by holding it with his left. You ask Cory to prepare the suction and BVM and place them nearby, ready for use if needed, while you begin to administer the Cincinnati Prehospital Stroke Scale. You ask Brian to look straight at you and smile, then show his teeth. The right side of his face droops downward. Next, you have the patient lift both arms outward and close his eyes and ask him to hold this position for 10 seconds. You notice his right arm drifts downward while the left remains in the outward position. Last, you ask Brian to repeat, "You can't teach an old dog new tricks." Brian repeats with a puzzled look on his face, "You train old sticks with new dogs." You can see that Brian is becoming frustrated.

While you are completing the Cincinnati Prehospital Stroke Scale, Cory positions the patient and proceeds with a rapid medical exam. You obtain a blood glucose level of 126 mg/dl with the glucometer. Cory shines a pocket penlight into Brian's eyes and remarks, "The left is midposition and reacts to light. The right is dilated and unreactive." He states, "Other than the facial droop, the face is unremarkable." There is no JVD, tracheal tugging, or subcutaneous emphysema to the neck. He quickly exposes the chest and palpates the chest and finds no evidence of trauma or scars. Auscultation reveals lung sounds that are clear bilaterally. The abdomen is soft and not tender. The lower extremities do not show edema, and distal pulses are felt in all four extremities. Cory notes that the right arm and leg both have no sensation to pain or movement while the left arm and leg are both normal. There is no noted edema to the small of the back in the lumbar area.

You obtain a set of baseline vital signs. The blood pressure is 230/124; the heart rate is 88 beats per minute and regular; the respiratory rate is 16 per minute; the skin is pink, warm, and dry; and the pupils remain the same. The SpO_2 reading is 98 percent.

You advise Brian's wife that you will be transporting soon and will meet the ALS unit en route. Cory helps to load the patient into the ambulance and then seats Brian's wife in the front seat, ensuring that her seatbelt is fastened. You quickly interview the wife to gain valuable information. You discover that Brian is 52 years of age, has a history of hypertension, and takes a multivitamin and high-blood-pressure medicine every day. He has no known drug allergies. She states he was watching his favorite team lose in the finals on television when he suddenly stood up from the couch and said he had a terrible headache. Shortly after, she noticed his speech was slurred and his face had drooped. You ask her exactly what time this was; she indicates it was 10 minutes before she called you. You contact dispatch to ascertain what time the call came in to dispatch. You add 10 minutes to the call time and document it, so as not to forget.

En route to the hospital you meet ALS Medic Four. The paramedic quickly steps into the rear of your ambulance, carrying her equipment. You recognize her as Lieutenant Meads. She quickly introduces herself to the patient and his wife. As she gathers the report and prepares to provide advanced life support, you begin to perform an ongoing assessment. You obtain the following vital signs: blood pressure 226/120, heart rate 80 beats per minute and regular, respiratory rate 16 per minute. The skin remains pink, warm, and dry. The pupils are unchanged. You ask the patient to describe the pain in his head, and he states, "It's the worst pain I've ever had, and it's all over my head." The patient remarks that his vision seems blurred. A few minutes later, Cory advises you that you have arrived at the emergency department.

1. What is the significance of the patient replying, "You train old sticks with new dogs"?
   a. This is a response that indicates a possible underlying diabetic condition.
   b. This response was normal; many patients, under stress, confuse these words.
   c. This was a normal response according to the Los Angeles Prehospital Stroke Screen.
   d. This was an abnormal response according to the Cincinnati Prehospital Stroke Scale.

2. Why is it important to obtain a blood-glucose level with the glucometer in a patient you suspect of having a stroke?
   a. Symptoms of a diabetic emergency can mimic those of the stroke patient.
   b. Blood-glucose levels in stroke patients can rapidly rise to dangerous levels.
   c. Ischemic strokes can be positively diagnosed by determining blood-glucose level.
   d. The Cincinnati Prehospital Stroke Scale requires the collection of this data.

3. Proper positioning is very important when treating the stroke patient. You have determined that this patient can protect his own airway. In what position should you place this patient?
   a. Supine with the head and chest elevated 15 to 30 degrees
   b. Right lateral recumbent with the head elevated 10 degrees
   c. Trendelenburg position with the knees slightly bent
   d. Left lateral recumbent with the head lower than the chest

4. This patient complained of a severe headache that came on suddenly. The signs and symptoms of stroke also developed rapidly. He has a history of hypertension treated with medication. All of these would lead you to believe your patient is suffering from which of the following?
   a. Ischemic stroke
   b. Hemorrhagic stroke
   c. Transient ischemic stroke
   d. Progressive stroke

5. Why was it important to determine the exact time that the symptoms were first noticed?
   a. Onset time is important to determine if the patient is a candidate for surgery.
   b. The time elapsed from first symptoms corresponds to probable recovery time.
   c. Time of onset is crucial in determining if clot-dissolving drugs can be administered.
   d. Onset-to-treatment time helps hospital personnel determine how symptoms will progress.

EMERGENCY TRIP SHEET

TRIP #	
MEDIC #	
BEGIN MILES	
END MILES	
CODE___/___ PAGE___/___	
UNITS ON SCENE	

NAME   SEX M F DOB ___/___/___

ADDRESS   RACE

CITY   STATE   ZIP

PHONE (   )   -   PCP DR.

RESPONDED FROM   CITY

TAKEN FROM   ZIP

DESTINATION   REASON

SSN   -   -   MEDICARE #   MEDICAID #

INSURANCE CO   INSURANCE #   GROUP #

RESPONSIBLE PARTY   ADDRESS

CITY   STATE   ZIP   PHONE (   )   -

EMPLOYER

DAY			
DATE			
RECEIVED			
DISPATCHED			
EN-ROUTE			
ON SCENE			
TO HOSPITAL			
AT HOSPITAL			
IN-SERVICE			

CREW	CERT	STATE #

TIME	ON SCENE (1)	ON SCENE (2)	ON SCENE (3)	EN-ROUTE (1)	EN-ROUTE (2)	AT DESTINATION
BP						
PULSE						
RESP						
KG						

IV THERAPY
SUCCESSFUL Y N # OF ATTEMPTS _____
ANGIO SIZE _____ga.
SITE _____
TOTAL FLUID INFUSED _____ cc
BLOOD DRAW Y N INITIALS

INTUBATION INFORMATION
SUCCESSFUL Y N # OF ATTEMPTS _____
TUBE SIZE _____ mm
TIME _____ INITIALS _____

MEDICAL HISTORY

MEDICATIONS

ALLERGIES

C/C

EVENTS LEADING TO C/C

ASSESSMENT

TREATMENT

EMS SIGNATURE

CONDITION CODES			

TREATMENTS

TIME	TREATMENT	DOSE	ROUTE	INIT

GCS	E___ V___ M___ TOTAL =	
GCS	E___ V___ M___ TOTAL =	

HOSPITAL CONTACTED

CPR BEGUN BY   B   P   TIME BEGUN

AED USED   Y   N   BY:

RESUSCITATION TERMINATED - TIME

(   ) OSHA REGULATIONS FOLLOWED

17 Seizures and Syncope

OBJECTIVES

Numbered objectives are from the United States Department of Transportation EMT-Basic National Standard Curriculum. Asterisked objectives, if any, pertain to material that is supplemental to the DOT curriculum.

Cognitive

* Explain the assessment and emergency care for a seizing patient.
* Recognize the common signs and symptoms of a generalized seizure.
* Recognize signs and symptoms of status epilepticus.
* Identify various conditions that cause seizures.
* Recognize the common signs and symptoms of syncope.
* Differentiate between syncope and seizures.

KEY IDEAS

This chapter focuses on seizures, their causes and characteristics, and their management in the prehospital setting. Syncope, or fainting, is also discussed.

■ A common cause of seizures is epilepsy, but seizures are caused by a variety of conditions.

■ The most common type of epileptic seizure is the generalized tonic-clonic seizure.

■ It is important to protect the airway in the seizing and postseizure patient.

■ Oxygen should be administered to the seizure patient. If breathing is inadequate, it may be necessary to assist breathing.

■ It is important to prevent injury to the seizing patient.

■ Syncope is a temporary loss of responsiveness and may be confused with a seizure. Among other distinctions between a seizure and syncope, the patient who has fainted usually becomes responsive and recovers almost immediately.

TERMS AND CONCEPTS

1. Write the number of the correct term next to each definition.

   1. Aura
   2. Epilepsy
   3. Generalized tonic-clonic seizure
   4. Postictal state
   5. Seizure
   6. Status epilepticus
   7. Syncope

   _____ a. An unusual sensory sensation that may precede a seizure episode

   _____ b. A sudden and temporary alteration in the mental status caused by massive electrical discharge in a group of nerve cells in the brain

   _____ c. Recovery period that follows the clonic phase of a generalized seizure

   _____ d. A medical disorder characterized by recurrent seizures

   _____ e. A seizure lasting longer than 10 minutes or seizures that occur consecutively without a period of responsiveness between them

   _____ f. A brief period of unresponsiveness due to a lack of blood flow to the brain

   _____ g. A common type of seizure that produces unresponsiveness and a generalized jerking muscle activity; a grand mal seizure

CONTENT REVIEW

1. A seizure is a sign of an underlying defect. Which of the following may be a cause of seizures?
   a. Head injury
   b. Abdominal aortic aneurisms
   c. Hypothermia
   d. Asthma

2. Select in order the five stages of a typical generalized tonic-clonic seizure.
   a. Aura, tonic, hypertonic, clonic, postictal
   b. Hypertonic, aura, postictal, clonic, tonic
   c. Aura, clonic, tonic, hypertonic, postictal
   d. Postictal, clonic, hypertonic, tonic, aura

3. You arrive on the scene of a seizure patient; in what state will you most often encounter the seizure patient?
   a. Aura phase
   b. Tonic phase
   c. Clonic phase
   d. Postictal phase

4. Since hypoglycemia is one possible cause of seizure, you should assess the blood-glucose level in a seizure patient, using a glucose meter. You should suspect the seizure is due to hypoglycemia if the blood-glucose level is
   a. below 60 mg/dl.
   b. below 70 mg/dl.
   c. between 80 and 120 mg/dl.
   d. above 120 mg/dl.

5. When you encounter a patient seizing with jerky body movements, to help prevent further injury, you should
   a. place a spoon in the mouth to stop the patient from swallowing his tongue.
   b. move objects away from the patient's area and guide his movements.
   c. physically restrain the patient's body movements until he becomes postictal.
   d. restrain the patient by securing him on a long spine board.

6. Following a generalized seizure, paralysis that affects one area or one side of the body that may indicate a space-occupying problem in the brain is known as
   a. Jackson paralysis.
   b. simple paralysis.
   c. Todd's paralysis.
   d. grand mal paralysis.

7. Which of the following is the most appropriate treatment for a patient suffering status epilepticus?
   a. Positive-pressure ventilation, transport after focused history and physical exam
   b. Positive-pressure ventilation, immediate transport to a medical facility
   c. Oxygen at 15 lpm via nonrebreather mask, transport after focused history and physical exam
   d. Oxygen at 15 lpm via nonrebreather mask, immediate transport to a medical facility

8. You are responding to a report of a child seizing. Which of the following is a common cause of seizures in infants and young children?
   a. Head injury
   b. Diabetes
   c. High fever
   d. Epilepsy

9. It is important to recognize when the seizure patient needs immediate transport. Which of the following patients is more stable, and thus transport can be delayed more than the other situations?
   a. The seizing patient who is pregnant, has a history of diabetes, or is injured.
   b. The patient whose seizure has occurred in the water, such as a swimming pool or lake.
   c. The patient who has suffered a seizure, regained responsiveness, then suffered another seizure an hour later.
   d. The patient who remains unresponsive following the seizure activity.

10. Which of the following signs and symptoms usually precedes the typical syncopal episode?
    a. Chest pain, breathing difficulty
    b. Yawning, diaphoresis, nausea
    c. Stuttering, hypertension, numbness
    d. Blurred vision, belching, cramping

11. You are preparing to ventilate your patient that is experiencing a grand mal seizure. Which of the following is the best way to ventilate this patient?
    a. Use the head-tilt/chin-lift maneuver, and ventilate with a bag-valve mask.
    b. Restrain the patient's head, and ventilate with a bag-valve mask.
    c. Insert an oropharyngeal airway, and ventilate with a bag-valve mask.
    d. Insert a nasopharyngeal airway, and ventilate with a bag-valve mask.

12. The postictal patient with no suspected spinal injury should be placed in which position?
    a. Semi-Fowler's
    b. Lateral recumbent
    c. Trendelenburg
    d. Prone

13. Which of the following is an unlikely sign or symptom of the patient who is experiencing a syncopal episode?
    a. The brain is briefly deprived of oxygen.
    b. The skin is usually warm, pale, and dry.
    c. The patient usually remembers feeling faint.
    d. The event usually begins in a standing position.

CASE STUDY

You and your partner, Sascha, are at a local grocery store picking up groceries for dinner when an elderly woman screams for help: "There's a man over here dying!" You ask Sascha to bring the ambulance closer to the building and bring the equipment and stretcher. You reach into your pocket for your extra pair of gloves and eye protection and put them on as you hurry to the patient's side. You find an elderly man on the ground, shaking uncontrollably. A closer look reveals the identity of the patient. You recognize him as Karl Louis, a local homeless man with a history of epilepsy and chronic alcoholism. The bystander states, "I found him lying on the ground shaking. I don't know how long he was like that, but he's been shaking for 3 or 4 minutes just since I found him!"

1. While you are waiting for Sascha to bring the equipment, you should
    a. guide the body movements, move obstacles.
    b. restrict the patient to limit movement.
    c. place the patient in a Fowler's position.
    d. place your finger into the mouth to position the tongue.

Sascha approaches with the stretcher and equipment. You advise him that it's a known patient, Karl Louis, and that you have never seen him this bad. The seizure stops, and you try to arouse Karl, but he remains unresponsive. As you are assessing his breathing, he begins to seize again, violently. You notice blood flowing from his mouth.

2. Which of the following is the most appropriate emergency care?
    a. Administer oxygen via nonrebreather mask at 15 lpm, wait for the seizure to end, and suction.
    b. Suction, administer oxygen via nonrebreather mask at 15 lpm, and transport immediately.
    c. Suction, begin positive-pressure ventilation with an oropharyngeal airway in place, and use rapid transport.
    d. Suction, begin positive-pressure ventilation with a nasopharyngeal airway in place, and use rapid transport.

3. Briefly explain why you might see blood coming from the mouth of a seizure patient and how you would treat this problem.

En route to the medical facility, Karl stops seizing. While you are reassessing Karl's mental status, you ask Sascha to obtain baseline vital signs. Karl responds to a painful stimulus by pulling away. Then he opens his eyes sluggishly and asks you to stop. He looks exhausted. Your physical exam reveals no injuries. The vital signs include heart rate 118 beats per minute, blood pressure 164/68, breathing adequate at 20 per minute.

4. Now that Karl is responsive, you recognize that he is in which phase?
   a. Aura phase
   b. Clonic phase
   c. Postictal phase
   d. Tonic phase

5. What should you now do for Karl?
   a. Place Karl in a supine position, administer positive-pressure ventilation with supplemental oxygen.
   b. Place Karl in a semisitting position, administer oxygen by bag-valve mask, and hyperventilate him at greater than 24 ventilations per minute.
   c. Place Karl in a full sitting position, administer oxygen by nonrebreather mask at 15 lpm.
   d. Place Karl in a lateral recumbent position and administer oxygen by nonrebreather mask at 15 lpm.

You arrive at the medical facility. Karl is feeling much better, although still somewhat confused and disoriented. You reassure him and give your report to the emergency-department nurse.

ENRICHMENT

1. You know that primary seizures are categorized as generalized or partial. Which of the following best describes the generalized seizure?
   a. Related to abnormal activity in one hemisphere and the patient usually remains conscious
   b. Related to abnormal activity in both hemispheres and the patient usually remains conscious
   c. Related to abnormal activity in one cerebral hemisphere and usually renders the patient unconscious
   d. Related to abnormal activity in both hemispheres and usually renders the patient unconscious

2. Which type of seizure generally produces jerky muscle activity in one area of the body, arm, leg, or face? (These patients cannot control the jerky movement but remain awake and aware of the seizure activity.)
   a. Simple partial seizure
   b. Complex partial seizure
   c. Absence or petit mal seizure
   d. Febrile seizure

3. You are treating a 4-year-old child who experienced a generalized seizure that lasted approximately 30 seconds. His mother states that the patient has been sick with a high fever all day. From this information, which of the following seizures is this child likely experiencing?
   a. Grand mal seizure
   b. Generalized tonic-clonic seizure
   c. Petit mal seizure
   d. Febrile seizure

SCENARIO 6: DOCUMENTATION EXERCISE

Read the following scenario, and think about how you would document this call if you were the EMT who responded to the scene. Then answer the multiple-choice questions and fill in the sample prehospital-care report, basing your documentation on information from the scenario.

While you and your partner, Jill, are cleaning the station, the alerting system sounds: "Unit 1 respond to 5555 Twentieth Street for a patient possibly having a seizure. Your ALS backup will be Medic Two." You acknowledge the call while Jill checks the location on the wall map. After a short emergency response, you arrive at a large retail store. You both quickly put on your gloves and eye protection. The store's manager meets you at the entrance and asks you to hurry—the patient is in the checkout area and is still seizing.

As you follow the manager to where the patient is located, you quickly scan the area for hazards and the best way to gain access to the patient. As you and Jill enter the checkout area, you find an approximately 30-year-old male lying supine on the floor. The patient's whole body is shaking with tonic-clonic movement. You radio your dispatch to advise that this is a priority call. The patient's body is up against shopping carts, and you ask the manager to carefully move the carts as you hold the patient's head and guide the patient's movements. Jill asks if anyone witnessed what happened. A checkout clerk says, "The man said he had a funny taste in his mouth, and then he sat down on the floor and went into a seizure."

Suddenly, the tonic-clonic movement ceases. You quickly assess the patient. You gently shake his shoulder and ask if he can hear you. There is no response. You assess the airway and note the patient is breathing approximately 20 times a minute with good air movement in and out of the lungs. There are no stridorous or crowing sounds with inhalation or exhalation. You check a radial pulse and find it to be strong at a rate of approximately 100 beats each minute and regular. The patient's general appearance is face flushed with slight cyanosis around the lips and nail beds. The skin is warm and diaphoretic. Jill places a nonrebreather mask on the patient, set at 15 liters per minute. Jill notices a medical alert bracelet on the patient's wrist. It reads that the patient has a history of epilepsy and takes Dilantin, which you know to be a seizure medication. You ask if there are any family or friends with the patient, and the checkout clerk states she thought the patient was alone. You quickly apply the pulse oximeter, which indicates 98 percent while on oxygen.

Before the patient becomes responsive, he slips back into a full-body seizure. Again, the body convulses with tonic-clonic movement. You and Jill quickly place the patient onto the stretcher and make your way toward the ambulance, which is close by. After placing the patient into the ambulance, you perform a rapid assessment and note the patient's breathing has decreased to approximately six times each minute with poor tidal volume. You open the airway using the head-tilt/chin-lift maneuver. You ask Jill to insert a nasopharyngeal airway and provide positive-pressure ventilations with the BVM with supplemental oxygen. The patient actively seizes for approximately 2 minutes before the activity once again subsides. Again the patient looks exhausted with slight cyanosis of the lips. You instruct Jill to continue to support the ventilations with the BVM. Jill notices a small amount of saliva and blood dripping from the patient's mouth, and she immediately suctions the secretions with the portable suction unit.

The patient responds with purposeful movement by trying to push the BVM from his face. Despite his efforts to remove the BVM, you continue to provide positive-pressure ventilations and reassure him. The patient now appears extremely sleepy, weak, and disoriented. You reassess his mental status. You ask him his name and he responds with a tired sigh, "Jim, my name is Jim." Jill proceeds with a medical exam. His pupils are equal and react briskly to light. The area around his mouth and nail beds are now pink. You find no jugular venous distention, tracheal tugging, or subcutaneous emphysema to the neck. You quickly inspect and palpate the chest and find no evidence of trauma or scars. Auscultation reveals normal lung sounds with good tidal volume. Jim's abdomen is soft and not tender. His lower extremities do not show any edema. Distal pulses are present in all four extremities. He obeys your commands to wiggle his toes and grasp your fingers. He states he can feel you touching his hands and feet. You do not note any edema to the small of the back in the lower lumbar area. Jill obtains vital signs. The blood pressure is 132/78, pulse 100 beats each minute and regular. The patient is breathing 20 times a minute with good tidal volume. The pulse oximeter reading remains 98 percent with oxygen. As the patient's breathing improves, you place him on a nonrebreather mask at 15 lpm, keeping the BVM close by.

You hear on the radio that Medic Two is now on-scene. As the paramedic lieutenant enters the rear of your ambulance, you begin to give him a report while Jill, using the glucometer, obtains a blood glucose level of 110 mg/dl. You instruct Jill to drive the ambulance, responding in the emergency mode so as to not delay transport. The patient becomes more awake and alert, and he tells you that he has not experienced a seizure for over a year. He thought his seizures were cured, so he stopped taking his Dilantin. You ask him if he has any drug allergies, and he states, "None that I know of." The paramedic starts an intravenous line in preparation for drug therapy. You obtain repeat vital signs, which are blood pressure 130/74, pulse 90 beats per minute, and respirations 16 each minute with good tidal volume. As you perform an ongoing assessment Jill advises that you have arrived at the emergency department.

1. You know that the kind of seizure this patient was experiencing, with the whole body shaking with tonic-clonic movement, is most likely which type of seizure?
   a. Focal motor seizure
   b. Grand mal seizure
   c. Febrile seizure
   d. Jacksonian motor seizure

2. The checkout clerk said that before the man went into a seizure he said he had a funny taste in his mouth. You recognize that the odd taste was likely a/an
   a. postictal.
   b. aura.
   c. epilepticus.
   d. aspiration.

3. The patient had been seizing for several minutes before you arrived on-scene and then had a second seizure without a period of responsiveness between seizures. Therefore, you recognized his condition as
   a. Jacksonian.
   b. syncopal.
   c. status epilepticus.
   d. postictal.

4. When the patient responded with purposeful movement and a sleepy, weak, disoriented appearance, he was likely in the
   a. postictal state.
   b. aura state.
   c. clonic state.
   d. tonic state.

5. Why did Jill obtain a blood-glucose level on this patient?
   a. The seizures may have been caused by hypoxia.
   b. The seizures may have been caused by an allergic reaction.
   c. The seizures may have been caused by hypoglycemia or hyperglycemia.
   d. The seizures may have been caused by eclampsia.

EMERGENCY
TRIP SHEET

TRIP #	
MEDIC #	
BEGIN MILES	
END MILES	
CODE___/___	PAGE___/___
UNITS ON SCENE	

BILLING USE ONLY				
DAY				
DATE				
RECEIVED				
DISPATCHED				
EN-ROUTE				
ON SCENE				
TO HOSPITAL				
AT HOSPITAL				
IN-SERVICE				

NAME   SEX M F DOB ___/___/___

ADDRESS   RACE

CITY   STATE   ZIP

PHONE ( ) -   PCP DR.

RESPONDED FROM   CITY

TAKEN FROM   ZIP

DESTINATION   REASON

SSN - -   MEDICARE #   MEDICAID #

INSURANCE CO   INSURANCE #   GROUP #

RESPONSIBLE PARTY   ADDRESS

CITY   STATE   ZIP   PHONE ( ) -

EMPLOYER

CREW	CERT	STATE #

TIME	ON SCENE (1)	ON SCENE (2)	ON SCENE (3)	EN-ROUTE (1)	EN-ROUTE (2)	AT DESTINATION
BP						
PULSE						
RESP						
EKG						

IV THERAPY
SUCCESSFUL Y N # OF ATTEMPTS _____
ANGIO SIZE _____ga.
SITE _____
TOTAL FLUID INFUSED _____ cc
BLOOD DRAW Y N INITIALS _____

INTUBATION INFORMATION
SUCCESSFUL Y N # OF ATTEMPTS _____
TUBE SIZE _____ mm
TIME _____ INITIALS _____

MEDICAL HISTORY

CONDITION CODES				

MEDICATIONS

TREATMENTS

TIME	TREATMENT	DOSE	ROUTE	INIT

ALLERGIES

C/C

EVENTS LEADING TO C/C

ASSESSMENT

TREATMENT

GCS | E___ V___ M___ TOTAL =

GCS | E___ V___ M___ TOTAL =

HOSPITAL CONTACTED

CPR BEGUN BY B P TIME BEGUN

EMS SIGNATURE

AED USED Y N BY:

RESUSCITATION TERMINATED - TIME

( ) OSHA REGULATIONS FOLLOWED

18 Allergic Reaction

OBJECTIVES

Numbered objectives are from the United States Department of Transportation EMT-Basic National Standard Curriculum. Asterisked objectives, if any, pertain to material that is supplemental to the DOT curriculum.

Cognitive

4-5.1 Recognize the patient experiencing an allergic reaction.

4-5.2 Describe the emergency medical care of the patient with an allergic reaction.

4-5.3 Establish the relationship between the patient with an allergic reaction and airway management.

4-5.4 Describe the mechanism of allergic response and implications for airway management.

4-5.5 State the generic and trade names, medication forms, dose, administration, action, and contraindications for the epinephrine auto-injector.

4-5.6 Evaluate the need for medical direction in the emergency medical care of the patient with an allergic reaction.

4-5.7 Differentiate between the general category of those patients having an allergic reaction and those patients having an allergic reaction and requiring immediate medical care, including immediate use of an epinephrine auto-injector.

KEY IDEAS

An allergic reaction can quickly be life-threatening. It is important for the EMT to rapidly assess and manage patients suffering an allergic reaction. Appropriate assessment and management techniques for allergic reactions are the focus of this chapter.

■ An allergic reaction is a misdirected or excessive response by the immune system to a foreign substance or allergen. An allergen can enter the body by injection, ingestion, inhalation, or contact.

■ Causes of allergic reactions include venom from bites or stings, foods, pollen, and medications. Medications taken orally or injected are the most common cause.

■ Hives and itching are hallmark signs and symptoms of an allergic reaction.

■ Most allergic reactions are mild. A severe form of allergic reaction is anaphylaxis, or anaphylactic shock.

■ In anaphylactic shock, the entire body is affected by the release of histamine by the immune system. There is swelling in the upper airway and bronchoconstriction and swelling in the lower airways. Blood vessels dilate and decrease the blood pressure. Anaphylaxis is a life-threatening condition that, without proper treatment, leads to death.

■ The two key categories of signs and symptoms that specifically indicate anaphylaxis are respiratory compromise and shock (hypoperfusion).

- Emergency medical care for anaphylaxis includes maintaining a patent airway, oxygen therapy, administering epinephrine by prescribed auto-injector, calling for advanced life support, and early transport. It may be necessary to provide positive-pressure ventilation to force air past the swollen upper airway.

TERMS AND CONCEPTS

1. Write the number of the correct term next to each definition.

   1. Allergen
   2. Allergic reaction
   3. Anaphylactoid reaction
   4. Anaphylactic shock
   5. Antibodies
   6. Histamine
   7. Hives
   8. Immune system
   9. Malaise
   10. Sensitization

   _____ a. The process by which antibodies are produced after exposure to an antigen

   _____ b. Misdirected and excessive response by the immune system to a foreign substance or an allergen

   _____ c. Raised, red blotches associated with some allergic reactions

   _____ d. Special proteins produced by the immune system that search out antigens, combine with them, and destroy them

   _____ e. The body's defense mechanism against invasion by foreign substances

   _____ f. A state of hypoperfusion that results from dilated and leaking blood vessels related to severe allergic reaction

   _____ g. A substance that enters the body by ingestion, injection, inhalation, or contact and triggers an allergic reaction

   _____ h. A general feeling of weakness or discomfort

   _____ i. Primary chemical mediator released from MAST cells and basophils

   _____ j. A reaction that requires no previous sensitization

CONTENT REVIEW

1. For each sign or symptom of an allergic reaction that is listed below, indicate if it is a sign or symptom of a mild (M) reaction or a severe (S) reaction.

    _____ a. Localized flushed skin

    _____ b. Cyanosis

    _____ c. Altered mental status

    _____ d. Watery eyes

    _____ e. Wheezing in all lung fields

    _____ f. Severe respiratory distress

2. The *most* common cause of allergic reactions and anaphylaxis is
    a. glue.
    b. pollen from ragweed.
    c. medications.
    d. mosquito bites.

3. Which of the following is a route by which an allergen may enter the body?
    a. Ulnar
    b. Excretion
    c. Contact
    d. Vagus

4. In an anaphylactoid reaction
    a. the second time an antigen is introduced into the body chemical mediators are released.
    b. bronchoconstriction, decreased capillary membrane permeability, and vasoconstriction occur.
    c. the treatment is significantly different from anaphylaxis.
    d. the patient will not have experienced a previous exposure to an antigen.

5. When assessing respiratory sounds, stridor or crowing indicates
    a. significant swelling to the upper airway, requiring positive pressure ventilation.
    b. significant swelling to the upper airway, requiring insertion of an airway adjunct.
    c. significant swelling to the bronchioles, requiring oxygen at 15 lpm by nonrebreather mask.
    d. possible collapse of the alveoli of the lungs, requiring endotracheal intubation.

6. You are providing positive-pressure ventilation to an anaphylaxis patient who is breathing inadequately. The bag-valve mask device's pop-off valve releases air with each squeeze of the bag. What is the *best* action to take?
    a. Deactivate the valve or place your thumb over it, and continue with ventilations.
    b. Continue ventilating the patient, and increase the rate of ventilations.
    c. Continue until ALS arrives, and report your finding to the crew.
    d. Reduce the pressure you are using to squeeze the bag to prevent the valve from opening.

7. Hives may be present all over the skin in a patient suffering an allergic reaction or anaphylaxis. Hives are usually accompanied by
   a. severe coughing.
   b. severe stuffy nose.
   c. severe itching.
   d. severe headache.

8. Most anaphylactic reactions are apparent within _____ minute(s) after exposure.
   a. 1
   b. 5
   c. 10
   d. 20

9. The two key categories of signs and symptoms that specifically indicate anaphylaxis are
   a. gastrointestinal compromise and shock.
   b. respiratory compromise and shock.
   c. central-nervous-system compromise and shock.
   d. respiratory compromise and gastrointestinal complaints.

10. Anaphylaxis can be mistaken for other conditions with similar signs and symptoms, such as
    a. an anxiety attack.
    b. a stroke.
    c. meningitis.
    d. epilepsy.

11. A common substance that causes an anaphylactoid reaction is
    a. pollen.
    b. nonsteroidal anti-inflammatory drug (NSAID).
    c. food additives.
    d. eggs.

12. Histamine release causes
    a. bronchodilation, vasodilation, and decreased capillary membrane permeability.
    b. bronchoconstriction, vasodilation, and increased capillary membrane permeability.
    c. bronchoconstriction, vasoconstriction, and decreased capillary membrane permeability.
    d. bronchodilation, vasodilation, and decreased capillary membrane permeability.

13. Anaphylaxis is a condition that
    a. is a minor medical problem with a low mortality rate.
    b. causes pulmonary hypertension and pulmonary emboli.
    c. causes blood vessels to constrict, increasing the blood pressure to dangerous levels.
    d. may make positive-pressure ventilation of the patient difficult.

14. The criteria that must be met before an EMT can administer epinephrine by auto-injector to a patient are (1) _____, (2) the medication has been prescribed to the patient, and (3) the EMT has received an order from medical direction.
    a. itching only
    b. headache and blurred vision
    c. respiratory distress and/or hypotension
    d. flushed, red skin and/or itching

15. You respond to a call for a patient that was stung by a bee. The patient's family reports that the patient is allergic to bee stings. As you approach the patient you note that the patient's face, neck, tongue, and lips are swollen. Given this information you know that it is most likely that

    a. the patient will complain of yellow vision.

    b. the patient will have peripheral edema.

    c. the patient is stable and will require limited care.

    d. the upper airway is also likely to be swollen.

CASE STUDY

You have responded to a call for a child who has been stung by a bee. The scene appears safe as you arrive at a small home. A frantic-looking woman meets you at the front of the house and asks you to "Please hurry up!" As you follow her to the backyard, you introduce yourself and your partner and ask, "Why did you call the ambulance?" She replies, "My daughter was just stung by a bee!"

The patient looks to be about 10 years old. She is sitting in a chair and looks up at you as you approach. Your general impression is that she looks well. Her skin color is red. She responds to your questions appropriately. She says her name is Caitlin. She tells you that she was stung by a bee about 5 minutes ago. She doesn't appear to have any difficulty breathing. She complains of a "lump" in her throat and her stomach feels "upset." Her pulse is strong and regular. There is no sign of trauma, and no bleeding is present.

You complete the OPQRST and SAMPLE history. You find out that she had an allergic reaction to a yellow jacket sting 1 year ago. She has a prescription for an EpiPen Jr. During the physical exam, you observe the small, red sting site on her arm but make no other findings.

1. Which of the following is true about the patient?

    a. She is not showing signs of anaphylaxis or allergic reaction. Caitlin does not require transport or additional treatment.

    b. She is not showing signs of anaphylaxis or allergic reaction. Caitlin should be transported by her mother for additional evaluation at a local hospital.

    c. She is not showing signs of anaphylaxis or allergic reaction. Place Caitlin on oxygen and closely evaluate her during transport.

    d. She is showing early signs of anaphylaxis or allergic reaction. Place Caitlin on oxygen, call for ALS backup, prepare for suction and to assist ventilations, and initiate early transport.

2. You should carefully monitor Caitlin for which of the following?

    a. Signs of developing hives and itching

    b. Signs of abdominal cramping

    c. Loss of bowel control

    d. Airway and breathing compromise and poor perfusion

3. En route to the hospital, Caitlin develops breathing that sounds noisy, with a rattling sound on inspiration and exhalation. These sounds are probably caused by

    a. swelling of the tongue.

    b. severe bronchoconstriction.

    c. excessive mucus in the upper airways.

    d. excessive mucus in the lower airways.

4. What additional signs and symptoms might you expect Caitlin to develop?

    a. Constipation

    b. Coughing and hoarseness

    c. Pinpoint pupils

    d. Hypertension

SCENARIO 7: DOCUMENTATION EXERCISE

Read the following scenario, and think about how you would document this call if you were the EMT who responded to the scene. Then answer the multiple-choice questions and fill in the sample prehospital-care report, basing your documentation on information from the scenario.

It is 11:00 AM on a bright summer day. You and your partner, Bill Jackson, have just completed a call for an elderly man who fell. You are returning to the station when dispatch calls: "Unit 2, respond to 425 East Lake Morton Drive, cross street McDonald, for a difficulty breathing. Time out 1100 hours." Bill advises dispatch that you are responding to the incident. You arrive on-scene in about 3 minutes.

When you arrive, you notice a small crowd of people standing and squatting next to a man on the ground. He is located in a grassy area next to a lake filled with ducks and swans. You observe a city Parks Department truck parked near the man. You park in a safe area and exit the emergency vehicle. With BSI precautions on, you and Bill walk toward the crowd and note that the man appears to be in his mid-30. He is on his knees, leaning forward, and is struggling to breathe. He is in obvious respiratory distress. Even as you approach, you can hear wheezing, and stridor is present on inspiration. He leans forward on his hands to breathe, his nostrils flare with each breath, and his respirations are rapid. His brow is covered with sweat. His color is flushed red, and there are hives on both arms as well as his neck and face. He begins scratching his arms and neck aggressively.

You quickly introduce yourself and your partner and say to the patient and bystanders, "Hello, my name is John, and this is Bill. We are EMTs, and we're here to help you. Does anyone know what happened today?" Simultaneously, Bill begins the initial assessment while you set up the oxygen equipment. A bystander states that the patient's name is Jack Kendrick and that he is a coworker with the Parks Department. He tells you that he and Jack were capturing swans to take for an annual veterinarian visit when a bee stung Jack on the forearm. He goes on to say that Jack has a history of similar episodes and that he has some kind of medication that he is supposed to take.

You quickly request paramedic backup. Dispatch confirms your request and tells you that paramedics are about 10 minutes out. The patient appears to be in severe respiratory distress as you set the oxygen flow rate to 15 lpm and attempt to place the non-rebreather mask on him. You ask the patient's co-worker to locate the patient's medication and bring it to you as quickly as possible. The patient refuses to allow you to place the nonrebreather face mask, so you hold the oxygen tubing close to his nose and mouth. Bill utters softly, "The patient's pulse is 160 per minute, regular and bounding; the skin is cool, clammy, and flushed; respirations are 30 per minute, shallow and labored. He responds to verbal stimuli appropriately. Pupils are equal and reactive. The SpO_2 is 88 percent, and his blood pressure is 90 by palpation."

The coworker returns with a prescribed epinephrine auto-injector and hands it to you. The label identifies the medication as the patient's, and the medication is not expired. You quickly expose the patient's thigh by cutting away the pants, administer the medication, and hold it in place for 10 seconds. You continue to administer oxygen and comfort the patient while the epinephrine takes effect. In about 2 minutes the patient's respiratory status has improved dramatically, and he is able to answer questions. He shows you the spot on his arm where the bee stung him. Bill had earlier removed the stinger while he was taking the patient's blood pressure. The patient states he feels sick to his stomach and has a horrible headache.

You hear a siren in the distance and know that the paramedic unit will arrive soon. You complete an ongoing assessment and have the following findings: The patient is alert and oriented and is breathing adequately; the pulse is 120 per minute, strong and regular; the skin is cool, moist, and slightly flushed; respirations are 22 per minute and normal; pupils are equal and reactive. The blood pressure is 100/76 by auscultation. The SpO_2 is 97 percent. You ask Jack if he has any allergies, and he advises that he is only allergic to bee stings. You go on to ask if he takes any additional medications, and he says only the epinephrine auto-injector. You ask, "Do you have any other medical conditions or problems?" Jack replies, "No, only the allergy to bee stings." You ask, "When was the last time you ate or drank anything?" He tells you, "It was about 3 hours ago. I ate a normal breakfast of frosted flakes and toast." You try to clarify the information presented to you by saying, "OK, Jack, let me make sure I understand what happened to you this morning. You were working here this morning capturing swans to take to the vet when a bee stung you on the arm. Is that correct?" "Yes," he says with a slight grin.

You hear the door of the ALS vehicle close and look up to see paramedic Janet Weinman walking toward you. You introduce Jack to Janet and provide a brief report of the patient's condition. You help place Jack on the cot and then into the ALS ambulance. You and Bill return your equipment to the vehicle and prepare the unit to respond to another call. You report to dispatch that you are available.

1. What sign(s) that Mr. Kendrick presented would be considered the hallmark sign(s) of an allergic reaction?
   a. Hives and severe itching
   b. Blood pressure of 90 mmHg
   c. Respiratory distress
   d. SpO_2 of 88 percent

2. Mr. Kendrick was in respiratory distress and had an SpO_2 of only 88 percent. What mechanism was the most likely cause of these signs and symptoms?
   a. Bronchoconstriction
   b. Blood-vessel dilation and leaking
   c. Psychogenic reaction
   d. Hypertension

3. When administering the epinephrine auto-injector, where is the preferred location to inject the contents?
   a. Proximal end of medial thigh
   b. Distal end of medial thigh
   c. Midpoint of lateral thigh
   d. Distal end of lateral thigh

4. Mr. Kendrick complains of a severe headache and nausea. This finding is most likely to indicate
   a. recurrence of the anaphylactic reaction.
   b. normal side effect of the epinephrine.
   c. hypoperfusion.
   d. nothing of significance.

5. Instead of cutting Mr. Kendrick's pants to administer the epinephrine, the EMT could have administered the epinephrine into
   a. the lateral aspect of his upper arm muscle.
   b. the medial aspect of his upper arm muscle.
   c. his lower leg with pants leg raised.
   d. his thigh through his pants.

EMERGENCY TRIP SHEET

TRIP #	
MEDIC #	
BEGIN MILES	
END MILES	
CODE___/___	PAGE___/___
UNITS ON SCENE	

NAME   SEX   M   F   DOB ___/___/___
ADDRESS   RACE
CITY   STATE   ZIP
PHONE (   )   -   PCP DR.
RESPONDED FROM   CITY
TAKEN FROM   ZIP
DESTINATION   REASON
SSN   -   -   MEDICARE #   MEDICAID #
INSURANCE CO   INSURANCE #   GROUP #
RESPONSIBLE PARTY   ADDRESS
CITY   STATE   ZIP   PHONE (   )   -
EMPLOYER

	DAY
	DATE
RECEIVED	
DISPATCHED	
EN-ROUTE	
ON SCENE	
TO HOSPITAL	
AT HOSPITAL	
IN-SERVICE	

CREW	CERT	STATE #

TIME	ON SCENE (1)	ON SCENE (2)	ON SCENE (3)	EN-ROUTE (1)	EN-ROUTE (2)	AT DESTINATION
BP						
PULSE						
RESP						
EKG						

IV THERAPY
SUCCESSFUL Y N # OF ATTEMPTS _____
ANGIO SIZE _____ga.
SITE _____
TOTAL FLUID INFUSED _____ cc
BLOOD DRAW Y N INITIALS

INTUBATION INFORMATION
SUCCESSFUL Y N # OF ATTEMPTS _____
TUBE SIZE _____ mm
TIME _____ INITIALS _____

MEDICAL HISTORY

MEDICATIONS

ALLERGIES

C/C

EVENTS LEADING TO C/C

ASSESSMENT

TREATMENT

EMS SIGNATURE

CONDITION CODES					

TREATMENTS

TIME	TREATMENT	DOSE	ROUTE	INIT

GCS E___ V___ M___ TOTAL =
GCS E___ V___ M___ TOTAL =
HOSPITAL CONTACTED

CPR BEGUN BY   B   P   TIME BEGUN
AED USED Y N BY:
RESUSCITATION TERMINATED - TIME

(   ) OSHA REGULATIONS FOLLOWED

19 Poisoning Emergencies

OBJECTIVES

Numbered objectives are from the United States Department of Transportation EMT-Basic National Standard Curriculum. Asterisked objectives, if any, pertain to material that is supplemental to the DOT curriculum.

Cognitive

4-6.1 List various ways that poisons enter the body.

4-6.2 List signs/symptoms associated with poisoning.

4-6.3 Discuss the emergency medical care for the patient with possible overdose.

4-6.4 Describe the steps in the emergency medical care for the patient with suspected poisoning.

4-6.5 Establish the relationship between the patient suffering from poisoning or overdose and airway management.

4-6.6 State the generic and trade names, indications, contraindications, medication form, dose, administration, actions, side effects, and reassessment strategies for activated charcoal.

4-6.7 Recognize the need for medical direction in caring for the patient with poisoning or overdose.

KEY IDEAS

This chapter focuses on the assessment and management of poisoning emergencies. Thousands of people become seriously ill or die each year due to accidental or intentional poisonings. As an EMT, you may encounter these patients in homes, at the workplace, or outdoors. It is important that you have a good understanding of the assessment and emergency care needed to effectively manage such patients. Key concepts include the following:

- A poison is any substance that impairs health or can cause death by its chemical effect when it enters the body or comes in contact with the skin.

- Poisons may enter the body via absorption, ingestion, inhalation, or injection.

- Children are the most frequent victims of accidental poisoning by ingestion of prescription or illicit drugs, cleaning agents, or cosmetics.

- The scene size-up must be carefully conducted to prevent the exposure of emergency response personnel to hazardous poisons that may be present on the emergency scene.

- The first priority of care in the management of poisoning emergencies is to ensure that any life-threatening findings to the airway, breathing, or circulation are immediately managed when discovered.

- Activated charcoal is an adjunct to the emergency management of ingested poisoning, since it inhibits the absorption of poisons. However, it is not effective for ingestions involving alcohol, kerosene, gasoline, caustics, or metals or for suspected food poisonings.

- All poisoned patients need to be evaluated by a physician.

TERMS AND CONCEPTS

1. Write the number of the correct term next to each definition.

   1. Absorption
   2. Ingestion
   3. Inhalation
   4. Injection
   5. Poison
   6. Toxin

   _____ a. Substance that can impair health or cause death

   _____ b. Exposure that results from breathing a substance

   _____ c. Passage of a substance through the skin surface upon contact

   _____ d. Exposure that results from swallowing a substance

   _____ e. A poison of animal, plant, or bacterial origin

   _____ f. Forceful introduction of a substance through the penetration of the skin surface

CONTENT REVIEW

1. Which statement is most correct related to poisoning emergencies?
   a. Approximately 1,000 poisonings occur each year in the United States.
   b. Most poisonings are intentional and result from homicide or suicide.
   c. Toxicology is the study of beneficial drugs and their effects on the body.
   d. Poisoning is commonly defined as exposure to a substance other than a drug or medication.

2. You have responded to an emergency scene where you suspect an environmental exposure hazard is present. What action should you next take?
   a. Contact the regional poison-control center.
   b. Immediately begin removal of patients from the scene.
   c. Request assistance from a trained hazardous materials team.
   d. Approach the scene, and try to identify the specific hazard present.

3. Which of the following indications that you may find at an emergency scene is a likely indicator of a poisoning emergency?
   a. Hazardous materials warning label on a locked cabinet
   b. Child safety locks on cabinets that contain cleaning supplies
   c. Chewed-up plants found near a child patient
   d. Cosmetic items placed out of reach of children

4. At the scene of a poisoning emergency, your medical priority is to
   a. identify the poisonous substance.
   b. contact the regional poison-control center.
   c. maintain the patient's airway.
   d. verify the type of exposure.

5. Inhaled poisons may cause airway and breathing compromise as a result of which three factors?
   a. Enhanced airway reactivity, respiratory depression, and direct damage to airway tissues
   b. Diminished bronchial cleansing, enhanced airway reactivity, and direct damage to airway tissues
   c. Alteration of mental status, respiratory depression, and direct damage to airway tissues
   d. Alteration of mental status, diminished bronchial cleansing, and direct damage to airway tissues

6. Inhaled poisonings
   a. cause millions of deaths each year in the United States.
   b. most frequently occur as a result of chemical spills in industrial settings.
   c. even with long exposure times are frequently successfully resuscitated.
   d. that are most common include carbon monoxide and carbon dioxide.

7. A young patient presents with an altered mental status and is found to have paint on his lips. This is mostly likely which type of poisoning?
   a. Injected poisoning
   b. Ingested poisoning
   c. Inhaled poisoning
   d. Absorption poisoning

8. From the following list, select the items that may indicate poisoning in children. Indicate yes (Y) if it is a possible indicator or no (N) if it is not a possible indicator.

   _____ a. Behavior changes (clumsiness, drowsiness, altered mental status)

   _____ b. Crackles on auscultation of the chest

   _____ c. Pupils normal in size and reaction

   _____ d. Excessive salivation

   _____ e. Normal skin and mucosa findings

   _____ f. No paralysis

9. Timmy is a 2-year-old who has ingested a corrosive acid. In addition to maintaining his airway and oxygenation, you should
   a. dilute the substance by giving large amounts of milk or water.
   b. prevent further injury by rinsing the substance from his mouth and lips.
   c. administer activated charcoal per local protocol or medical direction.
   d. talk seriously with his mother about child-safety issues.

10. Activated charcoal is the medication of choice in the emergency medical care of many poisonings because
   a. it is an antidote to most commonly ingested poisons.
   b. it neutralizes caustic and corrosive poisonous substances.
   c. it inhibits the absorption of poisons by the body.
   d. it reverses the toxic effects of drugs and alcohol.

11. When ordered by medical direction or the poison-control center, activated charcoal is indicated for the patient who has
   a. ingested poisons by mouth.
   b. inhaled toxic-chemical substances.
   c. made skin contact with corrosive powders.
   d. been bitten by a poisonous snake.

12. Activated charcoal is indicated for which of the following patients?
    a. A 16-year-old who is unresponsive from drug ingestion
    b. A 3-year-old who is responsive and crying after ingesting an unknown medication
    c. A 58-year-old who is incoherent after ingesting multiple medications
    d. A 30-year-old who is alert and has ingested bleach

13. The usual adult dosage of activated charcoal is
    a. 10 grams.
    b. 12–20 grams.
    c. 30–100 grams.
    d. 150 grams.

14. Activated charcoal is also known by the brand name
    a. CharAway.
    b. GoChar.
    c. Actidose.
    d. Toxi-aid.

15. Which patient is the most likely candidate for the use of activated charcoal?
    a. A patient who responds to verbal stimuli and has ingested ethanol.
    b. A patient who is alert and oriented and ingested an unknown plant.
    c. A patient who is alert and oriented and ingested ammonia.
    d. A patient who is confused and has potential food poisoning.

16. A common side effect seen with administration of activated charcoal is
    a. blackened stool.
    b. headache.
    c. rapid pulse.
    d. seizures.

17. The majority of toxic inhalations occur as a result of
    a. recreational use of inhalants.
    b. industrial accidents.
    c. fire-related incidents.
    d. hazardous materials incidents.

18. The primary symptom associated with toxic inhalation is
    a. altered mental status.
    b. difficulty breathing.
    c. increased tearing from the eyes.
    d. nausea.

19. An appropriate action in the management of a toxic inhalation is to
    a. perform the assessment where the patient is found.
    b. have the patient removed to fresh air as soon as possible.
    c. administer activated charcoal to minimize absorption.
    d. avoid positive-pressure ventilation of the patient.

20. As an EMT, when managing poisons due to absorption, one thing you should pay particular attention to is
    a. preventing the substance from contacting your own skin.
    b. avoiding irrigation of chemical burns to the patient's eyes.
    c. keeping the patient's clothing and jewelry intact and on the patient.
    d. flushing dry powder from the skin with copious amounts of water.

CASE STUDY

You have just returned the unit to service following a minor traffic accident call when you are dispatched to 1234 Early Lane for "one unconscious." You note no obvious hazards as you approach the house. Mrs. Johnson lets you in and reports she found her 50-year-old husband lying on the floor of his basement workshop when she returned from work. You are aware of a peculiar chemical odor as you descend the stairs.

1. What action should you take?
   a. Retreat to a safe area and call for personnel with self-contained breathing apparatus.
   b. Continue down the stairs until you can determine the source of the hazard.
   c. Continue down the stairs and quickly remove Mr. Johnson from the basement.
   d. Hold your breath as you quickly remove Mr. Johnson from the basement.

2. Following the removal of Mr. Johnson from the basement, which of the following best describes the care that should be provided before transport?
   a. Maintain spinal immobilization, ensure a patent airway, check for breathing, provide positive-pressure ventilation if required, and loosen tight clothing.
   b. Apply a nonrebreather mask with oxygen flowing at 15 lpm, place Mr. Johnson in a lateral recumbent position, and be prepared to suction.
   c. Maintain spinal immobilization, administer oxygen by nonrebreather at 15 lpm, and place the patient on a plastic-lined sheet.
   d. No care should be provided to Mr. Johnson until he is properly decontaminated.

You find Mr. Johnson to be unresponsive with rapid, shallow, labored breathing. His pulse is rapid. His skin is pale, cool, and sweaty. There are no signs of trauma.

3. From the following list of treatment descriptions, indicate yes (Y) if it is an appropriate treatment or no (N) if it is not an appropriate treatment for Mr. Johnson.

   _____ a. Inspect Mr. Johnson for any poison that may still be on his body or clothes.

   _____ b. Perform a rapid trauma assessment.

   _____ c. Perform a rapid medical assessment.

   _____ d. Have someone wearing self-contained breathing apparatus retrieve any containers that Mr. Johnson might have been using.

   _____ e. Give careful attention to Mr. Johnson's airway and breathing.

Mrs. Johnson reports that her husband has "never been sick a day in his life." He takes no medications and has no known allergies. She said that she left for work early and does not know when he last ate. Mrs. Johnson says that her husband enjoys refinishing furniture.

4. How often does Mr. Johnson require ongoing assessment en route to the hospital?
   a. Every 5 minutes
   b. Every 10 minutes
   c. Every 15 minutes
   d. Every 20 minutes

ENRICHMENT

1. Food poisoning
   a. commonly results in death.
   b. is decreasing in incidence from prior years in the United States.
   c. is often caused by tainted vegetables but seldom by tainted fish.
   d. is difficult to detect because the signs and symptoms vary greatly.

2. Carbon monoxide
   a. is generally easy to detect because of its foul smell.
   b. increases the amount of oxygen carried on the hemoglobin.
   c. inhibits the ability of body cells to utilize oxygen.
   d. is only rarely a cause of death in the United States.

3. Carbon monoxide poisoning should be suspected if
   a. the patient has a fever and a slower-than-normal respiratory rate.
   b. flulike symptoms are shared by people in the same environment.
   c. the patient's pupils are unequal in size and reactivity.
   d. chest pain and choking are experienced by people in the same environment.

4. This poison can enter the body through inhalation, absorption, injection, or ingestion. It is found in many household products, including rodent poisons and silver polish, and in cherry and apricot pits. Inhalation of this poison can occur in fires where plastics, silk, and synthetic carpets may be burning. The poison is
   a. carbon monoxide.
   b. carbon dioxide.
   c. chlorine.
   d. cyanide.

5. The smell of bitter almonds is most closely associated with _____ poisoning.
   a. carbon monoxide
   b. carbon dioxide
   c. chlorine
   d. cyanide

6. Strong acids
   a. have an extremely high pH.
   b. if ingested will cause the most severe burns in the esophagus.
   c. will typically burn for only 1–2 minutes.
   d. if ingested cause little if any abdominal pain.

7. Alkalis
   a. will produce burns that are not as deep as acid burns.
   b. will typically burn for only 1–2 minutes.
   c. if ingested will likely injure the stomach tissue.
   d. have an extremely low pH.

8. Hydrocarbon
   a. poisoning frequently involves elderly patients.
   b. toxicity is somewhat dependent upon the viscosity of the substance.
   c. poisoning can be safely treated with activated charcoal.
   d. products include most commercial drain cleaners.

9. Methanol
   a. is also known as domestic alcohol.
   b. is found in most alcoholic beverages.
   c. poisoning occurs only through ingestion.
   d. ingestion will produce large amounts of acid in the body.

10. Isopropanol
    a. acts as a cardiac depressant, causing bradycardia.
    b. is also known as isopropyl alcohol or rubbing alcohol.
    c. poisoning occurs most frequently by inhalation.
    d. is frequently found in antifreeze.

11. Ethylene glycol
    a. is found in detergents, radiator antifreeze, and windshield deicers.
    b. poisoning occurs infrequently in children due to its bitter taste.
    c. poisoning occurs in two distinct stages.
    d. poisoning is unresponsive to activated charcoal.

12. Which statement related to poisonous plants is most correct?
    a. About 5 percent of all Americans are allergic to urushiol.
    b. For a reaction to poison ivy to occur, direct contact is necessary.
    c. Poison sumac is found mostly in the Northeast and Southeast of the United States.
    d. Stinging nettle, crown of thorns, and buttercup can cause mild to severe dermatitis.

13. Poison-control centers
    a. are staffed and available for service from 8:00 AM to 5:00 PM 7 days a week.
    b. are able to provide information on a limited, small number of poisons.
    c. provide follow-up via telephone calls to monitor the patient's progress
    d. should not be consulted by EMTs on a routine basis.

SCENARIO 8: **DOCUMENTATION EXERCISE**

Read the following scenario, and think about how you would document this call if you were the EMT who responded to the scene. Then answer the multiple-choice questions and fill in the sample prehospital-care report, basing your documentation on information from the scenario.

It is 8:30 AM on an overcast Saturday morning. You are working with your partner, Laci Richard, when the alarm sounds: "Unit 1 respond to an unknown medical at 1621 Lake Hollingsworth Road, cross street Ingraham. Time out 0830 hours." Dispatch advises that the caller is hysterical and is unable to provide any information related to the patient.

You arrive on the scene in about 5 minutes. The home is located in a neighborhood of expensive homes in an exclusive area of town. You pull up in the driveway of a three-story home and park next to several bikes that are scattered across the driveway. As you are walking toward the door with your BSI precautions on, a boy of about 10 or 12 years of age comes running out of the house. He tells you that his younger brother ate some medicine and that his mom was "really upset." You introduce yourself and your partner and find out that his name is Jake and that his younger brother's name is Jimmy. Jimmy is about 2 years of age. You enter the house and proceed to a bathroom at the back, where a small boy is sitting on the floor on which some medicine containers are scattered. The mother grabs Laci and loudly screams, "You've got to do something for my son, NOW!"

Jimmy appears to be in minor distress. He looks at you as you enter. His skin color looks normal, with no abnormal respiratory sounds present, and he appears to be breathing normally. No signs of trauma are present. You reach down to check his pulse. His skin is warm and dry, and his pulse is rapid and strong. You say to the mother, "Hello, my name is John, and this is Laci. We are EMTs, and we are here to help your son. Can you tell us what happened today?" Laci begins an initial assessment and tells you she will obtain the vitals. You administer oxygen at 15 lpm via blow-by to the young boy. Meanwhile, the crying mother says, "I don't know how it happened. I was talking to my sister on the phone, and I thought Jimmy was next to me, but he got into the bathroom, and I guess he crawled up on the sink and got into the medicine cabinet. By the time I found him, he had all these bottles open, and I don't know what he swallowed." You ask, "What's your name, ma'am?" She says, "It's Mrs. Wilson."

You continue by saying, "Mrs. Wilson, we are going to do all we can to help Jimmy. How much does he weigh, and when did he get into the medicines?" She tells you, "He weighs about 28 pounds, and this happened about 10 or 15 minutes ago." You ask, "Has he complained of anything?" "No," she replies. "He doesn't know why I'm so upset." "Was your son sick to his stomach before we arrived?" "No," she says. You ask, "Does your son have any allergies?" The mother says, "No, he is not allergic to anything." "Is your son taking any medications?" "No," she replies. You continue the assessment. "Has your son ever been sick before or hospitalized?" "No," she quickly states. "When was the last time your son ate, and how much did he eat?" She says, "He ate a bowl of cereal about an hour ago . . . and some toast, too. I don't see what this all has to do with helping my son. Please do something!"

You ask the mother to please help by gathering up all the containers of medication that she thinks Jimmy could possibly have gotten into and bring them along to the hospital. Laci has established a good rapport with Jimmy by allowing him to participate in the evaluation. She advises that his respirations are normal at 28 per minute; pulse is strong and regular at 110; skin color is normal, warm, and dry; and pupils are equal, reactive, and respond briskly to light. Perfusion appears adequate; the SpO_2 is 99 percent on the blow-by oxygen. There is no abdominal tenderness. You quickly jot down the vitals and say that you are going to contact poison control. You explain to Mrs. Wilson that poison control will advise you of the very best and most up-to-date treatment for Jimmy.

You call poison control and advise the RN of the situation. You tell him Jimmy's age and weight, and you quickly summarize his general condition. You provide his vital signs and say that he seems to have ingested a medication, but there is presently no way to identify what medication it was. You tell him the child ate a bowl of cereal and some toast about an hour ago. The RN advises you to prepare a dose of 12.5 grams of activated charcoal in 6 to 8 ounces of water and administer it to Jimmy. The RN stays on the line while you prepare the activated charcoal. You prepare it in a colorful cup, shaking and stirring to be sure it is well mixed, then add a lid and a straw and coax Jimmy to sip it down. He makes a face, but his mother encourages him to keep sipping, and he finishes it as you and Laci and his mother praise him lavishly. You complete your assessment and transport Jimmy and his mother and brother and a paper bag containing all the medications from the bathroom to the local emergency department.

1. When Laci assessed Jimmy's vital signs
   a. she should have assessed the blood pressure early.
   b. she should have assessed the blood pressure by palpation.
   c. she was correct in not assessing the blood pressure, which is generally not assessed in children less than 3 years of age.
   d. she was correct in not assessing the blood pressure, which is generally not assessed in children less than 5 years of age.

2. Your treatment of Jimmy is primarily focused on
   a. preventing absorption of the medication he swallowed.
   b. providing an antidote to the medication he swallowed.
   c. speeding absorption of the medication to move it quickly through his system.
   d. reassuring his mother that something is being done for her son.

3. When a parent like Mrs. Wilson is extremely upset, what is the best thing to do?
   a. Send the parent out of the room so she doesn't upset the child.
   b. Keep the parent in the room because the child will be upset if she leaves.
   c. Tell the parent to "calm down."
   d. Ask the parent to step aside and let you do your job.

EMERGENCY TRIP SHEET

		BILLING USE ONLY			
TRIP #		DAY			
MEDIC #		DATE			
BEGIN MILES		RECEIVED			
END MILES		DISPATCHED			
CODE __/__ PAGE __/__		EN-ROUTE			

NAME _____ SEX M F DOB __/__/__

ADDRESS _____ RACE

CITY _____ STATE _____ ZIP

PHONE ( ) _____ - _____ PCP DR. _____

RESPONDED FROM _____ CITY

TAKEN FROM _____ ZIP

DESTINATION _____ REASON

SSN ___ - ___ - ___ MEDICARE # _____ MEDICAID # _____

INSURANCE CO _____ INSURANCE # _____ GROUP # _____

RESPONSIBLE PARTY _____ ADDRESS _____

CITY _____ STATE _____ ZIP _____ PHONE ( ) _____ - _____

EMPLOYER _____

	ON SCENE (1)	ON SCENE (2)	ON SCENE (3)	EN-ROUTE (1)	EN-ROUTE (2)	AT DESTINATION
TIME						
BP						
PULSE						
RESP						
EKG						

MEDICAL HISTORY _____

MEDICATIONS _____

ALLERGIES _____

C/C _____

EVENTS LEADING TO C/C _____

ASSESSMENT _____

TREATMENT _____

EMS SIGNATURE _____

Billing section (right column):

ON SCENE			
TO HOSPITAL			
AT HOSPITAL			
IN-SERVICE			

CREW	CERT	STATE #

IV THERAPY
SUCCESSFUL Y N # OF ATTEMPTS _____
ANGIO SIZE _____ ga.
SITE _____
TOTAL FLUID INFUSED _____ cc
BLOOD DRAW Y N INITIALS

INTUBATION INFORMATION
SUCCESSFUL Y N # OF ATTEMPTS _____
TUBE SIZE _____ mm
TIME _____ INITIALS _____

CONDITION CODES _____

TREATMENTS

TIME	TREATMENT	DOSE	ROUTE	INIT

GCS E__ V__ M__ TOTAL =

GCS E__ V__ M__ TOTAL =

HOSPITAL CONTACTED

CPR BEGUN BY B P TIME BEGUN

AED USED Y N BY:

RESUSCITATION TERMINATED - TIME

( ) OSHA REGULATIONS FOLLOWED

CHAPTER

20 Drug and Alcohol Emergencies

OBJECTIVES

Numbered objectives are from the United States Department of Transportation EMT-Basic National Standard Curriculum. Asterisked objectives, if any, pertain to material that is supplemental to the DOT curriculum.

Cognitive

4-6.3   Discuss the emergency medical care for the patient with possible overdose.
  *   Describe the steps in the assessment of a drug or an alcohol overdose patient.
  *   Explain how to determine if an emergency is drug or alcohol related.
  *   List six factors that may make a drug or an alcohol emergency life-threatening.
  *   Discuss the signs and symptoms that indicate a drug or alcohol emergency.
  *   Discuss the techniques for managing a violent drug or alcohol patient.

KEY IDEAS

This chapter focuses on the assessment and management of emergencies related to drug and alcohol use and abuse. Since drugs and alcohol are abused by a number of people in a variety of ways, you may encounter such patients in virtually any setting. In addition to the medical emergency created by drug or alcohol ingestion or withdrawal, these patients are also often victims of trauma and may exhibit aggressive or violent behavior toward the EMS crew. Key concepts include the following:

■   Safety must be a primary concern for the EMT at the scene of drug or alcohol emergencies, since these patients may exhibit aggressive or violent behavior and are also often infected with bloodborne or airborne diseases.

■   Overdose and withdrawal are potentially life-threatening emergencies.

■   Drug and alcohol emergency indicators include unresponsiveness or other altered mental status, respiratory difficulty, fever, abnormal pulse rates, vomiting, and seizures.

■   Management of drug and alcohol emergencies requires careful attention to the maintenance of airway, breathing, and circulation status as well as to controlling potentially volatile situations with unpredictable patients.

TERMS AND CONCEPTS

1. Write the number of the correct term next to each definition.

   1. Drug abuse
   2. Huffing
   3. Overdose
   4. Pharming
   5. Withdrawal

   _____ a. Physical syndrome that occurs after a period of abstinence from a substance to which a person's body has become accustomed

   _____ b. Self-administration of legal or illicit substances in a manner that is not in accord with approved medical or social patterns

   _____ c. An emergency that involves poisoning or toxicity caused by drugs or alcohol

   _____ d. Raiding parents' or friends' medicine cabinets for prescription medications

   _____ e. Inhaling paints or propellants in order to "get high"

CONTENT REVIEW

1. Which of the following are the goals at the scene of a drug or an alcohol emergency?
   a. Identify and reverse effects of the abused substance.
   b. Identify and treat potential life threats.
   c. Notify police of illegal drug use.
   d. Identify abused substance and control behavior of patient.

2. What are three common potential dangers at the scene of a drug or an alcohol emergency?
   a. Infectious disease, violent behavior, and weapons
   b. Violent behavior, weapons, and hazardous substances
   c. Infectious disease, violent behavior, and traffic
   d. Hazardous substances, weapons, and infectious disease

3. Your patient is found unresponsive on the living room floor, surrounded by nearly a dozen empty and partially filled pill bottles. What should be done with the bottles?
   a. Do nothing with the pill bottles; they are not important.
   b. Keep the pill bottles with the patient as a source of information.
   c. Turn the pill bottles over to the police; they may be a source of evidence.
   d. Return the pill bottles to the patient's family so they may be refilled.

4. In drug or alcohol emergencies, expect
   a. signs and symptoms that mimic only one or two medical disorders.
   b. to identify and treat the loss of vital functions caused by the drug or alcohol.
   c. scenes that seldom involve violent acts or physical abuse.
   d. scenes that do not require the use of body substance isolation precautions.

5. Upon completion of your initial assessment, you suspect that your unresponsive patient's condition may be due to drugs or alcohol. Which action is most appropriate to take next?
   a. Move the patient to the ambulance and transport immediately.
   b. Contact medical direction and seek additional guidance.
   c. With an ungloved hand, check the mouth for signs of pills or tablets.
   d. Ask bystanders for information about precipitating events.

6. From the following list, select those signs and symptoms that indicate a life-threatening drug or alcohol emergency. Mark those that indicate a life threat with a Y for yes and those that do not with an N for no.
   _____ a. Normal level of responsiveness
   _____ b. Respiratory difficulty
   _____ c. Vomiting with a normal level of responsiveness
   _____ d. Fever
   _____ e. Slow pulse rate
   _____ f. Seizures
   _____ g. Right-lower-quadrant abdominal pain
   _____ h. Lower-back discomfort

7. The most reliable indicators of a drug or alcohol emergency are likely to come from which two of the following phases of the patient assessment?
   a. Physical exam and vital signs
   b. Vital signs and patient history
   c. Scene size-up and patient history
   d. Physical exam and ongoing assessment

8. You are on-scene with a disoriented patient who reports taking an overdose of pain medication. Number the list below in the proper order from 1 to 5 to show the emergency-care steps for this patient.
   _____ Administer oxygen at 15 lpm by nonrebreather mask or positive-pressure ventilation with supplemental oxygen as necessary.
   _____ Transport the patient to the hospital.
   _____ Take measures to maintain body temperature and prevent shock.
   _____ Establish and maintain a patent airway.
   _____ If local protocol permits, assess the blood-glucose level.

9. Hallucinogenic substances
   a. such as PCP can cause paralysis, violence, and rage.
   b. are also known as "imbecilic drugs."
   c. are commonly derived from opiates and opioids.
   d. cause central-nervous-system depression and drowsiness.

10. The EMT pictured here is talking with a patient suffering a behavioral emergency. Which of the following is the most correct comment about the technique being demonstrated?
    a. Touch can be comforting; always touch the behavioral emergency patient.
    b. Touch can be comforting; however, never touch the patient without his permission.
    c. Pat the patient on the back to help clear his airway.
    d. Grasp the shoulder and forearm to initiate restraint.

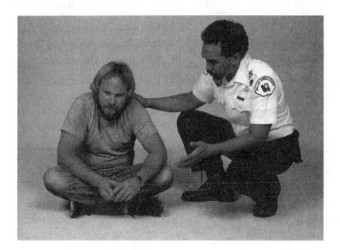

11. You are attempting to treat a drug-abuse patient experiencing a "bad trip." Which of the following is *not* an element of the "talk-down technique"?
    a. Transport the patient immediately and attempt to calm while en route to the hospital.
    b. Help the patient verbalize what is happening to him.
    c. Make simple statements to help orient the patient to time and place.
    d. Reassure the patient that his condition is caused by the drug.

12. Central-nervous-system-stimulant drugs typically cause
    a. constricted pupils.
    b. dilated pupils.
    c. have no effect on the patient's pupils.
    d. unequal pupils.

13. Bradycardia; hypotension; inadequate breathing rates and volume; cool, clammy skin; constricted pupils; and nausea are most commonly associated with
    a. central-nervous-system stimulants.
    b. central-nervous-system depressants.
    c. narcotics.
    d. hallucinogens.

CASE STUDY

You have just finished cleaning up the station kitchen following a great dinner prepared by your partner when the alarm sounds. You are dispatched to a call for an unresponsive patient. You arrive on-scene and find a 17-year-old female who was found unresponsive in her bedroom by her mother. She was last seen about 4 hours ago. Your initial assessment finds her unresponsive with snoring respirations of approximately 8 per minute. There is vomitus on the floor near her head. Her pulse is slow and irregular. Her skin is pale, cool, and dry.

1. What is your first priority in managing this patient?
   a. Cover the patient to maintain body temperature.
   b. Ensure that the airway is clear of vomitus.
   c. Quickly begin positive-pressure ventilation.
   d. Immobilize on a long spine board.

The mother reports that her daughter has been depressed since the death of her boyfriend in a car crash last month, but she has no medical problems or allergies. Your partner finds four empty pill bottles and a partially full wine bottle in the adjacent bathroom.

2. Your local protocol allows you to administer activated charcoal for ingestions. Should this patient be administered activated charcoal?
   a. Yes, at a dose of 3 g/kg
   b. Yes, at a dose of 1 g/kg
   c. No, because the patient has an altered level of consciousness
   d. No, because the patient has ingested alcohol

3. Which statement best describes the management of this patient?
   a. This is a life-threatening situation. The patient is a high priority for transport. Give the pill bottles and wine bottle to the police. Complete the physical exam and the baseline vital signs. Perform an ongoing assessment every 5 minutes during transport and closely monitor the airway and breathing.
   b. This is a life-threatening situation. The patient is a high priority for transport. Transport the pill bottles, wine bottle, and a sample of the vomitus to the emergency department. Complete the physical exam and the baseline vital signs. Perform an ongoing assessment every 5 minutes during transport and closely monitor the airway and breathing.
   c. This is a non-life-threatening situation. The patient is a low priority for transport. Complete the physical exam and the baseline vital signs. Perform an ongoing assessment every 15 minutes during transport.
   d. This is a non-life-threatening situation. The patient is a low priority for transport. Transport the pill bottles and wine bottle and a sample of the vomitus to the emergency department. Perform an ongoing assessment every 15 minutes during transport.

ENRICHMENT

1. The physically dependent drug user
   a. deals normally with problems and seldom thinks about using the drug.
   b. experiences a strong need to use the drug repeatedly.
   c. has no physiological consequences from drug withdrawal.
   d. may develop tolerance to a drug, in which smaller doses are needed.

2. Common signs and symptoms of drug withdrawal
   a. typically peak at 12–24 hours.
   b. include urinary retention, lower leg cramps, and dilated pupils.
   c. include excessive thirst, lower leg cramps, and indigestion.
   d. include nausea, abdominal cramping, and tremors.

3. A chronic brain syndrome resulting from the toxic effects of alcohol on the central nervous system combined with malnutrition is called
   a. Jackson-Pierce disease.
   b. Wernicke-Korsakoff syndrome.
   c. alcoholic nutritional syndrome.
   d. Perkins-Brower syndrome.

4. Which is the correct term for a combination of problem drinking (to relieve tension) and true addiction to alcohol (in which abstinence causes physical withdrawal symptoms)?
   a. Addiction syndrome
   b. Withdrawal syndrome
   c. Alcoholic syndrome
   d. Intoxication syndrome

5. Which is the correct term for the syndrome that occurs when the alcoholic's alcohol level falls below the amount usually ingested?
   a. Abstinence syndrome
   b. Hypoalcohol syndrome
   c. Addiction syndrome
   d. Withdrawal syndrome

6. Stage I of alcohol withdrawal occurs within about _____ and is characterized by nausea, insomnia, sweating, and tremors.
   a. 2 hours
   b. 4 hours
   c. 6 hours
   d. 8 hours

7. The last stage of alcohol withdrawal is a life-threatening condition with a mortality rate between 5 and 15 percent. This stage is called
   a. alcohol poisoning.
   b. delirium tremens.
   c. Jackson-Pierce syndrome.
   d. terminal alcohol toxicity.

8. Which of the following is a drug that is cheap to make and produces horrible psychological effects that can last for years? It is known by multiple names, such as angel dust, killer weed, supergrass, crystal cyclone, and many others.
   a. AGN
   b. Phencyclidine
   c. Amnioglycoside
   d. DHT

9. Cocaine
   a. use in the United States has been decreasing significantly in recent years.
   b. is taken only by inhalation through the nose.
   c. requires treatment that is very different from that for PCP.
   d. is now the drug most commonly involved in emergency-department drug-related visits.

10. The first priority of care for a patient under the influence of PCP is to
   a. begin the talk-down technique to manage the patient.
   b. quickly check for injuries that require attention.
   c. protect the safety of yourself and your response crew.
   d. monitor the vital signs and transport quickly.

11. Inhaled poisons intentionally inhaled commonly
   a. contain the chemical agent oban.
   b. improve oxygen movement across the alveolar membrane.
   c. have a more delayed onset of symptoms than injected poisons.
   d. accumulate in the regions of the brain responsible for feelings of pleasure.

12. Methamphetamine
   a. is a type of depressant drug.
   b. use is decreasing among teenagers.
   c. is commonly called crystal meth.
   d. can only be used by injection.

SCENARIO 9: **DOCUMENTATION EXERCISE**

Read the following scenario, and think about how you would document this call if you were the EMT who responded to the scene. Then answer the multiple-choice questions and fill in the sample prehospital-care report, basing your documentation on information from the scenario.

It is 11:30 PM on a cold winter night. You have just jumped into bed and are thinking about applying for the next Paramedic program when the alarm sounds: "Unit 1 respond to 350 North Crystal Lake Drive for patient who is 'hearing voices.' Cross street Longfellow Boulevard. Time out 2330 hours." You are working with Bob Clayton, who has been an EMT for 15 years. You have learned a lot from him and respect his emergency medical skills. Bob meets you at the vehicle, and you advise dispatch that you are responding.

You arrive at a run-down home located in a working-class neighborhood. The porch light is on, and a female, who appears to be in her 20s, waves you down. You stop, park the rescue vehicle, and with BSI in place approach the house. As you do so, the lady greets you with, "I'm sure glad you're here! It's my boyfriend. He took some LSD about 45 minutes ago, and he is just out of it. He hears voices and is acting weird." You say, "Good evening! My name is Bonnie, and this is Bob. Has your boyfriend been violent at all?" She asserts, "No, he is not the violent type at all. He is just acting strange." You ask her for her name and the patient's name. She tells you, "My name is April May and his name is Edward Bare."

You enter the home and are escorted to a bedroom located in the front of the house. When you go into the room, you see the patient sitting in a small chair next to the bed. He looks to be about 25 years of age. His eyes are open, and he is staring down at his lap. His hands are trembling. He does not acknowledge your presence. You say, "Good evening, Mr. Bare. This is Bob, and my name is Bonnie. We're EMTs, and we're here to help you. I'd like to talk with you." You maintain a distance of about 8 feet from the patient, who remains silent with his head lowered, continuing to stare at his lap. He is breathing adequately with no abnormal respiratory sounds noted. His skin color looks normal, and no signs of trauma are observed.

You continue by saying, "I'd like to try to help you understand what is happening to you." He looks up at you. You note that his pupils are dilated. He utters something that you can't understand. "Ed, I'm sorry, what did you say? I didn't understand you. Could you repeat what you said?" Ed replies, "What the X*%$ are you doing here? I didn't want you here or ask you to come! What? What's that you said? You think I'm a punk! Get out! Just get out!"

You and Bob calmly step outside and quickly request law-enforcement backup. The two of you wait outside for the police to arrive, explaining to April that you need to wait for law-enforcement assistance. They arrive on-scene in about 3 minutes. Now you reenter the scene with law enforcement at your side. You calmly approach Ed and say, "Ed, April is worried about you. She says that you took some LSD and that you've been hearing things. What's happening to you is caused by the LSD, and it won't last forever. It's temporary. You must try to focus on the fact that this is temporary."

Ed breaks in, saying, "Did you call me a punk?" "No, Ed. I didn't say that. You're hearing things that are caused by the LSD you took. It won't last forever, Ed. You must focus on that. It won't last forever." Ed quietly says, "It won't last? Hearing the voices, I mean." You reply calmly and just as quietly, "No, Ed. Focus on that. It won't last forever. Ed, I want you to also understand that as the drug wears off you may be confused at times and still hear voices. OK?" Ed says, "I'm hearing voices now, but I'm going to focus on it's not going to last!" You say, "Thanks, Ed!"

You continue, "Ed, we are going to take your blood pressure and pulse now and get you ready to go to the hospital. Bob is going to touch you. Is that OK?" Ed replies, "Yes, that's all right." Bob notes a red rash on Ed's arm and gathers the vital signs. His respirations are 18 per minute and normal; pulse of 100 per minute, strong, regular, and bounding; his skin color is normal, warm, and dry; his pupils are equal, dilated, and respond slowly to light; his blood pressure is 140/80; and the SpO_2 is 95 percent.

You speak with April to obtain additional information. You say, "April, I need to confirm some information with you. You said that Ed took some LSD about 45 minutes ago and that about 10 minutes ago he began acting strangely. Is that right?" She says, "That's right." "Did he have any other complaints?" "No," she states. "Does Ed have any allergies or take any medications?" you ask. "No," she says. You continue by asking, "Has Ed seen a doctor or been sick in the past?" She replies, "No, Ed has always been very healthy." "When did Ed last eat?" She says, "It was about an hour ago. He had a sandwich and a beer." You say, "Thanks, April, you've been a great help. We're going to take Ed to the hospital now." You place Ed on the cot and prepare him for transport.

1. The signs or symptoms of potential LSD use that Ed exhibited include
   a. red rash, dilated pupils, and blood pressure of 140/80.
   b. motor disturbance, dilated pupils, and hallucinations.
   c. SpO_2 of 95 percent, red rash, and dilated pupils.
   d. SpO_2 of 95 percent, motor disturbance, and dilated pupils.

2. The technique Bonnie used to communicate with and manage Ed is called the
   a. LSD-management technique.
   b. violent-patient technique.
   c. talk-down technique.
   d. drug-abuse technique.

3. The technique used to communicate with and manage Ed would not be used if he had taken
   a. PCP.
   b. PCB.
   c. marijuana.
   d. cocaine.

4. The technique for communicating with and managing a patient on hallucinogens includes the steps listed below. Did Bonnie accomplish each step with Ed? If she did, mark the step with a Y for yes. If she didn't, mark the step with an N for no.
   _____ a. Make the patient feel welcome.
   _____ b. Identify yourself clearly.
   _____ c. Reassure the patient that his condition is caused by the drug and will not last forever.
   _____ d. Reiterate simple and concrete statements.
   _____ e. Forewarn the patient about what will happen as the drug wears off.
   _____ f. Once the patient has been calmed, transport.

5. Was it appropriate for law-enforcement backup to be requested in this incident?
   a. Yes, law enforcement should have been requested as described.
   b. Yes, but the EMTs should not have left the patient's side.
   c. No, the patient can be managed without law-enforcement backup.
   d. No, law enforcement was not needed, as long as a way to safely exit the scene was anticipated.

EMERGENCY TRIP SHEET

IP #		
EDIC #		
GIN MILES		
D MILES		
DE___/___	PAGE___/___	
ITS ON SCENE		

ME   SEX M F DOB ___/___/___

DRESS   RACE

TY   STATE   ZIP

ONE ( )   -   PCP DR.

SPONDED FROM   CITY

KEN FROM   ZIP

STINATION   REASON

N   -   -   MEDICARE #   MEDICAID #

SURANCE CO   INSURANCE #   GROUP #

SPONSIBLE PARTY   ADDRESS

TY   STATE   ZIP   PHONE ( )   -

IPLOYER

ME	ON SCENE (1)	ON SCENE (2)	ON SCENE (3)	EN-ROUTE (1)	EN-ROUTE (2)	AT DESTINATION
LSE						
SP						
G						

EDICAL HISTORY

EDICATIONS

LERGIES

ENTS LEADING TO C/C

SESSMENT

EATMENT

S SIGNATURE

BILLING USE ONLY

DAY			
DATE			
RECEIVED			
DISPATCHED			
EN-ROUTE			
ON SCENE			
TO HOSPITAL			
AT HOSPITAL			
IN-SERVICE			

CREW	CERT	STATE #

IV THERAPY
SUCCESSFUL Y N # OF ATTEMPTS _____
ANGIO SIZE _____ga.
SITE _____
TOTAL FLUID INFUSED _____ cc
BLOOD DRAW Y N INITIALS

INTUBATION INFORMATION
SUCCESSFUL Y N # OF ATTEMPTS _____
TUBE SIZE _____ mm
TIME _____ INITIALS _____

CONDITION CODES | | | |

TREATMENTS

TIME	TREATMENT	DOSE	ROUTE	INIT

GCS | E___ V___ M___ TOTAL =

GCS | E___ V___ M___ TOTAL =

HOSPITAL CONTACTED

CPR BEGUN BY B P TIME BEGUN

AED USED Y N BY:

RESUSCITATION TERMINATED - TIME

( ) OSHA REGULATIONS FOLLOWED

21 Acute Abdominal Pain

OBJECTIVES

Numbered objectives are from the United States Department of Transportation EMT-Basic National Standard Curriculum. Asterisked objectives, if any, pertain to material that is supplemental to the DOT curriculum.

Cognitive

* Describe the structure and function of the organs contained within the abdominal cavity.
* Define the term "acute abdomen."
* Describe the assessment of a patient with acute abdominal pain.
* Describe the signs and symptoms of acute abdominal pain.
* Discuss the appropriate emergency medical care for a patient with acute abdominal pain.
* Discuss possible causes of acute abdominal pain.

KEY IDEAS

Acute abdominal pain may indicate a serious condition. This chapter reviews assessment and emergency care for the patient suffering from acute abdominal pain.

■ Acute abdominal pain, also called "acute abdomen" or "acute abdominal distress," is a common condition characterized by an acute onset of moderate to severe abdominal pain that may result from a variety of causes.

■ All patients with acute abdominal pain should be considered to have a life-threatening condition until proven otherwise.

■ Internal bleeding, peritonitis, and diarrhea are conditions that often involve considerable fluid loss, leading to shock (hypoperfusion). A top priority during the assessment of a patient with acute abdominal pain is to look for signs of shock.

■ Rapid transport should be considered for the acute abdomen patient who meets any of the following criteria: poor general impression, unresponsive, responsive but not following commands, shock (hypoperfusion), or severe pain.

■ Perform the examination of the abdomen carefully and gently. If the patient is a priority for rapid transport, the focused history and physical exam should be conducted en route to the hospital.

■ Emergency medical care for the patient with an acute abdomen includes maintaining a patent airway, placing the patient in a position of comfort, administering oxygen, not giving anything by mouth, calming and reassuring the patient, being alert for shock, and initiating a quick and efficient transport.

TERMS AND CONCEPTS

1. Write the number of the correct term next to each definition.

   1. Abdominal aorta
   2. Acute abdomen
   3. Guarded position
   4. Involuntary guarding
   5. Parietal pain
   6. Peritoneum
   7. Peritonitis
   8. Referred pain
   9. Rigidity
   10. Umbilicus
   11. Visceral pain
   12. Voluntary guarding

   _____ a. The navel

   _____ b. Abdominal-wall muscle contraction that the patient cannot control caused by inflammation of the peritoneum

   _____ c. The lining of the abdominal cavity

   _____ d. Pain that is felt in a body part removed from its point of origin

   _____ e. Moderate to severe abdominal pain with an acute onset

   _____ f. A position generally adopted by patients with acute abdominal pain: knees drawn up and hands clenched over the abdomen

   _____ g. A major division of the heart's primary artery that runs through the abdomen

   _____ h. Abdominal-wall muscle contraction that is controlled by the patient

   _____ i. A localized, intense, sharp, constant pain associated with irritation of the peritoneal lining

   _____ j. Inflammation or irritation of the peritoneum

   _____ k. Constant involuntary abdominal-muscle contraction that occurs as a result of peritonitis

   _____ l. Poorly localized, intermittent, crampy abdominal pain associated with ischemia or distention of an organ

2. Match the correct organs of the abdomen with their function.

1. Bladder
2. Duodenum
3. Gallbladder
4. Kidneys
5. Large intestine
6. Liver
7. Pancreas
8. Small intestine
9. Spleen
10. Stomach

_____ a. A saclike, stretchable pouch located below the diaphragm, which receives food from the esophagus (a tubelike structure from the throat)

_____ b. The first part of the small intestine that connects to the stomach

_____ c. A tubelike structure beginning at the distal end of the stomach and ending at the beginning of the large intestine. Its digestive function is to absorb nutrients from intestinal contents.

_____ d. A tubelike structure beginning at the distal end of the small intestine and ending at the anus. It reabsorbs fluid from intestinal contents, enabling the excretion of solid waste from the body.

_____ e. A large, solid organ located in the right upper quadrant (RUQ) just beneath the diaphragm with a slight portion extending to the left upper quadrant (LUQ). It filters the nutrients from blood as it returns from the intestines, stores glucose (sugar) and certain vitamins, plays a part in blood clotting, filters dead red blood cells, and aids in the production of bile.

_____ f. A pear-shaped sac that lies on the underneath right side of the liver. This organ holds bile, which aids in the digestion of fats.

_____ g. An elongated, oval, solid organ located in the LUQ behind and to the side of the stomach. It aids in the production of blood cells as well as in the filtering and storage of blood.

_____ h. A gland composed of many lobes and ducts located in both the RUQ and LUQ, just behind the stomach. It aids in digestion and regulates carbohydrate metabolism.

_____ i. Paired organs located behind the abdominal-wall lining (retroperitoneal), one on each side of the spine. These organs excrete urine and regulate water, electrolytes, and acid-base balance.

_____ j. A sac-like structure that acts as a reservoir for the urine received from the kidneys

CONTENT REVIEW

1. The abdomen is the area below the diaphragm to the top of the pelvis. It is helpful to reference the abdomen by dividing it into quarters, or quadrants. The central reference point is the umbilicus. Correctly identify the following terms on the figure below.

   Diaphragm
   Left lower quadrant (LLQ)
   Left upper quadrant (LUQ)
   Right lower quadrant (RLQ)
   Right upper quadrant (RUQ)
   Umbilicus

   A _____
   B _____
   C _____
   D _____
   E _____
   F _____

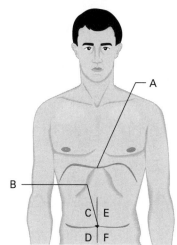

2. Dividing the abdominal cavity into regions is useful because the anatomical landmarks help identify the underlying organs' location. Correctly identify the following region on the figure below.

   _____ Hypogastric Region

   _____ Umbilical Region

   _____ Epigastric Region

   _____ Right Iliac Region

   _____ Right Lumbar Region

   _____ Right Hypochondriac Region

   _____ Left Hypochondriac Region

   _____ Left Lumbar Region

   _____ Left Iliac Region

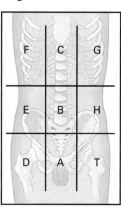

3. Abdominal pain that is sharp, knifelike, or pinpoint and associated with irritation and inflammation of the peritoneal lining affects which nerve fiber?
   a. Phrenic nerve
   b. Optic nerve fiber
   c. Visceral nerve fiber
   d. Parietal (somatic) nerve fiber

4. A patient experiencing a rapid onset of abdominal pain can also be reported as suffering from which of the following?
   a. Acute abdomen
   b. Visceral pain
   c. Gastritis
   d. Parietal pain

5. All patients with abdominal pain should be considered
   a. to have a bowel obstruction until proven otherwise.
   b. to have a life-threatening condition until proven otherwise.
   c. to be stable until proven otherwise.
   d. to have a digestive-system disorder until proven otherwise.

6. A person with an acute abdomen generally appears very ill. The patient will usually
   a. adopt a position on her side with her legs straight.
   b. adopt a position lying on her stomach with her legs flat.
   c. adopt a position lying flat on her back with her legs flat.
   d. adopt a position with her knees drawn up.

7. The acute-abdomen patient should be categorized as a priority for transport if she meets certain criteria. Which of the following should indicate a priority transport for the acute-abdominal patient?
   a. Poor general appearance, responsive but not following commands, hypoperfusion
   b. Awake and alert to time and place, blood pressure above 120 systolic, headache
   c. Grimacing facial expression, blood glucose of 60, pulse oximeter reading of 96 percent
   d. Dazed look, patient presents in a Fowler position, hypertensive, diarrhea for 2 days

8. Which statement is true regarding the scene size-up for the acute-abdomen patient?
   a. Patients experiencing abdominal pain are not likely to faint, and if they do, they usually faint in the bedroom.
   b. You should not worry about looking for mechanisms of injury to rule out trauma as the cause of abdominal pain.
   c. Bloody vomitus is always present in the acute-abdomen patient.
   d. Certain types of bleeding have a distinct smell that sometimes can be identified as you arrive at the patient's side.

9. When preparing to palpate the abdomen of the patient complaining of abdominal pain, you should
   a. have the patient point to the site of the pain and palpate this quadrant last.
   b. have the patient point to the site of the pain and palpate this quadrant first.
   c. have the patient point to the site of the pain and do not palpate this quadrant.
   d. palpate all four quadrants, always with the upper quadrants first, then the lower quadrants.

10. Which of the following signs or symptoms is most likely associated with an acute abdomen?
    a. Localized right-leg pain (referred pain)
    b. Soft abdomen that produces no pain on palpation
    c. Bloody vomitus or blood in the stool
    d. Normal vital signs and blood-glucose level

11. Which of the following is appropriate management for the patient with an acute abdomen?
    a. Palpate the most painful quadrant first, moving clockwise thereafter.
    b. Position the patient in a supine position with legs flat.
    c. Perform an ongoing assessment every 15 minutes for the unstable patient.
    d. Avoid giving anything to the patient by mouth.

12. Which of the following is a condition that can cause an acute abdomen?
   a. Cholecystitis
   b. Transient ischemic attack
   c. Bell's syndrome
   d. Pneumothorax

13. While assessing your patient that complains of abdominal pain, you perform a modified Markle ("heel jar") test by knocking the heels together while the patient is supine. The patient responds with a facial grimace and moans, "That hurts my stomach." This positive test for rebound tenderness indicates
   a. peritonitis.
   b. abdominal aortic aneurysm.
   c. ruptured diaphragm.
   d. hemothorax.

14. While assessing your patient that complains of abdominal pain, you observe that the pulse pressure is narrowing, the heart rate has increased, and the skin has become pale, cool, and diaphoretic. You suspect
   a. acute inflammation of the appendix.
   b. inflammation of the peritoneal lining.
   c. constipation from a blocked large intestine.
   d. internal bleeding within the abdomen.

CASE STUDY

You and your partner, Jill, are busy washing the unit when the alarm sounds. You respond to a call for a patient complaining of abdominal pain. The scene appears safe as you arrive at a well-kept one-story home. A man meets you at the curb and escorts you to the front door. As you follow him, you ask, "Why did you call the ambulance?" He replies, "My wife's stomach hurts really bad!" As you enter the house, you see the patient. She looks to be about 25 years old. She is lying on her side on the floor with her knees drawn up to her chest. She is holding her lower abdominal area. She doesn't look at you as you enter. Your general impression is that she looks ill. Her skin color is pale. She responds to your questions slowly but appropriately. She tells you, "My stomach started hurting about an hour ago. I think I'm going to throw up!" Her respirations are rapid and shallow. Her radial pulse is weak and rapid, and her skin is cool and moist. There is no sign of trauma, and no obvious bleeding is observed.

1. This patient
   a. is not showing serious signs. The patient does not require transport or additional treatment.
   b. is showing serious signs. However, the patient should be allowed to be transported by her husband to the hospital for additional evaluation.
   c. is not showing serious signs. However, the patient should be placed on oxygen and transported in a sitting-up position.
   d. is showing early signs of shock. The patient should be placed on oxygen, positioned with knees drawn up, and provided quick transport with suction unit ready.

2. When beginning the exam of the patient's abdomen, you should
   a. have the patient drink a glass of water to rehydrate.
   b. ask her to straighten her legs.
   c. ask her to point with one finger to the area that is most painful.
   d. reassure the patient that palpation of her abdomen will not hurt.

En route to the hospital, the patient vomits several times.

3. The patient's emesis (vomitus)
   a. should be saved for possible testing at the hospital.
   b. should be saved but only if it looks bloody or dark in color.
   c. should be disposed of immediately in an infectious-waste container.
   d. should not be considered a serious sign of acute abdomen.

4. An ongoing assessment of this patient should be performed every
   a. minute.
   b. 3 minutes.
   c. 5 minutes.
   d. 15 minutes.

SCENARIO 10: **DOCUMENTATION EXERCISE**

Read the following scenario, and think about how you would document this call if you were the EMT who responded to the scene. Then answer the multiple-choice questions and fill in the sample prehospital-care report, basing your documentation on information from the scenario.

It is 10:00 PM on a Monday night. You and your partner, Mike, are just returning to the station when dispatch calls: "Unit 3, respond to 2235 Combee Road, cross street Rotary Avenue, for a 70-year-old male patient with abdominal pain." You advise dispatch that you are responding to the call. In about 6 minutes you arrive on the scene. It is a residential area of mobile-home parks. You knock on the door of a tidy mobile home and wait for an answer. An elderly woman who appears to be in her mid-60s answers the door. With BSI precautions on, you and your partner enter. You introduce yourself and your partner, and you ask, "What's the problem today?" As you are walking toward a back bedroom, she tells you that her husband, Mr. Carter, has been complaining of severe abdominal pain.

You enter the room and observe Mr. Carter sitting up in bed, holding a small trashcan between his legs. He leans over the trashcan and retches but does not vomit. He briefly looks up at you as you enter the room. His skin looks pale, and you notice sweat on his forehead. He grabs his back and holds his flank area. He is breathing adequately with no audible abnormal respiratory sounds. Mike quickly begins to take the vital signs as you begin a focused history and physical exam.

You begin your assessment by saying, "Hello, Mr. Carter. My name is Bill, and this is Mike. We are EMTs, and we're here to help you. What is the prob-

lem today?" Mr. Carter replies, "My stomach hurts!" You continue by asking, "When did the pain start? What were you doing when it started? Did it start all of a sudden?" Mr. Carter replies, "I was taking the trash out about 2 hours ago, and it started, all of a sudden. It really hurts!" You quickly say, "We'll do everything we can, but we need to ask you some more questions. First, I'll give you some oxygen through this mask. It may help you feel better." You place a nonrebreather mask and oxygen on Mr. Carter and adjust the flow to 15 lpm. Mike finishes taking Mr. Carter's pulse and tells you it is 124 per minute, regular and weak. His skin is cool, clammy, and pale. Mike places the pulse oximeter, and you note his SpO_2 is 97 percent.

You determine that ALS backup is required, and you advise dispatch of the need. Mike continues with the vital signs while you continue with the focused history and physical exam. You ask Mr. Carter, "Does anything make the pain better or worse?" He says, "No, it just hurts. I can't make it go away! Nothing seems to help it!" "Can you describe the discomfort you are having? Is it sharp or dull, pressing or squeezing? What does it feel like?" He says, "It feels like a ripping pain in my back and stomach. I don't know how else to describe it." Mike says that the patient's respirations are 20 per minute, full and regular, and breath sounds are clear and equal bilaterally. You continue with, "Does the pain you are having move, or radiate, to any other part of your body?" He replies, "It starts in my lower gut and moves to my back. It hurts really bad." "Mr. Carter, I really appreciate your cooperation. Is the oxygen helping you?" "Well, no, it doesn't seem to be helping at all," he replies.

Mrs. Carter is visibly shaken by the events taking place. You look her in the eye, place your hand on her shoulder, and say, "Mrs. Carter, we're doing everything we can right now, but I really need your help. Could you help us by getting together any medicines that Mr. Carter is currently taking and bring them to me?" She says, "I'll get them for you. All he takes is something for his high blood pressure."

Mike tells you the blood pressure is 140/70, the pupils are equal and reactive. Mr. Carter's neck veins are flat. His abdomen is soft. You carefully palpate the abdomen and palpate a pulsating mass in the center of his lower abdomen. You quickly check for the equality of his femoral pulses. His right femoral pulse is stronger than his left. You don't see any swelling in his lower extremities or back region. You continue the focused history and physical exam. "Mr. Carter, have you ever had any pain like this before?" You wait for a response. "No, I don't think I have," he says. "On a scale of 1–10, with 10 being the worst pain you have ever had, how would you rate your current pain?" you ask. He replies, "It's at least a 9 or a 10. It really hurts." "Mr. Carter, when did this start? I know you told me it was about 2 hours ago. It's 10:10 PM now, so it started about 8:00 PM, right?" you ask. He responds by saying, "Yes, that's right; it started about 8:00 PM tonight."

Mrs. Carter returns to the room with his medication, a hypertension medication for his blood pressure. You ask Mr. Carter if he is allergic to any medications, and he shakes his head no. "When did you last eat or drink anything?" you inquire. He says, "About 7:30 PM I ate a small bowl of soup. That was it." You hear the doorbell ring and hear the ALS crew entering the home. Paramedic Ray Chatlos comes into the room. You introduce him to Mr. Carter and provide a patient report to Ray. You help move Mr. Carter to the ALS ambulance.

1. The most likely explanation for Mr. Carter's abdominal pain is
   a. intestinal obstruction.
   b. appendicitis.
   c. cholecystitis.
   d. abdominal aortic aneurysm.

2. Which statement best describes the inequality of Mr. Carter's femoral pulses?
   a. Acute appendicitis can result in obstruction of the aortic arch that limits blood flow.
   b. Cholecystitis results in inflammation and swelling of the aortic sheath limiting flow.
   c. Intestinal obstruction results in swelling that constricts the lower aorta.
   d. An aortic aneurysm can result in obstruction of blood flow to the femoral arteries.

3. Mr. Carter's abdomen was palpated carefully. Why was careful palpation important for Mr. Carter?
   a. Deep palpation can cause rupture of an acute appendix.
   b. Deep palpation can cause rupture of the gallbladder.
   c. Deep palpation can cause rupture of the lower colon.
   d. Deep palpation can cause rupture of the aorta.

4. The condition that Mr. Carter is experiencing
   a. occurs in 20 percent of men over 50 years of age.
   b. occurs frequently in women over 60 years of age.
   c. occurs commonly in both sexes and all age groups.
   d. occurs in 50 percent of men at any age.

TRIP #			
MEDIC #			
BEGIN MILES			
END MILES			
CODE___/___	PAGE___/___		
UNITS ON SCENE			

EMERGENCY
TRIP SHEET

DAY				
DATE				
RECEIVED				
DISPATCHED				

NAME	SEX M F DOB ___/___/___	EN-ROUTE
ADDRESS	RACE	ON SCENE
CITY STATE	ZIP	TO HOSPITAL
PHONE ( ) -	PCP DR.	AT HOSPITAL
RESPONDED FROM	CITY	IN-SERVICE

TAKEN FROM	ZIP	CREW	CERT	STATE #
DESTINATION	REASON			

SSN - -	MEDICARE #	MEDICAID #
INSURANCE CO	INSURANCE #	GROUP #
RESPONSIBLE PARTY	ADDRESS	
CITY STATE ZIP PHONE ( ) -		
EMPLOYER		

IV THERAPY
SUCCESSFUL Y N # OF ATTEMPTS _____
ANGIO SIZE _____ga.
SITE _____
TOTAL FLUID INFUSED _____ cc
BLOOD DRAW Y N INITIALS

TIME	ON SCENE (1)	ON SCENE (2)	ON SCENE (3)	EN-ROUTE (1)	EN-ROUTE (2)	AT DESTINATION
BP						
PULSE						
RESP						
EKG						

INTUBATION INFORMATION
SUCCESSFUL Y N # OF ATTEMPTS _____
TUBE SIZE _____ mm
TIME _____ INITIALS _____

MEDICAL HISTORY

CONDITION CODES

MEDICATIONS

TREATMENTS

TIME	TREATMENT	DOSE	ROUTE	INI

ALLERGIES

C/C

EVENTS LEADING TO C/C

ASSESSMENT

TREATMENT

GCS	E___ V___ M___ TOTAL =
GCS	E___ V___ M___ TOTAL =

HOSPITAL CONTACTED

CPR BEGUN BY   B   P   TIME BEGUN

EMS SIGNATURE

AED USED   Y   N   BY:

RESUSCITATION TERMINATED - TIME

(   ) OSHA REGULATIONS FOLLOWE

22 Environmental Emergencies

OBJECTIVES

Numbered objectives are from the United States Department of Transportation EMT-Basic National Standard Curriculum. Asterisked objectives, if any, pertain to material that is supplemental to the DOT curriculum.

Cognitive

4-7.1 Describe the various ways that the body loses heat.
4-7.2 List the signs and symptoms of exposure to cold.
4-7.3 Explain the steps in providing emergency medical care to a patient exposed to cold.
4-7.4 List the signs and symptoms of exposure to heat.
4-7.5 Explain the steps in providing emergency medical care to a patient exposed to heat.
4-7.8 Discuss the emergency medical care of bites and stings.

KEY IDEAS

Conditions brought on by interactions between people and the environment are reviewed in this chapter. The signs, symptoms, and expected emergency management of extremes of hot and cold and of bites and stings are addressed.

- Hypothermia occurs when the body loses more heat than it gains or produces. Heat loss occurs through five mechanisms: radiation, convection, conduction, evaporation, and respiration.

- Exposure to cold can cause two kinds of emergencies. The first is generalized cold emergency (generalized hypothermia), which is an overall reduction in body temperature affecting the entire body. The second is local cold injury (commonly called "frostbite") that results in damage to body tissues in a specific part or parts of the body.

- Signs and symptoms of generalized hypothermia include decreasing mental status, decreasing motor and sensory function, and changing vital signs.

- Emergency medical care for generalized hypothermia includes preventing further heat loss, rewarming the patient as quickly and safely as possible, and staying alert for complications. It is important to remove the patient from the cold environment, handle the patient gently, administer oxygen, and be prepared to resuscitate the patient if he or she goes into cardiac arrest.

- Local cold injury results from the freezing of body tissue. Local cold injury falls into two categories: early (superficial) or late (deep) injury.

- Signs and symptoms of early (superficial) cold injury include blanching of the skin and loss of feeling. The skin and tissue beneath it remain soft. There may be a tingling sensation during rewarming.

- Signs and symptoms of late (deep) cold injury include white, waxy skin; swelling; and blisters. The skin and tissues beneath the skin feel firm to frozen. If thawed, the skin may appear flushed or mottled.

- Emergency medical care for local cold injury includes removing the patient from the cold environment, avoiding thawing if there is danger of refreezing, administering oxygen, removing jewelry or wet or restrictive clothing if not frozen to the skin, covering the skin with dressings or dry clothing, avoiding rubbing, and not permitting the patient to walk on an injured extremity.

- Urban hypothermia occurs in individuals who have a predisposition, disability, illness, or medication usage that renders them more susceptible to hypothermia. It is subdivided into two general etiologies: internal and external causes. External hypothermia results from lack of protection from a cold environment, while internal hypothermia results chiefly from elderly patients' attempts to reduce their winter heating bills.

- Hyperthermia occurs when the amount of heat the body produces or gains exceeds the amount the body loses.

- Signs and symptoms of a heat emergency may include muscle cramps, weakness, dizziness, heartbeat becoming progressively weak and rapid, deep breathing that becomes progressively shallow and weak, headache, seizures, loss of appetite, nausea or vomiting, altered mental status, and possible unresponsiveness. The skin may be moist and pale with a normal-to-cool temperature, or the skin may be hot and either dry or moist.

- Emergency medical care for the patient with a heat emergency includes moving the patient to a cool place, administering oxygen, removing as much clothing as possible, and cooling the patient. The patient should be placed supine with elevated feet. If the patient is fully responsive and not nauseated, the patient may drink cool water. (If the patient has an altered mental status or is nauseated or vomiting, do *not* give fluids.)

- Hot skin (which may be either dry or moist, depending on how the sweat mechanisms are operating) represents a dire medical emergency. The patient requires rapid cooling and immediate transport.

- Emergency care for bites and stings includes removing the stinger by scraping, washing the area, removing jewelry or other constricting objects, lowering the injection site slightly below the heart, and applying cold packs (except for marine stings and snakebite). It is important to be alert for and prepared to treat anaphylaxis. Keep the patient calm and transport.

TERMS AND CONCEPTS

1. Write the number of the correct term next to each definition.

   1. Active rewarming
   2. Conduction
   3. Convection
   4. Evaporation
   5. Thermoreceptor
   6. Hyperthermia
   7. Hypothermia
   8. Local cold injury
   9. Myxedema coma
   10. Passive rewarming
   11. Radiation
   12. Urban hypothermia
   13. Water chill
   14. Wind chill

   _____ a. Technique of aggressively applying heat to a patient to rewarm the body

   _____ b. A sensory receptor that is stimulated by temperature

   _____ c. Transfer of body heat through direct physical contact with nearby objects

   _____ d. Abnormally low core body temperature

   _____ e. Helping the body to rewarm itself by simply placing the patient in a warm environment and covering with blankets

   _____ f. Conversion of a liquid or solid into a gas

   _____ g. The increase in rate of cooling in the presence of water or wet clothing

   _____ h. Loss of body heat to the atmosphere when air passes over the body

   _____ i. Transfer of heat from the surface of one object to the surface of another without physical contact between the objects

   _____ j. The combined effect of wind speed and environmental temperature

   _____ k. Abnormally high core body temperature

   _____ l. Damage to body tissues in a specific part of the body resulting from exposure to cold

   _____ m. A complication that occurs late in the progression of hypothyroidism

   _____ n. Occurs in individuals who have a predisposition, disability, illness, or medication usage that renders them more susceptible to hypothermia; is subdivided into two general etiologies—external and internal

CONTENT REVIEW

1. There are five basic mechanisms by which the body loses heat. Which mechanism results in a loss of body heat to the atmosphere when air passes over it?
   a. Respiration
   b. Conduction
   c. Consolidation
   d. Convection

2. Exposure to cold can cause which of the following two kinds of emergencies?
   a. Generalized cold emergency and generalized hypothermia
   b. Generalized hypothermia and local cold injury
   c. Generalized hypovolemia and local cold injury
   d. Generalized hypovolemia and generalized hypothermia

3. Which factor(s) may place a patient at greatest risk for developing generalized hypothermia?
   a. Drugs and alcohol
   b. Middle age
   c. Female gender
   d. Asian descent

4. The five stages of hypothermia are listed below. Next to each stage place a number from 1 to 5 (earliest to latest) to indicate which stage it represents.

   _____ a. Decreased vital signs

   _____ b. Death

   _____ c. Shivering

   _____ d. Decreased level of responsiveness

   _____ e. Apathy and decreased muscle function

5. Emergency care for generalized hypothermia should include
   a. careful and gentle handling of the patient.
   b. asking the patient to briskly walk about to raise his body temperature.
   c. administering oxygen by nonrebreather mask at 6 lpm.
   d. checking the patient's temperature with the EMT's hand on the patient's forehead.

6. Which statement best describes an appropriate technique for active rewarming?
   a. All unresponsive patients should be actively rewarmed.
   b. Increase the body temperature by no more than 1°F per hour.
   c. Immerse the patient in a hot tub of water or place in a hot shower.
   d. Apply heat first to the extremities, then the torso.

7. Immersion hypothermia should be considered in all cases of accidental immersion. Body temperature can drop to the water temperature in as little as
   a. 10 minutes.
   b. 15 minutes.
   c. 20 minutes.
   d. 25 minutes.

8. When managing the patient with immersion hypothermia be sure to
   a. lift the patient from the water in a vertical position.
   b. ask the patient to swim to you as quickly as possible.
   c. ask the patient to quickly remove all wet clothing.
   d. provide treatment similar to that for generalized hypothermia.

9. The stages of local cold injury are
   a. frostbite and hypothermia.
   b. early (superficial) and late (deep).
   c. frostnip and frostbite.
   d. generalized and local.

10. Appropriate management of local cold injuries includes
    a. rubbing or massaging the affected skin.
    b. removing clothing that is frozen to the skin.
    c. initiation of thawing, even if refreezing is possible.
    d. the careful removal of clothing and jewelry.

11. Guidelines for rapid rewarming of local cold injuries include
    a. maintaining the water temperature between 120 and 130°F.
    b. dressing the area with a nonsterile moist dressing and petroleum.
    c. rewarming all injuries regardless of transport times or temperatures.
    d. keeping the tissue in warm water until it is soft and the color returns.

12. The term that best describes a grouping of heat-related emergencies is
    a. hypothermia.
    b. hyperthermia.
    c. hyperpyrexia.
    d. hyperenviron.

13. Which of the following is a factor that can increase an individual's reaction to a heat-related injury?
    a. Heart disease
    b. Gastrointestinal disorders
    c. Cigarette smoking
    d. Psychological disorders

14. A patient represents a dire medical emergency if he or she has been exposed to heat and has which of the following signs or symptoms?
    a. Cool, pale, moist skin
    b. Dizziness
    c. Muscle cramps
    d. Hot skin, either moist or dry

15. When cooling a heat-emergency patient with hot skin, moist or dry,
    a. cooling takes priority over all other emergency-care procedures.
    b. one cooling method will generally be effective to cool the patient.
    c. be prepared to manage seizures and to prevent aspiration.
    d. place cold packs on the patient's hands and feet.

16. A heat-emergency patient with moist, pale, normal-to-cool skin who is responsive and vomiting should be given
    a. cool water to drink.
    b. nothing by mouth.
    c. a half glass of water every 15 minutes.
    d. warm water to drink.

17. A heat-emergency patient with moist, pale, normal-to-cool skin needs transport if the patient
    a. is sweating.
    b. has a temperature of 99°F.
    c. has a headache.
    d. has a history of medical problems.

18. The first step in the emergency medical care of any patient with a heat emergency is to
    a. administer oxygen at 15 lpm via a nonrebreather mask.
    b. place the patient supine and elevate the feet.
    c. move the patient to a cool place.
    d. remove as much clothing as possible.

19. Which of the following are grave indications that the heat-emergency patient is deteriorating?
    a. The blood pressure falls, and the patient feels exhausted.
    b. The capillary refill time decreases, and respirations are labored.
    c. The pulse rate changes rapidly, and the mental status declines.
    d. The patient begins to shiver, and the skin becomes pale.

20. Which statement is most correct related to bites and stings?
    a. Snake bites are common and annually result in a large number of fatalities.
    b. Exercise caution during the scene size-up to protect yourself.
    c. Complications associated with airway and breathing never occur.
    d. Most insect bites result in major anaphylactic reactions.

21. Urban hypothermia
    a. is limited to individuals who live outdoors and are unable to escape the cold environment.
    b. is limited to the elderly who attempt to reduce their home-heating bills.
    c. is limited to northern climates during the winter months.
    d. occurs in individuals with a predisposition to hypothermia.

CASE STUDY 1

You are standing by to provide medical coverage during a 10-kilometer running event on a hot summer day. You have responded to a call for a runner who is disoriented. The scene appears safe as you arrive at the finish line. As an event official leads you to the patient, you ask, "Why did you call the ambulance?" She replies, "This guy just finished the race, and he isn't acting right!"

As you approach the patient, you note that he looks to be about 25 years old. He is lying next to the finish line in full sunshine. He is wearing a polyester running suit. He is lying on his back, talking incoherently. He doesn't notice you as you kneel down beside him. Your general impression is that he looks ill. His skin color is red. He responds to your questions with inappropriate statements. His respirations are rapid and shallow, his radial pulse is weak and rapid, and his skin is hot to the touch and moist. There is no sign of trauma, and no bleeding is observed. You rapidly move the patient to the back of the ambulance, where the air conditioner is already turned on.

1. The next *best* action to take for this patient is to
    a. contact medical direction for treatment options.
    b. remove as much clothing as possible.
    c. fan the patient aggressively.
    d. give the patient cool water to drink.

You have removed the patient from the hot environment, performed the action taken above, and begun to administer oxygen at 15 lpm by nonrebreather mask.

2. The next *best* action to take for this patient is to
    a. radio a report on the patient's condition to the receiving facility.
    b. place the patient in a position of comfort.
    c. pour cool water over the patient's body.
    d. obtain a SAMPLE history.

You have begun rapid transport to the hospital.

3. The use of cold water should be avoided in this patient because it may
   a. stimulate the release of norepinephrine and increase the core temperature.
   b. stimulate central thermoreceptors and cause a reflex peripheral vasodilation.
   c. cause the acute onset of seizure activity.
   d. may produce vasoconstriction and shivering.

CASE STUDY 2

You are dispatched to the scene of a possible snakebite. The scene appears safe as you arrive at a hunting lodge in the woods. A man dressed in hunting clothing meets you at the gate and escorts you to the patient. As you follow him, you ask the hunter, "Why did you call the ambulance?" He replies, "Tony just finished for the day and was walking back to the lodge. He was walking across Crooked Creek and a cottonmouth got him! I blasted it and brought it and Tony back to the lodge. Then I called you."

As you approach the patient, you note that he looks to be about 35 years old. He is sitting in a chair, holding his leg. He looks at you as you enter the room. Your general impression is that he looks well, although he appears to be in pain. His skin color is normal. He responds to your questions appropriately. His respirations are normal. His radial pulse is strong and regular. His skin is warm and dry. You examine the bite and observe two distinct puncture wounds on the lower leg. The wound is red and moderately swollen. There are no other signs of trauma, and no bleeding is observed. The snake (which is obviously dead) is lying next to the patient. Tony's friend puts it into a box so you can take it along to the hospital. You are extremely careful in handling the box, even though you are sure the snake is dead.

1. Appropriate treatment for this patient should include
   a. application of a commercial cold pack to the area.
   b. washing the area with a mild agent or strong soap solution.
   c. encouraging the patient to move about to reduce stress and anxiety.
   d. application of a commercial hot pack to the area.

2. What additional treatments should be provided for this patient?
   a. Lower the injection site slightly below the level of the heart.
   b. Cut and then suction the venom from the bite site.
   c. Administer epinephrine and then cut and suction the bite.
   d. Elevate the site slightly above the level of the heart.

3. This patient should be observed closely for signs of
   a. respiratory distress.
   b. hives.
   c. hypotension.
   d. anaphylaxis.

CASE STUDY 3

You are dispatched to a call for a woman down. It is the middle of winter, and the temperature is in the mid-20s. The scene appears safe as you arrive at a single-story residence. A well-dressed man who introduces himself as a neighbor meets you at the ambulance and escorts you to the patient. As you follow him, you ask, "Why did you call the ambulance?" He replies, "Mary is in her 80s and lives by herself. I stop by to check on her when I can. I found her on the floor of her garage, and I can't wake her up!"

As you enter the garage, you note that it is quite cold inside. The patient is lying on her side next to her car. She is dressed in a nightgown and a light bathrobe and slippers. She doesn't respond as you kneel down next to her. You apply a painful stimulus, and she does not respond. Your general impression is that she looks ill. Her skin color is gray. Her respirations are slow and shallow. Her radial pulse is slow and barely palpable. There is no sign of trauma, and no bleeding is observed. You move the patient to the back of the ambulance where the heater is already on.

1. Assess the pulse in this patient for
   a. 10–20 seconds.
   b. 20–30 seconds.
   c. 30–45 seconds.
   d. 1–2 minutes.

2. This patient requires which of the following?
   a. Active rewarming
   b. Passive rewarming
   c. Immersion in a tub of hot water or in a hot shower
   d. Active rewarming if more than 30 minutes from the hospital

3. When moving this patient to the ambulance, you should
   a. move her as quickly as you can, using any possible method.
   b. try to keep her head elevated during movement, if possible.
   c. hyperventilate her during movement.
   d. handle her extremely gently.

CASE STUDY 4

You are dispatched to a call for a child with a local cold injury. It is mid-December and quite cold. The scene appears safe as you arrive at a small convenience store. Several children are standing next to the door as you arrive. You step out and ask, "Why did you call the ambulance?" One of the children replies, "I think my toes are frostbit! I called my mom and she's going to meet us here." The boy is 12 or 13 years old. He is dressed in a heavy coat and boots that look wet. He is alert and oriented to your questions. Your general impression is that he looks well. His skin color is normal. His respirations are normal. His radial pulse is strong and regular. There is no sign of trauma, and no bleeding is observed. You move the patient to the back of the ambulance where the heater is already on. You remove his shoes and socks. He tells you his right big toe is numb. You examine his toe, and it looks somewhat white.

1. You would expect which of the following signs or symptoms to be present if the patient has suffered an early, or superficial, local cold injury?
   a. Good feeling and sensation in the toe
   b. Firm-to-frozen feeling when the skin is palpated
   c. When you palpate the skin, the normal color does not return
   d. Swelling and blisters

2. Which of the following is an appropriate treatment for this patient?
   a. Remove wet or restrictive clothing.
   b. Gently massage the area to increase blood flow.
   c. Administer oxygen at 6 lpm.
   d. Avoid splinting the area; this would reduce blood flow.

The toe has thawed in the warm ambulance. The tissue is soft. The color and sensation have returned to the toe.

3. It is now *most* important to
   a. elevate the affected extremity.
   b. prevent the possibility of refreezing.
   c. dress the area with a dry, sterile dressing.
   d. dress the area with a moist, sterile dressing.

ENRICHMENT

1. Lightning-strike injuries
   a. result in about 50 deaths per year.
   b. occur most frequently on Wednesdays.
   c. occur mostly in work-related situations.
   d. most often involve multiple victims.

2. Lightning-strike patients
   a. are considered medical and trauma patients.
   b. do not routinely require spinal immobilization.
   c. are frequently talking on the telephone when struck.
   d. infrequently suffer damage to air-containing body cavities.

3. Dislocations and fractures associated with lightning strikes result from the
   a. thunder "blast wave" and the speed of the lightning strike.
   b. thunder "blast wave" and strong muscular contractions.
   c. burning effect of the lightning strike and strong muscular contractions.
   d. burning effect and the speed of the lightning strike.

4. What two types of poisonous snakes contribute to most snakebites in the United States?
   a. King cobras and coral snakes
   b. Coral snakes and pit vipers
   c. Pit vipers and king cobras
   d. King snakes and pit vipers

5. The signs and symptoms of a pit-viper bite are
   a. usually delayed for up to 8 hours.
   b. usually gauged by how much poison was injected.
   c. usually delayed for up to 1 hour.
   d. unrelated to the patient's size or weight.

6. Identify each of the following characteristics as belonging to either a poisonous (P) or a nonpoisonous (N) snake.

   _____ a. Triangular head

   _____ b. Pit between eye and mouth

   _____ c. Round head

   _____ d. Round pupils

   _____ e. Small teeth

   _____ f. Elliptical pupils

7. The black widow spider has a
   a. shiny black body, thin legs, and a crimson red hourglass on its abdomen.
   b. dull black body, thin legs, and a crimson red circle on its abdomen.
   c. shiny black body, short legs, and a white circle on its abdomen.
   d. dull black body, thin legs, and a red triangle on its back.

8. General signs and symptoms of a black widow spider bite include
   a. severe muscle spasms in the shoulders, back, chest, and abdomen.
   b. drooping eyelids with loss of eye movement and blinking.
   c. diminished saliva production and an inability to swallow.
   d. lower back pain and uncontrollable bowel movements.

9. This bite is usually painless for the first few hours. Several hours later, the site becomes bluish, surrounded by a red halo or "bull's-eye" pattern. The bite generally does not heal and may require surgical repair. These are characteristics of the bite of a
   a. southern fire ant.
   b. Rocky Mountain tick.
   c. brown recluse spider.
   d. scorpion.

10. The venom of aquatic organisms may be destroyed by the application of
   a. heat.
   b. rubbing alcohol.
   c. ice.
   d. tannic acid in the form of a tea bag.

11. Myxedema coma
   a. may make a person less susceptible to becoming hypothermic.
   b. occurs late in the progression of hyperthyroidism.
   c. occurs commonly in about 50 percent of all hyperthyroidism patients.
   d. is precipitated by exposure to cold, a recent illness, or infection and trauma

SCENARIO 11: DOCUMENTATION EXERCISE

Read the following scenario, and think about how you would document this call if you were the EMT who responded to the scene. Then answer the multiple-choice questions and fill in the sample prehospital-care report, basing your documentation on information from the scenario.

It is 3:30 PM in midsummer. It is a very hot day with the air temperature at 95°F and a humidity of 75 percent. You and your partner, Katy, just stopped to pick up a drink and are heading back to the station. The alert sounds: "Unit 6, respond to 500 Highlands Road for an altered mental status patient; cross street, Gachet Boulevard. Time out is 1530 hours." Katy tells dispatch that you are responding. You arrive in about 2 minutes at a small home that appears unkempt; the grass needs to be mowed, and the house is in need of basic repairs. Katy advises dispatch of arrival on-scene. With BSI precautions in place, you walk to the front of the home and knock. A girl of about 15 years of age answers the door and asks you to come in. You introduce yourself and Katy to her and find out that her name is Misty, and she is a friend of the elderly woman who lives in the home. The elderly woman's name is Mrs. Holland. Misty continues by telling you that she checked on Mrs. Holland this afternoon, and she was acting funny. Misty then called rescue for assistance.

It is quite hot in the house. The windows are open, but very little air is moving in the house. You walk to a back bedroom and see Mrs. Holland sitting in a chair next to her bed. She looks to be about 75 years of age. She is dressed in a long-sleeved shirt, a sweater, and long pants. She looks at you as you enter the room. Her skin looks flushed. She is breathing adequately with no audible, abnormal respiratory sounds heard. Your initial impression is that she looks ill. Katy quickly begins to take the vital signs as you begin a focused history and physical exam.

You begin your assessment by saying, "Hello, Mrs. Holland. My name is Roger, and this is Katy. We are EMTs, and we're here to help you. What's the problem today?" You place a nonrebreather mask on Mrs. Holland and set the oxygen flow rate at 15 lpm. She looks at you sleepily and replies, "Nothing. I'm just fine. Did you get my TV fixed?" You say, "Misty is concerned about you. She says that you seem confused about something." Mrs. Holland replies, "Well, Misty is a nice girl. I'm just glad you're here to get my TV fixed. Will it take you long? Misty, my head really hurts; will you get me some aspirin?" "Mrs. Holland, we are EMTs, and we are here to provide medical care for you. Misty is concerned about your health." You reach down to take her pulse and note that her skin is hot to the touch, and her pulse is rapid and bounding. Mrs. Holland retches as if to vomit. You hand her a small basin that is next to the bed. It is very warm in the room. You are sweating from the heat. You ask Misty if there is an air conditioner, and she says no, the house has no air-conditioning. You ask her to open some windows to try to get some air movement in the room.

You recognize that the situation is life-threatening and request ALS backup. You ask Misty about Mrs. Holland's medical history and if she takes any medications. She tells you that she doesn't know if she takes any medications but that she has a history of a thyroid disorder. You tell Katy to get the cot. As Katy heads out to the rescue vehicle, she hands you a report form with the vitals recorded. The respirations are 24 per minute and rapid, the pulse is 120 strong and bounding, the skin is flushed and hot and dry to the touch, the pupils are equal and reactive to light, the blood pressure is 164/92, and the SpO_2 is 98 percent. You help Mrs. Holland take off her heavy sweater, and you ask Misty to fan her. Katy, out at the ambulance, wets a sheet with tepid water, places it on the cot, and turns the air-conditioning on high. She removes the cot from the ambulance, closes the rear doors, and returns to the room with the cot. Katy and Misty remove all of Mrs. Holland's clothing and place two towels to cover her genitals and breasts. You move her to the cot and place cold packs in her armpits, on either side of her neck, and behind her knees. You encourage Misty to continue to fan Mrs. Holland aggressively.

The ALS crew arrives just as you are exiting the front door. Paramedic Darleen Brooks introduces herself to Mrs. Holland and looks to you for a report. You provide a quick report and help place Mrs. Holland in the ALS vehicle. You clean up your vehicle and advise dispatch that you are available for another call.

1. Mrs. Holland is mostly likely suffering from _____, which has a mortality rate ranging from _____ to _____.
   a. heat cramps, 5 to 50 percent
   b. heat exhaustion, 30 to 60 percent
   c. heat stroke, 20 to 80 percent
   d. high fever, 15 to 60 percent

2. The cooling of Mrs. Holland
   a. was appropriately performed.
   b. should have been performed by pouring ice water over Mrs. Holland's body.
   c. should have been performed by surrounding Mrs. Holland's torso with ice packs.
   d. should have included placing Mrs. Holland's hands and feet in ice water.

3. What information that Roger obtained made him *most* likely to believe that Mrs. Holland was a priority patient who required rapid transport and ALS management?
   a. Environmental factors
   b. Mrs. Holland's confusion
   c. Mrs. Holland's headache
   d. Mrs. Holland's hot and dry skin

4. Roger and Katy did not provide any cool water for Mrs. Holland to drink. Was this appropriate?
   a. Yes, Mrs. Holland was nauseated and had an altered level of consciousness.
   b. Yes, Mrs. Holland had a headache and is over 65 years of age.
   c. No, Mrs. Holland should have been given a half glass of water every 15 minutes.
   d. No, Mrs. Holland should have been given one full glass of water.

5. An air temperature of 95°F and a relative humidity of 75 percent would represent a
   a. moderate danger on the heat-and-humidity risk scale.
   b. severe danger on the heat-and-humidity risk scale.
   c. caution status on the heat-and-humidity risk scale.
   d. safe area on the heat-and-humidity risk scale.

EMERGENCY TRIP SHEET

TRIP #	
MEDIC #	
BEGIN MILES	
END MILES	
CODE___/___ PAGE___/___	
UNITS ON SCENE	

BILLING USE ONLY			
DAY			
DATE			
RECEIVED			
DISPATCHED			
EN-ROUTE			
ON SCENE			
TO HOSPITAL			
AT HOSPITAL			
IN-SERVICE			

NAME   SEX   M   F   DOB ___/___/___

ADDRESS   RACE

CITY   STATE   ZIP

PHONE ( )   -   PCP DR.

RESPONDED FROM   CITY

TAKEN FROM   ZIP

DESTINATION   REASON

SSN   -   -   MEDICARE #   MEDICAID #

INSURANCE CO   INSURANCE #   GROUP #

RESPONSIBLE PARTY   ADDRESS

CITY   STATE   ZIP   PHONE ( )   -

EMPLOYER

CREW	CERT	STATE #

TIME	ON SCENE (1)	ON SCENE (2)	ON SCENE (3)	EN-ROUTE (1)	EN-ROUTE (2)	AT DESTINATION
BP						
PULSE						
RESP						
EKG						

IV THERAPY
SUCCESSFUL   Y   N   # OF ATTEMPTS _____
ANGIO SIZE _____ga.
SITE _____
TOTAL FLUID INFUSED _____ cc
BLOOD DRAW   Y   N   INITIALS

INTUBATION INFORMATION
SUCCESSFUL   Y   N   # OF ATTEMPTS _____
TUBE SIZE _____ mm
TIME _____ INITIALS _____

MEDICAL HISTORY

CONDITION CODES | | | |

MEDICATIONS

TREATMENTS

TIME	TREATMENT	DOSE	ROUTE	INIT

ALLERGIES

C/C

EVENTS LEADING TO C/C

ASSESSMENT

TREATMENT

GCS	E___ V___ M___ TOTAL =				
GCS	E___ V___ M___ TOTAL =				

HOSPITAL CONTACTED

CPR BEGUN BY   B   P   TIME BEGUN

EMS SIGNATURE

AED USED   Y   N   BY:

RESUSCITATION TERMINATED - TIME

( ) OSHA REGULATIONS FOLLOWED

23 Drowning and Diving Emergencies

OBJECTIVES

Numbered objectives are from the United States Department of Transportation EMT-Basic National Standard Curriculum. Asterisked objectives, if any, pertain to material that is supplemental to the DOT curriculum.

Cognitive

4-7.6 Recognize the signs and symptoms of water-related emergencies.
4-7.7 Describe the complications of submersion.

KEY IDEAS

Drowning is often assumed to be the major cause of death from water-related emergencies. Drowning actually accounts for only one in 20 water-related deaths. Drowning- and diving-emergency statistics, signs, symptoms, and management are reviewed in this chapter.

- Many drownings could be prevented if personal flotation devices (PFDs) were utilized in and around water, adult supervision were provided around swimming pools, and pools were fenced and locked.

- Always suspect a spinal injury in any swimmer that is found unresponsive in or out of the water, has injury or alcohol-intoxication signs, or has used a water slide or has been into the water.

- Never enter the water to rescue a patient unless you meet all of the following criteria: you are a good swimmer, you are specially trained in water-rescue techniques, you are wearing a personal flotation device, and you are accompanied by other rescuers.

- Use the reach, throw, row, and go strategy to reach a responsive, close-to-shore swimmer who requires rescue.

- All drowning patients require transport even if you think they are stable.

- Attempt resuscitation on any pulseless, nonbreathing patient who has been submerged in cold water (41°F) for an extended time period.

- For the water-related-emergency patient, look for signs and symptoms of any of the following: airway obstruction, absent or inadequate breathing, pulselessness, spinal or head injury, soft-tissue injuries, musculoskeletal injuries, external or internal bleeding, shock, hypothermia, or alcohol or drug abuse.

- The emergency care for drowning patients includes the following: If spinal injury is suspected, immobilize the patient. If no spinal injury is suspected, position the patient on the left side, suction as needed, rapidly establish an airway, begin positive-pressure ventilation with supplemental oxygen (if pulseless and apneic, proceed with AED protocol), watch for gastric distention, and transport quickly.

TERMS AND CONCEPTS

1. Write the number of the correct term next to each definition.

    1. Drowning
    2. Gastric distention
    3. Mammalian diving reflex
    4. Surfactant

    _____ a. A substance responsible for maintaining surface tension in the alveoli

    _____ b. The body's natural response to submersion in cold water in which breathing is inhibited, the heart rate decreases, and blood vessels constrict in order to maintain cerebral and cardiac blood flow

    _____ c. A person is submerged or immersed in a liquid that prevents the person from breathing.

    _____ d. The filling of the stomach with water and/or air, causing an enlarged abdomen, which makes ventilation difficult

CONTENT REVIEW

1. Deaths from drowning
    a. occur only in deep water.
    b. are often associated with the use of alcohol.
    c. are not affected by the wearing of personal flotation devices.
    d. are not affected by adult supervision at swimming pools.

2. The two major age groups that are most at risk of death from drowning are
    a. children less than 2 years of age and young adults age 18–24.
    b. children less than 5 years of age and teenagers.
    c. children less than 8 years of age and adolescents age 15–18.
    d. children less than 10 years of age and adults age 65 and over.

3. Between 10 and 20 percent of drowning patients aspirate no water into their lungs during submersion. This is referred to as a
    a. hemostatic drowning.
    b. pernicious drowning.
    c. dry drowning.
    d. surfactant drowning.

4. Drowning patients may be placed into one of the four categories listed below. Into which category should you place a patient with an altered mental status and a persistent cough?
    a. Asymptomatic
    b. Symptomatic
    c. Class I
    d. Near drowning

5. Abdominal thrusts should be used in the drowning victim
    a. routinely during resuscitation efforts.
    b. never because it may lead to vomiting and aspiration.
    c. only if a foreign body airway obstruction is suspected.
    d. only in salt-water immersion incidents.

6. If the drowning patient is close to shore, the strategy you should use is
   a. reach, go, row, and tow.
   b. call, throw, tow, and go.
   c. reach, throw, row, and go.
   d. go, throw, reach, and row.

7. A patient is found unresponsive, floating in shallow water. Your *primary* suspicion should be that
   a. the patient has a spinal injury.
   b. the patient is a poor swimmer.
   c. the patient was struck by a boat.
   d. the patient had a seizure.

8. You are evaluating a young patient who, you learn, has been submerged in cold water (<41°F) for 30 minutes. You should
   a. not attempt resuscitation on this patient.
   b. not attempt resuscitation until ALS arrives on-scene.
   c. attempt resuscitation of the patient with full efforts.
   d. provide a brief resuscitative effort for the benefit of the family.

9. Differences between salt-water and fresh-water drowning
   a. pertain to whether or not surfactant is washed out.
   b. explain why there are more drownings in salt water than in fresh water.
   c. result in different degrees of respiratory distress suffered by the patient.
   d. do not play a major role in resuscitation of submersion victims.

10. When a person dives into water colder than 68°F, which controversial reflex may prevent death even after prolonged submersion?
    a. Human diving reflex
    b. Beck's diving reflex
    c. Mammalian diving reflex
    d. Momentary submersion reflex

CASE STUDY 1

You are dispatched to a call for a drowning. You arrive at a small home located just outside of town. The scene appears safe as you arrive. A woman is frantically motioning to you. She screams at you as you exit the ambulance, "Please! Please! Hurry! My daughter! I just found her floating in the pool!" You follow the distraught mother to a backyard pool. As you approach the patient, you note that she looks to be about 4 years old. She is lying supine on the pool deck. CPR is being performed by a neighbor. The patient is located next to the shallow end of the pool. Your general impression is that she looks ill. Her skin color is cyanotic. She is unresponsive to pain. She has no respirations and no palpable carotid pulse. There is a small laceration on the front of her forehead with minor bleeding.

1. Which of the following is the appropriate *initial* treatment for this patient?
   a. Determine the "down time" before beginning resuscitation.
   b. Determine the "down time" and the temperature of the water before beginning resuscitation.
   c. Begin resuscitation efforts after performing a detailed assessment.
   d. Begin resuscitation efforts immediately.

2. *Immediate* treatment for this patient should include which of the following?
   a. Checking for gastric distention
   b. Treating the patient for a possible spinal injury
   c. Controlling the bleeding from the laceration
   d. Administering oxygen by nonrebreather mask

3. You have been providing positive-pressure ventilation to the patient for a few minutes. You notice that the patient's abdomen is distended, and you cannot effectively ventilate the patient. You should
   a. reduce the volume and pressure delivered during your ventilations.
   b. continue with the ventilations and advise the ALS crew of the condition when they arrive.
   c. increase the volume and pressure delivered during your ventilations.
   d. turn the patient on her left side and apply pressure over the epigastric region; have suction available.

CASE STUDY 2

You are dispatched to the city pool for a drowning. Upon arrival you observe a small crowd of people standing around a young boy who is sitting up in a chair. The scene appears safe as you walk to the patient. A lifeguard approaches and tells you, "I found this kid on the bottom of the pool. He couldn't have been under very long. I pulled him out and gave him one breath. He coughed, and then he woke up. I called his mom to come and get him. She should be here in a few minutes." As you approach the patient, you note that he looks to be about 11 years old. He looks up at you as you approach. He is coughing occasionally. Your general impression is that he looks well. His skin color is normal. He answers your questions appropriately. His respirations are normal. His radial pulse is strong and regular. There is no sign of trauma, and no bleeding is observed. No other findings are made during the focused history and physical exam.

1. Should this patient be allowed to return home with his mother?
   a. Yes. The patient is stable. Allow him to return home.
   b. Yes, but only after you have described to his mother potential complications that can occur and what to watch for.
   c. No. Observe the patient at the scene for at least 30 minutes before making a decision.
   d. No. Fatal complications from a submersion can occur as long as 72 hours after the incident. He must be transported for evaluation by a physician.

2. Your care and treatment for this patient should include which of the following?
   a. No care is required. The patient will be allowed to return home.
   b. Administer oxygen, monitor carefully, and transport on his left side.
   c. Monitor carefully, and transport sitting up.
   d. Administer oxygen, reevaluate his condition, and reach a decision following further observation.

3. This patient would be placed into which category?
   a. Asymptomatic
   b. Symptomatic
   c. Cardiac arrest
   d. Obviously dead

ENRICHMENT

1. Scuba-diving emergencies
   a. never involve drowning.
   b. occur only in areas near the ocean.
   c. are increasing in incidence.
   d. can be managed only by a paramedic.

2. Which law of physics states that, at a constant temperature, the volume of a gas is inversely related to the pressure?
   a. Boyle's law
   b. Dalton's law
   c. Henry's law
   d. Charles's law

3. Decompression sickness
   a. occurs as a result of bubbles formed from the expansion of nitrogen.
   b. has two primary effects: acting as emboli and reducing oxyhemoglobin loading.
   c. will be temporarily relieved by getting to a high altitude, as in an airplane.
   d. is more likely to occur while diving in warm rather than cold water.

4. The joint in which pain associated with decompression sickness is most commonly experienced is the
   a. hip.
   b. knee.
   c. shoulder.
   d. elbow.

5. Decompression sickness can be divided into three categories. Complete the following chart by indicating with an X or a check mark if the sign or symptom is most likely associated with Type 1 decompression sickness (DCS), Type 2 decompression sickness (DCS), or arterial gas embolism (AGE). Since each may be associated with more than one category, one, two, or three check marks may be used for each sign or symptom.

Sign or Symptom	Type 1 DCS	Type 2 DCS	AGE
Pain in joints or tendons			
Low back pain			
Skin rash, itching			
Altered mental status			
Substernal burning sensation on inhalation			
Dyspnea			
Headache, visual disturbance			
Bloody sputum			
Nausea and vomiting			

6. The "squeeze" or barotrauma
   a. results from too rapid a descent.
   b. occurs during either ascent or descent.
   c. commonly occurs in divers with hypertension.
   d. results in a staggering gait or lack of coordination.

SCENARIO 12: **DOCUMENTATION EXERCISE**

Read the following scenario, and think about how you would document this call if you were the EMT who responded to the scene. Then answer the multiple-choice questions and fill in the sample pre-hospital-care report, basing your documentation on information from the scenario.

It's 6:30 PM on a Thursday evening. You and your partner are just sitting down to supper when the alarm sounds: "Unit 5, respond to a vehicle accident at 3211 North Lucerne Park Road; cross street, Old Crossover Road. Time out 1830 hours." You take a bite of biscuit, grab your jacket, and quickly move to the vehicle. Your partner, Brent, advises dispatch that you are responding. Dispatch tells you that a vehicle has plunged down a steep embankment; the local fire department, ALS backup, and law enforcement are responding.

You arrive on-scene in 6 minutes. A police officer directs you to the side of the road. A group of people are crowded around a person lying on his side. With BSI precautions in place, you and Brent approach the crowd, and you say, "Good evening. My name is Jennifer, and this is Brent. We are EMTs. What happened?" The police officer replies, "The best I can make out at this time is that this guy was driving a car that went down that embankment. He was going too fast for the curve, and his car just lost it." A bystander quickly chimes in, "I saw the car flip at least three times, and I found it lying upside down in about 5 feet of water. These two guys [he points to two young men who are wet and have blankets draped around their shoulders] pulled him out of the car, started CPR, and carried him to the top of the hill."

Brent is performing an initial assessment. He notes that the patient appears to be about 17 years of age. He is unresponsive to voice or pain; has a small laceration on his forehead; is breathing adequately with no abnormal respiratory sounds audible; has a strong, regular radial pulse; and his skin is cold and wet. Oxygen via a nonrebreather mask at 15 lpm is placed. Brent asks a trained Emergency Medical Responder to stabilize the cervical spine. You quickly inspect the neck for trauma and then place the cervical-spine-immobilization collar. Brent checks the airway for secretions or foreign material and finds the airway is clear. You quickly cut the clothing off the young man, inspect his back, position the spine board behind him, and carefully roll him onto the board. You place a heavy blanket on the patient.

Brent begins taking the vital signs while you begin a rapid trauma assessment. Your rapid trauma assessment reveals a 3-inch laceration on his forehead, a large bruise on his left lateral chest, an intact pelvis, and a fracture of his left ankle. You check for a distal pulse and sensation in his ankle before and after you splint it.

Suddenly, the patient begins coughing and opens his eyes. You tell him, "Hi. You've been in an accident. I'm Jennifer, and my partner is Brent. We've immobilized you just in case you may have other injuries. Please try to remain still. Could you tell me where you hurt?" The patient looks at you but does not respond. His coughing continues for about 30 seconds before it begins to diminish. Brent has completed the vitals and reports that the patient's respirations are 20 per minute; the breath sounds are equal and clear; the pulse is 90 per minute, strong and regular; the skin is pale and cold; the pupils are equal and reactive and respond briskly to light; the blood pressure is 124/74; and the SpO_2 is 97 percent.

The police officer now tells you that the patient's name is Billy Wilson. He was on the way home from basketball practice and didn't make the curve. The officer also tells you that the two young men who pulled Billy from the car reported that he was in the water for at least 10 or 15 minutes before they were able to get him out of the car. The young man who pulled him free is standing behind the policeman and says, "We were coming back from the movies when we saw someone standing beside the road screaming and waving. We turned around and came back to help. He said a car went down the embankment. We found the spot where the car went off the road, and we went down to find the car. I can't believe how cold the water was. It came up to my chest. The car was turned over. I pulled the door open and kept grabbing till I felt something; I could feel it was a person, but he was jammed inside. I took my buddy's knife and cut the seatbelt. We were pulling and pulling and finally he came out. We pulled him to the bank, and we started CPR. After a few minutes he coughed and started breathing. So then we pulled him up the bank to the road. He was in the water for at least 10 or 15 minutes."

You look up and see the ALS unit arriving on-scene. It is a new paramedic whom you don't recognize. You quickly provide a report and assist with placing the patient in the ALS ambulance.

1. Treatment and management of Billy should be focused on
   a. hypothermia and traumatic injuries.
   b. drowning and traumatic injuries.
   c. drowning, hypothermia, and traumatic injuries.
   d. traumatic injuries only.

2. Billy's breath sounds on auscultation were clear and equal. How is this possible, given his submersion?
   a. Spasm and tight closing of the larynx
   b. Relaxation of the laryngeal structures following hypoxia
   c. Upper bronchial tree spasm and contraction
   d. Alveolar spasm and massive production of surfactant

3. What effect did the very cold water temperature possibly have on Billy's condition?
   a. May have triggered aspiration of water via the mammalian diving reflex
   b. May have caused development of severe peripheral acidosis
   c. May have helped prevent brain damage while the brain cells were deprived of oxygen
   d. May have caused an increase in the heart rate and dilation of blood vessels

4. Management of Billy's condition should include
   a. removal from the cold environment.
   b. performance of a thermal rub.
   c. immediate immersion in hot water.
   d. placement of the AED.

5. Deaths due to complications of drowning occur. What is the likelihood that a patient such as Billy will die as a result of these complications?
   a. 5 percent
   b. 10 percent
   c. 15 percent
   d. 20 percent

EMERGENCY TRIP SHEET

TRIP #	
MEDIC #	
BEGIN MILES	
END MILES	
CODE___/___ PAGE___/___	
UNITS ON SCENE	

NAME _____ SEX M F DOB ___/___/___
ADDRESS _____ RACE
CITY _____ STATE _____ ZIP
PHONE ( ) ___ - ___ PCP DR.
RESPONDED FROM _____ CITY
TAKEN FROM _____ ZIP
DESTINATION _____ REASON
SSN ___ - ___ - ___ MEDICARE # _____ MEDICAID #
INSURANCE CO _____ INSURANCE # _____ GROUP #
RESPONSIBLE PARTY _____ ADDRESS
CITY _____ STATE ___ ZIP ___ PHONE ( ) ___ - ___
EMPLOYER

TIME	ON SCENE (1)	ON SCENE (2)	ON SCENE (3)	EN-ROUTE (1)	EN-ROUTE (2)	AT DESTINATION
BP						
PULSE						
RESP						
EKG						

MEDICAL HISTORY

MEDICATIONS

ALLERGIES

C/C

EVENTS LEADING TO C/C

ASSESSMENT

TREATMENT

EMS SIGNATURE

BILLING USE ONLY

DAY			
DATE			
RECEIVED			
DISPATCHED			
EN-ROUTE			
ON SCENE			
TO HOSPITAL			
AT HOSPITAL			
IN-SERVICE			

CREW	CERT	STATE #

IV THERAPY
SUCCESSFUL Y N # OF ATTEMPTS _____
ANGIO SIZE _____ ga.
SITE _____
TOTAL FLUID INFUSED _____ cc
BLOOD DRAW Y N INITIALS

INTUBATION INFORMATION
SUCCESSFUL Y N # OF ATTEMPTS _____
TUBE SIZE _____ mm
TIME _____ INITIALS _____

CONDITION CODES				

TREATMENTS

TIME	TREATMENT	DOSE	ROUTE	INIT

GCS E___ V___ M___ TOTAL =
GCS E___ V___ M___ TOTAL =

HOSPITAL CONTACTED

CPR BEGUN BY B P TIME BEGUN
AED USED Y N BY:
RESUSCITATION TERMINATED - TIME

( ) OSHA REGULATIONS FOLLOWED

24 Behavioral Emergencies

OBJECTIVES

Numbered objectives are from the United States Department of Transportation EMT-Basic National Standard Curriculum. Asterisked objectives, if any, pertain to material that is supplemental to the DOT curriculum.

Cognitive

4-8.1 Define the term "behavioral emergency."
4-8.2 Discuss the general factors that may cause an alteration in a patient's behavior.
4-8.3 State the various reasons for psychological crises.
4-8.4 Discuss the characteristics of an individual's behavior that suggest the patient is at risk for suicide.
4-8.5 Discuss the special medical/legal considerations for managing behavioral emergencies.
4-8.6 Discuss the special considerations for assessing a patient with behavioral emergencies.
4-8.7 Discuss the general principles of an individual's behavior that suggest he or she is at risk for violence.
4-8.8 Discuss methods to calm behavioral emergency patients.

KEY IDEAS

This chapter focuses on the assessment and management of behavioral emergencies. Behavioral emergencies may be manifested in a variety of ways and require special considerations from the EMT. Key concepts include the following:

■ A behavioral emergency is one in which the patient exhibits behavior that may pose a danger to the patient or others and is intolerable to the patient, the family, or the community.

■ The precipitating factor in a behavioral emergency may be extremes of emotion, a physical condition, or a psychological condition.

■ The priority of the EMT at the scene of a behavioral emergency is to manage the patient's injuries or illness.

■ Acts of violence against oneself or others are often associated with behavioral emergencies.

■ Every suicidal act or gesture should be taken seriously, and the patient should be transported for evaluation by a physician.

■ When managing behavioral emergencies, the EMT should remember that interpersonal communications may have more impact on the outcome of the situation than emergency medical skills.

■ Behavioral emergencies require special assessment and medical legal considerations on the part of the EMT.

TERMS AND CONCEPTS

1. Write the number of the correct term next to each definition.

   1. Behavior
   2. Behavioral emergency
   3. Bipolar disorder
   4. Humane restraints
   5. Paranoia
   6. Phobia
   7. Reasonable force
   8. Schizophrenia
   9. Suicide

   _____ a. The minimum amount of force required to prevent the patient from harming himself or others

   _____ b. The way a person acts or performs

   _____ c. A willful act designed to end one's own life

   _____ d. Padded leather or cloth straps used to keep the patient from hurting herself or others

   _____ e. A situation in which a person exhibits "abnormal" behavior

   _____ f. Causes a patient to swing to opposite sides of the mood spectrum

   _____ g. The name given to a group of mental disorders

   _____ h. Irrational fears of specific things, places, or situations

   _____ i. A highly exaggerated or unwarranted mistrust or suspiciousness

CONTENT REVIEW

1. For each of the following signs or symptoms indicate if it is potentially a clue of a physical (rather than a psychological) problem. Indicate yes (Y) if it is a potential clue for a physical problem. Indicate no (N) if it is not a potential clue for a physical problem.

   _____ a. The patient has auditory hallucinations.

   _____ b. The pupils are dilated.

   _____ c. The patient has intact memory and responsiveness.

   _____ d. The patient is incontinent.

   _____ e. The onset of symptoms was gradual.

   _____ f. The patient has excessive salivation.

   _____ g. The patient has an unusual breath odor.

2. _____ often presents with an overwhelming fear that is accompanied by rapid breathing, palpitations, dizziness, and carpal-pedal spasms.
   a. A panic attack
   b. Paranoia
   c. Bipolar disorder
   d. Schizophrenia

3. Deep feelings of sadness and worthlessness that are accompanied by fatigue, loss of appetite, and a sense of hopelessness may be due to which psychiatric disorder?
   a. Paranoia
   b. Schizophrenia
   c. Depression
   d. Anxiety

4. Which of the following best describes the name given to a group of mental disorders that are debilitating and present with bizarre delusions, hallucinations, and social withdrawal?
   a. Paranoia
   b. Schizophrenia
   c. Bipolar disorder
   d. Depression

5. For each of the following patients, indicate yes (Y) if the patient is in a high-risk category for suicide and no (N) if the patient is not in a high-risk category for suicide.

   _____ a. A 45-year-old man with a history of depression and other mental disorders

   _____ b. A 17-year-old who is recently married

   _____ c. A 20-year-old who has previously attempted suicide

   _____ d. A 30-year-old female with a history of child abuse

   _____ e. A 75-year-old patient who recently had a stroke and is unable to care for herself

   _____ f. A 65-year-old female who recently took a new job

   _____ g. A 55-year-old male who is recently widowed

   _____ h. A 40-year-old female who recently lost a job she had held for 20 years

6. When dealing with behavioral emergencies, it is important to understand that
   a. only certain people are susceptible to emotional injury.
   b. people have a more limited ability to cope with a crisis than they may think.
   c. primarily women and children are affected by disaster or injury.
   d. an emotional injury is just as real as a physical injury.

7. Your best protection against legal problems or false accusations when dealing with emotionally disturbed patients is
   a. careful documentation.
   b. use of restraints.
   c. a credible witness.
   d. use of a calm, reassuring voice.

8. Which of the following best describes the guidelines that apply when restraining a combative patient?
   a. Use as much force as possible to quickly subdue the patient.
   b. Never attempt restraint until you have sufficient help and an appropriate plan.
   c. Once you have determined that restraint is necessary, move slowly to avoid agitating the patient.
   d. Police-style metal handcuffs are a good way to restrain a combative patient to the stretcher.

9. The *first* priority in dealing with a behavioral emergency is to
   a. determine if the behavior is caused by a medical condition.
   b. establish and maintain an airway and oxygenation.
   c. protect yourself and others at the scene from harm.
   d. restrain the patient to protect him from harming himself.

10. Potential treatments are listed below. Mark an X beside each treatment that would be appropriate for a behavioral emergency. Leave the other blanks unmarked.

   _____ a. Avoid speaking directly to the patient.

   _____ b. Stay as close as you can to the patient.

   _____ c. Avoid making eye contact with the patient.

   _____ d. Avoid making any quick movements.

   _____ e. Do not play along with visual or auditory hallucinations.

   _____ f. Let the patient decide whether to involve family or friends.

   _____ g. Avoid spending long amounts of time on the scene.

   _____ h. Never leave the patient alone.

   _____ i. Force the patient to make decisions.

CASE STUDY

You have been called to a dormitory at a local college. Your patient is a 20-year-old male who is cowering in the corner of the lobby. Bystanders report that his name is Jim and that just before your arrival he was shouting, "Go away, leave me alone," and gesturing at someone or something that isn't there.

1. Your *first* action should be to do which of the following?
   a. Speak with authority and ask the patient to stand.
   b. Approach the patient to gain his trust.
   c. Stand directly in front of the patient to make eye contact.
   d. Scan the scene for potential hazards.

After asking if you can come closer, Jim allows you to come within 3 feet of his location. You notice that he seems frightened. His hands are trembling slightly, and his breathing is rapid. You note that his skin is pink and dry, and you observe no obvious injuries. He tells you that he's hearing voices that are telling him to do "bad things."

2. Which technique would best help gain the trust of this patient?
   a. Maintain eye contact and speak calmly.
   b. Play along with visual or auditory disturbances.
   c. Leave the patient alone so he can rationalize his thoughts.
   d. Tell the patient what he wants to hear even if it is not truthful.

3. What actions should your partner take?
   a. Keep you in his line of sight, move quickly to talk to bystanders, avoid eye contact with the patient, try to obtain additional information, and try to disperse bystanders
   b. Keep you in his line of sight, speak in a loud and rapid voice, avoid eye contact with the patient, try to obtain information, and try to disperse bystanders
   c. Keep you in his line of sight, be alert that Jim may become violent, try to obtain additional information, and try to disperse bystanders
   d. Be alert that Jim may become violent, leave the room, and try to find witnesses who can provide additional information.

After 15 minutes of quiet conversation, you find that Jim has no past medical history but has had trouble concentrating and sleeping over the past several weeks. He denies that he has been injured recently. You ask Jim if he'll let you take him to the hospital to see the doctor. Jim agrees to accompany you. You help Jim to his feet and lead him out of the lobby and to your ambulance.

4. What should you do while en route to the hospital?

SCENARIO 13: **DOCUMENTATION EXERCISE**

Read the following scenario, and think about how you would document this call if you were the EMT who responded to the scene. Then answer the multiple-choice questions and fill in the sample pre-hospital-care report, basing your documentation on information from the scenario.

It is 10:30 PM on a Saturday night. You and your partner, LaToya, are at the station watching TV. The alarm tone sounds: "Rescue 5, respond to 1626 Leighton Street, cross street Chatfield Street, for a possible suicide. Police are responding. Time out 2230 hours." You and LaToya quickly move to the rescue vehicle and advise dispatch that you are responding. Dispatch tells you that police are on the scene and that the patient is a 60-year-old female who is depressed. You arrive in about 5 minutes. LaToya tells dispatch, "Rescue Five on-scene." Dispatch responds, "Rescue Five on-scene at 2235 hours."

The home is a large block home in a pleasant, well-kept neighborhood. A police car, with parking lights on, is parked in front of the home. LaToya parks in the driveway. The door to the home is open, and you hear a TV blaring loudly. With BSI precautions on, you carefully enter and see a woman in her mid- to late 60s sitting in a chair. She is crying softly while leaning forward with her head in her hands. Your general impression is that she looks physically well. Two

women are kneeling next to her and consoling her. A police officer is standing next to the front door holding a notepad.

You quickly introduce yourself to the police officer and ask what happened. He tells you, "This lady's name is Mrs. Raunecker; she called the police department about 20 minutes ago and said that she was going to kill herself. I've been on-scene for about 10 minutes. The two ladies are neighbors who came over when they saw my car. She seems to be pretty depressed." LaToya turns down the TV while you walk toward the patient and say, "Mrs. Raunecker, good evening. My name is Ted, and this is LaToya. We are EMTs, and we are here to help you." She lifts her head from her hands and quietly says, between sobs, "I just can't do it anymore. I can't take it. My husband died last year, I just found out that I'm going to be laid off at my job, and the police are here, so I guess I'm about to be arrested! I just can't keep going on."

You and LaToya are about 6 feet from Mrs. Raunecker. You kneel down, look her in the eyes, and say softly, "Mrs. Raunecker, we're concerned about your well-being. You called the police department and made a suicide threat. I can see that you're very depressed. We're here to help you. Would it be OK if LaToya took your vital signs?" Mrs. Raunecker nods her head yes. You move closer to Mrs. Raunecker, and LaToya begins to take her vital signs. One of the women consoling

Mrs. Raunecker catches your eye and moves her head toward the kitchen. She heads to the kitchen, and you follow. She tells you that her name is Juanita Black and that she has lived next door to Mrs. Raunecker for many years. She tells you that Mrs. Raunecker has been depressed for the last 3 months. Juanita tried to get her to seek professional help, but she refused. Mrs. Black continues by saying that the patient has been drinking heavily since her husband died last year and that she made a similar suicide threat just last month. Mrs. Black says that she didn't take the threat seriously, and she told her to "go ahead and do it." She felt that this would shock her into reality.

You thank Mrs. Black for this information and head back to where the policeman is standing. You ask the policeman to accompany you on a quick search of the home. You find nothing out of the ordinary except for two full pill bottles of a medication, prescribed for her husband, that was recently refilled. The containers were sitting on her nightstand. You return to the front of the house where Mrs. Raunecker is located. LaToya hands you a vitals report form. You quickly scan the sheet and review her vitals. She is alert and oriented to person, place, and time; respirations are normal at 14 per minute; pulse is 88, strong and regular; skin color is normal, warm, and dry; pupils are equal and reactive; the blood pressure is 138/78; SpO_2 reads 96 percent.

LaToya tells you that she obtained a SAMPLE history and found out that the patient has no allergies, takes no medicines, and has no prior medical history. She last ate at about 6:00 PM. Mrs. Raunecker says, "I don't think all this is necessary. I'm much better now. Thank you all for coming. I will be all right. I really don't need to go to the hospital." You reply, "Mrs. Raunecker, you called the police and made a threat to commit suicide; I found two bottles of pills next to your bed; and Mrs. Black told me that you made a similar suicide threat some months ago. All this must be taken very seriously. We are really concerned about your well-being. We can't leave you here under these circumstances. You must go to the hospital." She sobs and says, "Well, if you really think that I should, I guess I will." You place Mrs. Raunecker in the ambulance and transport her without incident.

1. When managing a patient who has made a suicide attempt, the EMT's primary concern is to
   a. manage the psychological aspects of the patient's condition.
   b. manage the well-being of the family and any bystanders.
   c. manage any injuries or medical conditions related to the suicide attempt.
   d. provide accurate documentation of the events.

2. Mrs. Raunecker appeared to improve and initially refused to be transported to the hospital. Was the action that Ted took to encourage her transport appropriate?
   a. Yes, Mrs. Raunecker was at great risk for following through on her threats.
   b. Yes, but Mrs. Raunecker should have been restrained for transport.
   c. No, Mrs. Raunecker is alert and oriented and should be allowed to refuse.
   d. No, Mrs. Raunecker should be placed under arrest and transported.

3. In questioning Mrs. Raunecker, what technique did Ted use?
   a. He avoided the use of yes or no questions.
   b. He used the OPQRST method.
   c. He made use of closed-ended questions.
   d. He used a technique of rapid questioning.

4. The interview with Mrs. Raunecker
   a. was appropriately conducted and performed professionally.
   b. should have been concluded by challenging her suicide gesture.
   c. should have taken place at the hospital rather than at her home.
   d. should have been conducted in a quiet surrounding with limited people.

5. The search of Mrs. Raunecker's home
   a. should not have been performed.
   b. should only have been conducted by law enforcement.
   c. was appropriate, given the circumstances.
   d. was inappropriate and required a search warrant.

EMERGENCY TRIP SHEET

TRIP #
MEDIC #
BEGIN MILES
END MILES
CODE___/___	PAGE___/___
UNITS ON SCENE

BILLING USE ONLY				
DAY				
DATE				
RECEIVED				
DISPATCHED				
EN-ROUTE				
ON SCENE				
TO HOSPITAL				
AT HOSPITAL				
IN-SERVICE				

NAME	SEX M F DOB ___/___/___
ADDRESS	RACE
CITY	STATE	ZIP
PHONE ( ) -	PCP DR.
RESPONDED FROM	CITY
TAKEN FROM	ZIP
DESTINATION	REASON
SSN - -	MEDICARE #	MEDICAID #
INSURANCE CO	INSURANCE #	GROUP #
RESPONSIBLE PARTY	ADDRESS
CITY	STATE	ZIP	PHONE ( ) -
EMPLOYER

CREW	CERT	STATE #

TIME	ON SCENE (1)	ON SCENE (2)	ON SCENE (3)	EN-ROUTE (1)	EN-ROUTE (2)	AT DESTINATION
BP						
PULSE						
RESP						
EKG						

IV THERAPY
SUCCESSFUL Y N # OF ATTEMPTS ____
ANGIO SIZE _____ ga.
SITE _____
TOTAL FLUID INFUSED _____ cc
BLOOD DRAW Y N INITIALS

INTUBATION INFORMATION
SUCCESSFUL Y N # OF ATTEMPTS ____
TUBE SIZE _____ mm
TIME _____ INITIALS ____

MEDICAL HISTORY

MEDICATIONS

ALLERGIES

C/C

EVENTS LEADING TO C/C

ASSESSMENT

TREATMENT

CONDITION CODES					

TREATMENTS

TIME	TREATMENT	DOSE	ROUTE	IN

GCS	E___ V___ M___ TOTAL =
GCS	E___ V___ M___ TOTAL =

HOSPITAL CONTACTED

CPR BEGUN BY   B   P   TIME BEGUN

AED USED   Y   N   BY:

RESUSCITATION TERMINATED - TIME

EMS SIGNATURE

(   ) OSHA REGULATIONS FOLLOWE

25 Obstetric and Gynecological Emergencies

OBJECTIVES

Numbered objectives are from the United States Department of Transportation EMT-Basic National Standard Curriculum. Asterisked objectives, if any, pertain to material that is supplemental to the DOT curriculum.

Cognitive

4-9.1 Identify the following structures: uterus, vagina, fetus, placenta, umbilical cord, amniotic sac, perineum.

4-9.2 Identify and explain the use of the contents of an obstetrics kit.

4-9.3 Identify predelivery emergencies.

4-9.4 State indications of an imminent delivery.

4-9.5 Differentiate the emergency medical care provided to a patient with predelivery emergencies from a normal delivery.

4-9.6 State the steps in the predelivery preparation of the mother.

4-9.7 Establish the relationship between body substance isolation and childbirth.

4-9.8 State the steps to assist in the delivery.

4-9.9 Describe care of the infant as the head appears.

4-9.10 Describe how and when to cut the umbilical cord.

4-9.11 Discuss the steps in the delivery of the placenta.

4-9.12 List the steps in the emergency medical care of the mother post-delivery.

4-9.13 Summarize neonatal resuscitation procedures.

4-9.14 Describe the procedures for the following abnormal deliveries: breech birth, prolapsed cord, limb presentation.

4-9.15 Differentiate the special considerations for multiple births.

4-9.16 Describe special considerations of meconium.

4-9.17 Describe special considerations of a premature baby.

4-9.18 Discuss the emergency medical care of a patient with a gynecological emergency.

KEY IDEAS

This chapter focuses on the assessment and management of obstetric and gynecological emergencies. The EMT does not frequently encounter emergencies related to the reproductive organs, so these are often stressful calls. In this chapter, you will learn how to recognize and provide emergency care for obstetric and gynecological emergencies. Key concepts include the following:

■ The anatomical structures associated with pregnancy include the uterus, placenta, amniotic sac, umbilical cord, cervix, and vagina.

■ The three stages of labor are dilation, expulsion, and placental.

- Recognition of a predelivery emergency is based on information obtained from the focused history and physical exam that relates to the reported abnormality, such as pain, discomfort, or bleeding.

- The priorities for care do not change at the scene of an obstetric or a gynecological emergency. Use the same assessment and treatment techniques as you would use on any patient who is not pregnant.

- Imminent delivery is recognized by crowning, the frequency and duration of contractions, and the sensation of bowel movement (urge to push).

- The role of the EMT during childbirth is to assist in the delivery and to recognize and treat life-threatening problems for the mother or baby.

- Gravida refers to pregnancy while par refers to a woman who has given birth. When a Roman numeral is added it indicates the number for each. For example, a patient who is pregnant for the third time is reported as gravida III and a woman who has given birth as para I (or primapara).

- Delivery emergencies include abnormal presentation, prematurity, meconium staining, and multiple births.

- The APGAR score is performed 1 minute and 5 minutes after birth. Assessed are the newborn's Appearance (0–2), Pulse (0–2), Grimace (0–2), Activity (0–2), and Respiration (0–2). A newborn with a score of 7–10 should be active and requires routine care. A score of 4–6 indicates a moderately depressed newborn that requires stimulation and oxygenation. A score of 0–3 points indicates a severely depressed newborn that requires bag-valve-mask ventilation and CPR.

- The essential emergency care of the newborn includes the establishment and maintenance of an adequate airway, breathing, oxygenation, and circulation and the prevention of heat loss.

- The goals for the emergency management of gynecological emergencies are to ensure an adequate airway, breathing, oxygenation, and circulation; to control vaginal bleeding; and to treat for shock (hypoperfusion).

TERMS AND CONCEPTS

1. Write the number of the correct term next to each definition.

   1. Amniotic sac
   2. Braxton-Hicks contractions
   3. Fetus
   4. Perineum
   5. Placenta
   6. Primagravida
   7. Prolapsed cord
   8. Umbilical cord

   _____ a. Unborn infant

   _____ b. Placental extension that supplies nourishment to the fetus

   _____ c. Organ of pregnancy for the exchange of oxygen and waste products

   _____ d. When the umbilical cord is the presenting part

   _____ e. Transparent membrane forming the sac that holds fluid and the fetus

   _____ f. Area of skin between a female's vagina and anus

   _____ g. Woman who is pregnant for the first time

   _____ h. Painless, short duration, irregular contractions

CONTENT REVIEW

1. Which of the following is the lowest portion of the birth canal?
   a. Cervix
   b. Uterus
   c. Vagina
   d. Perineum

2. Uterine contractions that expel the fetus and placenta are referred to as
   a. labor.
   b. the placental phase.
   c. the dilation phase.
   d. fetal expulsion.

3. The final stage of labor is generally described as the
   a. dilation stage.
   b. expulsion stage.
   c. placental stage.
   d. fundal stage.

4. A woman who is gravida III is a woman who
   a. is pregnant for the fourth time.
   b. has delivered three times.
   c. is pregnant for the third time.
   d. has delivered for the fourth time.

5. Which of the following is a sign or a symptom of a predelivery emergency?
   a. Altered mental status or seizures
   b. Right-arm pain with numbness
   c. Calf-muscle cramping and discomfort
   d. Urinary retention and fever

6. Your supine, third-trimester pregnant patient is noted to have low blood pressure. You suspect that this may be due to which of the following?
   a. Supine hypotensive syndrome
   b. Lateral emergent syndrome
   c. Prone hypertensive syndrome
   d. Supine hyperglycemic syndrome

7. Management specific to the situation noted in item 6 should include
   a. placing the patient in the Trendelenburg position.
   b. beginning chest compressions.
   c. positioning the patient on her side.
   d. applying the AED (automated external defibrillator).

8. Your 30-year-old female patient is 4 months pregnant. She complains of cramping, abdominal pain, and bright red vaginal bleeding. Your treatment should include
   a. packing the vagina with sanitary pads to control bleeding.
   b. elevation of the patient's head to prevent aspiration.
   c. the administration of oxygen at 6 lpm.
   d. providing general management for shock.

9. Your 20-year-old patient is 8 months pregnant. Prior to your arrival, she had a seizure that lasted about 2 minutes. You find her to have an altered mental status with a patent airway and adequate respirations and perfusion. Care of this patient should include
   a. administration of low-flow oxygen by nonrebreather mask.
   b. withholding positive-pressure ventilation to such a patient.
   c. transporting the patient in a supine position.
   d. minimization of noise, light, and movement to prevent further seizures.

10. Which of the following is a sign of an imminent delivery?
    a. Contractions that occur every 2 minutes and last 60–90 seconds
    b. Contractions that occur every 2 minutes and last 30–60 seconds
    c. Contractions that occur every 4 minutes and last 30–60 seconds
    d. Contractions that occur every 4 minutes and last 60–90 seconds

11. Number the list below in the proper order from 1 to 5 to show, after taking appropriate BSI precautions and positioning the patient, the emergency care of a patient during active labor for a normal delivery.

    _____ Suction the infant's mouth and nose. Support the body as the infant delivers, then again suction the mouth and nose. Dry and wrap the infant.

    _____ Observe for the delivery of the placenta. As it delivers, grasp it gently. Place in a plastic bag for transport to the hospital.

    _____ Support the bony part of the infant's skull and exert gentle pressure against the perineum as the head delivers. Determine the position of the umbilical cord.

    _____ Keep the infant level with the vagina. Have your partner assume care of the infant. When the pulsations cease, clamp, tie, and cut the umbilical cord.

    _____ Place one or two sanitary pads at the vaginal opening. Record the time of delivery and then transport. Keep mother and infant warm en route.

12. Your patient has just delivered a healthy baby boy. Following the delivery of the placenta, her vaginal bleeding seems to increase. Which of the following best describes what you should do to provide emergency care for this patient?
    a. Massage the uterus, and position your patient on her side.
    b. Administer oxygen, and firmly massage the uterus.
    c. Massage the uterus, and pack the vagina to control bleeding.
    d. Administer oxygen, and pack the vagina with sanitary pads.

13. Which of the following is a sign of an abnormal delivery emergency?
    a. Fetal presentation of the head
    b. Colorless amniotic fluid
    c. Labor before the 46th week of pregnancy
    d. Recurrence of contractions after the infant is born

14. Management of a breech-birth presentation includes
    a. positioning the mother in a supine head-down position.
    b. administering low-flow oxygen by nonrebreather mask.
    c. placing a hand in the vagina to delay delivery.
    d. delaying transport for safe delivery on the scene.

15. Which of the following *best* describes an abnormal delivery situation where there may be compression of the cord against the walls of the vagina and the bony pelvis by the pressure of the infant's head or buttocks?
    a. Crowning
    b. Limb presentation
    c. Breech
    d. Prolapsed cord

16. How should you manage the situation in item 15?
    a. Immediately push the cord back into the vagina.
    b. Insert a gloved hand into the vagina to relieve pressure on the cord.
    c. Cover the cord with a dry, sterile towel to prevent infection.
    d. Push on the mother's abdomen to expedite delivery.

17. Meconium staining of the amniotic fluid should be managed by
    a. immediate transport to the hospital for evaluation by a physician.
    b. administration of oxygen to the mother to resolve fetal distress.
    c. suctioning mouth and nose before the infant takes the first breath.
    d. stimulating the infant to cough to clear meconium from the airway.

18. In addition to the usual care for a newborn, care of the premature infant requires
    a. vigorous suctioning to maintain the airway.
    b. direct administration of supplemental oxygen by a face mask.
    c. immediate transport for resuscitation.
    d. vigilant attention to prevent heat loss or contamination.

19. The APGAR scoring assessment of the newborn
    a. ranges from 0 to 10.
    b. includes assessment of the newborn's affect.
    c. ranges from 3 to 10.
    d. is performed at 1 and 2 minutes following birth.

20. Which of the following is a sign of a severely depressed newborn?
    a. Respiratory rate over 50 per minute
    b. APGAR score of 7–10 points
    c. Cyanotic body
    d. Heart rate over 120 per minute or under 80 per minute

21. You have just assisted with the delivery of a baby girl. She has shallow, gasping respirations and a heart rate that is less than 90 beats per minute. Which of the following best describes your emergency care for this patient?
    a. Administer "blow-by" oxygen and monitor pulse for 60 seconds.
    b. Assist ventilations with a bag-valve mask and reassess in 30 seconds.
    c. Administer high-flow oxygen with a nonrebreather mask.
    d. Assist ventilations with a bag-valve mask and begin chest compressions.

22. You have responded to the scene of a sexual assault. After taking appropriate BSI precautions and completing the initial assessment, your focused history and physical exam should include
    a. direct examination of the genitalia to verify injury.
    b. cleaning and dressing the patient's wounds.
    c. questioning the patient about other potential injuries.
    d. placing any clothing that is removed in one bag to preserve evidence.

23. The APGAR score is initially performed at _____ after birth and repeated at _____ after birth.
  a. 30 seconds, 3 minutes
  b. 60 seconds, 5 minutes
  c. 90 seconds, 6 minutes
  d. 30 seconds, 4 minutes

24. Irregular contractions that vary in intensity and duration are called
  a. Braxton-Hicks contractions.
  b. normal predelivery contractions.
  c. Braddock-McKoy contractions.
  d. post-delivery contractions.

CASE STUDY

You have been dispatched to the scene of a single vehicle accidentally driven into the river. A jogger and another bystander dove into the river and were able to rescue the driver. Your patient is a woman in her 30s who is obviously pregnant. By the size of her abdomen, you suspect that she is near term. Your initial assessment reveals an unresponsive female with rapid, shallow respirations. Her pulse is slow and irregular. Her skin is cool and dry. There are no obvious signs of injury.

1. Initial management of this patient should first include
  a. assisting respirations by bag-valve mask with oxygen.
  b. completing a trauma assessment.
  c. covering with a blanket to maintain body heat.
  d. immobilization on a long spine board.

2. The patient is immobilized on a long spine board. How should the potential for supine hypotensive syndrome be managed in this patient?
  a. Keep the spine board in a flat position.
  b. Position a blanket or pillow under the side of the spine board.
  c. Position a blanket or pillow under the head of the spine board.
  d. Position a blanket or pillow under the foot end of the board.

Two blocks from the hospital your patient stops breathing and becomes pulseless.

3. What is the best action to take?
  a. Start CPR.
  b. Start modified CPR.
  c. Contact the hospital for instructions.
  d. Speed your response time to the hospital.

Your patient is successfully resuscitated at the hospital and undergoes surgical delivery of a baby girl.

ENRICHMENT

1. Placenta previa results from
  a. uterine trauma and subsequent placental separation from the uterine wall.
  b. rupture of blood vessels under the placenta and subsequent separation.
  c. an abnormal implantation of the placenta.
  d. hypertension and separation of the placenta from the uterine wall.

2. A predisposing factor for the development of placenta previa is
   a. less than two deliveries.
   b. less than 20 years of age.
   c. no history of vaginal bleeding.
   d. bleeding following intercourse.

3. The hallmark sign of placenta previa is
   a. second-trimester painless vaginal bleeding.
   b. third-trimester painless bright red vaginal bleeding.
   c. third-trimester painless vaginal bleeding.
   d. third-trimester painless dark red vaginal bleeding.

4. Abruptio placenta results from
   a. uterine trauma and subsequent placental separation from the uterine wall.
   b. rupture of blood vessels under the placenta and subsequent separation.
   c. an abnormal implantation of the placenta.
   d. hypertension and separation of the placenta from the uterine wall.

5. Predisposing factors for an abruptio placenta are
   a. history of fewer than two deliveries.
   b. an abnormally long umbilical cord.
   c. fever and use of psychotropic drugs.
   d. smoking and hypertension.

6. The hallmark sign of abruptio placenta is
   a. vaginal bleeding that is associated with constant abdominal pain.
   b. lower abdominal pain without vaginal bleeding.
   c. lower-back pain and cramping.
   d. signs and symptoms of hypovolemic shock.

7. Preeclampsia
   a. is a common condition that affects one in five women.
   b. occurs most frequently in the first trimester of pregnancy.
   c. frequently affects pregnant women over the age of 40.
   d. chiefly affects women with a history of hypertension or diabetes.

8. The primary clinical signs of preeclampsia are
   a. vomiting and pulmonary edema.
   b. hypertension and swelling in the extremities.
   c. abdominal pain and severe headache.
   d. reactive airway disease and pulmonary edema.

9. The leading cause of maternal death in the first trimester of pregnancy is
   a. abruptio placenta.
   b. placenta previa.
   c. preeclampsia/eclampsia.
   d. ectopic pregnancy.

10. Factors that predispose an individual to develop an ectopic pregnancy include
    a. smoking.
    b. urinary tract infection.
    c. pelvic inflammatory disease.
    d. inactivity.

11. A sign or symptom of an ectopic-pregnancy emergency is
    a. an intense urge to urinate.
    b. sharp, knifelike lower abdominal pain localized to one side.
    c. a bluish discoloration around the umbilicus immediately following rupture.
    d. bilateral lower abdominal pain that is described as a tearing pain.

SCENARIO 14: DOCUMENTATION EXERCISE

Read the following scenario, and think about how you would document this call if you were the EMT who responded to the scene. Then answer the multiple-choice questions and fill in the sample pre-hospital-care report, basing your documentation on information from the scenario.

It is 3:30 AM. You are sleeping soundly when the alarm sounds: "Unit 3, respond to 1451 US Highway 98 South, cross street Highway 540A, for an unknown medical emergency." You climb out of bed, get dressed, and meet your partner in the rescue vehicle. Dispatch tells you that your patient is in a car parked on the northbound lane of Highway 98 and is a female patient in labor. You advise dispatch that you are responding. You arrive on-scene in about 8 minutes. You pull up behind a car with its hood up, and you park. A young man is in the back seat of the car and motions you to hurry.

You walk toward the car with your BSI precautions on. You look inside and observe a young woman lying in a supine position in the back seat of the car. She is lying with her legs spread apart and her head against the door. She is covered by a small blanket and is moaning loudly as you approach the car. You tell the young man, "Hello! My name is Barb, and this is Jack, and we are EMTs. We're here to help. What's the problem tonight?" He anxiously says, "I was taking Mary to the hospital when my car broke down. She has been in labor for about 2 hours. She's going to have the baby! You've got to help us!" You reply, "We will do everything we can."

You quickly jump into the back seat to evaluate Mary. Mary, who appears to be about 30 years old, is alert and screaming, "It's coming! It's coming!" You administer oxygen via nonrebreather mask and set the flow rate at 15 lpm. You quickly remove the blanket and cut off her underpants so you can examine the vaginal area. Crowning is present with each contraction.

Mary says, "I feel like I have to move my bowels. I really need to push." You tell her to try not to push until you can get things set up. You place a folded sheet under her hips and open up the sterile obstetrical kit that Jack brings you. You create a sterile area by placing a sterile sheet under her buttocks and place a sterile sheet on her lower abdomen. You then put the OB kit within easy reach.

She yells once again, "I've gotta push now!" You tell her to go ahead and push. You place your gloved spread fingers on the infant's skull and exert gentle, steady pressure. The head is bulging from the vagina and is covered with a thin semitransparent membrane. You quickly use a clamp from the OB kit to tear the membrane and push it away from the infant's head and face. The head delivers quickly and is positioned in a "nose down" position. You use two fingers to check down the neck of the infant. The head is completely delivered and has rotated in such a manner as to now be facing the mother's right leg. You suction the mouth free and then the nose of fluid and express it onto a spare towel. The fluid is clear and odorless. The infant's torso is expelled. You support the head and torso with your hands and grasp the infant's feet as the delivery proceeds. You clear the mouth and nose again as the infant begins to cry.

You tell Mary, "It's a girl!" You dry the infant with a sterile towel, and place it on its side with the neck in an extended position on the car seat even with the mother's vagina. You place two clamps on the umbilical cord and use a sterile scalpel to cut the cord between the clamps. You hand the baby to Jack to manage. Jack wraps the baby in a warm receiving blanket, shows it to the ecstatic father, and takes the baby to the ambulance to keep warm and evaluate. You continue to manage the mother. You clean her up while preparing for delivery of the placenta. You observe some bleeding from the vagina and control it with sanitary pads. You take the vital signs on the mother.

You ask Mary if she has been under prenatal care. She states, "Yes, Dr. Menendez has been taking care of me. Everything has been quite normal, up to now. He is at the hospital waiting for us." Mary is alert and oriented; her respirations are 14 per minute and of normal depth; the pulse is 100 per minute, strong and regular; the skin is warm and dry; pupils are equal and reactive and respond briskly to light; the blood pressure is 130/80; her SpO_2 is 96 percent. In about 10 minutes the placenta appears at the vagina, and you take hold of it and gently support it as it is expelled. You place the placenta in a plastic bag. You inspect the perineum for tearing and place sanitary pads over the vaginal opening. You ask the mother to put her legs together and you record the time of birth.

You find out that Mary has had four pregnancies and has delivered three live births, including this new-born. Jack has been managing the infant baby girl. He obtained the following findings from the 1-minute APGAR: *appearance*—blue hands and feet with pink skin at the body core; *pulse*—140 per minute; *grimace*—stimulation causes a cry; *activity*—newborn moves around; *respiration*—good respirations and strong cry. He maintains the infant's warmth and repeats the APGAR at 5 minutes. The following findings are noted: *appearance*—the skin of the extremities as well as the trunk is pink; *pulse*—150 per minute; *grimace*—stimulation causes a cry; *activity*—newborn moves around; *respiration*—good respirations and strong cry.

You transport mother and daughter to the hospital while continuing to monitor both closely. The father rides along in the front of the ambulance, planning to call the car-repair service from the hospital.

1. Immediately after cutting and clamping the umbilical cord Barb should
   a. document the time on the run report.
   b. place a second umbilical clamp on the mother.
   c. place a second umbilical clamp on the infant.
   d. check to make sure no bleeding is taking place.

2. What physical findings or symptoms let Barb know that delivery was imminent?
   a. Her age and general attitude
   b. Need to push and crowning
   c. Prior number of births
   d. Length of time in labor for prior births

3. What is the 1-minute APGAR score?
   a. 6
   b. 7
   c. 8
   d. 9

4. What is the 5-minute APGAR score?
   a. 7
   b. 8
   c. 9
   d. 10

5. The bleeding that occurs following the birth of Mary's baby girl is normal and expected. Bleeding, however, should typically not exceed _____.
   a. 200 ml (cc)
   b. 300 ml (cc)
   c. 400 ml (cc)
   d. 500 ml (cc)

EMERGENCY TRIP SHEET

TRIP #	
MEDIC #	
BEGIN MILES	
END MILES	
CODE___/___ PAGE___/___	
UNITS ON SCENE	

NAME	SEX M F DOB ___/___/___
ADDRESS	RACE
CITY STATE ZIP	
PHONE ( ) - PCP DR.	
RESPONDED FROM	CITY
TAKEN FROM	ZIP
DESTINATION	REASON
SSN - - MEDICARE #	MEDICAID #
INSURANCE CO INSURANCE #	GROUP #
RESPONSIBLE PARTY ADDRESS	
CITY STATE ZIP PHONE ( ) -	
EMPLOYER	

TIME	ON SCENE (1)	ON SCENE (2)	ON SCENE (3)	EN-ROUTE (1)	EN-ROUTE (2)	AT DESTINATION
BP						
PULSE						
RESP						
EKG						

MEDICAL HISTORY

MEDICATIONS

ALLERGIES

C/C

EVENTS LEADING TO C/C

ASSESSMENT

TREATMENT

EMS SIGNATURE

BILLING USE ONLY

DAY				
DATE				
RECEIVED				
DISPATCHED				
EN-ROUTE				
ON SCENE				
TO HOSPITAL				
AT HOSPITAL				
IN-SERVICE				

CREW	CERT	STATE #

IV THERAPY
SUCCESSFUL Y N # OF ATTEMPTS ___
ANGIO SIZE _____ga.
SITE _____
TOTAL FLUID INFUSED _____cc
BLOOD DRAW Y N INITIALS

INTUBATION INFORMATION
SUCCESSFUL Y N # OF ATTEMPTS ___
TUBE SIZE _____ mm
TIME _____ INITIALS ___

CONDITION CODES				

TREATMENTS

TIME	TREATMENT	DOSE	ROUTE	IN

GCS E___ V___ M___ TOTAL =

GCS E___ V___ M___ TOTAL =

HOSPITAL CONTACTED

CPR BEGUN BY   B   P   TIME BEGUN

AED USED   Y   N   BY:

RESUSCITATION TERMINATED - TIME

( ) OSHA REGULATIONS FOLLOWE

MEDICAL EMERGENCIES: CHAPTERS 12–25

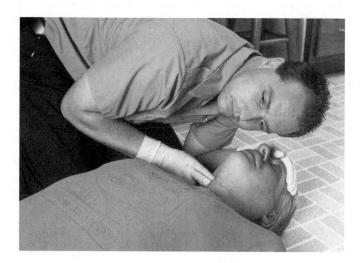

Medical emergencies are usually the result of something that goes wrong inside the body—as opposed to trau-matic injuries, which are usually the result of some outside force.

Q   **Why is it important to look for a mechanism of injury at the scene of a medical call?**

A   It is important to rule out trauma. Sometimes, the only clue that the patient's signs and symptoms are due to a medical cause is the absence of a mechanism of injury. It is also possible that a patient with a medical condition may be suffering from trauma. For example, the patient may have become dizzy because of a breathing problem, then fallen and sustained an injury. (Conversely, a patient who has sustained an injury may also be suffering from a medical condition; for example, a heart attack brought on by the trauma.) Never assume that this is "only" a medical call until you have ruled out any mechanism of injury or sign of trauma.

Q   **Why is there so much emphasis on altered mental status for a wide variety of medical conditions?**

A   An altered mental status, which may range from confusion to complete unresponsiveness, is emphasized because it may be a sign of a serious condition. Mostly, however, it is important because a patient with an altered mental status may lose the ability to protect his own airway, and as you learned in the Airway module, without a patent airway, all other assessments and treatments are worthless. So mental status and airway must be monitored on every medical call.

Q   **Why does the emergency care for almost any medical condition include providing oxygen?**

A   The body requires oxygen to function. In many conditions, something is preventing enough oxygen from entering the body or the bloodstream or is preventing it from being carried adequately to all the body's cells, and especially to the brain. Even if the body is receiving its normal supply of oxygen, extra oxygen can help to support the functions of body and brain and will help to prevent many conditions from getting worse. In other words, oxygen is a medication that is almost always good for any medical condition and will almost never be harmful if given to the patient.

Q   **What other medications, besides oxygen, are EMTs allowed to administer to patients?**

A   Oral glucose (used in certain diabetic emergencies) and activated charcoal (administered in some ingested poisonings) and aspirin are carried on the ambulance and may be administered by the EMT under certain circumstances with on-line or off-line approval from medical direction. Three medications that may have been prescribed to the patient and may be found in his possession may also be administered by the EMT under certain circumstances with on-line or off-line approval of medical direction. These are the metered-dose inhaler (for certain respiratory emergencies), nitroglycerin (for chest pain), and epinephrine (administered by auto-injector for severe allergic reactions). *Detailed information on these medications is found on the Medication Cards at the back of this book.*

Q   **What are the chief functions of the EMT at the scene of a medical emergency?**

A   The chief functions are to assess the patient, gathering as much information as possible from the environment and the SAMPLE history; to monitor the patient's mental status and protect the airway; to administer oxygen or positive-pressure ventilation as appropriate; to administer medications as appropriate and permitted by medical direction; to position the patient (often in a position of comfort); and to transport.

Q   **What are the key functions of the EMT in a behavioral emergency?**

A   The key functions are to protect your safety and that of your partner, to treat the patient's medical condition or injuries, to calm and reassure the patient to the degree possible, and to transport the patient, with humane restraints if necessary.

Q   **What are the key functions of the EMT at the scene of an obstetric or gynecological emergency?**

A   The key functions are to treat the medical condition or injuries of the patient as for any patient, to transport a pregnant patient if delivery is not imminent, to assist the mother in delivering the baby if transport cannot be accomplished before delivery, and to care for both the mother and the newborn (or newborns).

26 Mechanisms of Injury: Kinetics of Trauma

OBJECTIVES

Numbered objectives are from the United States Department of Transportation EMT-Basic National Standard Curriculum. Asterisked objectives, if any, pertain to material that is supplemental to the DOT curriculum.

Cognitive

3-1.4 Discuss common mechanisms of injury/nature of illness.

* Explain how the following affect the force of impact: mass and velocity, acceleration and deceleration, energy changing form and direction.
* Describe the three main impacts that occur in a vehicle collision.
* Discuss the following mechanisms of injury and their effects on the human body: motor vehicle collisions, vehicle-pedestrian collisions, motorcycle collisions, falls, penetrating injuries, and blast injuries.
* Discuss the steps of patient assessment, including the priority decision, as they relate to and are guided by the mechanism of injury.

KEY IDEAS

Maintaining a high index of suspicion for hidden injuries in the trauma patient is just as important as identifying obvious injuries. An understanding of the mechanism of injury (how the patient was injured) is the chief component of this crucial assessment skill.

- The amount of kinetic energy contained in a moving body depends on the body's mass (weight) and velocity (speed). Velocity is a much more significant factor than mass when evaluating the mechanism of injury.

- Motor vehicle collisions can be classified as frontal, rear-end, lateral, or rotational rollover. Each type involves characteristic injuries.

- In a vehicle–pedestrian collision, the extent of injury depends on the speed of the vehicle, what part of the pedestrian's body was struck, how far she was thrown, the surface she lands on, and the body part that first impacts the ground. Also, children and adults will display different injury patterns.

- Motorcycle collisions are classified as head-on impact, angular impact, or ejection. Incidence of injury and death is greatly increased when the rider does not wear a helmet.

- Falls are the most common mechanism of injury. The severity of injury depends on the falling distance, landing surface, and the body part that impacts first. A fall of 15 feet or more onto an unyielding surface is considered severe for an adult. A fall greater than 10 feet is considered severe for a child.

- Penetrating injuries are classified as low-velocity (knives), medium-velocity (shotgun and handgun pellets or bullets), or high-velocity (high-velocity rifles). Assess the patient for both entrance and exit wounds.

- Blast injuries are classified as primary-phase (injuries due to the pressure wave), secondary-phase (injuries due to flying debris), and tertiary-phase (patient is thrown from source of blast) injuries. Keep a high index of suspicion for all three types of injuries when a patient has been involved in a blast.

- Start to evaluate the mechanism of injury during your scene size-up. Rely on it when making decisions regarding patient priorities; determine what injuries are possible, even when they are not apparent. During patient assessment, the mechanism of injury will help you determine if manual in-line stabilization of the patient's head and neck is necessary, how to proceed with the focused history and physical exam, and what problems may arise during transport. Be sure to give the hospital staff all relevant information about the patient's mechanism of injury.

TERMS AND CONCEPTS

1. Write the number of each term next to its definition.
    1. cavitation
    2. dissipation of energy
    3. drag
    4. kinetic energy
    5. kinetics of trauma
    6. mechanism of injury
    7. profile
    8. trajectory

    _____ a. A cavity formed by a pressure wave resulting from the kinetic energy of a bullet traveling through body tissue; also called pathway expansion

    _____ b. Refers to the size and shape of a bullet's point of impact; the greater the point of impact, the greater is the injury

    _____ c. The energy contained by an object in motion

    _____ d. The factors and forces that cause traumatic injury

    _____ e. The factors that slow a projectile

    _____ f. The path of a projectile during its travel; it may be flat or curved

    _____ g. The science of analyzing mechanisms of injury

    _____ h. The way energy is transferred to the human body by the forces acting upon it

CONTENT REVIEW

1. The amount of kinetic energy a moving body contains depends on which of the following two factors?
    a. Mass and weight
    b. Drag and mass
    c. Rate of acceleration and velocity
    d. Mass and velocity

2. Which of the following factors is most significant when evaluating the mechanism of injury?
   a. Mass
   b. Rate of acceleration
   c. Velocity
   d. Rate of deceleration

3. The rate at which a body in motion increases its speed is known as which of the following?
   a. Mass
   b. Deceleration
   c. Velocity
   d. Acceleration

4. The typical vehicular collision involves which of the following?
   a. One impact (vehicle)
   b. Two impacts (vehicle and body)
   c. Three impacts (vehicle, body, and organs)
   d. Four impacts (vehicle, body, organs, and vessels)

5. Which of the following is the most common mechanism of injury, accounting for over half of all trauma incidents?
   a. Vehicular collisions
   b. Falls
   c. Penetrating gunshots
   d. Explosions

6. Which of the following is the most lethal mechanism of injury, responsible for over one-third of all trauma deaths?
   a. Vehicular collisions
   b. Falls
   c. Penetrating gunshots
   d. Explosions

7. Which grouping is most likely to suffer injury from air-bag deployment?
   a. Middle-age adults
   b. Tall adults
   c. Short adults
   d. 14- to 18-year-olds

8. In a motor vehicle collision, the "up and over" and "down and under" pathways are examples of injury patterns associated with a _____ impact.
   a. frontal
   b. medial
   c. lateral
   d. rotational

9. When a passenger's head strikes the car windshield, the glass may crack in a typical _____ pattern.
   a. "cracked ice"
   b. "broken egg"
   c. "spider web"
   d. "halo"

10. The automobile driver's neck whips back, and the body is propelled forward even while the head seems to remain at rest. This best describes which of the following?
    a. A rotational impact
    b. A rear-end impact
    c. A lateral impact
    d. A frontal impact

11. In this type of motor vehicle collision, the body is struck from the side. This best describes which of the following?
    a. A rotational impact
    b. A rear-end impact
    c. A lateral impact
    d. A frontal impact

12. Which statement best describes injuries due to rotational or rollover impact?
    a. Multiple-system injury and possible ejection if the patient was unrestrained.
    b. Head and neck are whipped back.
    c. Head injuries are common when passenger heads collide with one another.
    d. "Up and over" or "down and under" path.

13. A child who is about to be struck by an auto generally
    a. turns away from the oncoming auto.
    b. turns to the side of the oncoming auto.
    c. turns to face the oncoming auto.
    d. does not turn at all.

14. A common pattern of injuries to a child struck by an auto is injuries to the
    a. upper and lower extremities.
    b. femur, chest, abdomen, and head.
    c. phalanges, radius, and ulna.
    d. pelvis, chest, skull, and face.

15. Which of the following is correct regarding motor vehicle restraints?
    a. In a collision, a seatbelt worn too low can cause lower-leg fractures.
    b. Properly applied lap belts and shoulder straps prevent lateral head movement.
    c. Air bags work well in multiple-collision events.
    d. A deployed air bag should be lifted from the steering wheel.

16. Which injury listed below is most likely the result of "laying the bike down," an evasive action meant to prevent ejection or separation of a motorcycle rider from his bike.
    a. Femur fracture
    b. Closed-head injury
    c. Dislocated shoulder
    d. Leg burns

17. A fall of _____ feet onto an unyielding surface is considered severe for an adult. A fall of more than _____ feet can cause severe injuries to a child.
    a. 5, 10
    b. 10, 5
    c. 15, 10
    d. 10, 15

18. Experts say that a patient in a feet-first fall who falls _____ or more will likely have a spinal injury.
   a. 2 times his height
   b. 3 times his height
   c. 4 times his height
   d. 5 times his height

19. In a gunshot incident, the EMT should suspect both thoracic and abdominal injury if the entrance wound is
   a. between the nipple line and the waist.
   b. between the navel and the waist.
   c. between the trachea and the clavicle.
   d. between the nipple line and the sternum.

20. Primary-phase, secondary-phase, and tertiary-phase injuries are related to
   a. motor vehicle collisions.
   b. blasts and explosions.
   c. low- and medium-velocity weapons.
   d. head-first falls.

CASE STUDY 1

You are at the scene of a one-car, high-speed motor vehicle collision. The driver is dead, ejected from the vehicle sometime during several rollovers. A woman about 20 years old approaches you and identifies herself as a passenger in the vehicle. She tells you she walked to a gas station to call for help, then returned. Your general impression is that she looks well, although she has a small laceration over her left eye. She is holding her left upper abdominal and chest region. Her skin color appears to be normal. She responds to your questions appropriately, although somewhat slowly.

1. Which of the following describes the most appropriate treatment for the patient?
   a. The patient should be assessed for any injuries.
   b. The patient should be advised of potential serious signs and symptoms to watch for and released.
   c. The patient should be assessed, immobilized, monitored carefully, and transported.
   d. The patient should be transported by a family member for evaluation at a local hospital.

2. Which of the following regarding the patient's mental status is correct?
   a. Should concern you but only if her mental status deteriorates further
   b. Should concern you, since an altered mental status is one of the earliest signs of brain injury
   c. Should not concern you, since it appears to be normal or only slightly altered
   d. Should not concern you, since the mechanism of injury has been identified

CASE STUDY 2

You have been dispatched to a residential area to assist a worker who fell from a tree. The 35-year-old patient is lying on his right side in a soft, grassy area. His eyes are open. You ask him, "What happened?" He tells you that he was trimming the tree when the branch he was standing on gave way.

1. Which of the following questions is most important in determining the patient's potential injuries?
   a. How long have you been lying here?
   b. Where do you hurt the most?
   c. What is your doctor's name?
   d. How did you land?

2. The patient tells you that he landed feet first with his knees locked and then broke his forward fall with his hands. What potential injuries should you suspect?
   a. Spine injury in the lumbar, midthoracic, and cervical regions; and head trauma
   b. Injuries to the femur, hips, pelvis, spine, midthoracic and cervical regions, and wrists
   c. Spinal injury in the cervical and lumbar region, plus chest and shoulder injury
   d. Injuries to the hands and knees

CASE STUDY 3

A teenage gunshot victim is lying on her back next to the front door of her house. Her eyes are open. You ask, "What happened?" She replies, "I was just standing here, and these guys drove by and shot me." There is noticeable bleeding to her left lower chest, and she is holding the area with her right hand. Her skin is pale, cool, and moist. Respirations are normal, and radial pulse is weak, rapid, and regular.

1. Given this description of the patient's injury, which of the following statements is correct?
   a. Lung tissue is intolerant of cavitation caused by projectiles.
   b. Pneumothorax is an uncommon result of injury to the chest and/or lung.
   c. Evaluate the patient for both thoracic and abdominal injury.
   d. The presence of associated rib fractures is unlikely.

2. You dress the wound to the patient's lower chest. What have you forgotten to do?
   a. Look for and treat any additional (entrance or exit) wounds.
   b. Probe the wound to see if the bullet has lodged in the body.
   c. Pour an antiseptic solution into the wound prior to bandaging.
   d. Provide oxygen therapy via nasal cannula at 6 lpm.

CHAPTER

27 Bleeding and Shock

OBJECTIVES

Numbered objectives are from the United States Department of Transportation EMT-Basic National Standard Curriculum. Asterisked objectives, if any, pertain to material that is supplemental to the DOT curriculum.

Cognitive

5-1.1 List the structure and function of the circulatory system.
5-1.2 Differentiate between arterial, venous, and capillary bleeding.
5-1.3 State methods of emergency medical care of external bleeding.
5-1.4 Establish the relationship between body substance isolation and bleeding.
5-1.5 Establish the relationship between airway management and the trauma patient.
5-1.6 Establish the relationship between mechanism of injury and internal bleeding.
5-1.7 List the signs of internal bleeding.
5-1.8 List the steps in emergency medical care of the patient with signs and symptoms of internal bleeding.
5-1.9 List signs and symptoms of shock (hypoperfusion).
5-1.10 State the steps in the emergency medical care of the patient with signs and symptoms of shock (hypoperfusion).

KEY IDEAS

This chapter focuses on the emergency management of bleeding and shock (hypoperfusion). As an EMT, you must be able to recognize the signs and symptoms of internal and external bleeding. Failure to rapidly recognize and treat bleeding of either type has the potential to lead to rapid patient deterioration, shock, and death.

- It is imperative that the EMT always take all appropriate BSI precautions and practice good hand-washing when caring for any patient.

- Differentiation of the type of bleeding (arterial, venous, or capillary) is based on the color of the blood and the nature of blood flow. Each type can be life threatening.

- Only airway and breathing have a higher priority than the control of severe bleeding.

- Control of severe external bleeding is performed during the initial assessment, while the treatment of internal bleeding and shock is accomplished immediately following the initial assessment.

- External bleeding may be controlled by a variety of methods including direct pressure, elevation, pressure points, splints, pressure splints, and tourniquets.

- Always suspect internal bleeding in cases of unexplained shock.

©2008 by Pearson Education, Inc.

- The goal of emergency medical care for internal bleeding is to recognize its presence quickly, maintain the body's perfusion, and provide rapid transport to an appropriate medical facility.

- Shock is the direct result of inadequate perfusion. If allowed to persist, cell failure, organ failure, and death will follow.

- No matter what kind of bleeding has caused shock, rapid transport to a medical facility is a critical element of the emergency medical care.

MEDICAL TERMINOLOGY

Term	Prefix	Word Root Combining Form	Suffix	Definition
epistaxis (ep-uh-STAKS-is)	epi- (upon, over, above)		-staxis (dripping, trickling)	Bleeding from the nose; a nosebleed
hemophilia (hee-moh-FEEL-yuh)		hem/o (blood)	-philia (attraction)	Disease that prevents activation of the normal clotting mechanism
hypertension (high-per-TEN-shun)	hyper- (above, beyond, excessive)	tens (tension)	-ion (process)	A higher-than-normal blood pressure
hypoperfusion (high-poh-per-FYU-zhun)	hypo- (below, under, deficient)	perfusion (supplying an organ with nutrients and oxygen)		The insufficient supply of oxygen and other nutrients to some of the body cells that results from inadequate circulation of blood
hypovolemic (high-poh-vo-LEE-mik)	hypo- (below, under, deficient)	volem (volume)	-ic (pertaining to)	Diminished blood volume
systolic (sis-TOL-ik)		systole (contraction)	-ic (pertaining to)	The part of the heart cycle when the heart is contracting; pertaining to the top number of a blood pressure reading
vasoconstriction (VAYZ-oh-kon-STRIK-shun)	vas/o- (vessel)	constriction (narrowing)		The narrowing of a blood vessel's diameter
vasodilation (VAYZ-oh-dye-LAY-shun)	vas/o- (vessel)	dilation (widening)		The widening of a blood vessel's diameter

1. The medical term *epistaxis,* referring to a nosebleed, contains the suffix *-staxis.* You know this means
   a. flowing, rushing.
   b. dripping, trickling.
   c. uncontrolled.
   d. surge, flood.

2. The medical term *hemophilia* contains the word root *hem/o,* which refers to
   a. blood.
   b. heart.
   c. clotting.
   d. vessel.

3. The medical term *hypertension* refers to a higher-than-normal blood pressure. The word root *tens* means
   a. the number 10.
   b. high, above.
   c. blood.
   d. tension.

4. The medical term *systolic* contains the word root *systole.* You know this means
   a. system.
   b. contraction.
   c. upper.
   d. pressure.

5. The medical term *vasoconstriction* contains the prefix *vas/o-,* which means
   a. heart.
   b. blood.
   c. cell.
   d. vessel.

TERMS AND CONCEPTS

1. _____ is the insufficient supply of oxygen and other nutrients to the body's cells, which results from inadequate circulation of blood.

2. The medical term for a nosebleed is _____.

3. By compressing an artery at a _____ _____, arterial blood flow can be reduced in an extremity.

CONTENT REVIEW

1. The circulatory system provides
   a. blood to the human body.
   b. nutrients to the human body.
   c. nutrients and filters the blood.
   d. nutrients and blood to the human body.

2. The three main components of the circulatory system are
   a. heart, arteries, and veins.
   b. heart, capillaries, and veins.
   c. arteries, capillaries, and veins.
   d. heart, vessels, and blood.

3. For adequate tissue perfusion at the level of the capillaries, it is necessary that the body maintain certain functions. Which of the following is *not* required to maintain tissue perfusion at the level of the capillaries?
   a. Adequate blood volume
   b. Adequate kidney function
   c. Adequate pumping of the heart
   d. Adequate vessel size

4. The vital organs that are particularly sensitive to a decrease in perfusion (and that play a major role in attempting to reverse shock) are the heart, brain, lungs, and
   a. bowels
   b. spleen
   c. kidneys
   d. liver

5. Write the number of the correct term beside its description.
   1. Arterial bleeding
   2. Venous bleeding
   3. Capillary bleeding

   _____ a. Dark red blood that flows steadily from a wound

   _____ b. Dark red blood that slowly oozes from a wound

   _____ c. Bright red blood that spurts from a wound

6. Your patient is not breathing and has life-threatening bleeding from a large open wound. What is the treatment priority?
   a. Airway, breathing, and then bleeding control.
   b. Breathing, airway, and then bleeding control.
   c. Bleeding, airway, and then breathing control.
   d. This patient is critical; there is no priority of sequence.

7. Your patient has a large wound to his right lower leg, which is bleeding profusely. There is no deformity of the extremity. Which of the following best describes the *first* steps in emergency management of this injury?
   a. Use a tourniquet and elevation
   b. Use a sling, swathe, and elevation
   c. Use direct pressure, elevation
   d. Use the femoral pressure point and elevation

8. You are treating a patient who has a large laceration. You note that the vessels have been cut across, or perpendicular to, the vessel. You know that a vessel that has been cut in this manner has a tendency to
   a. retract and clot off.
   b. spasm and dilate.
   c. open and hemorrhage.
   d. contract, then expand.

9. Label each photograph with the name of the major pressure point that is illustrated.

A. _____

B. _____

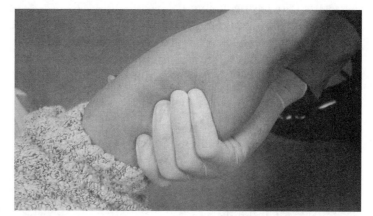
A

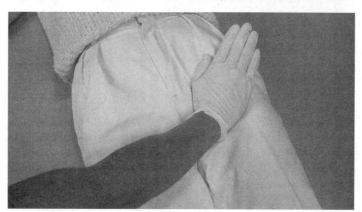
B

10. The only circumstance in which a tourniquet should be considered as a way to control bleeding is
    a. when there is spurting arterial bleeding.
    b. when there is an amputated extremity.
    c. when nerves, muscles, and blood vessels are damaged.
    d. when pressure is also needed to stabilize bones.

11. You are treating a patient who has sustained a large wound and has an altered mental status. You apply direct pressure to the wound and assess the patient. The patient's breathing is adequate, so you should
    a. apply oxygen via nasal cannula at 6 lpm.
    b. administer oxygen via simple face mask at 8 lpm.
    c. provide oxygen via a nonrebreather mask at 15 lpm.
    d. deliver positive-pressure ventilations by bag-valve mask.

12. List at least three mechanisms of injury that can cause internal bleeding.

13. Which of the following is considered inappropriate emergency medical care for the patient you suspect of having an internal bleed?
    a. Administer high-flow oxygen
    b. Splint painful, swollen, or deformed extremities
    c. Increase fluids by administering water by mouth
    d. Place patient in a Trendelenburg position

14. Shock (hypoperfusion) should be suspected in patients who have suffered which of the following injuries?
    1. Penetrating injury
    2. Burns
    3. Organ rupture or laceration
    4. Crush injury
    5. Blunt trauma
    a. 2, 3
    b. 1, 3, 4
    c. 1, 2, 4, 5
    d. 1, 2, 3, 4, 5

15. You are treating the victim of a shooting. You recognize which of the following as a *late* sign of shock?
    a. Low blood pressure
    b. Anxiety
    c. Altered mental status
    d. Restlessness

16. The following items reflect the progressive nature of shock (hypoperfusion). Number the list below in the proper general order from 1 to 5 in which they occur.

    _____ Leaking capillaries cause loss of vital blood plasma; unresponsiveness and death may result.

    _____ Blood vessels constrict in extremities to conserve blood, causing cold, clammy skin.

    _____ Low oxygen levels to breathing-control centers of the brain make respirations rapid and shallow; nervous system reaction results in profuse sweating.

    _____ Vasoconstriction fails, and blood pressure drops.

    _____ Blood loss causes rapid heart rate and weak pulse.

17. The body has a defensive mechanism that causes the peripheral blood vessels to constrict to shunt blood to the core of the body and the vital organs. You know this defensive mechanism is provided by the
    a. sympathetic nervous system.
    b. compensatory nervous system.
    c. peripheral nervous system.
    d. cardiovascular nervous system.

18. Describe the emergency medical care of shock.

19. A tourniquet applied to an extremity that does not completely stop arterial blood flow will likely
  a. reduce the bleeding by acting as a constricting band.
  b. increase arterial bleeding by decreasing arterial pressure in the wound.
  c. reduce the amount of venous pressure and decrease bleeding from the wound.
  d. build up arterial and venous pressure in the wound and increase bleeding.

20. Which of the following will cause the skin of the traumatic patient to become pale, diaphoretic, and cool?
  a. Inhibiting the release of delta properties by limiting the amount of epinephrine and norepinephrine stimulation from the brain
  b. Stimulation of the adrenal glands to secrete epinephrine and norepinephrine alpha properties constricting the vessels
  c. Inhibiting the release of epinephrine and norepinephrine, which helps to dilate the vessels stimulating clotting factors
  d. Stimulation of beta properties from the release of epinephrine and norepinephrine that constrict the bronchiole smooth muscles

21. You are assessing a trauma patient. Which of the following would you likely observe as the patient blood volume depletes?
  a. The diastolic blood pressure increases and the diastolic blood pressure maintains, then drops, causing a widening pulse pressure.
  b. The systolic and diastolic blood pressure drops, causing the pulse pressure to widen.
  c. The systolic blood pressure maintains or increases as the diastolic blood pressure decreases, causing a narrowing pulse pressure.
  d. The systolic blood pressure drops and the diastolic blood pressure maintains or increases, creating a narrowing pulse pressure.

22. Which of the following factors may interfere with the clotting process of your trauma patient and lead to an increase of bleeding?
  a. Medication such as asprin and ibuprofen
  b. Immobilizing the extremity from moving
  c. Normal or higher body temperture (fever)
  d. Applying direct digital pressure to the bleeding site

23. Which of the following statements is correct pertaining to an infant or child with a traumatic injury?
  a. Infants and children compensate for blood loss for a longer period of time than do adults, then deteriorate rapidly once they begin to decompensate.
  b. Infants and children deteriorate rapidly after blood loss, then begin to compensate and the blood pressure stabilizes.
  c. Infants and children compensate for blood loss for a longer period of time than do adults and then maintain an adequate blood pressure.
  d. Infants and children deteriorate rapidly, with a decreasing blood pressure, and continue to deteriorate until impending cardiac arrest.

CASE STUDY

You are on-scene with a 28-year-old male who put his hands through a window while attempting to open it. Your initial assessment reveals that he is responsive and alert, with a patent airway and adequate respirations. He has numerous lacerations on both hands and forearms, which are bleeding steadily, as well as a very large wound on the inside of his right wrist, which is spurting bright red blood. His skin is pale, cool, and clammy.

1. To control the arterial bleeding you should
   a. place a sterile gauze over the large wound and apply fingertip pressure to the site.
   b. apply a wide tourniquet below the laceration site, ensuring adequate perfusion of the hand.
   c. elevate the wound above the level of the heart and apply a cold compress.
   d. apply an occlusive dressing over the wound site and secure with a tight gauze bandage.

After taking the steps you have just described, you note that the patient seems more anxious and restless than when you arrived several minutes ago. He continues to talk coherently and answers your questions.

2. What is the significance of his increasing agitation?
   a. This agitation may indicate the patient has been drinking.
   b. An agitated state may indicate the patient is mentally unstable.
   c. His increasing agitation may be an early sign of shock.
   d. Agitation in this case likely indicates a decreased mental capacity.

You move him to your ambulance and prepare to begin transport. You have learned that he has no allergies and he takes AZT because he is HIV-positive. He says that he has been feeling fine and has no other medical problems. He ate a sandwich and had a soft drink for lunch about an hour ago. He says that the window was stuck and he was trying to pull it open when he lost his balance, put his hands up to catch himself, and shattered the window.

3. While transporting your patient, you notice the bandage has become soaked through with blood. You should
   a. remove the bandage and replace with a new sterile dressing.
   b. place a new sterile bandage over the blood-soaked bandage.
   c. apply a constricting band over the wound to decrease blood flow.
   d. apply an ice pack over the blood-soaked bandage and elevate.

ENRICHMENT

1. You are treating a trauma patient. Of the following signs, which of the following is considered a late sign of shock?
   a. Narrow pulse pressure
   b. Weaker pulse
   c. Slightly pale and cool skin
   d. Low blood pressure

2. The main indicator that your patient has progressed from compensatory shock to decompensated, or progressive, shock is a
   a. decrease in respiratory rate.
   b. widening of the pulse pressure.
   c. decrease in the heart rate.
   d. drop in systolic blood pressure.

3. Your patient is in late decompensated, or progressive, shock. Which of the following signs and symptoms is an indicator of this late-shock state?
   a. Unresponsiveness
   b. Slightly pale skin
   c. Bounding peripheral pulses
   d. Increase in body temperature

4. In the irreversible stage of shock, the compensatory mechanisms have all been exhausted. Highly acidic, cold, sludged blood dumps into the core circulation. Which of the following signs and symptoms would indicate your patient is in irreversible shock?
   a. The patient will become agitated.
   b. The patient may bleed from all orifices.
   c. The patient's blood pressure will return to near normal.
   d. The patient's skin becomes flushed, warm, and dry.

5. This type of shock is usually the result of a spinal or head injury, which causes the nervous system to lose control over the vascular system, dilating the blood vessels. It is known as
   a. hypovolemic shock.
   b. vasogenic shock.
   c. cardiogenic shock.
   d. septic shock.

SCENARIO 15: DOCUMENTATION EXERCISE

Read the following scenario, and think about how you would document this call if you were the EMT who responded to the scene. Then answer the multiple-choice questions and fill in the sample prehospital-care report, basing your documentation on information from the scenario.

It's 0800 hours on a sultry Saturday morning. You and your partner, Mim, are performing your daily cleaning and inspection of your ambulance when a car pulls into the driveway. The frantic driver runs toward you screaming, "They stabbed my friend!" As you try to calm the driver to gain information, the station alerting system sounds. "Unit 1, EMS Battalion Chief, respond to 1600 14th Avenue for a patient stabbed. Law enforcement is on-scene, and the scene is safe." The frantic man in your driveway has overheard the call. "That's my friend!" he interjects. Mim acknowledges the call, and you recognize the address as two blocks down the street. You both apply gloves and eye protection before leaving the station.

As you approach the scene, you see many police cars and officers. One officer is pointing toward a particular police car. You mark on-scene with dispatch. Upon exiting the ambulance, you see the patient lying on his left side next to the police car with an officer bending over him. You and Mim quickly pull the stretcher from the ambulance, making sure to bring your oxygen bag and trauma box.

As you and Mim approach the patient, you advise dispatch that you have made patient contact. The officer crouching by the patient says, "He got stabbed twice, once on the right side and once in the inner-thigh area." The officer is holding direct pressure with a small bandage to the right lower lateral flank area and another to the right inner thigh. As you quickly open two large trauma dressings, you ask the officer to gently lift the bandages so you can inspect the wounds. You see two large puncture wounds. The wound to the right lower lateral flank area is bleeding freely with dark red blood. The wound to the inner thigh is spurting bright red blood. You quickly place the trauma dressings over the wounds and instruct the officer to apply firm, direct pressure over both wounds.

The patient is awake, alert, and talking to the officer. You ask if he was stabbed anywhere else on his body, and he says, "No, I don't think so." You ask him his name, and he replies, "Frank." You respond, "My name is Lee. Mim and I will be your EMTs, and we're going to take good care of you." Mim quickly asks the patient if he has any medical history or takes any medication, and he replies, "No." She asks if he is allergic to anything, and he replies, "Not that I know of." Mim performs a quick initial assessment. There are no stridorous or crowing sounds with inhalation or exhalation. She indicates that Frank's breathing is normal at an approximate rate of 18 per minute. She also notes that his chest appears to be rising and falling, with adequate air flowing in and out of his mouth and nose and without use of accessory muscles. Mim applies high-flow oxygen via nonrebreather mask at 15 lpm. She radios dispatch to notify the trauma center of a trauma alert and to launch the helicopter. She explains to Frank that he must go to a specialized trauma center in a neighboring town, and he will get there by helicopter. He states, "I trust you both. Please don't let me die." You recognize the wounds to be very serious. You ask the police officer if he has the knife or knows how long it was, and he replies, "The knife hasn't been located yet."

Mim feels for a radial pulse and finds a weak pulse at 90 beats per minute; the skin is warm and slightly diaphoretic; the capillary blanch is less than 2 seconds. She begins a rapid trauma assessment. The head reveals no deformities; the pupils are equal and react briskly to light. The nose, mouth, and ears are all clear of blood or fluid. The neck is soft without any obvious injuries or subcutaneous emphysema. The trachea is midline, and there is no deformity or pain to the posterior neck. She palpates the chest and notes equal chest rise and fall, finding no signs of trauma or use of accessory muscles. She carefully inspects the axillary area by lifting the arms, looking for hidden injuries. No trauma is noted.

Inspection of the abdomen reveals only the puncture wound located during the initial assessment. The abdomen is distended with slight discoloration around the umbilicus and bilateral flank areas. She palpates the abdomen, and Frank responds with a grimaced face and remarks, "Ouch, that really hurts." Mim says she is sorry and that she is almost done. She notes that the pain is in all four quadrants and that the patient guards the area. She then turns to you and says, "The abdomen is distended and rigid with slight discoloration and pain on palpation." Mim quickly inspects the pelvis for deformity, contusions, abrasions, or penetrating injuries, and none are found. She rapidly assesses the extremities and finds no injuries other than the previously noted right-inner-thigh puncture wound. Frank indicates he can feel her touching each extremity, and he has good movement in all extremities. Mim remarks to you, "I can't find any distal pulses." She immediately feels for a femoral pulse, locates it, and reports it is strong. She examines the posterior

body and finds no trauma or sacral edema. She does note slight discoloration to the small of the back. The patient does not complain of any pain when the spine is palpated.

You position the cot next to the patient and, with Mim's assistance, you place the patient on the cot. The patient is placed in a supine position and Mim lifts the foot end of the cot and locks it, which places the patient into the Trendelenburg position. You both wheel the cot to the ambulance while talking reassuringly to Frank. Your battalion chief arrives on-scene and asks, "What do you have?" You briefly give him a size-up of Frank's condition. He asks, "How can I help you?" You inform him that you have a police officer assisting you and that you are in good shape right now. He informs you that he will set up the helicopter landing zone at a nearby park. You ask another police officer to drive your ambulance to the landing zone so that you and Mim can both care for Frank in the patient compartment. You notify dispatch that you are en route to the LZ area.

While en route to the landing zone, you assess the vital signs. You notice the patient's breathing rate has increased to 28 times a minute, is shallow, with use of accessory muscles. Frank appears more restless and anxious, and you reassure him. You immediately insert a nasopharyngeal airway and provide positive-pressure ventilation with the BVM attached to oxygen. The carotid pulse is 130 beats per minute. The skin has become cool, sweaty, and pale. The blood pressure is 96/80 and difficult to hear. The capillary blanch is now delayed at 4 seconds.

As the police officer pulls the ambulance near the landing zone, you see that the helicopter is just touching down. You hear your battalion chief advise dispatch that the helicopter is on the ground. You hear a gentle knock on the rear door of the ambulance, and as it opens, you recognize flight medics Doug and Mike. Doug asks you what you have, and you give him a brief but thorough report. Mike notifies the pilot of the helicopter that they will be doing a "hot load." Frank is quickly loaded onto the helicopter. Less than a minute later, the helicopter lifts from the LZ and advises the battalion chief that the patient will be at the trauma center in approximately 10 minutes.

You and Mim gather your thoughts while decontaminating your equipment and ambulance in preparation for the next call. Your battalion chief meets you at the ambulance and asks how you're doing. He coordinates a critique of the call for quality-improvement purposes.

1. During the initial assessment, the stab wound to the right lower lateral flank area produced a dark red blood that was flowing freely. Which type of bleeding would you suspect?
   a. Arterial
   b. Arteriolar
   c. Venous
   d. Capillary

2. The bleeding to the right inner-thigh area produced bright red spurting blood. Which type of bleeding would you suspect?
   a. Arterial
   b. Venous
   c. Venular
   d. Capillary

3. While assessing the patient, Mim noticed the abdomen was distended with slight discoloration around the umbilicus. You know this to be an indication that
   a. blood is being shunted to the extremities as a compensatory response.
   b. severe hypoxia has occurred, and cardiac arrest is imminent.
   c. the patient is having a severe allergic reaction to an unknown antigen.
   d. a significant amount of blood has collected in the abdomen.

4. When Mim felt for distal pulses and could not locate any, she immediately felt for a femoral pulse and found it to be strong. What does this indicate?
   a. Blood is being pushed into the extremities.
   b. A severe state of hypoperfusion (shock) exists.
   c. Respiratory effort has increased.
   d. The patient is in the early stages of shock.

5. You know this patient has entered the late, decompensated stage of shock. Which of the following signs indicates that your patient has progressed into this stage?
   a. The patient developed bradycardia (abnormally slow heart rate).
   b. The patient developed bradypneia (abnormally slow respirations).
   c. The peripheral pulses became absent.
   d. The patient had a widening pulse pressure.

6. The police officer applied firm, direct pressure to the right inner-thigh wound. If the bleeding remains uncontrolled, your next immediate action should be to
   a. apply a wide tourniquet to the upper right thigh.
   b. apply firm, direct pressure to the abdominal aorta pressure point.
   c. apply firm, direct pressure to the right brachial pressure point.
   d. apply firm, direct pressure to the right femoral pressure point.

EMERGENCY TRIP SHEET

TRIP #	
MEDIC #	
BEGIN MILES	
END MILES	
CODE___/___	PAGE___/___
UNITS ON SCENE	

BILLING USE ONLY				
DAY				
DATE				
RECEIVED				
DISPATCHED				
EN-ROUTE				
ON SCENE				
TO HOSPITAL				
AT HOSPITAL				
IN-SERVICE				

NAME   SEX M F DOB ___/___/___

ADDRESS   RACE

CITY   STATE   ZIP

PHONE ( )   -   PCP DR.

RESPONDED FROM   CITY

TAKEN FROM   ZIP

DESTINATION   REASON

SSN   -   -   MEDICARE #   MEDICAID #

INSURANCE CO   INSURANCE #   GROUP #

RESPONSIBLE PARTY   ADDRESS

CITY   STATE   ZIP   PHONE ( )   -

EMPLOYER

CREW	CERT	STATE #

TIME	ON SCENE (1)	ON SCENE (2)	ON SCENE (3)	EN-ROUTE (1)	EN-ROUTE (2)	AT DESTINATION
BP						
PULSE						
RESP						
EKG						

IV THERAPY
SUCCESSFUL Y N # OF ATTEMPTS _____
ANGIO SIZE _____ga.
SITE _____
TOTAL FLUID INFUSED _____ cc
BLOOD DRAW Y N INITIALS

INTUBATION INFORMATION
SUCCESSFUL Y N # OF ATTEMPTS _____
TUBE SIZE _____ mm
TIME _____ INITIALS _____

MEDICAL HISTORY

CONDITION CODES

MEDICATIONS

TREATMENTS

TIME	TREATMENT	DOSE	ROUTE	INIT

ALLERGIES

C/C

EVENTS LEADING TO C/C

ASSESSMENT

TREATMENT

GCS | E___ V___ M___ TOTAL =
GCS | E___ V___ M___ TOTAL =

HOSPITAL CONTACTED

CPR BEGUN BY   B   P   TIME BEGUN

AED USED   Y   N   BY:

RESUSCITATION TERMINATED - TIME

EMS SIGNATURE

( ) OSHA REGULATIONS FOLLOWED

28 Soft Tissue Injuries

OBJECTIVES

Numbered objectives are from the United States Department of Transportation EMT-Basic National Standard Curriculum. Asterisked objectives, if any, pertain to material that is supplemental to the DOT curriculum.

Cognitive

5-2.1 State the major functions of the skin.

5-2.2 List the layers of the skin.

5-2.3 Establish the relationship between body substance isolation (BSI) and soft tissue injuries.

5-2.4 List the types of closed soft tissue injuries.

5-2.5 Describe the emergency medical care of the patient with a closed soft tissue injury.

5-2.6 State the types of open soft tissue injuries.

5-2.7 Describe the emergency medical care of the patient with an open soft tissue injury.

5-2.8 Discuss the emergency medical care considerations for a patient with a penetrating chest injury.

5-2.9 State the emergency medical care considerations for a patient with an open wound to the abdomen.

5-2.10 Differentiate the care of an open wound to the chest from an open wound to the abdomen.

5-2.21 List the functions of dressing and bandaging.

5-2.22 Describe the purpose of a bandage.

5-2.23 Describe the steps in applying a pressure dressing.

5-2.24 Establish the relationship between airway management and the patient with chest injury, burns, blunt injuries, and penetrating injuries.

5-2.25 Describe the effects of improperly applied dressings, splints, and tourniquets.

5-2.26 Describe the emergency medical care of a patient with an impaled object.

5-2.27 Describe the emergency medical care of a patient with an amputation.

KEY IDEAS

A soft tissue injury is an injury to skin, muscles, nerves, blood vessels, or organs. The general goals of the emergency medical care of such injuries are to control bleeding, prevent further injury, and reduce the risk of infection.

■ Soft tissue injuries are categorized as closed, open, single, or multiple.

■ In general, emergency care of closed injuries includes taking BSI precautions; ensuring an open airway and adequate breathing; treating for shock; and splinting painful, swollen, or deformed extremities.

- In general, emergency care of open injuries includes taking BSI precautions; ensuring an open airway and adequate breathing; exposing the wound; controlling bleeding; preventing further contamination; and treating for shock.

- Special considerations for the emergency care of soft tissue injuries include using occlusive dressings on open chest wounds, abdominal eviscerations, and large open neck injuries; securing objects impaled in the body (except the cheek); and caring for amputated parts.

- Dressings cover open wounds, and bandages hold dressings in place. A pressure (or bulky) dressing can be used to control bleeding. General principles of dressing and bandaging include using materials that are sterile or at least clean; bandaging only when bleeding has stopped; adequately covering the entire wound with a dressing and the entire dressing with a bandage; applying a bandage from distal to proximal; removing all jewelry from injured parts; bandaging not too loosely or tightly (checking distal pulses, motor, and sensory function before and after bandage application); on an extremity, bandaging a larger area than the wound to avoid creating a pressure point; and applying a tourniquet only as a last resort.

MEDICAL TERMINOLOGY

Term	Prefix	Word Root Combining Form	Suffix	Definition
abrasion (uh-BRAY-zhun)	ab- (away from)	ras (to scrape)	-ion (process)	An open injury to the epidermis caused by a scraping away, rubbing, or shearing away of the tissue
avulsion (uh-VUL-shun)	a- (no, not, without, lack of)	vuls (to pull)	-ion (process)	An open injury characterized by a loose flap of skin and soft tissue that has been torn loose or pulled off
dermis (DER-miss)		derm (skin)	-is (pertaining to)	The second layer of skin; the layer of skin below the epidermis
embolism (EM-boh-lizm)		embol (to cast, to throw)	-ism (condition of)	Obstruction of a blood vessel by a foreign substance
epidermis (ep-uh-DER-miss)	epi- (upon, over, above)	derm (skin)	-is (pertaining to)	The outermost or top layer of skin; the layer above the dermis
hematoma (hee-muh-TOH-muh)		hemat (blood)	-oma (tumor)	A closed injury to the soft tissues characterized by swelling and discoloration caused by a mass of blood below the epidermis
pneumothorax (nu-moh-THOR-aks)		pneumo/o (lun, air) thorax (chest)		Collection of air or gas in the pleural cavity
subcutaneous (sub-kyu-TAY-nee-us)	sub- (below, under, beneath)	cutane (skin)	-ous (pertaining to)	The third layer of skin; the layer below the dermis

1. The medical term *abrasion* refers to an open injury to the epidermis caused by scraping. You know the prefix *ab-* means
   a. skin.
   b. toward.
   c. away from.
   d. scrape.

2. The medical term *avulsion* contains the word root *vuls*, which means
   a. to pull.
   b. to cut.
   c. flap.
   d. skin.

3. You use the medical term *dermis* in your patient-care report. You know that the word root *derm* means
   a. skin.
   b. blood.
   c. above.
   d. toward.

4. The medical term *hematoma* contains the word root *hemat*. You partner asks what this root means, and you answer
   a. cut.
   b. bump.
   c. tumor.
   d. blood.

5. The medical term *subcutaneous* contains the word root *cutane*, which means
   a. lung.
   b. skin.
   c. below.
   d. finger.

TERMS AND CONCEPTS

1. Write the number of the correct term next to each definition.

   1. Abrasion
   2. Air embolism
   3. Avulsion
   4. Contusion
   5. Crush injury

   6. Evisceration
   7. Hematoma
   8. Laceration
   9. Occlusive dressing
   10. Penetration/puncture

   _____ a. An open injury usually caused by forceful impact with a sharp object and characterized by a wound whose edges may be linear or stellate in appearance

   _____ b. A protrusion of organs from a wound

   _____ c. A closed or an open injury to soft tissues and underlying organs that is the result of a crushing force applied to the body

   _____ d. An open injury to the outermost layer of the skin caused by a scraping, rubbing, or shearing away of the tissue

   _____ e. An open injury caused by a sharp, pointed object being forced into the soft tissues

   _____ f. An air bubble that obstructs a blood vessel

   _____ g. A closed injury to the cells and blood vessels contained within the dermis that is characterized by discoloration, swelling, and pain; a bruise

   _____ h. A closed injury to the soft tissues characterized by swelling and discoloration caused by a mass of blood beneath the epidermis

   _____ i. A dressing that can form an airtight seal over a wound

   _____ j. An open injury characterized by a loose flap of skin and soft tissue that has been torn loose or pulled completely off

CONTENT REVIEW

1. The layers of the skin from the outermost to the innermost are
   a. Dermis, epidermis, and subcutaneous layer
   b. Subcutaneous, epidermis, and dermis layer
   c. Subcutaneous, dermis, and epidermis layer
   d. Epidermis, dermis, and subcutaneous layer

2. Which of the following descriptions are considered functions of the skin?
   1. Aids in the elimination of water and various salts
   2. Serves as a receptor organ
   3. Produces white blood cells
   4. Protects the body from the environment

   a. 1, 2, 3
   b. 1, 2, 4
   c. 1, 3, 4
   d. 2, 3, 4

3. Which of the following injuries is considered an open injury?
   a. Contusion
   b. Amputation
   c. Hematoma
   d. Crush injury

4. Which of the following dressings contain fibrinogen and thrombin on the surface, which promotes clotting when applied to wounds?
   a. Occlusive dressing
   b. Hemostatic dressing
   c. Hemorrhagic dressing
   d. Tamponade dressing

5. Which of the following is the correct order for treatment of closed soft tissue injuries?
   a. Airway and breathing, BSI precautions, shock, injured extremities
   b. BSI precautions, shock, airway and breathing, injured extremities
   c. BSI precautions, airway and breathing, shock, injured extremities
   d. Injured extremities, BSI precautions, airway and breathing, shock

6. You are treating a patient who has sustained a chest wound. Which of the following dressings is used to prevent air from entering the chest cavity?
   a. Nonelastic, self-adhering
   b. Multitrauma
   c. Bulky
   d. Occlusive

7. While treating a patient who has sustained an open chest wound, how should you tape the dressing?
   a. On the top and bottom only
   b. On three sides only
   c. On all four sides
   d. Down the middle only

8. Which of the following amputation injuries is usually associated with severe bleeding?
   a. Circumferential abrasions of the appendage
   b. A clean cut through the vessels and tissues
   c. Jagged or crushing-type injuries to a vessel
   d. Laceration that cuts through the epidermis

9. Which of the following is the correct order of steps for emergency care of a patient with an impaled object?
   1. Use a bulky dressing to help stabilize the object.
   2. Manually secure the object.
   3. Control bleeding.
   4. Expose the wound area.
   a. 2, 4, 3, 1
   b. 4, 3, 2, 1
   c. 3, 1, 2, 4
   d. 4, 2, 3, 1

10. Which of the following is considered an inappropriate treatment for an amputated part and may cause further tissue damage?
    a. Immerse the part in cool, sterile water.
    b. Wrap the part in dry, sterile dressing.
    c. Wrap or bag the part in plastic.
    d. Keep the part cool.

11. Bleeding control and prevention of an air embolism are the major goals of emergency care of a large open neck wound. What type of dressing would help to prevent an air embolism?
    a. Occlusive
    b. Trauma
    c. Porous
    d. Bulky

12. List the steps for applying a pressure dressing.

13. For circumferential bandages, which of the following should you check before and after bandaging?
    a. Distal pulses, skin color, and temperature
    b. Capillary refill, skin color, and temperature
    c. Distal pulses, motor function, and sensory function
    d. ABCs, motor function, and sensory function

14. Which of the following are the proper dressings for an abdominal evisceration?
    a. Sterile, moist gauze, then an occlusive dressing
    b. Self-adhering roller bandage, then an occlusive dressing
    c. Any sterile absorbent material, then an occlusive dressing
    d. Bulky dressing, then an occlusive dressing

15. You have ruled out potential spinal injury in a patient with abdominal evisceration. Your partner asks you to flex the patient's hips and knees during transport. Why?
    a. It helps stabilize the abdominal organs.
    b. It will prevent the development of an embolism.
    c. It reduces the tension on the abdominal muscles.
    d. It helps to increase oxygen to the vital organs.

CASE STUDY 1

You are dispatched to a local bar for a stabbing. The patient is a female, about 25 years old. She is sitting at a table, her hand to her neck, with dark red blood flowing steadily through her fingers. Your general impression of her is good; however, her skin is pale, warm, and slightly moist. As your partner begins to control the bleeding, you find that respirations are adequate with good tidal volume. The radial pulse is strong and regular. There are no other obvious signs of trauma or bleeding present.

1. The bleeding from the patient's neck wound is likely which of the following?
   a. Capillary bleeding
   b. Arterial bleeding
   c. Venous bleeding
   d. Combination of arterial/capillary bleeding

2. Which of the following lists the correct procedures in the correct order for emergency care for this wound?
   a. Gloved hand over the wound, then an occlusive dressing, and finally a pressure dressing
   b. Occlusive dressing over the wound, then a pressure dressing, and finally your gloved hand
   c. Pressure dressing over the wound, then an occlusive dressing, and finally your gloved hand
   d. Gloved hand over the wound, then a pressure dressing, and finally an occlusive dressing

CASE STUDY 2

You are at the scene of a shooting. The 20-year-old patient is supine and responsive. A law-enforcement officer has told you that three shots were fired, the weapon was a .357-caliber handgun, and the patient was shot from 30 to 40 yards away. There is obvious bleeding coming from the patient's right upper-chest region and a sucking sound is heard with each breath. As your partner proceeds to control bleeding, you find that the patient is cyanotic; respirations are shallow and rapid; radial pulse is weak and regular; and the skin is cool and slightly moist.

1. In addition to this patient's obvious injury, you should suspect which of the following?
   a. Ring avulsion
   b. Spinal injury
   c. Lower airway obstruction
   d. Cardiac tamponade

2. In addition to treatment for this patient's obvious injury, treatment also includes
   a. splinting of upper extremities.
   b. care of large, open neck injuries.
   c. methodically assessing for closed wounds.
   d. assessing for other entry and exit wounds.

ENRICHMENT

1. You are called to a patient who has been bitten by a large dog. You know the most dangerous bites are those in which the injury occurs
   a. over nerve tissue.
   b. over fat tissue.
   c. over vascular areas.
   d. over bone or joints.

2. You are treating a 5-year-old patient who has placed his hand into the mouth of a small jar and now is unable to remove it. Which of the following would be considered part of the inappropriate treatment for this situation?
   a. Apply lubricant and try to remove the hand.
   b. Raise the hand and the jar above the patient's head.
   c. Transport the patient with the hand in the jar to the hospital.
   d. Wrap a towel around the jar and gently break it to remove the hand.

SCENARIO 16: **DOCUMENTATION EXERCISE**

Read the following scenario, and think about how you would document this call if you were the EMT who responded to the scene. Then answer the multiple-choice questions and fill in the sample prehospital-care report, basing your documentation on information from the scenario.

It's 1800 hours. You and your partner, Lt. Rodriguez, are preparing a healthful dinner at your station. The workday has been steady with typical medical calls. As you prepare the salad, the station alerting system sounds. "Squad 7, Engine 7, EMS Battalion Chief, respond to an industrial accident at 1215 82nd Avenue for a possible amputated arm." You acknowledge the call, and ask dispatch to notify the trauma center and to place the helicopter on standby. En route to the scene, Lt. Rodriguez double-checks the address in the map book. After a short emergency response, you arrive on-scene at a large manufacturing plant. As you both scan for obvious hazards, you apply gloves, mask, and eye protection. You pull the stretcher from the ambulance, place all the equipment you may need on it, and walk briskly toward the building.

You approach the entryway and are met by an anxious manager of the facility, who says, "You must hurry. His whole arm has been cut off by the equipment." Lt. Rodriguez asks the manager if the patient is entrapped and if the equipment has been shut down. He answers, "He's not trapped, and all of the equipment has been shut down and secured with lockout locks so the equipment cannot be restarted inadvertently."

As you and Lt. Rodriguez approach, you see the middle-aged male patient lying supine on the floor with a coworker holding a towel over the end of a right arm severed at about the mid-shaft area of the humerus. The patient also has a deep laceration to the right side of the neck, which is bleeding profusely with a steady flow of dark red blood. The patient's eyes meet yours with a terrified look.

You ask the patient his name as you apply a large sterile trauma dressing to the amputated site. He responds, "Bill." You quickly introduce yourself and Lt. Rodriguez and reassure him that you are going to take good care of him. Lt. Rodriguez places his gloved hand directly over the wound on the patient's neck. Bill is quite restless. You explain that, since he has a serious injury, he will be transported to the trauma center in a nearby town by helicopter. You ask Bill what his age is and if he has any medical history or takes any medications. He replies, "I'm 48, and I haven't been to a doctor in 10 years." You ask him if he is allergic to anything, and he states, "Not that I know of."

Lt. Rodriguez asks dispatch to launch the helicopter and issue a trauma alert to the trauma center so they can prepare for the arrival of a serious patient. Lt. Rodriguez performs a quick initial assessment. There are no stridorous or crowing sounds with inhalation or exhalation. Bill's breathing is normal at about 20 breaths per minute. His chest is rising and falling with adequate air flowing in and out of the mouth without the use of accessory muscles. You apply high-flow oxygen with a nonrebreather mask at 15 lpm.

You ask the manager what happened, and he says that Mary, a coworker, witnessed the incident. The manager calls Mary over. She is visibly upset. You explain that it is very important that she quickly explain what happened. She says, "Bill was working on the conveyor belt when his hand got pulled into the mechanisms. He got pulled hard against the conveyor belt when his arm was cut off, and that's how his neck got slashed." You ask her if he was knocked out, and she states, "No, he has remained awake the whole time."

The firefighters arrive on the scene and ask what they can do to help. You instruct the firefighter lieutenant to see if they can locate the severed arm. You instruct another firefighter to maintain in-line stabilization of the spine while you apply a dressing to the neck.

You feel for a radial pulse and find a weak pulse at 110 beats per minute. The skin is cool and diaphoretic, and the capillary blanch is delayed at 4 seconds. Lt. Rodriguez begins a rapid trauma assessment. The head reveals no deformities; the pupils are equal and react briskly to light. The nose, mouth, and ears are all clear of blood or fluid. The neck is soft with a large, deep laceration to the right side; there is no noted subcutaneous emphysema. The trachea is midline, and there is no deformity or pain to the posterior neck. He palpates the chest and notes equal chest rise and fall with no signs of trauma or use of accessory muscles. He inspects the axillary area, and no trauma is noted. Inspection of the abdomen reveals no obvious injuries, distention, or pain with palpation. Lt. Rodriguez quickly inspects the pelvis for deformity, contusions, abrasions, or penetrating injuries, and none are found. He rapidly assesses the extremities and finds no injuries to the other arm or legs. The amputated arm is a clean cut with little bleeding. Bill indicates he can feel him touching each of the unaffected extremities, and he has good movement. Lt. Rodriguez remarks, "I have good distal pulses." He examines the posterior body and finds no trauma or sacral edema. The patient does not complain of any pain when the spine is palpated.

You and Lt. Rodriguez maintain in-line stabilization and place the patient on a backboard, using a c-collar, then secure him with straps. As you place the patient into the Trendelenburg position, the fire lieutenant approaches you and says, "We found it. We found the missing arm." With a squeamish look on his face, he hands the detached arm to you, wrapped in a towel. You ask Lt. Rodriguez and the firefighters to load the patient into the ambulance while you prepare the severed arm for transport.

With the severed arm in the ambulance, you instruct the firefighter to carefully drive in an emergency-response mode to a local baseball field where your battalion chief has instructed the helicopter to land. En route to the landing zone, you obtain baseline vital signs: pulse 124 beats per minute, weak but regular; blood pressure 102/86; respirations 20 each minute with good tidal volume; skin pale, cool, and diaphoretic, no cyanosis noted; pupils equal and slightly sluggish; pulse-oximeter reading at 99 percent on high-flow oxygen. You arrive at the landing zone area and are met by the flight crew, Missy and Dave. You give a quick report to Missy and help to transfer the patient to the waiting helicopter. Missy thanks you and says, "We'll have Bill at the trauma center in approximately 15 minutes." With a thumbs-up gesture, she slides the door closed on the helicopter and lifts off en route to the trauma center.

1. The neck wound is bleeding profusely with a dark red blood that flows steadily. You suspect the patient has sustained what type of injury?
   a. Laceration to the carotid artery
   b. Laceration to the pulmonary artery
   c. Laceration to the jugular vein
   d. Laceration to the pulmonary vein

2. Why did Lieutenant Rodriguez place his gloved hand directly over the wound on the patient's neck?
   a. There was a danger of air being sucked into the neck vein.
   b. This prevents clots from forming and occluding the airway.
   c. He was assessing the blood flow through the severed vessel.
   d. The gloved hand will prevent the area from becoming infected.

3. You recognize the laceration to the patient's neck to be very serious. Which of the following dressings is appropriate for this type of injury?
   a. An all-purpose sterile cotton bandage held in place with circumferential rolled meshed gauze
   b. A universal or multitrauma dressing that is sterile and usually bulky, taped on two sides
   c. A commercially wrapped sterile gauze pad that is the same size as the wound and is self-adhering
   d. An occlusive dressing that extends beyond the edge of the laceration, taped on all four sides

4. If the bleeding soaks through the original pressure dressing that was applied to the severed right arm, indicating continued severe bleeding, what should you do?
   a. Without removing the original bandage, apply additional bandages on top of the previous ones and then rewrap the wound.
   b. Remove the bandages and apply direct fingertip pressure. Once the bleeding is controlled, apply a dressing and bandage to cover the wound again.
   c. Remove all of the original bandages, apply a wide tourniquet proximal to the severed site, and tighten until the bleeding has stopped.
   d. Without removing the original bandages, apply a circumferential constricting band and tighten until the bleeding has slowed.

5. Prior to loading the patient and his severed arm onto the helicopter, you prepared the arm for transport. You know the proper handling of the amputated arm can have a significant impact on the success of surgical reattachment. Which of the following is the appropriate treatment for an amputated body part?
   a. Wrap the amputated part in a pressure dressing and place on ice.
   b. Place the amputated part into a plastic bag and fill the bag with ice.
   c. Wrap in sterile gauze, place in a plastic bag, and keep the amputated part cool.
   d. Place the amputated part directly on ice or chemical ice pack, then wrap with gauze.

EMERGENCY TRIP SHEET

TRIP #
MEDIC #
BEGIN MILES
END MILES
CODE___/___ PAGE___/___
UNITS ON SCENE

NAME   SEX M F DOB ___/___/___

ADDRESS   RACE

CITY   STATE   ZIP

PHONE (   )   -   PCP DR.

RESPONDED FROM   CITY

TAKEN FROM   ZIP

DESTINATION   REASON

SSN   -   -   MEDICARE #   MEDICAID #

INSURANCE CO   INSURANCE #   GROUP #

RESPONSIBLE PARTY   ADDRESS

CITY   STATE   ZIP   PHONE (   )   -

EMPLOYER

TIME	ON SCENE (1)	ON SCENE (2)	ON SCENE (3)	EN-ROUTE (1)	EN-ROUTE (2)	AT DESTINATION
BP						
PULSE						
RESP						
EKG						

MEDICAL HISTORY

MEDICATIONS

ALLERGIES

C/C

EVENTS LEADING TO C/C

ASSESSMENT

TREATMENT

EMS SIGNATURE

BILLING USE ONLY

DAY				
DATE				
RECEIVED				
DISPATCHED				
EN-ROUTE				
ON SCENE				
TO HOSPITAL				
AT HOSPITAL				
IN-SERVICE				

CREW	CERT	STATE #

IV THERAPY
SUCCESSFUL Y N # OF ATTEMPTS _____
ANGIO SIZE _____ ga.
SITE _____
TOTAL FLUID INFUSED _____ cc
BLOOD DRAW Y N INITIALS

INTUBATION INFORMATION
SUCCESSFUL Y N # OF ATTEMPTS _____
TUBE SIZE _____ mm
TIME _____ INITIALS _____

CONDITION CODES [ ][ ][ ][ ]

TREATMENTS

TIME	TREATMENT	DOSE	ROUTE	INIT

GCS E___ V___ M___ TOTAL =

GCS E___ V___ M___ TOTAL =

HOSPITAL CONTACTED

CPR BEGUN BY B P TIME BEGUN

AED USED Y N BY:

RESUSCITATION TERMINATED - TIME

(   ) OSHA REGULATIONS FOLLOWED

29 Burn Emergencies

OBJECTIVES

Numbered objectives are from the United States Department of Transportation EMT-Basic National Standard Curriculum. Asterisked objectives, if any, pertain to material that is supplemental to the DOT curriculum.

Cognitive

5-2.1 State the major functions of the skin.
5-2.2 List the layers of the skin.
5-2.11 List the classifications of burns.
5-2.12 Define superficial burns.
5-2.13 List the characteristics of a superficial burn.
5-2.14 Define a partial-thickness burn.
5-2.15 List the characteristics of a partial-thickness burn.
5-2.16 Define a full-thickness burn.
5-2.17 List the characteristics of a full-thickness burn.
5-2.18 Describe the emergency medical care of a patient with a superficial burn.
5-2.19 Describe the emergency medical care of a patient with a partial-thickness burn.
5-2.20 Describe the emergency medical care of a patient with a full-thickness burn.
5-2.24 Establish the relationship between airway management and the patient with chest injury, burns, blunt injuries, and penetrating injuries.
5-2.28 Describe the emergency care for a chemical burn.
5-2.29 Describe the emergency care for an electrical burn.

KEY IDEAS

Burn injuries can do more than burn the skin. They can impair the body's fluid and chemical balance, its temperature regulation, and its musculoskeletal, circulatory, and respiratory functions. In order to care for burns properly, you need to have a basic understanding of the kinds of burns; how burn injuries are classified; and how they affect adult, child, and infant patients.

- Burns are classified according to the depth of the injury. A superficial burn affects the epidermis. A partial-thickness burn affects the epidermis and portions of the dermis. A full-thickness burn involves all layers of the skin and can extend into the muscle, bone, or organs below.

- Burns are also classified by severity of injury—critical, moderate, or minor. The most important factors in determining burn severity are percentage and location of body surface area involved, the patient's age, and preexisting medical conditions.

- Assessment and emergency care of burn patients includes removing the patient from the source of the burn and stopping the burning process, being especially alert for compromise of the airway, estimating severity of the burns, and determining whether or not the patient is a priority for transport.

- When called to care for chemical burns, be prepared to protect yourself from exposure to hazardous materials. Remember to flush chemicals from the patient, when appropriate, for at least 20 minutes. Brush off dry chemicals before flushing.

- Special considerations for care of electrical burns include making sure power sources have been shut down before rescue and emergency care, monitoring the patient for respiratory and cardiac arrest, and assessing for both entrance and exit wounds.

TERMS AND CONCEPTS

1. Write the number of each term next to its definition.

   1. Circumferential burn
   2. Eschar
   3. Full-thickness burn
   4. Partial-thickness burn
   5. Rule of nines
   6. Superficial burn

   _____ a. Standardized format used to quickly identify the amount or percentage of skin or body surface area that has been burned

   _____ b. Burn that involves all of the layers of the skin and can extend beyond the subcutaneous layer into the muscle, bone, or organs below

   _____ c. The hard, tough, leathery, dead soft tissue formed as a result of a full-thickness burn

   _____ d. A burn that encircles a body area

   _____ e. A burn that involves only the epidermis

   _____ f. A burn that involves the epidermis and portions of the dermis

CONTENT REVIEW

1. List six functions of the skin.

2. In discussing burn assessment, the letters "BSA" stand for
   a. body surface area.
   b. burn severity assessment.
   c. blistered surface area.
   d. burn surface analysis.

3. Which of the following classifications of burns is usually caused by a flash flame, a hot liquid, or the sun?
   a. Superficial burn (first-degree)
   b. Eschar burn
   c. Full-thickness burn (third-degree)
   d. Circumferential burn

4. You are treating a patient who has sustained a burn. Which of the following would indicate that the patient has most likely sustained a deep partial-thickness burn?
   a. Thin-walled blisters
   b. Skin is red and blanched white
   c. Skin is soft and tender to touch
   d. Capillary refill is normal to the burn site

5. Which one of the following kinds of burns damages the blood vessels, causing plasma and tissue fluid to collect between layers of the skin?
   a. Superficial burn (first-degree)
   b. Partial-thickness burn (second-degree)
   c. Eschar burn
   d. Circumferential burn

6. Burns to the face are considered
   a. minor.
   b. moderate.
   c. critical.
   d. fatal.

7. You are treating a patient who has sustained an electrical injury with a deep burn that extends into the muscle, blood vessels, and nerves. This type of burn can be categorized as which of the following?
   a. Neuromuscular burn
   b. Partial-thickness, second-degree burn
   c. Circumferential burn
   d. Fourth-degree burn

8. In a child, partial-thickness burns of 10–20 percent BSA are considered
   a. minor.
   b. moderate.
   c. critical.
   d. fatal.

9. Which of the following age groups are less tolerant of burn injuries?
   a. Children under age 3 and adults over age 33
   b. Children under age 4 and adults over age 44
   c. Children under age 5 and adults over age 55
   d. Children under age 6 and adults over age 66

10. Briefly list the steps of emergency medical care of burn injuries.

11. When treating a burn patient, you know it is inappropriate to apply the rule of nines to which type of burn?
   a. Superficial burns
   b. Superficial partial-thickness burns
   c. Deep partial-thickness burns
   d. Full-thickness burns

12. Separate burned fingers or toes with dry, sterile dressings to prevent
   a. scarring of burned areas.
   b. adherence of burned areas.
   c. further contamination of burned areas.
   d. potential blistering of burned areas.

13. Your patient has sustained a burn to his right eye. Which of the following is an appropriate treatment for this patient?
   a. Apply firm pressure to the right eye.
   b. Treat the burn by applying burn ointment.
   c. Apply a dry sterile dressing to both eyes.
   d. Cover the burned eye with a moist sterile dressing.

14. Which of the following statements pertaining to the care of a patient that has sustained a chemical burn is considered inappropriate?
   a. Chemical burns may involve hazardous materials, so protect yourself first.
   b. Dry chemicals should be immediately flushed off the patient.
   c. Some chemicals may produce combustion when in contact with water.
   d. Chemical burns require immediate care.

15. You are treating a patient that has sustained a superficial partial-thickness burn from touching a hot exhaust pipe on a vehicle. What type of mechanism caused this burn?
   a. Flame burn
   b. Gas burn
   c. Flash burn
   d. Contact burn

16. Which of the following is correct about the assessment and care of an electrical burn patient?
   a. Always assume that the power source has been shut down.
   b. Rescue all victims in contact with an electrical source.
   c. All tissues between the entrance and exit wounds may be injured.
   d. Injuries caused by an electrical burn always have a rapid onset.

CASE STUDY

You are called to the scene of a burned child. You note that the patient's pajamas are still smoldering. The patient is crying loudly.

1. After soaking the pajamas with water, you try to remove them. However, the plastic booties have adhered to the patient's feet. You should
   a. gently try to remove the plastic from the skin.
   b. gently cut around the area with bandage scissors.
   c. transport to the hospital with the clothes left on.
   d. call medical direction for help with this situation.

2. Your partner notices singed nasal hairs in the patient. After requesting ALS backup, you should provide
   a. oxygen via nasal cannula at 6 lpm.
   b. oxygen via simple mask at 8 lpm.
   c. oxygen via nonrebreather mask at 15 lpm.
   d. positive-pressure ventilations with oxygen.

The mother tells you that she heard the 4-year-old child's screams and found him on fire in the garage. She suspects that lighter fluid may have been involved. You determine that the burns are all partial-thickness burns that cover the entire right leg and foot. You begin to transport the patient to the hospital, which is also a burn center.

3. What is the estimated body surface area affected by the burn, and what is the severity classification?
   a. 1 percent and moderate
   b. 9 percent and critical
   c. 14 percent and critical
   d. 18 percent and moderate

4. You continue the emergency care en route to the hospital. Which of the following is most appropriate?
   a. Cover the burned area with a sterile, dry dressing, and keep the patient cool.
   b. Cover the burned area with a sterile, dry dressing, and keep the patient warm.
   c. Cover the burned area with a sterile, moist dressing, and keep the patient cool.
   d. Cover the burned area with a sterile, moist dressing, and keep the patient warm.

ENRICHMENT

1. You are treating a patient who has been severely burned. You know that the burns will
   a. cause fluid to leak into the cells.
   b. increase capillary permeability.
   c. increase blood flow to the kidneys.
   d. protect against fluid loss.

2. Which one of the following conditions is incorrect and unlikely to be seen in the burn patient?
   a. Leakage of fluid from body cells will cause severe edema (swelling).
   b. Circumferential burns can interfere with respiration by preventing chest expansion.
   c. Scarring from burns can cause long-term muscle wasting and joint dysfunction.
   d. Gastrointestinal dysfunction is caused by increased blood flow to the gastrointestinal system.

SCENARIO 17: DOCUMENTATION EXERCISE

Read the following scenario, and think about how you would document this call if you were the EMT who responded to the scene. Then answer the multiple-choice questions and fill in the sample prehospital-care report, basing your documentation on information from the scenario.

It's near dinnertime on your shift duty day. You and your partner, Julie, are picking up groceries from the store for tonight's dinner. Suddenly your portable radio squawks: "Unit 4, respond to a possible burned child at 1500 Ninth Street South West." You and Julie quickly place the groceries at the front counter, telling the cashier you have a call and will return later. You both walk briskly toward the ambulance and, after confirming the address location in the map book, you mark en route.

After a short emergency response, you arrive at a modest home. You quickly scan the area, looking for hazards, as you both put on your gloves and eye protection. You are pulling the stretcher and equipment from the rear of the ambulance when a frantic mother, carrying her daughter, meets you at the back of the ambulance. Her daughter is wearing shorts and a T-shirt with socks and tennis shoes. Quickly you lower the stretcher and help the mother to lay the injured child supine on the stretcher. The visibly upset mother tells you, "I was frying chicken in a pan of hot oil when the whole pan caught fire. I tried to carry the flaming pan outside the house when my daughter came in to see what was the matter. I bumped into her, and the hot oil spilled all down the front of her. Please help her."

The patient gazes into your eyes with a frightened look and says, "I hurt real bad." You quickly introduce Julie and yourself to the patient and ask her how old she is and what her name is. She replies with a trembling voice, "My name is Ashley, and I'm 9 years old." You quickly place Ashley into the ambulance with the mother sitting by her side. Julie explains that you will be doing a lot of things quickly to help her, and if she has any questions she should just ask.

Julie explains to Ashley that she will need to cut off all of her clothes and place cool water on her burns. She also describes how she will place special bandages on her burns. Julie carefully cuts the clothing off and you find that the burned area has thick-walled blisters, some of which have ruptured. The burned area is red with blanched white patches. You gently press on an area of the burn and find that the capillary refill is delayed, but the patient can feel pressure at the site. You begin to cool the burns with sterile saline while Julie performs an initial assessment.

The burns encompass the patient's anterior trunk, bilateral anterior legs, and genitalia area. You advise the mother that you will be transporting her daughter to a local hospital that specializes in the treatment of burn patients. There are no stridorous or crowing sounds with inhalation or exhalation. Ashley's breathing is slightly shallow and rapid at approximately 24 breaths per minute. The chest is rising and falling, with adequate air flowing in and out of the mouth, without the use of accessory muscles. Julie applies high-flow oxygen with a nonrebreather mask with 15 lpm. You feel for a radial pulse and find a strong, rapid pulse at 120 beats per minute. The unaffected skin is warm and dry with a capillary blanch less than 2 seconds.

You begin a rapid trauma assessment. Ashley's head reveals no injuries or deformities; the pupils are equal and react briskly to light. The nose, mouth, and ears are all clear of blood, fluid, or burns. The neck is soft and free of any burns, and there is no noted subcutaneous emphysema. The trachea is midline, and there is no deformity or pain to the posterior neck. The chest and abdomen reveal the burns found in the initial assessment. You remember to inspect the axillary area, and no trauma or burns are noted. The same type of burn extends down from the chest and abdomen and covers the pelvis and genital area. You assess the extremities and find no injuries to the arms, but the anterior portions of both legs are burned. The patient's feet were protected from the hot oil by her socks and shoes, and no burns are found on her feet. You remark, "I have good distal pulses in all extremities." You promptly examine the posterior body and find no burns, trauma, or sacral edema. The patient does not complain of any pain when her spine is palpated.

You say to Julie, "Let's get going. I'll finish the rest en route." Julie moves to the driver's seat and marks en route to the burn center with dispatch. On the way to the burn center, you apply dressings to the burns. Ashley says she feels cold, so you cover her and adjust the interior temperature of the ambulance to keep her warm and comfortable. You now have time to gather additional information, including a SAMPLE history that will be helpful to the burn-center team. Ashley's mother tells you that Ashley has no known allergies, takes no medications, and has no past medical history. You notify the burn center by radio that you are en route with an approximately 10-minute arrival time, and you brief the burn team on your patient's condition.

After a short emergency response, you arrive at the burn center. Ashley once again looks into your eyes for reassurance. You tell her that she is at a special hospital, and they will take good care of her. She cracks a small smile, acknowledging that she understands. You and Julie whisk her through the emergency-department doors with her mother still by her side.

1. This burn was caused by hot oil that was spilled onto the patient. What type of burn resulted from this type of incident?
   a. Flash burn
   b. Steam burn
   c. Gas burn
   d. Scald

2. When you assessed the burn area, you found thick-walled blisters, some of which have ruptured. The burned area was red with blanched white patches. When you gently pressed on the area of the burn you found that the capillary refill was delayed and the patient could feel pressure at the site. From this description you would suspect that the patient is suffering from which classification of burn?
   a. Superficial partial-thickness burn (second degree)
   b. Deep partial-thickness burn (second degree)
   c. Full-thickness burn (third degree)
   d. Full-thickness burn (fourth degree)

3. This patient's burns cover her anterior trunk, bilateral anterior legs, and genitalia area. By the rule of nines, what percentage of the total body surface area (BSA) best represents this patient's burns?
   a. 19 percent
   b. 28 percent
   c. 37 percent
   d. 55 percent

4. Which statement best describes this patient's condition?
   a. The patient's burns are critical because they comprise over 20 percent partial-thickness burns.
   b. The patient's burns are critical because they comprise over 10 percent full-thickness burns.
   c. The patient's burns are moderate because they comprise 10–20 percent partial-thickness burns.
   d. The patient's burns are moderate because they comprise 15–25 percent full-thickness burns.

5. For treating this patient's burns, which of the following dressings would be considered appropriate?
   a. Wet, sterile, particle-free dressing
   b. Dry, sterile, particle-free dressing
   c. Dry, sterile dressing with burn cream
   d. Moist cotton-batting-type dressing

EMERGENCY TRIP SHEET

TRIP #	
MEDIC #	
BEGIN MILES	
END MILES	
CODE___/___ PAGE___/___	
UNITS ON SCENE	

NAME _____ SEX M F DOB ___/___/___

ADDRESS _____ RACE

CITY _____ STATE _____ ZIP

PHONE ( )____-_____ PCP DR. _____

RESPONDED FROM _____ CITY

TAKEN FROM _____ ZIP

DESTINATION _____ REASON

SSN ____-____-_____ MEDICARE # _____ MEDICAID #

INSURANCE CO _____ INSURANCE # _____ GROUP #

RESPONSIBLE PARTY _____ ADDRESS

CITY _____ STATE ____ ZIP ____ PHONE ( )____-____

EMPLOYER

BILLING USE ONLY			
DAY			
DATE			
RECEIVED			
DISPATCHED			
EN-ROUTE			
ON SCENE			
TO HOSPITAL			
AT HOSPITAL			
IN-SERVICE			
CREW	CERT	STATE #	

TIME	ON SCENE (1)	ON SCENE (2)	ON SCENE (3)	EN-ROUTE (1)	EN-ROUTE (2)	AT DESTINATION
BP						
PULSE						
RESP						
EKG						

MEDICAL HISTORY

MEDICATIONS

ALLERGIES

C/C

EVENTS LEADING TO C/C

ASSESSMENT

TREATMENT

EMS SIGNATURE

IV THERAPY
SUCCESSFUL Y N # OF ATTEMPTS _____
ANGIO SIZE _____ ga.
SITE _____
TOTAL FLUID INFUSED _____ cc
BLOOD DRAW Y N INITIALS

INTUBATION INFORMATION
SUCCESSFUL Y N # OF ATTEMPTS _____
TUBE SIZE _____ mm
TIME _____ INITIALS _____

CONDITION CODES				

TREATMENTS

TIME	TREATMENT	DOSE	ROUTE	INIT

GCS	E___ V___ M___ TOTAL =
GCS	E___ V___ M___ TOTAL =

HOSPITAL CONTACTED

CPR BEGUN BY   B   P   TIME BEGUN _____

AED USED   Y   N   BY:

RESUSCITATION TERMINATED - TIME _____

( ) OSHA REGULATIONS FOLLOWED

30 Musculoskeletal Injuries

OBJECTIVES

Numbered objectives are from the United States Department of Transportation EMT-Basic National Standard Curriculum. Asterisked objectives, if any, pertain to material that is supplemental to the DOT curriculum.

Cognitive

5-3.1 Describe the function of the muscular system.
5-3.2 Describe the function of the skeletal system.
5-3.3 List the major bones or bone groupings of the spinal column, the thorax, the upper extremities, and the lower extremities.
5-3.4 Differentiate between an open and a closed painful, swollen, and deformed extremity.
5-3.5 State the reasons for splinting.
5-3.6 List the general rules of splinting.
5-3.7 List the complications of splinting.
5-3.8 List the emergency medical care for a patient with a painful, swollen, and deformed extremity.

KEY IDEAS

Musculoskeletal injuries are frequently encountered in the field. Most of these injuries are simple and not life threatening. Appropriate management can prevent further painful injury and even prevent permanent disability or death. This chapter provides a review of the musculoskeletal system and discusses musculoskeletal injuries and their appropriate management.

- The functions of the musculoskeletal system are to give the body shape, to protect the internal organs, and to provide for movement.
- The six basic components of the skeletal system are the skull, spinal column, thorax, pelvis, lower extremities, and upper extremities.
- The forces that may cause bone and joint injuries are direct, indirect, and twisting forces.
- Bone and joint injuries can be either open or closed.
- Any painful, swollen, or deformed extremity should be immobilized.
- Splinting prevents movement of bone fragments, bone ends, or dislocated joints, thereby reducing the chance for further injury, and it reduces pain and minimizes complications.
- The general rules of splinting include the following: Check pulse, motor function, and sensation (PMS) before and after splinting; immobilize the joints above and below a long-bone injury site, or immobilize the bones above and below a joint injury; remove clothing and jewelry; cover all

wounds before splinting; never replace bone ends; splint before moving the patient; when in doubt, splint the injury and pad splints.

- If there is severe deformity or the distal extremity is cyanotic or pulseless, then make one attempt to realign the limb. If pain, resistance, or crepitus increase, stop and transport immediately.

- If a patient shows signs of shock, align the patient in the normal anatomical position, treat for shock, and transport immediately without taking the time to apply a splint.

- The general types of splints are rigid, traction, pressure, improvised, and sling and swathe.

TERMS AND CONCEPTS

1. Write the number of each term next to its definition.

1. Crepitus
2. Direct force
3. Indirect force
4. Paresthesia
5. Splint
6. Twisting force

_____ a. A force that rotates a bone while one end is held stationary

_____ b. The sound or feel of broken fragments of bone grinding against each other

_____ c. A force that causes injury some distance away from the point of impact

_____ d. A force that causes injury at the point of impact

_____ e. Any device used to immobilize a body part

_____ f. A prickling or tingling feeling that indicates some loss of sensation

CONTENT REVIEW

1. Three of the following are functions of the musculoskeletal system and one is the function of the circulatory system. Which is a function of the circulatory system?
   a. Gives the body shape
   b. Produces platelets
   c. Protects the internal organs
   d. Provides for movement

2. List the six basic components of the skeletal system.

3. Which of the following are forces that cause bone and joint injury?
   a. Direct, partial, and indeterminate
   b. Direct, indirect, and frontal
   c. Direct, indirect, and twisting
   d. Direct, primary, and secondary

4. Which of the following distal to an injured extremity is considered to be a serious condition?
   a. Swelling and tenderness
   b. Coolness and paleness
   c. Pain and flushing
   d. Pulselessness and cyanosis

5. If a fracture is suspected, which of the following is considered to be a critical injury that must be managed in a manner that not only immobilizes but also reduces the associated bleeding?
   a. Radius or ulna
   b. Tibia or fibula
   c. Scapula or clavicle
   d. Femur or pelvis

6. A patient has an injured extremity. The patient is unresponsive and has a suspected spinal injury and other life-threatening injuries unrelated to the extremity injury. You and your partner have established manual in-line stabilization of the head and spine, assured an open airway and adequate breathing, controlled major bleeding, and completed a rapid trauma assessment. There is no one at the scene that can provide a history, and you will assess vital signs en route. In addition, you perform the steps listed below. Number the list below in the proper order from 1 to 4 to show the order of priority for performing these steps.

   _____ Splint the injured extremity.

   _____ Perform further management of the life-threatening injuries and ongoing assessments every 5 minutes.

   _____ Immobilize the patient to a spine board.

   _____ Initiate transport.

7. The skin over the fracture site has been broken, and the bone may or may not protrude through the skin. Which type of injury does this statement best describe?
   a. A spiral injury
   b. An open injury
   c. A closed injury
   d. A simple injury

8. List at least five signs and symptoms of bone or joint injury.

9. Which of the following, if fractured, can easily cause the loss of one to two liters of blood around the bone?
   a. Humerus
   b. Mandible
   c. Femur
   d. Radius

10. If an injured extremity is painful, swollen, and deformed, which of the following should you do?
    a. Apply warm packs to the site
    b. Restrict blood flow
    c. Splint the extremity
    d. Position the extremity below the heart

11. The patient's distal pulses, motor function, and sensation should be checked
    a. before splinting.
    b. after splinting.
    c. before and after splinting.
    d. just before arrival at the hospital.

12. A general rule for the immobilization of an injury to a long bone is to immobilize
    a. the joints above and below the injury site.
    b. the joint above the injury site only.
    c. the joint below the injury site only.
    d. only the bone, not the adjacent joint.

13. In a patient who may have sustained a fracture to the pelvis, the pneumatic antishock garment (PASG) performs two functions. One function is to stabilize the fracture; the other is to
    a. decrease the compartment into which the pelvis can bleed.
    b. apply direct pressure to the anterior olecranon.
    c. pull the femur away from the pelvic girdle.
    d. apply downward and lateral pressure to the pelvis.

14. If there is severe deformity in an extremity, the distal pulses are absent, or the extremity is cyanotic, you should
    a. make no attempt to align the extremity.
    b. make one attempt to align the extremity.
    c. persist until the extremity is aligned.
    d. apply the splint before attempting to align.

15. Which of the following is considered an inappropriate action when splinting an injured extremity?
    a. Maintain manual traction until after the splint has been applied.
    b. Push protruding bones back into the skin.
    c. Cover all open wounds before splinting.
    d. Cut clothing away and remove jewelry from the site.

16. When forced to use an improvised splint, ensure that the splint is
    a. heavy but flexible and soft.
    b. short, extending just the length of the bone.
    c. narrower than the thickest part of the injured limb.
    d. well padded on the inner surface.

17. A sling and swathe is commonly used to provide stability to a painful and tender
    a. leg injury.
    b. shoulder injury.
    c. cervical-spine injury.
    d. pelvic injury.

18. When splinting an extremity, the hand or foot must be immobilized in the position of function. The position of function for the hand can be attained by
    a. extending the hand over the end of the splint.
    b. securing the hand to the splint in a palm-up position.
    c. bandaging the hand in a clenched-fist position.
    d. putting a roll of bandage in the patient's hand.

19. In which of the following situations should you use a traction splint?
    a. The injury is within 1 or 2 inches of the knee.
    b. The knee has been injured.
    c. The thigh is painful, swollen, or deformed.
    d. The hip or pelvis has been injured.

20. Which statement describes how the traction splint achieves stabilization?
    a. It applies circumferential pressure to the femur.
    b. It stabilizes the bone ends by producing negative torque.
    c. It pulls on the thigh and realigns the broken femur.
    d. It pushes the bones together and "resets" the fracture.

21. Your patient injured her right ankle and foot when she stepped off a curb while crossing the street. Which of the following assessment techniques will give you the same results as if the entire foot was tested?
    a. Checking pulses, motor, and sensory (PMS)
    b. Having the patient push and pull back the great (big) toe
    c. Palpating for a brachial pulse
    d. Pushing upward on the bottom (plantar) of the patient's foot

22. Which of the following splints can be used to help stabilize a suspected fractured pelvis?
    a. Bipolar traction splint
    b. Sling and swathe
    c. Short padded-board splint
    d. Pneumatic antishock garment (PASG)

23. The condition that occurs when the pressure in the space around the capillaries exceeds the pressure needed to perfuse the tissues, then causes the blood flow to be cut off, leading to cellular hypoxia is known as
    a. compartment syndrome
    b. extremity-necrosis syndrome
    c. system-dysfunction syndrome
    d. capillary-pressure syndrome

CASE STUDY 1

You are dispatched to a high school to assist a 17-year-old soccer player who is injured. The patient is sitting on a bench on the sideline of the field, holding his left shoulder and leaning forward. You sit down next to him and ask, "What happened?" He replies, "I was moving down to score and tripped in a hole. I put my arm out to catch myself, and I felt something snap in my shoulder." Your general impression is a noncritical injured patient. He responds to your questions appropriately and is alert and oriented. His respirations are normal; radial pulse is strong and regular; and skin is a good color, warm, and dry. You examine his shoulder and observe deformity over his left clavicle. The area is tender to touch and obviously swollen. He denies any other complaints or injuries.

1. The immediate action to take for this patient should be to
   a. immobilize the shoulder with an air splint, splinting the entire arm.
   b. evaluate the pulse, motor function, and sensation.
   c. splint the shoulder with a sling and swathe.
   d. immobilize the shoulder with a rigid splint on the entire arm.

2. What is the best way to evaluate this patient's sensory function?
   a. Ask if he can feel you pinch him on the back.
   b. Ask him to wiggle his fingers without looking.
   c. Ask him to tell you which finger you are touching without looking.
   d. Ask him if he can feel you prick him with a sharp object.

3. This patient's injury is most likely due to what type of force?
   a. Direct
   b. Indirect
   c. Twisting
   d. Secondary

CASE STUDY 2

You are at the scene of a motorcycle collision with a car. About 20 yards from the vehicles, a male biker is sitting holding his right leg. He looks to be about 30 years old. You ask, "What happened?" He replies, "That car stopped in front of me. I hit the rear, flew off the bike, and landed on my leg." Respirations are normal; radial pulse is strong and regular; skin is a good color, warm, and dry. You cut away his pant leg so you can evaluate his injury. The thigh region is deformed, swollen, and tender to touch. He denies any other complaints or injuries. You ask your partner to initiate manual traction to the right leg.

1. Manual traction on the patient's leg
   a. should be continued until you arrive at the hospital.
   b. should be continued until you are ready to position the splint.
   c. should be continued until the splint is applied.
   d. should not have been initiated.

2. When checking the pulse distal to the injury site on this patient, use which of the following?
   a. Pedal or posterior tibial pulse
   b. Radial or brachial pulse
   c. Popliteal or femoral pulse
   d. Carotid or femoral pulse

CASE STUDY 3

You are dispatched to a call for an elderly patient who is lying on the kitchen floor. She is 70 years old and in severe pain. She tells you that when she fell she heard a "loud pop." There is bruising to the right hip region, and the patient complains of severe pain there upon palpation. She also tells you that her leg feels numb and is tingling. She denies any additional complaints or injuries. You apply a padded rigid splint that extends from below the foot to above the hip.

1. The patient's complaint of numbness and tingling in her right leg
   a. may indicate some loss of sensation.
   b. may indicate an additional injury to the lower leg.
   c. may require the application of a full leg air splint.
   d. is to be expected after this type of injury.

2. The patient's foot should be immobilized in a position of function. Which statement best describes the position of function for the foot?
   a. Toes curled toward the sole of the foot
   b. Foot bent at a normal angle to the leg
   c. Foot pushed downward to align with the shin
   d. Foot bent upward toward the shin

3. To evaluate this patient's motor function, ask her to do which of the following?
   a. Lift the leg and rotate it outward
   b. Rotate the leg outward and tense the foot
   c. Tighten the kneecap and move the foot up and down
   d. Tighten the buttocks and lift the leg

SCENARIO 18: DOCUMENTATION EXERCISE

Read the following scenario, and think about how you would document this call if you were the EMT who responded to the scene. Then answer the multiple-choice questions, and fill in the sample prehospital-care report, basing your documentation on information from the scenario.

You and your newly promoted partner, Lt. Downs, are working as the EMT crew at a local horse show. A show official runs up to your ambulance and tells you that a horse in a barn kicked a person. Lt. Downs notifies dispatch of the possible injury as you drive the ambulance to the barn. While putting on your eyewear and gloves, you both scan the general area looking for obvious hazards, but none are observed. As you are removing the stretcher from the rear of the ambulance, the show official runs up to you, saying in a stern voice, "You must hurry. She is in a lot of pain." You reassure her and walk briskly toward the barn door. As you enter the large open door, you once again scan the area for hazards. The official leads you toward an open stall door. You ask if the horse has been removed and secured in another area,

and she replies, "The horse has been removed to a corral outside."

As you enter the stall area, you find a young adult female lying supine on the floor. She is holding her right leg above the knee and is screaming in agony. She appears slightly pale and extremely anxious. You approach her and quickly introduce yourself and Lt. Downs. You reassure her and explain that you are there to help her. Lt. Downs asks her name and what happened, and she says, "My name is Annie, and I was cleaning the stall when the horse spooked and kicked me in the thigh. It really hurts!" You mention to your partner that a kick from a horse can be violent, with potential for other injuries. Lt. Downs positions himself to maintain in-line stabilization of the patient's head, neck, and spine. You observe that the patient is breathing approximately 22 times each minute. Her chest is rising and falling, with adequate air flowing in and out of the mouth, and without the use of accessory muscles. You feel for a radial pulse and find a strong, rapid pulse at 100 beats per minute. Her skin is warm and dry. You quickly apply high-flow oxygen with a nonrebreather mask at 15 lpm. You notice a small blood spot on the patient's jean. The spot is on the right thigh midway between knee and hip.

Because of the potential for other injuries, you begin a rapid trauma assessment. You quickly expose the patient by cutting the clothes, being careful to protect her modesty. The head reveals no injuries or deformities, and the pupils are equal and react briskly to light. The nose, mouth, and ears are all clear of blood or fluid. The neck is soft with no trauma or subcutaneous emphysema noted. The trachea is midline, and there is no deformity or pain to the posterior neck. You palpate the chest and note equal chest rise and fall. There is no sign of trauma or use of accessory muscles. You inspect the axillary area, noting that it is without injury. Inspection of the abdomen reveals no obvious injuries, distention, or pain with palpation. You quickly inspect the pelvis for deformity, contusions, abrasions, or penetrating injuries, and none are found.

You assess the lower extremities and find that the left leg is not injured, but the right has a large contusion and open wound that is oozing blood. The injury is to the anterior mid-position of the thigh. You do not observe any bone ends protruding from the open wound. When you palpate the affected leg, you feel broken bone fragments grinding against each other, which sends an uncomfortable shiver up your spine. The right leg appears to be having muscle spasms, and it appears to be larger than the unaffected left leg. The upper extremities are uninjured. You ask Annie if she can feel you touching her extremities, and she replies, "Yes." You then ask her to wiggle her toes and fingers, and she does. Next, you check all four distal pulses and find them to be strong and regular.

This appears to be an isolated injury to the right leg. However, you and Lt. Downs agree to maintain in-line stabilization of the spine as a precaution. You apply a cervical collar and solicit assistance from two bystanders to help with moving the patient onto the backboard. While placing the patient on the backboard, you support the affected leg and examine the posterior body, finding no injuries or sacral edema. The patient does not complain of any pain when the spine is palpated. She is quickly secured to the backboard.

Lt. Downs repositions himself and tells the patient that he will help to relieve the pain to her right leg by applying manual traction. She replies in a stern, loud voice, "Don't touch my leg. It hurts too bad!" He reassures her that it is necessary and the pain should decrease when traction is pulled. Lt. Downs reassesses the PMS of the injured leg and then stabilizes the injured leg by applying manual traction. Annie grimaces and says, "Ouch! Oh! That does feel much better!" You prepare and apply the bipolar traction splint. After the leg has been placed in the splint, you attach the "S" hook and start to apply mechanical traction. After the splint has been applied, the patient states that she still feels the pain but it is more tolerable now. After you apply a dressing to the open wound site, you place cold packs on and around the injury.

You and Lt. Downs lift the backboard and place the patient on the stretcher, then make your way toward the ambulance. You advise the patient that it will take about 25 minutes to reach the hospital and you will try to give her a smooth ride. The show official asks Annie if there is anyone she should notify to inform them that she has been taken to the hospital, and Annie gives her the contact information. You both load the patient into the back of the ambulance, and Lt. Downs positions himself in the driver's seat.

While en route to the hospital, you gather additional information, including a SAMPLE history. Annie tells you that she is allergic to penicillin and takes Albuterol through a metered-dose inhaler for her asthma. You obtain vital signs, which are blood pressure 118/60, pulse rate 94 and regular; respirations are now 18 each minute with good tidal volume. The pulse oximeter reveals an SpO_2 of 98 percent on oxygen. You notify the hospital by radio that you are en route with an approximately 20-minute arrival time and quickly brief them on the patient's condition.

1. When you palpated the affected leg, you felt the broken fragments of bone grinding against each other. What is the medical term for this finding?
   a. Atelectasis
   b. Kyphosis
   c. Eupnea
   d. Crepitus

2. When Lt. Downs applied manual traction, the pain to the affected leg decreased. In addition to reducing pain, application of manual traction also
   a. reduces the diameter of the thigh, which increases pressure on the bleeding bones, slowing bleeding.
   b. pulls the arteries, which decreases the size of the vessel, reducing the associated bleeding.
   c. applies direct pressure to the fractured ends of the femur, cutting off the flow of blood.
   d. slows bleeding by circumferential direct, as well as indirect, pressure from the snug ischial strap.

3. If this patient were to become unresponsive, how would you know when full traction was achieved when applying mechanical traction with the bipolar traction splint?
   a. The injured leg will be 3 to 5 centimeters longer than the uninjured leg.
   b. The injured leg should be the same length as the uninjured leg.
   c. The size of the injured thigh will increase slightly over that of the uninjured thigh.
   d. The unresponsive patient will grimace when full traction has been achieved.

4. Which of the following actions would be considered inappropriate for this patient?
   a. Application of ice packs to the injury site
   b. Pulling traction to a suspected open fracture
   c. Pulling manual traction while the splint is readied
   d. Elevating the injured extremity to reduce swelling

5. It was proper to evaluate the pulse, motor function, and sensation distal to the injury before and after the splint was applied. How often should you reevaluate the PMS after the splint is applied?
   a. Every 2 minutes
   b. Every 5 minutes
   c. Every 10 minutes
   d. Every 15 minutes

EMERGENCY TRIP SHEET

BILLING USE ONLY			
DAY			
DATE			
RECEIVED			
DISPATCHED			
EN-ROUTE			
ON SCENE			
TO HOSPITAL			
AT HOSPITAL			
IN-SERVICE			

CREW	CERT	STATE #

P #

EDIC #

GIN MILES

D MILES

DE___/___ PAGE___/___

ITS ON SCENE

ME   SEX M F DOB ___/___/___

DRESS   RACE

TY   STATE   ZIP

ONE ( )   -   PCP DR.

SPONDED FROM   CITY

KEN FROM   ZIP

STINATION   REASON

N   -   -   MEDICARE #   MEDICAID #

SURANCE CO   INSURANCE #   GROUP #

SPONSIBLE PARTY   ADDRESS

TY   STATE   ZIP   PHONE ( )   -

MPLOYER

ME	ON SCENE (1)	ON SCENE (2)	ON SCENE (3)	EN-ROUTE (1)	EN-ROUTE (2)	AT DESTINATION
LSE						
SP						
G						

EDICAL HISTORY

EDICATIONS

LERGIES

C

ENTS LEADING TO C/C

SESSMENT

EATMENT

MS SIGNATURE

IV THERAPY
SUCCESSFUL Y N # OF ATTEMPTS _____
ANGIO SIZE _____ ga.
SITE _____
TOTAL FLUID INFUSED _____ cc
BLOOD DRAW Y N INITIALS

INTUBATION INFORMATION
SUCCESSFUL Y N # OF ATTEMPTS _____
TUBE SIZE _____ mm
TIME _____ INITIALS _____

CONDITION CODES				

TREATMENTS

TIME	TREATMENT	DOSE	ROUTE	INIT

GCS	E___ V___ M___ TOTAL =	
GCS	E___ V___ M___ TOTAL =	

HOSPITAL CONTACTED

CPR BEGUN BY B P TIME BEGUN

AED USED Y N BY:

RESUSCITATION TERMINATED - TIME

( ) OSHA REGULATIONS FOLLOWED

31 Injuries to the Head

OBJECTIVES

Numbered objectives are from the United States Department of Transportation EMT-Basic National Standard Curriculum. Asterisked objectives, if any, pertain to material that is supplemental to the DOT curriculum.

Cognitive

5-4.1 State the components of the nervous system.
5-4.2 List the functions of the central nervous system.
5-4.3 Define the structure of the skeletal system as it relates to the nervous system.
5-4.4 Relate mechanism of injury to potential injuries of the head and spine.
5-4.11 Establish the relationship between airway management and the patient with head and spine injuries.

KEY IDEAS

Injury to the skull, which contains the brain, can have severe consequences for the patient. Since head injuries may occur weeks before signs and symptoms appear, it is important to recognize both potential and actual injury at the scene.

- The brain and spinal cord make up the central nervous system, which controls the body's systems.

- The skull, which protects the brain, is made up of the cranial skull, the facial bones, and the basilar skull. Cerebrospinal fluid and the meninges help protect the brain inside the skull.

- The brain is made up of three parts: the cerebrum (conscious and sensory functions), the cerebellum (muscle movement and coordination), and the brain stem (most autonomic and vital functions).

- Head injuries may involve the scalp, skull, and/or the brain and are classified as open or closed. Both open and closed injuries of the head may involve extensive damage to the brain.

- Brain injury may be direct (from penetrating trauma), indirect (from a blow to the skull), or secondary (for example, from lack of oxygen, buildup of carbon dioxide, or a change in blood pressure).

- Unresponsiveness or an altered mental status, especially in trauma patients, should always suggest the possibility of head injury. Nontraumatic injury may be caused by clots or hemorrhaging and also may result in an altered mental status.

- Emergency medical care of head injury includes in-line stabilization of the spine; maintaining a patent airway, adequate breathing, and oxygenation (consider ventilation at 20 breaths/min in a patient with severe head injury); closely monitoring airway, breathing, and mental status for changes or deterioration; and immediate transport.

TERMS AND CONCEPTS

1. Write the number of each term next to its definition.

1. Anterograde amnesia	7. Cushing's reflex
2. Battle's sign	8. Extension or decerebrate posturing
3. Cerebellum	9. Flexion or decorticate posturing
4. Cerebrospinal fluid	10. Meninges
5. Concussion	11. Raccoon sign
6. Coup–contrecoup injury	12. Subarachnoid hemorrhage

_____ a. The patient extends arms and legs and sometimes arches the back, which may be a sign of serious brain injury.

_____ b. The patient is unable to remember circumstances after the incident.

_____ c. Three layers of tissue that enclose the brain

_____ d. Discoloration of the mastoid, suggesting basilar skull fracture

_____ e. Discoloration of tissue around the eyes

_____ f. Sometimes called the "little brain"; it controls equilibrium and coordinates muscle activity

_____ g. Serous substance that protects the brain

_____ h. Hypertension, bradycardia, and altered respiratory pattern

_____ i. The patient flexes arms across the chest and extends legs, which may be a sign of serious brain injury.

_____ j. Damage at the point of a blow to the head and/or damage on the side opposite the blow as the brain is propelled against the opposite side of the skull

_____ k. Temporary loss of brain function

_____ l. Bleeding that occurs between the arachnoid membrane and the surface of the brain

CONTENT REVIEW

1. Injury to the brain that results from shearing, tearing, and stretching of nerve fibers is called
   a. diffuse axonal injury.
   b. cerebral contusion.
   c. cerebral hematoma.
   d. cerebral laceration.

2. The single most important sign in cases of suspected head injury is
   a. decreasing blood pressure.
   b. altered respiratory pattern.
   c. decreasing mental status.
   d. increasing pulse rate.

3. This is a tool that uses numerical values to carefully monitor a patient's level of consciousness. It is called the
   a. Common Coma Scale.
   b. AVPU Scale.
   c. Glasgow Coma Scale.
   d. Bond Responsiveness Scale.

4. Which technique should be used to maintain the airway of a patient with a possible head injury who has a decreased level of responsiveness?
   a. Head-tilt/chin-lift maneuver
   b. Jaw-thrust maneuver
   c. Crossed-finger technique
   d. Two-rescuer ventilation

5. The mental-status response that is likely to indicate the most serious head injury is
   a. alertness.
   b. responsiveness to verbal stimulus.
   c. responsiveness to painful stimulus.
   d. unresponsiveness.

6. Any patient whose mental status worsens at any stage of the assessment or treatment process needs
   a. treatment for anaphylactic shock.
   b. palpation of the head and neck.
   c. immediate transport and monitoring.
   d. SAMPLE history and rapid trauma assessment.

7. A flexion response or decorticate posturing
   a. indicates a lower-brainstem injury.
   b. results in extension of the arms and arching of the back.
   c. is also called a purposeful response.
   d. results in flexing of arms across the chest and extension of the legs.

8. When managing a patient with a suspected head injury
   a. a lowered SpO_2 is always an indication of a head injury.
   b. oxygenation and ventilation are not of critical importance.
   c. it is critical to determine a baseline mental status.
   d. who had a brief period of unconsciousness, evaluation is not necessary.

9. Mark an X beside each of the following signs that is a potential sign of increasing intracranial pressure.
   _____ a. Systolic blood pressure is high or rising.
   _____ b. Systolic blood pressure is low or dropping.
   _____ c. Pulse is slow or decreasing.
   _____ d. Pulse is fast or increasing.
   _____ e. Respiratory pattern is altered.
   _____ f. Respiratory pattern remains unchanged.

10. Emergency care of a patient with a severe head injury should include
   a. ventilation at 12/min.
   b. application of a snug pressure dressing to any open skull injury.
   c. scant or little attention to airway and breathing status.
   d. anticipation of potential seizure activity.

CASE STUDY 1

You have been called to the scene of a four-wheeler ATV accident. The patient is a 16-year-old male who hit a small hole and was thrown from the vehicle. A bystander who witnessed the accident states that the driver was thrown about 30 feet and that he landed on his back and struck his head on the ground. As you approach the patient, his eyes are closed and he appears to be in critical condition. His skin color is normal, and his respirations appear to be rapid, deep, and full without any audible abnormal respiratory sounds. His pulse is slow, regular, and weak. His blood pressure is 130/80; the pulse is 60/min, weak and regular; his respirations are 24/min, deep and full; his pupils are unequal and slow to respond to light; the SpO$_2$ is 96 percent. The vital signs are repeated in 5 minutes and are as follows: respirations 24/min and irregular; pulse 50, weak and regular; skin color normal, warm, and dry; pupils remain unequal and slow to respond to light; and blood pressure is 140/86.

1. This patient is exhibiting signs of _____ reflex, which is a sign of a severe head injury.
   a. Bank's
   b. Histonic
   c. Cushing's
   d. Corral's

2. The reflex described in the above answer consists of a "triad" of signs. These three signs are
   a. decrease in blood pressure, increasing pulse, and rapid respirations.
   b. increasing blood pressure, slowing pulse, and alteration in respirations.
   c. increasing blood pressure, increasing pulse, and alteration in respirations.
   d. decrease in blood pressure, slowing pulse, and rapid respirations.

3. This patient would best be managed by ventilations delivered at a rate of _____.
   a. 10 per minute
   b. 12 per minute
   c. 20 per minute
   d. 28 per minute

CASE STUDY 2

You have been called to the scene of a fall. The caller, the patient's neighbor, says he found a 70-year-old female, Mrs. McDonald, lying at the bottom of her basement stairs. He has not moved her. She is unresponsive with good skin color, skin that is warm and dry, and the pulse is slow and regular. You observe a large deformity at the back of Mrs. McDonald's head. Her pupils are dilated and slow to respond to light. She has bruising around both eyes and over the mastoid process. You find no blood or fluid in the nose, but a clear fluid is draining from her left ear. She is unresponsive to painful stimuli. There is no other evidence of injury. Baseline vitals are blood pressure 178/72, pulse 68, respirations regular and full at 18/min, and SpO$_2$ 95 percent.

1. The bruising around Mrs. McDonald's eyes is a late sign of a skull fracture and is called
   a. Battle's sign.
   b. raccoon sign.
   c. orbital bruising.
   d. Barry's sign.

2. The bruising over the mastoid area is also a late sign of a skull fracture and is called
   a. Battle's sign.
   b. raccoon sign.
   c. mastoid bruising.
   d. Barry's sign.

3. Mark an X next to each treatment below that should be provided for Mrs. McDonald.

   _____ a.   Manual in-line spinal stabilization

   _____ b.   Cervical spine immobilization collar (CSIC)

   _____ c.   Head-tilt/chin-lift to open the airway

   _____ d.   Placement of an oropharyngeal airway

   _____ e.   Administer oxygen at 15 lpm

   _____ f.   Consider ventilation at 20 per min

   _____ g.   Immobilize to a spine board

   _____ h.   Pack gauze into her left ear

   _____ i.   Continued evaluation of mental status

   _____ j.   Pressure applied to the head deformity

ENRICHMENT

1. Complete the following chart by indicating with an X or a check mark if each listed sign or symptom is associated with each brain injury (concussion, contusion, subdural hematoma, or epidural hematoma). You may use one or up to four check marks for each sign or symptom.

Sign or Symptom	Concussion	Contusion	Subdural Hematoma	Epidural Hematoma
Momentary confusion				
Abnormal respiratory pattern				
Retrograde and anterograde amnesia				
Loss of responsiveness followed by a return of responsiveness and then rapid deterioration				
Weakness or paralysis on one side of the body				
Dilation of one pupil				
Fixed and dilated pupil				
Posturing (withdrawal or flexion)				
Repeated questioning about what happened				
Increasing blood pressure				
Decreasing pulse rate				
Seizures				
Cushing's reflex				
Vomiting				

2. A mild form of diffuse axonal injury, that presents with an altered mental status that progressively improves, is called a
   a. concussion.
   b. contusion.
   c. epidural hematoma.
   d. subdural hematoma.

3. A contusion of the brain is usually caused by two types of injuries. They are
   a. blunt lateral injury and anterior/posterior injury.
   b. coup–contrecoup injury and acceleration/deceleration injury.
   c. medial–central injury and acceleration/deceleration injury.
   d. explosive–implosive injury and radical/conservative injury.

4. This brain injury is typically the result of low-pressure venous bleeding that occurs above the tissue of the brain. This is called a
   a. concussion.
   b. contusion.
   c. epidural hematoma.
   d. subdural hematoma.

5. A subdural hematoma
   a. is the least common type of head injury.
   b. occurs in 10 percent of all severe head injuries.
   c. is more common in patients older than 80 years of age.
   d. is more likely in patients with abnormally long blood-clotting times.

SCENARIO 19: DOCUMENTATION EXERCISE

Read the following scenario, and think about how you would document this call if you were the EMT who responded to the scene. Then answer the multiple-choice questions and fill in the sample prehospital-care report, basing your documentation on information from the scenario.

It is 5:00 PM on a Thursday. You are backing into the station after completing a call for an elderly woman with respiratory distress when the alarm sounds. "Unit 3, respond to 1186 US Highway 92 East for a car that struck a bicycle. Time out 1700 hours." Your partner, Susan, advises dispatch that you are responding. You arrive on the scene in about 6 minutes. As you prepare to park, you observe a man who appears to be in his mid-30s lying supine on the side of the roadway. You exit the rescue vehicle with BSI in place and walk toward the patient. A mangled bicycle is lying in the roadway underneath a pickup truck. The truck is about 75 feet from where the patient is lying. As you and Susan walk by the truck, you notice that the front of the hood has significant damage. You quickly confirm that ALS backup has been dispatched.

As you approach the patient you observe three bystanders kneeling next to him. One is holding a towel on the man's forehead while the other two motion for you and Susan to hurry. Your initial impression is that the patient is in critical condition. A woman kneeling next to him identifies herself as an Emergency Medical Responder and quickly says, "I saw the accident happen!" The patient's eyes are closed as you approach, and he has gurgling respirations that seem shallow and slow. You quickly tell your partner, "Susan, we need to roll him on his side and suction the mouth!" "OK, Jack," she replies. You ask Susan to maintain the cervical spine and enlist the help of the bystanders to quickly roll the patient on his side.

You suction a small amount of vomitus from his nose and mouth. You quickly size and place an oropharyngeal airway, and no gag reflex is observed.

You position the spine board behind the patient, cut off his clothing, and roll him onto the board. You ask the Emergency Medical Responder on the scene to once again assume manual cervical-spine control so that Susan can strap the patient to the board. You quickly assess the patient's breathing and note that the respirations are shallow and rapid. His skin color is cyanotic. You attach the bag-valve-mask device to 15 lpm of oxygen and begin to ventilate the patient at 20 respirations per minute. The Emergency Medical Responder is helping to maintain the head in neutral alignment. You ask her what she saw. She tells you, "I was driving along behind the pickup truck that struck him. The truck veered right off the road and struck him. It threw him about 60 or 70 feet. He landed on the top of his head. He wasn't wearing a helmet. I stopped to help, and he was unconscious when I got to him."

Susan performs a rapid trauma assessment and finds a depressed area of his skull on the right parietal region, blood in his right ear, a fracture of his left ankle, and a large bruise on his upper right abdomen. The abdomen appears to be slightly distended. His right pupil is fixed and dilated, and the left is slow to respond to light. His skin is cool and clammy; he has a weak and rapid radial pulse; the breath sounds are clear and equal bilaterally; his SpO_2 is 95 percent. Susan checks for a pain response. The patient responds by moving his arms across his chest, and his hands rotate inward, his back arches, and his feet extend. You are relieved to look up and see Paramedic Ed Nixon and his partner Connie Buck approaching. You give a report to Ed and quickly help place the patient in the ALS ambulance. You return to the station, clean up your ambulance, and prepare for another call.

1. Rolling the patient quickly on his side to suction his airway
   a. should have been delayed until after the oropharyngeal airway was placed.
   b. should not have been performed until after ALS took over management.
   c. was an appropriate and important action to take.
   d. should have been delayed until he was immobilized on the long spine board.

2. This patient is most likely suffering from
   a. a high-level brainstem injury.
   b. injury to the lateral cerebrum.
   c. a low-level brainstem injury.
   d. injury to the cerebral cortex.

3. The patient should be ventilated at _____ ventilations/minute.
   a. 12
   b. 14
   c. 18
   d. 20

4. This patient is likely suffering from
   a. hypoperfusion from bleeding into a body cavity.
   b. hypoperfusion from bleeding into the head.
   c. shock from the fractured left ankle.
   d. spinal shock from the head injury.

5. The patient's fractured ankle
   a. should have been immobilized prior to placement on the long spine board.
   b. should have been immobilized with a splint prior to transport by ALS.
   c. should not have been immobilized because it would delay transport.
   d. should have been stabilized with sandbags and tape.

EMERGENCY TRIP SHEET

		BILLING USE ONLY

TRIP #	
MEDIC #	
BEGIN MILES	
END MILES	
CODE___/___	PAGE___/___
UNITS ON SCENE	

BILLING USE ONLY				
DAY				
DATE				
RECEIVED				
DISPATCHED				
EN-ROUTE				
ON SCENE				
TO HOSPITAL				
AT HOSPITAL				
IN-SERVICE				

NAME	SEX M F DOB ___/___/___
ADDRESS	RACE
CITY	STATE	ZIP
PHONE ( ) -	PCP DR.
RESPONDED FROM	CITY
TAKEN FROM	ZIP
DESTINATION	REASON
SSN - -	MEDICARE #	MEDICAID #
INSURANCE CO	INSURANCE #	GROUP #
RESPONSIBLE PARTY	ADDRESS
CITY	STATE	ZIP	PHONE ( ) -
EMPLOYER	

CREW	CERT	STATE #

TIME	ON SCENE (1)	ON SCENE (2)	ON SCENE (3)	EN-ROUTE (1)	EN-ROUTE (2)	AT DESTINATION
BP						
PULSE						
RESP						
EKG						

IV THERAPY
SUCCESSFUL Y N # OF ATTEMPTS ___
ANGIO SIZE _____ga.
SITE _____
TOTAL FLUID INFUSED _____ c
BLOOD DRAW Y N INITIALS

INTUBATION INFORMATION
SUCCESSFUL Y N # OF ATTEMPTS ___
TUBE SIZE _____ mm
TIME _____ INITIALS ___

MEDICAL HISTORY

CONDITION CODES				

MEDICATIONS

TREATMENTS

TIME	TREATMENT	DOSE	ROUTE	IN

ALLERGIES

C/C

EVENTS LEADING TO C/C

ASSESSMENT

TREATMENT

GCS E___ V___ M___ TOTAL =

GCS E___ V___ M___ TOTAL =

HOSPITAL CONTACTED

CPR BEGUN BY   B   P   TIME BEGUN

EMS SIGNATURE

AED USED   Y   N   BY:

RESUSCITATION TERMINATED - TIME

(   ) OSHA REGULATIONS FOLLOWE

32 Injuries to the Spine

OBJECTIVES

Numbered objectives are from the United States Department of Transportation EMT-Basic National Standard Curriculum. Asterisked objectives, if any, pertain to material that is supplemental to the DOT curriculum.

Cognitive

5-4.1 State the components of the nervous system.
5-4.2 List the functions of the central nervous system.
5-4.3 Define the structure of the skeletal system as it relates to the nervous system.
5-4.4 Relate mechanism of injury to potential injuries of the head and spine.
5-4.5 Describe the implications of not properly caring for potential spine injuries.
5-4.6 State the signs and symptoms of a potential spine injury.
5-4.7 Describe the method of determining if a responsive patient may have a spine injury.
5-4.8 Relate the airway emergency medical care techniques to the patient with a suspected spine injury.
5-4.9 Describe how to stabilize the cervical spine.
5-4.10 Discuss indications for sizing and using a cervical spine immobilization device.
5-4.11 Establish the relationship between airway management and the patient with head and spine injuries.
5-4.12 Describe a method for sizing a cervical spine immobilization device.
5-4.13 Describe how to log roll a patient with a suspected spine injury.
5-4.14 Describe how to secure a patient to a long spine board.
5-4.15 List instances when a short spine board should be used.
5-4.16 Describe how to immobilize a patient using a short spine board.
5-4.17 Describe the indications for the use of rapid extrication.
5-4.18 List steps in performing rapid extrication.
5-4.19 State the circumstances when a helmet should be left on the patient.
5-4.20 Discuss the circumstances when a helmet should be removed.
5-4.21 Identify different types of helmets.
5-4.22 Describe the unique characteristics of sports helmets.
5-4.23 Explain the preferred methods to remove a helmet.
5-4.24 Discuss alternative methods to remove a helmet.
5-4.25 Describe how the patient's head is stabilized to remove the helmet.
5-4.26 Differentiate how the head is stabilized with a helmet compared to without a helmet.

KEY IDEAS

As an EMT, you may encounter patients with potential spinal injuries in a wide variety of settings. Each encounter must be grounded in the recognition that improper movement and handling of such patients could easily lead to permanent disability or even death. This chapter focuses on the assessment and management of spinal injuries.

- The spinal column, which serves to protect the spinal cord, is the principal support system of the body. It is made up of 33 vertebrae, each pair of vertebrae separated by a disc.

- Common mechanisms of spinal injury include compression, flexion, extension, rotation, lateral bending, distraction, and penetration, which may occur as a result of collisions, falls, diving accidents, and so on.

- Even in the absence of obvious trauma or patient complaints, when the mechanism of injury suggests possible spinal injury, every care must be taken, and immediate manual in-line spinal stabilization must be established.

- Once established, manual stabilization must not be released until the patient is securely strapped to a backboard with head and neck immobilized.

- The goal of emergency management of suspected spinal cord injury is to ensure that life-threatening conditions are cared for, that the possibility of further injury is reduced through careful handling, and that the patient is properly immobilized and expeditiously transported.

- The tools associated with spinal immobilization include cervical-spine immobilization collars, full-body spinal-immobilization devices, and short spinal-immobilization devices.

TERMS AND CONCEPTS

1. Write the number of each term next to its definition.

    1. Autonomic nervous system
    2. Central nervous system
    3. Peripheral nervous system
    4. Voluntary nervous system

    _____ a. The portion of the nervous system that influences deliberate muscle movement

    _____ b. The structures of the nervous system located outside the brain and spinal cord

    _____ c. The portion of the nervous system that influences involuntary muscles and glands

    _____ d. The portion of the nervous system consisting of the brain and the spinal cord

2. Label the diagram with the following spinal column divisions:

Cervical spine

Coccyx

Lumbar spine

Sacral spine

Thoracic spine

CONTENT REVIEW

1. Mark an X beside each mechanism of injury/type of emergency scene that should make you especially alert to the possibility of spinal injury.

_____ a. Electrical injury

_____ b. Blunt trauma

_____ c. Fall

_____ d. Heart attack victim

_____ e. Motorcycle crash

_____ f. Gunshot wound to the head, neck, chest, abdomen, back, or pelvis

_____ g. Acute asthmatic attack

_____ h. Hanging

_____ i. Diving accident

_____ j. Unresponsive trauma patient

2. Which of the following would apply to a patient who is found lying unresponsive in an alley beside an apartment building?
   a. Assume the patient has a psychological problem.
   b. Maintain a high index of suspicion for spinal injury.
   c. If the patient can move her extremities, there is no spinal injury.
   d. Quickly place her in a lateral recumbent position.

3. This mechanism of spinal injury occurs when the vertebrae and spinal cord are stretched or pulled apart and is common in hangings. It is called
   a. flexion.
   b. lateral bending.
   c. extension.
   d. distraction.

4. Which statement is correct regarding signs and symptoms associated with spinal injury?
   a. Diaphragmatic breathing is indicative of a thoracic spine injury.
   b. The patient should move about to try and locate the area of spinal pain.
   c. Priapism, if present, is a classic sign of cervical spine injury.
   d. Obvious deformity of the spine upon palpation is a common finding.

5. When assessing for pulses, motor function, and sensory function in the patient with a spine injury
   a. bilaterally check the brachial and popliteal pulses for strength and equality.
   b. assess motor function by having the patient lift his shoulders and feet slightly.
   c. check the sensory function by lightly touching both knees and elbows.
   d. if unresponsive, pinch the foot and hand to determine a sensory response.

6. When positioning the patient for manual spinal stabilization, the nose should be aligned with the navel, and the head should be
   a. slightly flexed forward in a "sniffing" position.
   b. slightly extended with chin pointing up.
   c. neither flexed nor extended.
   d. both flexed and extended.

7. Which of the following regarding cervical-spine immobilization collars is correct?
   a. Soft collars permit needed lateral movement.
   b. The collar provides complete immobilization of the spine.
   c. The size of the collar is important but not critical.
   d. The collar should be applied by two rescuers.

8. For each type of patient listed below, indicate with an X or a check mark the appropriate device or technique required to properly immobilize the patient.

Patient type	Standing immobilization technique	Rapid extrication	Apply vest-type immobilization device	Immobilize to backboard
Standing patient				
Seated patient with critical injuries				
Seated patient with no critical injuries				
Supine or prone patient				

9. Mark an X beside each treatment that would be an appropriate management technique for a patient with a spine injury

_____ a. The EMT must attempt to diagnose the condition and locate the exact site of spinal injury.

_____ b. If in doubt as to whether a spinal injury is present, always immobilize the patient.

_____ c. Manual in-line spinal stabilization should be established as soon as patient contact is made.

_____ d. If the patient complains of severe neck or spine pain or the head does not easily move, the patient's head should be immobilized in the position found.

_____ e. Use the head-tilt/chin-lift airway maneuver to maintain the airway.

_____ f. Following immobilization, reassess, record, and document the pulses, motor function, and sensory function in all extremities.

10. When performing the log-roll technique of spinal immobilization
    a. you must always use four rescuers.
    b. avoid placing padding on the board to prevent slipping.
    c. the cervical-spine immobilization collar should be placed before movement.
    d. immobilize the patient's head to the board before the torso is immobilized.

11. The steps below describe the procedure for immobilizing a supine or prone patient. Number the list in the proper order from 1 to 7.

_____ Place pads in the spaces between the patient and the board.

_____ Establish and maintain in-line manual stabilization.

_____ Apply a cervical-spine immobilization collar.

_____ Immobilize the patient's torso to the board with straps.

_____ Log roll the patient onto the long spine board.

_____ Secure the patient's legs to the board.

_____ Immobilize the patient's head to the board.

12. Identify the best description of immobilization of a standing patient.
    a. Walk him to the cot, and have him lie on the backboard placed there.
    b. Immobilize him from a standing position while maintaining alignment.
    c. Have him sit on the backboard, and then carefully help him lie down.
    d. Patients who are able to stand or walk do not require immobilization.

13. A short spinal immobilization device
    a. is chiefly used to immobilize a critical sitting patient with a spinal injury.
    b. does not require the use of a long spine board.
    c. does not generally require the use of a cervical-spine immobilization collar.
    d. requires that the torso be secured prior to the head.

14. Rapid extrication is indicated if
    a. the patient's condition is stable.
    b. the patient is on a scene that is safe.
    c. the patient blocks access to a critical patient.
    d. the patient complains of severe pain.

15. Safe and effective rapid extrication requires which of the following?
    a. Constant cervical spine stabilization
    b. Application of a short spine board or vest-type immobilization device
    c. Application of only a cervical-spine immobilization collar with no manual stabilization
    d. At least one rescuer

16. Removal of a helmet
    a. should, generally, not be attempted if the helmet fits well.
    b. is always required, even if the patient is breathing adequately.
    c. can be adequately performed by one rescuer working carefully.
    d. should be performed only on motorcycle helmets, not football helmets.

17. Which of the following describes what is generally the *best* care for a football player with potential spinal injury?
    a. Leave the helmet and shoulder pads in place.
    b. Remove the helmet, but leave the shoulder pads in place.
    c. Cut away and remove all clothing and equipment.
    d. Remove both the helmet and the shoulder pads.

18. Number the list below in the proper order from 1 to 5 to identify the sequence of steps necessary to immobilize an infant in a car seat.

    _____ Transport in the normal seated position after securing the car seat to the ambulance seat.

    _____ Assess the infant to ensure there are no life-threatening injuries or other reasons for removal from the car seat.

    _____ Determine if padding is required between the infant's body and the car seat.

    _____ Apply manual in-line spinal stabilization.

    _____ Support the head in a neutral position, using towel rolls and tape.

CASE STUDY

You have been dispatched for a young woman injured in a softball game. You arrive at a local college softball complex and observe a 20-year-old female softball player lying supine on the ground next to home base. The coach tells you that she was the catcher and was accidentally struck in the head with a bat. She was unconscious for about a minute. She regained consciousness and is now alert and oriented. She complains of neck and head pain.

1. When immobilizing this patient
   a. only prevention of lateral movement is required.
   b. pad voids under the head and torso.
   c. use a vest-type device in addition to the long spine board.
   d. carefully pad behind the cervical-spine immobilization collar.

2. Manual in-line stabilization can be released
   a. following application of the cervical-spine immobilization collar.
   b. just prior to movement onto the long spine board.
   c. following placement of the patient on the long spine board but just prior to immobilization of the head to the board.
   d. following immobilization of the head to the long spine board.

3. A minimum of _____ straps should be used to ensure proper immobilization.
   a. 2
   b. 3
   c. 4
   d. 5

ENRICHMENT

1. Spinal shock usually results from injury of the _____ region of the spine.
   a. cervical
   b. thoracic
   c. lumbar
   d. sacral

2. Which of the following findings are commonly associated with neurogenic shock?
   a. Moist, cool, clammy skin
   b. Pulse rate of 60–100/min
   c. Irregular respirations of 12–20/min
   d. Pale skin color

3. Neurogenic shock results in
   a. a "relative" hypovolemia.
   b. massive vasoconstriction.
   c. excessive fluid loss.
   d. a temporary fluid overload.

SCENARIO 20: DOCUMENTATION EXERCISE

Read the following scenario, and think about how you would document this call if you were the EMT who responded to the scene. Then answer the multiple-choice questions and fill in the sample prehospital-care report, basing your documentation on information from the scenario.

It is 2:45 AM on a Saturday night—or actually Sunday morning. You have been asleep since 1:00 AM, when you returned from a call for a hit pedestrian. The alarm sounds and wakes you from a deep sleep. "Unit 4, respond to 6th Street NW and Avenue D NW for a two-car collision. Time out 0245 hrs." You jump from bed and arrive at the rescue vehicle at the same time as your partner, Carly. You advise dispatch that you are responding, and dispatch advises that Engine One and law enforcement are also responding. You arrive on-scene in about 3 minutes.

Two cars are involved, a silver Cadillac and a white Toyota Camry. The Cadillac struck the Camry in the passenger-side door. The Cadillac does not appear to be damaged. The impact broke the glass in the

Camry's door and pushed the door about a foot into the passenger compartment. The airbags deployed in both vehicles. The firefighters on-scene advise you that the driver of the Cadillac fled the scene, and the driver of the Camry is the only patient. Jack, a burly firefighter, waves you over to the Camry where the driver of the vehicle is sitting behind the steering wheel with his seatbelt on. Jack walks around to the rear driver-side door and positions himself behind the driver. He establishes manual in-line stabilization of the driver's cervical spine, explaining to the driver who he is and why he is holding his head. You and Carly circle the car quickly to check for additional hazards and mechanisms of injury. No other damage is noted to the car other than the damage on the passenger side.

The driver appears to be about 25 years old. His eyes are open. He has a small laceration on his forehead. His skin color is normal, and he appears to be in stable condition. You introduce yourself to the driver by saying, "Hello! My name is Don, and this is Carly. We are EMTs, and we're here to help you. Where do you hurt?" You reach down and feel his radial pulse, which is rapid and strong. His skin is warm and dry. He is breathing adequately, and there are no audible, abnormal respiratory sounds. You quickly place a nonrebreather mask on him and set the oxygen flow rate at 15 lpm. The patient is keeping his head and neck very still as he says, "My neck. It really hurts! It started just after the accident. That idiot! He ran the red light! I was just driving along, and he slams into me. Then he jumps out of his car and takes off. What a jerk! . . . My neck really hurts!" You say, "Do you hurt anyplace else?" "No," he says.

"What is your name?" you ask. "Wardell Johnson," he replies. "Wardell, I need you to keep your head and neck still and don't move at all. I know Jack told you that's why he's holding your head, to help you keep still. Carly and I are going to take some vital signs and ask you some additional questions. Then we are going to place you in a special immobilization device that will help to keep your head and neck from moving. We are concerned that you may have damaged your spine, and—again—it is important to keep your head and neck still. Do you understand this? Do you have any questions?" He moves his eyes to look at you and says, "Yes, I understand. I'll keep my head as still as I can. I really appreciate you guys helping me!" You say, "We're glad to help you, Wardell."

Carly climbs in the passenger side of the car and performs a rapid trauma assessment. She tells you she finds nothing and quickly checks the neck again before placing a cervical-spine immobilization collar on Wardell. She begins to take vital signs while you begin a SAMPLE history. You ask, "Wardell, you don't hurt anyplace else? Is that correct?" "That is right," Wardell says. "Are you allergic to any medications?" "Not a thing!" Wardell replies. "Are you taking any medications, or have you ever been injured or sick before?" Wardell quickly responds, "Nope!" You continue by saying, "OK, so when was the last time you ate or drank something?" "Well, I guess it was about 1:00 AM or so. I stopped at The Clock restaurant and grabbed something to eat after I got off work. I had a burger, a soda, and some fries." Carly reports Wardell's vital signs. He is alert and oriented to person, place, and time; his respirations are normal at 14 per minute; his skin is warm, dry, and of normal color; his pupils are equal and reactive and respond briskly to light; his blood pressure is 124/68; and his SpO_2 is 95 percent.

You ask Carly to get the cot, the short spinal immobilization device, and the long spine board while you continue with your assessment. "Wardell, don't try to, but can you move your hands and feet?" "Yes, I can," he says. "Do you have any numbness or tingling sensations in any of your arms or legs?" you ask. "Well, I do have some numbness in both arms but not my legs," Wardell states in a tentative voice. "Did you move about after the accident?" you continue. "No, I knew that I was hurt. I didn't move a bit," Wardell replies.

"All right, Wardell, I'm going to ask you to perform some tasks for me. It involves checking for pulses, ability to move your fingers and toes, and sensation in both your arms and legs. I'm going to start with your hands." You assess for pulses in each extremity, for sensation (pain and light touch) in each extremity, and for motor movement. Wardell's pulses are present and equal, he has good sensation in each extremity (to pain and light touch), and he is able to perform all tests for motor function appropriately. Carly returns with the equipment, and you prepare to immobilize Wardell. You carefully immobilize him with the short spine immobilization device and move him to the cot for transport to the hospital.

1. The injury sustained by Wardell is most likely the result of
   a. compression.
   b. flexion.
   c. extension.
   d. lateral bending.

2. Improper management and stabilization of Wardell's injury could produce complications. Three major complications of spinal injury are
   a. inadequate breathing effort, hemiplegia, and inadequate circulation.
   b. cerebral hypoxia, hemiplegia, and inadequate circulation.
   c. inadequate breathing effort, paralysis, and inadequate circulation.
   d. cerebral hypoxia, paralysis, and circulatory overload.

3. The presence of numbness and tingling in Wardell's arms is
   a. not an important physical finding.
   b. a significant finding of a spinal injury.
   c. not generally important unless accompanied by paralysis.
   d. most likely the result of a stress reaction.

4. Following immobilization of Wardell in the short spinal immobilization device, Don and Carly
   a. rapidly transport Wardell to the hospital.
   b. now reevaluate the pulse, motor, and sensory function.
   c. place Wardell on the long spine board.
   d. tie Wardell's hands together.

5. When securing Wardell to the long spine board, straps (at a minimum) should be positioned at the
   a. hips and above the knees.
   b. hips, above the knees, and below the knees.
   c. arms, hips, and below the knees.
   d. chest, hips, and above the knees.

TRIP #		EMERGENCY TRIP SHEET		BILLING USE ONLY				

EMERGENCY TRIP SHEET

TRIP #		
MEDIC #		
BEGIN MILES		
END MILES		
CODE___/___	PAGE___/___	
UNITS ON SCENE		

BILLING USE ONLY				
DAY				
DATE				
RECEIVED				
DISPATCHED				

NAME	SEX M F DOB ___/___/___	EN-ROUTE
ADDRESS	RACE	ON SCENE
CITY	STATE	ZIP	TO HOSPITAL
PHONE ( ) -	PCP DR.	AT HOSPITAL
RESPONDED FROM	CITY	IN-SERVICE

TAKEN FROM	ZIP	CREW	CERT	STATE #
DESTINATION	REASON			
SSN - -	MEDICARE #	MEDICAID #		
INSURANCE CO	INSURANCE #	GROUP #		
RESPONSIBLE PARTY	ADDRESS			
CITY	STATE ZIP PHONE ( ) -			

EMPLOYER

IV THERAPY
SUCCESSFUL Y N # OF ATTEMPTS _____
ANGIO SIZE _____ga.
SITE _____
TOTAL FLUID INFUSED _____ cc
BLOOD DRAW Y N INITIALS

INTUBATION INFORMATION
SUCCESSFUL Y N # OF ATTEMPTS _____
TUBE SIZE _____ mm
TIME _____ INITIALS _____

TIME	ON SCENE (1)	ON SCENE (2)	ON SCENE (3)	EN-ROUTE (1)	EN-ROUTE (2)	AT DESTINATION
BP						
PULSE						
RESP						
EKG						

MEDICAL HISTORY

CONDITION CODES				

TREATMENTS

MEDICATIONS

TIME	TREATMENT	DOSE	ROUTE	INIT

ALLERGIES

C/C

EVENTS LEADING TO C/C

ASSESSMENT

TREATMENT

GCS E___ V___ M___ TOTAL =

GCS E___ V___ M___ TOTAL =

HOSPITAL CONTACTED

CPR BEGUN BY   B   P   TIME BEGUN

EMS SIGNATURE

AED USED   Y   N   BY:

RESUSCITATION TERMINATED - TIME

( ) OSHA REGULATIONS FOLLOWED

33 Eye, Face, and Neck Injuries

OBJECTIVES

Numbered objectives are from the United States Department of Transportation EMT-Basic National Standard Curriculum. Asterisked objectives, if any, pertain to material that is supplemental to the DOT curriculum.

Cognitive

* List the major anatomical structures of the eye, face, and neck.
* Describe the relationship between eye, face, and neck injuries and the personal protection and safety of the EMT-Basic.
* List the overall assessment procedures for eye, face, and neck injuries.
* Describe the general assessment procedures for eye injuries, including use of the penlight.
* List the basic rules for emergency medical care for eye injuries.
* List specific common eye injuries and describe their appropriate emergency medical care.
* Describe emergency medical care for patients with an eye injury wearing contact lenses.
* Describe the general assessment and care guidelines for face injuries.
* List the signs and symptoms and describe the emergency medical care for injuries to the mid-face, upper jaw, and lower jaw.
* Describe the emergency medical care for an object impaled in the cheek.
* Describe the emergency medical care for injuries to the nose and ear.
* List special signs and symptoms of injury to the neck.
* Describe the emergency medical care for injuries to the neck.

KEY IDEAS

Injuries to the eyes, face, or neck have a high probability of causing airway compromise, severe bleeding, and shock. Injuries to the face and neck also are associated with spinal injury. When the potential for these life-threatening conditions exists, establish manual stabilization of the head and neck, open the airway with the jaw-thrust maneuver, and suction as needed. Consider ALS backup for advanced airway care, and provide oxygen.

■ Basic rules for emergency care of eye injuries include the following: Consult medical direction before irrigating foreign objects from the eye and before removing contact lenses; do not remove blood or blood clots from the eye; do not apply salve or medicine; do not try to force the eyelid open unless chemicals must be flushed out; flush a chemically burned eye for at least 20 minutes; stabilize an impaled object of the eye; cover both an injured eye and uninjured eye to prevent unnecessary movement; give the patient nothing by mouth; and always transport for evaluation by a physician.

- Injuries to the face include injury to the mid-face, jaw, nose, ear, and objects impaled in the cheek. For severe injuries to the face, suspect and treat for cervical-spine injury and immediately manage airway, breathing, and circulation problems. Consider advanced life support to provide advanced airway care. An object impaled in the cheek should be stabilized with bulky dressings. If the object has penetrated the cheek all the way and it may obstruct the airway, remove the object.

- With any blunt or penetrating trauma to the neck, maintain a high index of suspicion for cervical-spine injury. Due to the possibility of swelling, crushed airway structures, debris, and clotted blood, maintaining an airway also is extremely important.

TERMS AND CONCEPTS

1. Write the number of each term next to its definition.

1. Aqueous humor
2. Conjunctiva
3. Cornea
4. Iris
5. Pupil
6. Lens
7. Retina
8. Sclera
9. Vitreous humor

_____ a. Portion of the eye that covers the pupil and the iris

_____ b. Fluid that fills the anterior chamber of the eye

_____ c. Clear jelly that fills the large chamber of the eye

_____ d. Back of the eye

_____ e. Outer coating of the eye; the white of the eye

_____ f. Colored portion of the eye that surrounds the pupil

_____ g. Thin covering of the inner eyelids and exposed portion of the sclera of the eye

_____ h. The dark center of the eye

_____ i. The portion of the eye that focuses light on the retina

2. Label the diagram of the eye with the appropriate terms from the list in item 1.

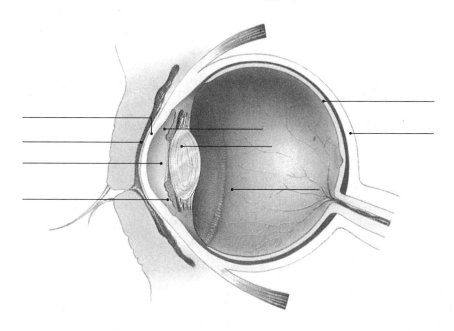

CONTENT REVIEW

1. When conducting the focused history and physical exam on a patient with an eye injury
   a. evaluate the pupils for size by applying direct pressure to the globe.
   b. check for appropriate eye movement up and down only.
   c. check the lids for bruising, swelling, and laceration by direct visualization.
   d. check the globe for redness and abnormal coloring by pulling the eyelid open.

2. During the initial assessment of a patient with facial trauma, establish manual stabilization of the head and neck
   a. after assessing the facial trauma.
   b. on first contact with the patient.
   c. following application of oxygen.
   d. while examining the eye with a penlight.

3. Suspect significant damage to the eye if
   a. vision improves only after blinking.
   b. the field of vision increases.
   c. there is an injury to the forehead or cheek.
   d. there is unusual sensitivity to light.

4. Which of the following is considered appropriate when treating an injured eye?
   a. Remove blood clots from the sclera with a sterile dressing.
   b. Force the eyelids open, if necessary, to examine the pupils.
   c. Have the patient walk to distract him from the pain.
   d. Transport the patient for evaluation covering both eyes.

5. Only attempt to remove foreign particles that are lodged in which of the following?
   a. Conjunctiva
   b. Cornea
   c. Globe
   d. Retina

6. You are treating a patient with a lacerated eyelid. Your treatment and management of this patient should include
   a. covering the eye with a dry sterile dressing.
   b. application of direct pressure to control bleeding.
   c. frequently checking for visual acuity in the uninjured eye.
   d. preserving any avulsed skin and transporting with the patient.

7. Your patient who presents with double vision (diplopia), a marked decrease in vision, and loss of sensation above the eyebrow, over the cheek, or in the upper lip is most likely suffering from a/an
   a. chemical eye burn.
   b. orbital fracture.
   c. laceration to the eyelid.
   d. laceration of the globe.

8. When should you begin treatment of a suspected chemical burn of the eye?
   a. During the initial assessment
   b. After a rapid trauma assessment
   c. After the focused history and physical exam
   d. During the ongoing assessment

9. You are treating a patient with a chemical burn to the eyes. You know the eyes should be flushed from the inside corner to the outside edge for at least
   a. 5 minutes.
   b. 10 minutes.
   c. 15 minutes.
   d. 20 minutes.

10. In which of the following positions would you place the patient with an impaled or extruded eye injury?
    a. Fowler's position
    b. Lateral recumbent position
    c. Supine position
    d. Prone position

11. Contact lenses
    a. are never worn by people who wear glasses.
    b. are always worn in both eyes.
    c. can be clearly seen by using a penlight.
    d. should not be removed in chemical burns to the eye.

12. You are treating a patient that has sustained an eye injury and is wearing soft contacts. Which of the following is the correct way to remove a soft contact lens?
    a. Pinch the lens between your thumb and index finger.
    b. Press the lower eyelid under the bottom edge of the lens.
    c. Apply a moistened suction cup.
    d. Slide a fingernail under the edge of the lens and lift.

13. Your patient presents with a painful, deformed, and swollen jaw and has dentures that are still intact and in place. How should this be managed?
    a. Leave the dentures in place.
    b. Remove if the patient requests it.
    c. Contact medical direction for instructions.
    d. They should always be removed.

14. Your patient is suffering from facial trauma with exposed nerves and tendons. You should do which of the following?
    a. Apply a moist, sterile dressing to the injury.
    b. Apply a dry, sterile dressing to the injury.
    c. Do not cover; it may damage the nerves.
    d. Cover exposed tissues with an occlusive dressing.

15. Your patient has presented you with an avulsed tooth resulting from facial trauma. You should
    a. scrub it with water, and place it in a saline solution.
    b. rinse it with saline, and place it in a saline solution.
    c. scrub it with saline, and place it in dry gauze.
    d. rinse it with water, and place it in an alcohol solution.

16. Your patient has an impaled nail that has penetrated the cheek all the way through and is loose. What should you do?
    a. Stabilize it, and be prepared to remove it from the airway.
    b. Stabilize it with bulky dressings, and transport.
    c. Pull it out in the same direction from which it entered.
    d. Push it out in the direction opposite to the way it entered.

17. To prevent a patient from swallowing a dressing that is packed between the teeth and cheek, you should do which of the following?
    a. Place a gloved index finger into the mouth to hold the dressing.
    b. Have the patient hold onto one end of the dressing.
    c. Tape some of the dressing material to the outside of the mouth.
    d. Never place dressings into the mouth because it may block the airway.

18. You suspect your patient has a nasal fracture. Which of the following is the most appropriate for treating this type of injury?
    a. Gently pull to align the nose, and transport.
    b. Apply cold compresses, and transport.
    c. Apply a pressure dressing, and transport.
    d. Pack the nostrils, and transport.

19. You are assessing your patient and notice a clear fluid draining from the ear. You should do which of the following?
    a. Pack the ear with dressings.
    b. Apply pressure dressings.
    c. Apply direct pressure.
    d. Place a loose dressing across the opening.

20. Your patient has a severed blood vessel of the neck. You should
    a. apply pressure to both sides of the neck at the same time.
    b. use a loosely placed, moist sterile dressing.
    c. use a figure-eight wrap to secure the dressing.
    d. position the patient on his left side, head up.

21. You are assessing your patient that has an eye injury and notice blood in the anterior chamber of the eye. You know this condition as
    a. bipolar.
    b. hyphema.
    c. hemophilia.
    d. myopia.

22. You are preparing to treat a critically injured patient with a mid-facial injury. Your initial management priorities should be
    a. spinal stabilization with a cervical collar, bleeding control, ensure a patent airway, assist breathing.
    b. ensure a patent airway, stabilization of cervical spine, support breathing, ensure a patent airway.
    c. manual spinal stabilization, ensure a patent airway, support breathing, control life-threatening bleeding.
    d. manage life-threatening bleeding, manage the cervical spine, ensure a patent airway, and support breathing.

CASE STUDY

You and your partner are at the scene of an overturned car. Your patient is a 22-year-old male. He is responsive and supine with battery acid burns to the eyes and a deep laceration to the left side of the neck that is bleeding heavily. An EMR will maintain manual stabilization of the head and neck.

1. Should you consider advanced life support backup for this patient? Explain your answer.

2. Which of the following best describes the sequence that should be followed?
    a. Assess the patient, provide emergency care, then transport.
    b. Assess the patient, provide emergency care, and wait for the paramedics.
    c. Provide emergency care for life-threatening injuries first, assess and treat other injuries, and then transport.
    d. Transport immediately, and provide emergency care en route.

3. Which of the following describes the best treatment for this patient's injuries?
    a. Immediately begin flushing the eyes with saline. Simultaneously, place a gloved hand over the neck wound to control bleeding and administer high-flow oxygen.
    b. Immediately begin flushing the eyes with saline. Probe the neck wound to locate and apply pressure to the carotid artery, then administer high-flow oxygen.
    c. Immediately stop the profuse bleeding from the neck wound. Then begin flushing the eyes with saline. Administer high-flow oxygen as soon as you can.
    d. Once bleeding is under control and you have administered oxygen, check with medical control to find out if you can flush the patient's eyes with saline.

Read the following scenario, and think about how you would document this call if you were the EMT who responded to the scene. Then answer the multiple-choice questions and fill in the sample prehospital-care report, basing your documentation on information from the scenario.

It's about 10:30 PM on a warm summer evening. You and your partner, Ali, are completing a continuing education program homework assignment. The alarm sounds and startles you. "Unit 7, respond to the Wild Buck Club at 8204 Bush Boulevard, cross street Lincoln Avenue, for a fight. Law enforcement is responding. Time out 2230 hours." You meet your partner at the vehicle, quickly remove the shoreline (the electrical connection from the station to the ambulance that provides electrical power to run heaters, computers, lights, etc., and charge batteries), and advise dispatch that you are responding. Dispatch tells you law enforcement advises the scene is secure and one patient has been stabbed. You arrive in front of a nightclub that is located in a formerly abandoned strip shopping center. The parking lot is full of patrons. A large crowd is milling about near two police cars parked in front of the club. You tell dispatch of your arrival on-scene. Dispatch responds, "Affirmative. Unit 7 on-scene at 2237 hours."

With BSI precautions in place, you exit the vehicle and walk toward the crowd. A police officer waves you over to his location. The crowd moves so that you can get to the patient. You observe what looks to be a 20-year-old male patient lying in a supine position. A bystander is holding a towel on the left side of the patient's neck. There is a large pool of blood next to the patient. The patient's left eye is swollen shut. The right eye is open, and the patient acknowledges your presence by moving his right hand. His skin color is good, and he appears to be breathing adequately with no obvious respiratory sounds heard. You and Ali kneel down next to the patient. You reach down and feel his radial pulse, which is rapid and weak. You say, "My name is Pat and this is Ali. We are EMTs, and we're here to help you. Can you tell me what happened?"

You note a strong odor of alcohol as the patient says, "I was trying to talk to this girl that I just met, and this guy runs up to me and hits me in the face with his fist, and then he stabs me in my neck! I'm really worried about my eye. I was seeing double before my eye got so swollen." You ask his name. He tells you it is Richard Martz. You quickly place a nonrebreather face mask on Richard at 15 lpm. Ali quickly inspects the neck wound and finds bleeding from a laceration on Richard's left neck about an inch lateral to the trachea at the level of the larynx. Ali quickly covers the wound with a dressing and applies direct pressure to control the bleeding. You tell dispatch that you need an ALS unit. Dispatch lets you know that they are responding and are about 5 minutes away from the scene. Ali asks a bystander, who identified himself as an EMR, to assume direct pressure on the neck wound while another EMR stabilizes the neck. Ali then takes the vital signs while you prepare to immobilize the patient to the long spine board.

You quickly begin a rapid trauma assessment. Your assessment reveals that the left eye is swollen shut and that the patient complains of numbness just above the left eye. The bleeding from the wound on the patient's neck is controlled; the trachea is midline; breath sounds are clear and equal bilaterally; and a small laceration is found on his right hand. You place a cervical-spine immobilization collar on the patient, cut his clothing away, and roll him onto the long spine board. You obtain a SAMPLE history from Richard and determine that he is complaining of pain in the eye and neck and denies any other pain or complaint. He has no allergies and doesn't take any medications. He has no prior medical history. He last ate about 7:00 PM and had a large meal. Ali reports the vital signs: Respirations are 20 per minute, full and normal; the pulse is 98 per minute, weak and regular; the skin color is pale, warm, and moist; the right pupil responds normally to light; the blood pressure is 100/80; and the SpO_2 is 96 percent.

You place Richard on the stretcher just as the ALS unit arrives. You provide a brief patient report to the paramedic and assist in placing the patient in the ALS unit.

1. When assessing Richard's pupils, Ali should
   a. perform a normal pupil check.
   b. carefully check both eyes for visual acuity.
   c. cover both eyes and not check the pupils.
   d. check the pupil in the right eye and then cover both eyes.

2. Which of the following best describes how to secure a figure-eight bandage over the neck wound?
   a. Over the dressing, around the neck, under the armpit on the side of the injury, back around the neck, and anchored at the shoulder
   b. Over the dressing, across one shoulder, across the back, under the opposite armpit, and anchored at the shoulder
   c. Over the dressing, continue around the neck, and anchored at the neck
   d. Over the dressing, continue around the neck, under the armpit on the side of the injury, and anchored at the shoulder

3. Richard complained about numbness over his left eye and double vision (diplopia). These complaints are most likely the result of
   a. the injury to the neck.
   b. an injury to the orbit of the eye.
   c. trauma to the globe of the eye.
   d. hypoperfusion.

4. Ali should have applied what kind of dressing to Richard's neck injury?
   a. Gauze
   b. Self-adhering
   c. Porous
   d. Occlusive

5. Richard's neck injury
   a. is not serious since Richard is alert and oriented.
   b. is not serious unless Richard has difficulty in speaking or a loss of voice.
   c. is not serious since the trachea remains at midline.
   d. must be carefully observed for swelling and airway compromise.

TRIP #		EMERGENCY

EMERGENCY
TRIP SHEET

TRIP #
MEDIC #
BEGIN MILES
END MILES
CODE___/___   PAGE___/___
UNITS ON SCENE

NAME	SEX M F DOB ___/___/___
ADDRESS	RACE
CITY STATE	ZIP
PHONE ( ) - PCP DR.	
RESPONDED FROM	CITY
TAKEN FROM	ZIP
DESTINATION	REASON
SSN - - MEDICARE #	MEDICAID #
INSURANCE CO INSURANCE #	GROUP #
RESPONSIBLE PARTY ADDRESS	
CITY STATE ZIP PHONE ( ) -	
EMPLOYER	

BILLING USE ONLY
DAY
DATE

RECEIVED					
DISPATCHED					
EN-ROUTE					
ON SCENE					
TO HOSPITAL					
AT HOSPITAL					
IN-SERVICE					

CREW	CERT	STATE #

TIME	ON SCENE (1)	ON SCENE (2)	ON SCENE (3)	EN-ROUTE (1)	EN-ROUTE (2)	AT DESTINATION
BP						
PULSE						
RESP						
EKG						

IV THERAPY
SUCCESSFUL Y N # OF ATTEMPTS _____
ANGIO SIZE _____ ga.
SITE _____
TOTAL FLUID INFUSED _____ cc
BLOOD DRAW Y N INITIALS _____

INTUBATION INFORMATION
SUCCESSFUL Y N # OF ATTEMPTS _____
TUBE SIZE _____ mm
TIME _____ INITIALS _____

MEDICAL HISTORY

CONDITION CODES				

MEDICATIONS

TREATMENTS

ALLERGIES

C/C

TIME	TREATMENT	DOSE	ROUTE	INIT

EVENTS LEADING TO C/C

ASSESSMENT

TREATMENT

GCS	E___ V___ M___ TOTAL =
GCS	E___ V___ M___ TOTAL =

HOSPITAL CONTACTED

CPR BEGUN BY B P TIME BEGUN

EMS SIGNATURE

AED USED Y N BY:

RESUSCITATION TERMINATED - TIME

(   ) OSHA REGULATIONS FOLLOWED

OBJECTIVES

Numbered objectives are from the United States Department of Transportation EMT-Basic National Standard Curriculum. Asterisked objectives, if any, pertain to material that is supplemental to the DOT curriculum.

Cognitive

5-2.8   Discuss the emergency medical care considerations for a patient with a penetrating chest injury.
5-2.9   State the emergency medical care considerations for a patient with an open wound to the abdomen.
5-2.10 Differentiate the care of an open wound to the chest from an open wound to the abdomen.
   * Review the anatomy of the chest cavity as it pertains to chest injuries.
   * Identify signs and symptoms of possible life-threatening chest injuries.
   * Describe emergency medical care for life-threatening chest injuries.
   * Review the anatomy of the abdomen.
   * Recognize the common signs and symptoms of abdominal injuries.
   * Describe the emergency medical care for a suspected abdominal injury.
   * Describe the emergency medical care for genitalia injuries.

KEY IDEAS

Injuries to the chest and abdomen can be easily overlooked in the physical assessment because clothing hides potential physical findings, unless the areas are exposed for examination. Injury to vital organs in the chest and abdomen can quickly cause lethal disturbances in respiration, oxygen exchange, and circulation. The EMT must rely on the mechanism of injury, a high index of suspicion, and careful physical examination in order to anticipate and manage these potential life threats.

■   A closed chest injury is the result of blunt trauma to the chest, and an open chest wound is the result of a penetrating injury, both of which can cause extensive damage to ribs and internal organs.

■   Points to remember when assessing the patient with a chest injury: Establish and maintain in-line spinal stabilization and administer oxygen; quickly expose the chest and examine it; note any sign of respiratory distress; immediately seal any open wound with a gloved hand; if there is paradoxical movement, immediately splint it with your hand. A patient with a sucking chest wound sealed with an occlusive dressing requires careful respiratory-status monitoring. Patients with chest injuries are a high priority; immediate transport with assessment and care continuing en route is required. Early recognition and prompt transport is key.

■   Emergency care of an open chest injury includes the points described above and, additionally, quickly sealing the wound with an occlusive dressing, positioning the patient to ease breathing, and continually assessing respiratory status.

- Significant findings for a chest injury include a mechanism of injury involving either blunt or penetrating trauma, signs of trauma, early signs and symptoms of shock, cyanosis, dyspnea, absent or decreased breath sounds, tachypnea or bradypnea, hemoptysis, pulsus paradoxus, and tracheal deviation.

- Abdominal injuries are broadly classed as open or closed injuries. Open wounds to the abdomen include evisceration, in which organs protrude through the skin. Closed abdominal injuries can crush, tear, or rupture a large number of organs, causing severe internal bleeding.

- Assessment of abdominal injury includes recognizing that such injury can cause excruciating pain, so much so that other injuries or problems may not be noticed by the patient. A mechanism of injury that involves either blunt or penetrating trauma, signs of trauma, early signs and symptoms of shock, shallow and rapid respirations, and abdominal pain and rigidity is showing significant signs of serious abdominal injury.

- Emergency care of both open and closed abdominal injury includes aggressive management of the airway, breathing, and circulation. Early recognition and prompt transport is key. In abdominal evisceration, apply a moist dressing over protruding organs, cover with an occlusive dressing, and add a second dressing over that. Secure the dressings in place with tape, cravats, or a bandage.

- While injuries to the genitalia are rarely life threatening, they are typically extremely painful and embarrassing. They may have a number of causes, including sexual assault. Treat such injuries as you would any soft tissue injury.

MEDICAL TERMINOLOGY

Term	Prefix	Word Root Combining Form	Suffix	Definition
atelectasis (at-uh-LEK-tuh-sis)		atel (imperfect)	-ectasis (dilation, distention)	Condition in which the lungs have collapsed or are airless
eupnea (yoop-NEE-uh)	eu- (good, normal)	-pnea (breathing)		Good or normal breathing
hemopneumothorax (HEE-moh-NEW-moh-THOR-aks)		hem/o (blood); pneum/o (lung, air); thorax (chest)		Accumulation of blood and air in the thoracic cavity, causing collapse of a portion of the lung
hemoptysis (hee-MOP-tuh-sis)		hem/o (blood)	-ptysis (to spit, spitting)	Spitting up of blood
hemorrhage (HEM-uh-rij)		hem/o (blood)	-rrhage (to burst forth, bursting forth)	Excessive bleeding
hemothorax (hee-moh-THOR-aks)		hem/o (blood); thorax (chest)		Accumulation of blood in the thoracic cavity, causing collapse of a portion of the lung
orthopnea (or-THOP-nee-uh)		orth/o (straight)	-pnea (breathing)	Inability to breathe unless in an upright position
pneumothorax (new-moh-THOR-aks)		pneum/o (lung, air); thorax (chest)		Accumulation of air in the thoracic cavity, causing collapse of a portion of the lung

Term	Prefix	Word Root Combining Form	Suffix	Definition
pulmonectomy (pull-moh-NEK-tuh-mee)		pulmon (lung)	-ectomy (surgical excision)	Surgical removal of the lung or part of the lung (synonym: pneumo-nectomy)
tracheostomy (tray-kee-OSS-tuh-mee)		trache/o (trachea)	-stomy (new opening)	New opening created into the trachea
visceral (VISS-er-ul)		viscer (body organs)	-al (pertaining to)	Pertaining to a body organ

1. The home-health nurse tells you that your patient had an episode of hemoptysis. You know that the word root *hemo* means "blood" and the suffix *-ptysis* refers to
   a. vomiting.
   b. spitting.
   c. artery.
   d. lung.

2. In your patient care report, you describe your patient's breathing as *eupnea*. What does the prefix *eu-* mean?
   a. Clear, unremarkable
   b. Loud, noisy
   c. Difficult, labored
   d. Good, normal

3. Your patient is suffering from a hemothorax. You know that the word root *thorax* refers to
   a. chest.
   b. blood.
   c. air, lung.
   d. abdomen.

4. While transferring your patient to the hospital staff, you hear the nurse state that the patient suffers from orthopnea. You know that the parts of this word—the word root *ortho* and the suffix *-pnea*—mean
   a. blood, lung.
   b. damaged, lung.
   c. difficult, breathing.
   d. straight, breathing.

5. While reviewing your patient's medical records at a local care facility, you note the patient has a tracheostomy. You know the word root *trache/o* means trachea and the suffix *-stomy* means
   a. inflammation of.
   b. new opening.
   c. surgical removal.
   d. constriction, closing.

TERMS AND CONCEPTS

1. Write the number of each term beside its definition.

1. Flail segment
2. Paradoxical movement
3. Pneumothorax
4. Sucking chest wound
5. Tension pneumothorax

_____ a. A segment of the chest wall that moves inward during inhalation and outward during exhalation

_____ b. An open wound to the chest that permits air to enter the thoracic cavity during inhalation

_____ c. Two or more consecutive ribs that are fractured in two or more places

_____ d. Air in the chest cavity, outside the lungs

_____ e. A condition in which the buildup of air and pressure in the thoracic cavity on the injured side is so severe that it begins to shift the lung on that side to the uninjured side, resulting in compression of the heart, vessels, and the uninjured lung

CONTENT REVIEW

1. List each of the following terms under the correct heading below.

Aorta	Spleen
Heart	Stomach
Intestines	Superior vena cava
Liver	Trachea
Lungs	Urinary bladder

Chest Cavity	Abdominal Cavity

2. The pleura consist of the visceral pleura and parietal pleura. Which statement describes the parietal pleura?
 a. The parietal pleura is the outermost layer of the pleura.
 b. The parietal pleura is in contact with the lungs.
 c. The parietal pleura lines the abdominal cavity.
 d. The parietal pleura is where gas is exchanged in the lungs.

3. Jugular veins that engorge during inhalation may be a sign of a
 a. developing flail segment.
 b. pericardial tamponade.
 c. simple pneumothorax.
 d. hemothorax.

4. You are treating a patient who has been stabbed in the chest. There is a puncture wound that penetrates the parietal and visceral pleura, with air being sucked into the pleural space. As the pleural space expands, you would suspect which of the following to occur?
   a. The expanding pressure will cause a hemothorax.
   b. The space will expand, resulting in a hematoma.
   c. A pneumothorax develops, leading to a collapsed lung.
   d. The internal and external pressures equalize, causing a flail chest.

5. While treating your patient, you find that the ribs are separated from both sides of the sternum. You identify this as a
   a. complex flail segment.
   b. posterior flail segment.
   c. lateral flail segment.
   d. central flail segment.

6. The mechanism of injury suggests an open chest injury. You should quickly expose and examine the patient's chest during which phase of the patient assessment?
   a. Initial assessment
   b. Rapid trauma assessment
   c. Focused history and physical exam
   d. Ongoing assessment

7. Some patients with chest-wall injury will breathe with extremely shallow, rapid breaths. What is the probable reason?
   a. The patient is hyperventilating.
   b. It is an attempt to reduce pain.
   c. It is an attempt to relieve hypoxia.
   d. The patient is hyperglycemic.

8. In subcutaneous emphysema, air is trapped under the skin. When found around the neck and upper chest, what is the usual cause?
   a. Air expelled from the carotid artery
   b. The progressive nature of hypoperfusion
   c. Gravity's causing the air to flow upward
   d. Tracheal deviation or jugular distention

9. Which of the following is the correct way to identify tracheal deviation?
   a. Palpate the trachea immediately above the cricoid cartilage.
   b. Palpate immediately above the suprasternal notch.
   c. Inspect the trachea visually above the cricoid cartilage.
   d. Inspect visually just inferior to (below) the suprasternal notch.

10. Your patient is exhibiting signs and symptoms of a flail segment with paradoxical movement of the chest. What is the ideal way to treat this condition?
    a. Place a nonporous dressing over the site.
    b. Place the patient on the uninjured side.
    c. Provide positive-pressure ventilation.
    d. Place a gloved hand over the injured site.

11. Which of the following best describes lung sounds produced during a tension pneumothorax?
    a. Absent breath sounds on the uninjured side; decreased breath sounds on the injured side
    b. Absent breath sounds at the lower lobes; decreased breath sounds at the upper lobes
    c. Absent breath sounds on the injured side; decreased breath sounds on the uninjured side
    d. Absent breath sounds at the upper lobes; decreased breath sounds at the lower lobes

12. Which of the following is considered appropriate treatment for an open chest wound?
    a. Seal the open wound with your gloved hand during the ongoing assessment.
    b. Apply an occlusive dressing taped on three sides, and lift the untaped corner occasionally.
    c. Apply an occlusive dressing taped on four sides, and do not remove.
    d. Apply an occlusive dressing taped on three sides. and do not lift it at all.

13. Which organ is considered to be a hollow organ?
    a. Liver
    b. Gallbladder
    c. Spleen
    d. Pancreas

14. The major complication associated with the laceration, or tearing, of a solid organ is
    a. major bleeding.
    b. diaphragmatic rupture.
    c. the release of highly acidic gastric juices.
    d. intense pain.

15. Often abdominal injuries produce only subtle signs and symptoms. Therefore, you must base your treatment and transport decisions on which of the following?
    a. The patient's chief complaint
    b. The patient's sensory response
    c. The mechanism of injury
    d. Bystander information

16. When assessing a patient with abdominal pain, start palpating the abdomen
    a. without regard to the pain.
    b. at the upper-right quadrant.
    c. closest to or directly over the pain.
    d. farthest from the pain.

17. If no injury to the lower extremities, hips, pelvis, or spine is suspected, place a patient with a closed abdominal injury in a
    a. lateral recumbent position with both legs flexed.
    b. Trendelenburg position with legs flexed at hips.
    c. supine position with legs flexed at knees.
    d. Fowler's position with legs straight.

18. Which of the following dressings is most appropriate to use with an abdominal evisceration?
    a. Sterile, dry paper dressing, covered with plastic wrap or aluminum foil
    b. Sterile, absorbent cotton soaked in saline and covered with an occlusive dressing
    c. Sterile dressing soaked in saline and covered with plastic wrap as an occlusive dressing
    d. Sterile dressing soaked in saline and covered by a bulky dressing

19. Which of the following is the best method of transporting an amputated body part?
    a. Wrap it in a dry, sterile dressing and put in a plastic bag with ice chips or cubes.
    b. Wrap it in a dry, sterile dressing; cover with an occlusive dressing; and place on ice.
    c. Wrap it in a saline-moistened, sterile dressing and cover with an occlusive dressing.
    d. Wrap it in a saline-moistened, sterile dressing; put in a plastic bag; and place the bag on a cold pack.

20. You are treating a female who has a laceration to her external genitalia. Which of the following is the correct way to control the bleeding?
    a. Apply direct pressure, using a moistened sterile compress.
    b. Apply direct pressure, using your gloved hand.
    c. Pack the vagina with a sterile moist dressing.
    d. Place a moist dressing on the laceration and cover with plastic wrap.

CASE STUDY

You and your partner are on the scene of a fall. The injured tree trimmer is lying on the ground among fallen branches. You immediately take in-line spinal stabilization. You introduce yourself and your partner. The patient can only speak a word or two at a time and must breathe in between. Your partner hears a sucking sound, and she quickly exposes the patient's body to find an open chest wound under the left breast and an eviscerated abdomen with protruding bowel. You immediately call for advanced life support backup.

1. Which of the following is the correct immediate treatment for the sucking chest wound?
    a. Place an occlusive dressing on the wound during the initial assessment.
    b. Place an occlusive dressing on the wound during the rapid trauma assessment.
    c. Seal the wound with a gloved hand during the initial assessment.
    d. Seal the wound with a gloved hand during the rapid trauma assessment.

2. You apply a dressing to the abdominal evisceration. Which of the following is appropriate regarding dressing the open abdominal wound?
    a. The dressing should be a dry sterile dressing
    b. The dry dressing should be covered by an occlusive dressing.
    c. The dressing should be secured on three sides only to allow air to escape.
    d. The dressing should be secured with tape, cravats, or bandages.

The patient is now unresponsive and requires ventilatory assistance. Your partner states that it is becoming increasingly harder and harder to squeeze the bag-valve-mask device to ventilate the patient. You note cyanosis of the fingertips and quickly palpate the trachea through the examination hole in the cervical-spine immobilization collar. The trachea appears to be deviated or shifted to the right side. Further examination reveals jugular-vein distention. You quickly auscultate the lungs and find that breath sounds are absent on the left and decreased on the right.

3. The changes in respiratory status of this patient indicate which possible condition, and what steps should be taken to rectify the problem?
    a. Flail segment with paradoxical movement, support with pressure from your hand.
    b. Flail segment with paradoxical movement, roll the patient onto the injured side.
    c. Tension pneumothorax, transport immediately.
    d. Tension pneumothorax, lift the corner of the occlusive dressing on the chest wound to allow air to escape.

ENRICHMENT

1. The serious condition often caused by blunt trauma, which causes bleeding to occur in and around the alveoli and into the interstitial space that separates the capillaries and alveoli, is known as
   a. pulmonary contusion.
   b. pneumatic hematoma.
   c. pneumohemorrhage.
   d. pulmonic tension.

2. Which traumatic injury may result in a narrowing pulse pressure?
   a. Cardiac contusion
   b. Traumatic asphyxia
   c. Hemothorax
   d. Pericardial tamponade

3. Your patient presents with severe chest pain upon movement and breathing. There is tenderness and crepitus on palpation of the right lateral chest, and you suspect simple rib fractures. Which of the following is considered an appropriate technique for managing this injury?
   a. Apply a sling and swathe to the arm located on the opposite side of the chest injury.
   b. The patient holds a book firmly over the site, applying heavy pressure.
   c. The patient guards the injury by placing his arm tightly over the injury site.
   d. Apply a swathe or tape circumferentially, snugly and completely, around the chest.

SCENARIO 22: DOCUMENTATION EXERCISE

Read the following scenario, and think about how you would document this call if you were the EMT who responded to the scene. Then answer the multiple-choice questions and fill in the sample prehospital-care report, basing your documentation on information from the scenario.

While receiving the report from the previous shift's crew, you and your partner, EMT Parker, are preparing to inventory the ambulance when the station alerting system sounds: "Unit 4, respond to 3344 Ocean Drive for a person who fell from a ladder. ALS backup is not, repeat not, available." Parker acknowledges the call as you both walk to the front of the ambulance. Parker confirms the location in the map book as you pull from the station. While en route to the call, you approach the railroad track and notice that the guard gates are down with an approaching train. You advise dispatch that you will have a train delay. After the short train has passed, you advise dispatch that you are back en route to the call.

You soon arrive on the scene of a construction site and notify dispatch. As you and Parker quickly scan the area for obvious hazards, you see a bystander motioning you to the area where the patient is lying. After you pull up, you both put on eye protection and protective gloves and proceed to the rear of the am-

bulance. You place all of the equipment that you may need on the stretcher and quickly make your way toward the patient. You find the patient lying on his left side on the ground next to a tall ladder. A worker states, "Fred was up on the ladder about 12 feet when he and the ladder fell to the ground." Parker positions himself at the patient's head and maintains in-line stabilization of the spine as he asks the patient his name and age. The patient responds, "Fred. I'm 22." Parker introduces you and himself to Fred, then asks him where he hurts. Fred replies, "My left chest and stomach hurt a lot!"

Parker says, "He is breathing about 26 times a minute with shallow breathing. There is adequate air flowing in and out of the mouth." You quickly apply high-flow oxygen via nonrebreather mask set at 15 lpm. A quick check of the pulse reveals a strong pulse at approximately 100 beats per minute. You notice the front of Fred's shirt has a blood stain to the center of the abdominal area. The skin is warm and dry with a capillary blanch less than 2 seconds. You palpate the neck. It is soft with no trauma or subcutaneous emphysema noted. The trachea is palpated and found to be midline, and there is no deformity or pain to the posterior neck. As you place the cervical collar on the patient, Parker explains how you will be placing him on the backboard. Because the patient is already lying on his left side, you quickly cut his shirt to expose the back. No deformities are noted or felt. You place the backboard next to the patient and carefully roll him onto the board with the assistance of two coworkers. The patient is quickly secured to the backboard, and you and Parker begin a rapid trauma assessment.

You quickly cut away the clothing to the patient's anterior body. To your horror, you see an open wound just below the umbilicus. The patient's abdominal organs are protruding through the skin. There is little bleeding. You reassure the patient and ask dispatch to notify the local trauma center of a trauma alert and to send an engine crew for a driver.

Parker states the head reveals no injuries or deformities; the pupils are equal and react briskly to light. The nose, mouth, and ears are all clear of blood or fluid. The neck was assessed prior to application of the c-collar. Parker palpates the chest and notes an area of the left chest that moves inward when the patient inhales and outward when the patient exhales. The patient is breathing with small, fast breaths and says, "It hurts when I take a deep breath." Lung sounds are diminished but equal. You inspect the axillary area. It is without injury. You quickly inspect the pelvis for deformity, contusions, abrasions, or penetrating injuries, and none are found. You assess the upper and lower extremities, and there is no deformity or pain on palpation. You proceed to check pulse, motor, and sensory function, asking Fred if he can feel you touching his extremities. He replies, "Yes." You then ask him to wiggle his fingers and toes, and he does. Next, you check all four distal pulses and find them to be strong and regular.

Parker immediately begins to provide positive-pressure ventilation with the bag-valve mask with sup-

plemental oxygen. You attend to the open abdominal wound by applying a dressing over the wound. The engine arrives, and the fire lieutenant approaches you and asks how they can help. You advise him that you will need their assistance moving the patient to the ambulance. You request one of their crew to drive the ambulance while both you and Parker tend to the patient. The fire lieutenant is glad to help. The patient is moved to the ambulance, and the driver marks en route to the trauma center with dispatch.

You apply a folded towel over the flail segment to help stabilize the area. Next, you obtain vital signs while Parker continues to ventilate the patient. The blood pressure is 128/68; the pulse is 104 and regular. Respirations are supported at about 20 breaths each minute. The pulse oximeter reveals an SpO_2 at 98 percent with the BVM. Reassessment of the PMS reveals no changes. You ask Fred if he has any medical history or is on any medication or is allergic to anything, and he responds, "No." You ask him what happened that caused him to fall; he explains that he lost his footing on the ladder, and it just went out from under him. You ask when his last oral intake was, and he states, "I had breakfast cereal about 2 hours ago."

You reassure Fred and explain what he should expect at the trauma center. Parker states that he feels increased resistance to positive-pressure ventilation. Fred's breathing becomes more labored with severe tachypnea. You check but do not note any tracheal tugging or deviation. You quickly auscultate his chest and find diminished lung sounds on the left side. You notice slight cyanosis around his lips. A quick check of the pulse oximeter reveals a SpO_2 of 84 percent. After a short emergency response you arrive at the trauma center.

1. When Parker palpated the chest, he noted an area of the left chest that moved inward when the patient inhaled and outward when the patient exhaled. What type of injury did Parker discover?
    a. Pneumothorax
    b. Flail segment
    c. Pericardial tamponade
    d. Hemothorax

2. What type of dressing should you apply to the abdominal evisceration?
    a. Sterile dressing soaked with saline covered with an occlusive dressing
    b. Dry sterile absorbent cotton covered with a pressure dressing
    c. Saline-soaked sterile dressing covered with aluminum foil
    d. Occlusive dressing covered with a saline-soaked sterile dressing

3. Which action would be considered inappropriate treatment for this patient?
   a. Splint the unstable chest segment in an inward position with the gloved hand.
   b. Place a pillow beneath the patient's left arm to support the unstable area of the chest.
   c. Continue to provide positive pressure ventilations with the BVM while transporting.
   d. Flex the legs up toward the chest to relieve pressure on the abdominal muscles.

4. Parker stated that he felt increased resistance while providing positive-pressure ventilation. You should suspect which of the following?
   a. The patient has developed pericardial tamponade.
   b. A rupture of the diaphragm has occurred.
   c. A tension pneumothorax has likely developed.
   d. The evisceration has limited diaphragm movement.

5. Which of the following best describes a flail segment?
   a. Two or more consecutive ribs have been fractured in two or more places.
   b. A single rib has been fractured in two or more places.
   c. Three or more successive ribs have been fractured in one place, producing crepitus.
   d. Two or more ribs on the affected side have at least one fracture each.

EMERGENCY TRIP SHEET

TRIP #	
MEDIC #	
BEGIN MILES	
END MILES	
CODE___/___ PAGE___/___	
UNITS ON SCENE	

DAY				
DATE				
RECEIVED				
DISPATCHED				
EN-ROUTE				
ON SCENE				
TO HOSPITAL				
AT HOSPITAL				
IN-SERVICE				

NAME   SEX M F DOB ___/___/___

ADDRESS   RACE

CITY   STATE   ZIP

PHONE ( ) -   PCP DR.

RESPONDED FROM   CITY

TAKEN FROM   ZIP

DESTINATION   REASON

SSN - -   MEDICARE #   MEDICAID #

INSURANCE CO   INSURANCE #   GROUP #

RESPONSIBLE PARTY   ADDRESS

CITY   STATE   ZIP   PHONE ( ) -

EMPLOYER

	CREW	CERT	STATE #

TIME	ON SCENE (1)	ON SCENE (2)	ON SCENE (3)	EN-ROUTE (1)	EN-ROUTE (2)	AT DESTINATION
BP						
PULSE						
RESP						
EKG						

IV THERAPY
SUCCESSFUL Y N # OF ATTEMPTS _____
ANGIO SIZE _____ ga.
SITE _____
TOTAL FLUID INFUSED _____ cc
BLOOD DRAW Y N INITIALS

INTUBATION INFORMATION
SUCCESSFUL Y N # OF ATTEMPTS _____
TUBE SIZE _____ mm
TIME _____ INITIALS _____

MEDICAL HISTORY

CONDITION CODES

TREATMENTS

MEDICATIONS

TIME	TREATMENT	DOSE	ROUTE	INI

ALLERGIES

C/C

EVENTS LEADING TO C/C

ASSESSMENT

TREATMENT

GCS E___ V___ M___ TOTAL =

GCS E___ V___ M___ TOTAL =

HOSPITAL CONTACTED

CPR BEGUN BY B P TIME BEGUN

EMS SIGNATURE

AED USED Y N BY:

RESUSCITATION TERMINATED - TIME

( ) OSHA REGULATIONS FOLLOWED

35 Agricultural and Industrial Emergencies

OBJECTIVES

Numbered objectives are from the United States Department of Transportation EMT-Basic National Standard Curriculum. Asterisked objectives, if any, pertain to material that is supplemental to the DOT curriculum.

Cognitive

* Describe the general guidelines for emergency care of agricultural injuries and related industrial injuries.
* Identify the mechanisms of injury responsible for the majority of agricultural accidents.
* List the general guidelines for stabilizing and shutting down agricultural equipment and other machinery.
* List the common accidents/mechanisms of injury associated with various types of agricultural machinery, storage devices, and livestock.
* List the general guidelines for industrial rescue.

KEY IDEAS

This chapter focuses on the types of accidents and injuries that you may encounter in agricultural or industrial settings involving heavy machinery and specialized equipment. Such accidents can present unique challenges to the EMT, so it is important to have an understanding of how to approach these situations safely.

■ Agricultural and industrial accidents often involve unique mechanisms of injury and tremendous kinetic energy resulting in severe trauma. In addition, suffocation, inhalation injuries, and submersion are common.

■ The agricultural and industrial emergency scene is never safe until machinery is stabilized and shut down and any other hazards are controlled. If necessary, wait for fire personnel or specialized hazardous materials teams to control the scene.

■ Never enter any structure (confined space) without the help of other rescuers, without being tied to a lifeline, and without wearing appropriate protective equipment or a self-contained breathing apparatus.

1. List three hazards that might be found at the scene of an agricultural or industrial accident.

2. You are at the scene of a rollover tractor accident. Which of the following is the best approach to this situation?
   a. Due to the potential for severe and extensive traumatic injury, patient extrication and treatment must always be your first priority.
   b. The rescue requires two teams—one to handle the potential fire hazard and one to provide patient extrication and treatment.
   c. Such situations require a physician on-scene because amputation is usually necessary to rescue the patient.
   d. Due to potential hazards, you should not enter the scene without full "turnout" gear.

3. "Rules" that apply to rescue scenes involving silos or grain tanks include which of the following?
   a. Extricate the patient immediately to minimize exposure to toxic gases.
   b. Anticipate the need for decontamination activities.
   c. Never attempt rescue alone or without a lifeline.
   d. Use any method available to speed up patient access.

4. If your patient was exposed to chemicals or manure, your actions should include
   a. removing all of the patient's clothing.
   b. flushing the patient's body with a weak bleach solution or alcohol.
   c. having the patient move upwind and downhill.
   d. place the patient in the Trendelenburg position.

5. Your patient has suffered a pinch-point injury that has severed and mangled the right hand. You should
   a. preserve the avulsed body part, however mangled the appearance.
   b. place the mangled hand in a plastic bag with ice covering the body part.
   c. leave the entangled body part in the machinery; this is evidence needed for the investigation.
   d. delay transport of the patient until the body part is disentangled and transport together.

6. You are treating a patient who has become entangled with the power takeoff (PTO) shaft of tractor. The patient is critically injured, and you are unable to free him by cutting the clothing from the shaft. You should next
   a. remove the PTO shaft from the equipment.
   b. use the self-reversing feature on the equipment.
   c. release the stored energy within the equipment.
   d. uncouple the hydraulic hoses to decrease pressure.

7. Write the number of each mechanism of injury beside its definition.

    1. Crush points
    2. Pinch points
    3. Shear points
    4. Stored energy
    5. Wrap points

  _____ a. Hazards remain after the machinery is shut down.

  _____ b. Aggressive component of machinery moves in a circular motion.

  _____ c. Two objects meet to cause a squeezing or pulling action.

  _____ d. Two large objects come together to cause a mashing action.

  _____ e. Two objects move close enough together to cause a cutting action.

8. Which of the following is considered inappropriate when stabilizing agricultural equipment?
   a. Block or chock the vehicle.
   b. Tie it to another vehicle.
   c. Turn off the ignition switch.
   d. Set the parking brake.

9. If the patient is in a life-threatening situation and all other attempts at equipment shutdown have failed, you should
   a. discharge a fire extinguisher into the air intake.
   b. use the shut-off valve on the bottom of the fuel tank.
   c. clamp the fuel line, using Vise Grip–type pliers.
   d. slow the engine down with the throttle.

10. In addition to injuries, you should assume that a patient who has been buried in a grain tank is also
    a. hypovolemic.
    b. hypothermic.
    c. hypoglycemic.
    d. hypoallergenic.

11. Which of the following signs is unlikely to be found in a "silo gas" environment?
    a. Yellowish or reddish vapor
    b. Dead birds or insects near the silo
    c. Signs of illness in nearby livestock
    d. Corn or freshcut-grass-like odor

12. Never enter a livestock building or livestock area
    a. without the owner's permission and guidance.
    b. with brightly colored clothing.
    c. until every animal is secured.
    d. until the animals have been fed.

13. Which of the following guidelines used for an industrial rescue is considered dangerous and may lead to further injury to the patient and rescuers?
    a. Check with the staff to determine potential hazards specific to this situation.
    b. Assume the machine is locked and secured to prevent movement.
    c. Wait for a specialized confined-space team to arrive prior to entering the space.
    d. Limit the number of rescuers in a potentially dangerous area.

14. An aggressive component of machinery that moves in a circular motion is known as a
    a. pinch point.
    b. crush point.
    c. shear point.
    d. wrap point.

15. Your patient is caught in a crush point of a machine. You should
    a. secure the equipment by shutting off the electric power at the power source.
    b. instruct a person who knows how to operate the machine what you need to be done.
    c. release the stored energy prior to attempting to disentangle your patient.
    d. instruct other rescuers how to operate and secure the machine prior to disentanglement.

CASE STUDY

You have arrived on-scene at the Wilson farm. John, a 16-year-old, was accidentally impaled in the abdomen by one of the tines of a forklift and is apparently "pinned" to the wall of the barn. The forklift has been secured and shut down. You find John awake and alert. Your partner initiates in-line manual spinal stabilization. You note that although the tine of the forklift enters the right side of his abdomen, John is moving air adequately. His breathing is rapid, pulse is strong and regular, and skin is warm and slightly diaphoretic. There is very little bleeding coming from the wound. The patient denies any other injuries and has pulses, motion, and sensation in all four extremities.

1. Your first action should be to
    a. administer oxygen by nonrebreather mask at 15 lpm.
    b. immediately remove the patient from the forklift tine.
    c. wait for the arrival of an ALS backup crew.
    d. apply dressings and cold packs to the entry wound.

2. Regarding the impaled tine on the forklift, what should be your next action?
    a. First remove the tine from the forklift, and then remove it from the patient.
    b. Locate a physician to respond to the scene and remove the tine from the patient.
    c. Leave the tine in place, and surround the wound and abdomen with ice packs.
    d. Do not remove the impaled tine but stabilize it by applying dressings around the wound.

3. How should you extricate this patient?
    a. Remove the patient from the tine, and transport the patient lying on the injured side.
    b. Remove the tine from the forklift, and transport the tine with the patient to the hospital.
    c. Back up the forklift to aid in removing the patient, and transport while maintaining direct pressure.
    d. Remove the tine, and place your gloved hand into the wound to control the bleeding during transport.

TRAUMA EMERGENCIES: CHAPTERS 26–35

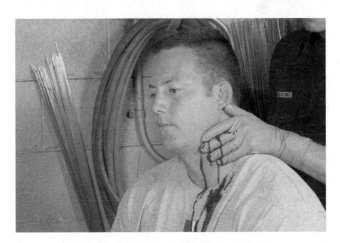

Trauma is an injury or injuries resulting from some outside force, such as a fall, a blow, a motor vehicle collision, a stabbing, or a gunshot. Whether the injury is open (the skin has been broken and, perhaps, an object has penetrated the body) or closed (from a blow that does not break the skin or penetrate the body), the injuries sustained, including injuries to internal organs of the body, may be severe.

Q **Why are mechanism of injury and index of suspicion so important?**

A Many injuries cannot be observed. There may be damage to internal organs from a blow that has left only minor marks on the exterior body. In almost any injury, spinal injury should also be suspected, even though the patient may not yet be showing any signs of spinal injury. It is also possible to be distracted by a dramatic-looking injury, such as a deep laceration or a deformed extremity, and be unaware of a far more serious injury that is not visible. Often, the mechanism of injury—how the patient was injured, such as by falling from a height or being struck by a car—is the only clue to hidden injuries the patient may have sustained and how severe these injuries may be. Based on the mechanism of injury, you must maintain a high index of suspicion for injuries that you cannot observe and/or that the patient is unaware of. For example, if the mechanism of injury was one that could cause spinal injury—whether or not the patient shows signs of spinal injury—take in-line manual stabilization of the head and neck on first contact with the patient and maintain it until the patient is secured to a backboard for transport.

Q **What are the chief concerns of the EMT at a trauma emergency, in addition to the need for spinal stabilization and immobilization?**

A Airway, airway, and airway! Many mechanisms of injury can cause airway compromise through injury to structures of the airway, broken teeth, dentures, bone fragments, blood, and secretions. In addition, the injury may cause an altered mental status, which can prevent the patient from protecting his airway. Since all other assessments and treatments are of no use if the patient does not have a patent airway, the airway must be the chief concern with any trauma emergency. Also, be alert for any signs of inadequate breathing and be prepared to provide positive-pressure ventilation with supplemental oxygen, if needed.

Q   What about bleeding and shock?

A   Bleeding is a concern whenever there is trauma. Severe external bleeding must be controlled. You must also be alert for signs of internal bleeding. Whether internal or external, blood loss can cause a life-threatening reduction of perfusion known as shock (hypoperfusion). If shock is suspected, keep the airway open, administer oxygen, keep the patient warm, position with feet elevated, and transport without delay.

Q   Are open injuries considered dangerous?

A   Yes. Open injuries to the chest and abdomen are always considered life threatening, as are severe lacerations to the neck. Immediately cover any open injury to the chest or neck with a gloved hand. Then apply dressings, including occlusive dressings. An occlusive dressing to an open chest injury should be taped on only three sides to allow trapped air to escape when the patient exhales, preventing a life-threatening buildup of air in the chest cavity known as tension pneumothorax.

Q   What are the major elements of care at a burn emergency?

A   Remove clothing and jewelry in the area of the burn, cool the burn with water, apply dressings, keep the patient warm, and transport. Flush a chemical burn with water for at least 20 minutes. If the burn is from a dry chemical, first brush off the chemical before flushing.

Q   We have learned that it is important to look for a mechanism of injury or signs of trauma at a medical emergency. Is it also important to assess for signs and symptoms of a medical emergency at the trauma scene?

A   Yes. A patient may be suffering from a medical condition as well as from trauma. For example, when a car has gone off the road and the driver is injured, might he have lost control because he was suffering from a medical condition such as a heart attack or diabetic emergency? Or might a medical condition have been brought on or aggravated by the injury? Always keep in mind that the patient may be a trauma patient and a medical patient at the same time.

36 Infants and Children

OBJECTIVES

Numbered objectives are from the United States Department of Transportation EMT-Basic National Standard Curriculum. Asterisked objectives, if any, pertain to material that is supplemental to the DOT curriculum.

Cognitive

6-1.1 Identify the developmental considerations for the following age groups:
- Infant
- Toddler
- Preschooler
- School age
- Adolescent

6-1.2 Describe the differences in anatomy and physiology of the infant, child, and adult patient.

6-1.3 Differentiate the response of the ill or injured infant or child from that of an adult.

6-1.4 Indicate various causes of respiratory emergencies.

6-1.5 Differentiate between respiratory distress and respiratory failure.

6-1.6 List the steps in the management of foreign body airway obstruction.

6-1.7 Summarize emergency medical care strategies for respiratory distress and respiratory failure.

6-1.8 Identify the signs and symptoms of shock (hypoperfusion) in the infant and child patient.

6-1.9 Describe the method of determining end organ perfusion in the infant and child patient.

6-1.10 State the usual causes of cardiac arrest in infants and children versus adults.

6-1.11 List the common causes of seizures in the infant and child patient.

6-1.12 Describe the management of seizures in the infant and child patient.

6-1.13 Differentiate among the injury patterns in adults, infants, and children.

6-1.14 Discuss the field management of the infant and child trauma patient.

6-1.15 Summarize the indicators of possible child abuse and neglect.

6-1.16 Describe the medical legal responsibilities in suspected child abuse.

6-1.17 Recognize the need for EMT-Basic debriefing following a difficult infant or child transport.

KEY IDEAS

This chapter focuses on the unique assessment and emergency medical management considerations that the EMT must take into account when providing care to ill or injured infants and children. Most EMS providers find such situations among the most stressful of any emergency call they encounter. A good understanding of the basics about caring for infants and children will go a long way toward increasing your confidence and decreasing your stress.

- The ill or injured infant or child is not your only patient. You must remember that the caregiver will also need your attention.

- The developmental classifications of the infant or child patient include neonate, infant, toddler, preschooler, school age, and adolescent. The developmental characteristics related to age will affect your assessment and treatment activities. Management of most infant and child emergencies is identical to the management of the adult patient; however, modifications may need to be made based on anatomical, physiological, and psychological development of the infant or child.

- The primary goal in treating any infant or child patient is to anticipate and recognize respiratory problems and to support any function that is compromised or lost.

- The skin color, temperature, and condition and capillary-refill time provide valuable information about the perfusion status of infants and children.

- Fever is a common emergency for infants and children and may be due to infection or heat exposure. Sudden infant death syndrome (SIDS) is the leading cause of death among infants from 1 month to 1 year old. Blunt trauma is the most common injury in children.

- Child abuse may take a variety of forms, including physical, emotional, and sexual abuse and neglect.

- Infant and child patients with special needs are often cared for at home and may be encountered by EMS personnel as a result of problems with tracheostomies, ventilators, venous access devices, or feeding tubes.

- The EMT can alleviate some of the personal stress of caring for children through advance preparation and by seeking out help when necessary.

TERMS AND CONCEPTS

1. Fill in the chart below. Include at least two characteristics for each stage.

Developmental Stage	Age Group	Characteristics
a. Neonate		
b. Infant		
c. Toddler		
d. Preschooler		
e. School Age		
f. Adolescent		

CONTENT REVIEW

1. Which of the following is a generally helpful method of dealing with caregivers at the scene of an emergency for an infant or a child?
   a. The use of technical terms will reassure caregivers that you are qualified to care for their child.
   b. Acknowledge caregivers' concerns and, when appropriate, allow them to assist you in caring for their child.
   c. Immediately remove the child from the scene so that caregivers cannot interfere with your care.
   d. Even if the child is seriously injured, reassure caregivers that "everything will be fine" to help keep them calm.

2. Which statement best describes the anatomical difference between a child and an adult airway?
   a. Newborns and infants are obligate mouth breathers.
   b. Infants have proportionally smaller tongues than adults when compared to the size of the mouth.
   c. The smallest level of the airway in the child is at the level of the vocal cords.
   d. The epiglottis is much higher in the child airway than in the adult airway.

3. The child's skin surface is large compared to its body mass, thus making children more susceptible to which of the following?
   a. Hyperventilation
   b. Hyperglycemia
   c. Hypothermia
   d. Hypovolemia

4. Infants and children have faster _____ rates than adults; therefore, they use oxygen from the bloodstream faster than adults do.
   a. lymphatic
   b. metabolic
   c. abdominal musculature
   d. central nervous system

5. The primary goal in treating any infant or child patient is the anticipation and recognition of _____ problems and support of any compromised or lost function.
   a. central nervous system
   b. cardiovascular system
   c. respiratory system
   d. urinary system

6. Which is a sign of early respiratory distress?
   a. Warm skin temperature
   b. Nasal flaring
   c. Flushed skin color
   d. SpO_2 reading of 96 percent

7. Your infant patient is lethargic, has decreased muscle tone, grunting respirations at 80 per minute with obvious use of accessory muscles, and head bobbing. You suspect which of the following?
   a. Early respiratory distress
   b. Supraclavicular retractions
   c. Decompensated respiratory failure
   d. Cardiopulmonary arrest

8. Which of the following occurs when the compensatory mechanisms designed to maintain oxygenation of the blood have failed and the body is just moments away from complete cardiopulmonary arrest?
   a. Decompensated respiratory failure
   b. Early cardiopulmonary arrest
   c. Respiratory arrest
   d. Hypotension

9. Which item is most correct regarding the initial assessment of the infant or child?
   a. Normal respiration ranges from 30 to 50/min in an infant.
   b. Normal respiration ranges from 15 to 30/min in a child.
   c. Measure respiratory rate by counting for 15 seconds and multiplying by 4.
   d. Adults generally breathe faster than children and infants.

10. When assessing breath sounds in an infant or child, auscultate in the
   a. midclavicular line on the anterior chest.
   b. midscapular line on the posterior chest.
   c. midaxillary line on the lateral chest.
   d. midsternal line on the anterior chest.

11. If perfusion is adequate, pulses, skin color and temperature, capillary refill, mental status, and _____ will be normal.
   a. respiratory effort
   b. urinary output
   c. motor function
   d. intercostal motion

12. Number the list below in the proper order from 1 to 5 to show the steps for managing a foreign body airway obstruction in an infant. The following assumes that your attempts to ventilate the infant have failed.

   _____ Support the infant in a prone, head-down position on your forearm.

   _____ Attempt to ventilate; if unsuccessful, repeat sequence.

   _____ Look in the mouth; if object is visible, sweep it out with your finger.

   _____ Deliver five sharp back slaps between the shoulder blades.

   _____ Transfer the patient to a supine position, and deliver five chest thrusts using two fingertips.

13. Regarding seizures in infants and children, which of the following is correct?
   a. Seizures are generally not caused by conditions that cause seizures in adults.
   b. Children over age 12 have an especially high risk for seizures.
   c. Seizures are caused by fever in about 50 percent of cases.
   d. Seizures can result in loss of bladder and bowel control.

14. Status epilepticus is defined as a seizure that lasts for
   a. at least 20 minutes with a recovery period.
   b. longer than 10 minutes or that recurs without a recovery period.
   c. at least 2 minutes with a recovery period and a recurrence.
   d. any period of time over 15 minutes with or without a recovery period.

15. Management of the infant or child with a fever includes
    a. suctioning secretions for at least 30 seconds.
    b. administering antipyretics.
    c. cooling by sponging with ice or cold water.
    d. removal of clothing and sponging with tepid water.

16. Regarding shock or hypoperfusion in children, which of the following is correct?
    a. It is common in children because their blood vessels are unable to constrict efficiently.
    b. It can occur in older children due to loss of body heat and an immature thermoregulatory system.
    c. When it leads to cardiac arrest in a child, it is generally due to cardiac compromise.
    d. In the pediatric patient, it occurs faster and is more serious than in adults

17. Management of an infant or a child in shock includes
    a. keeping the patient warm.
    b. performing an ongoing assessment every 10 minutes.
    c. administering oxygen at 6 lpm via nonrebreather mask or blow-by.
    d. providing positive-pressure ventilation with supplemental oxygen at 6/min.

18. Sudden infant death syndrome (SIDS)
    a. is also known as "sleeping death."
    b. is the leading cause of death in infants age 12 to 18 months.
    c. occurrence cannot be predicted.
    d. is easy to diagnose in the field.

19. Management of SIDS should include
    a. avoiding resuscitation efforts until law enforcement is present.
    b. not providing false reassurances to the family.
    c. discouraging the caregivers from talking and telling their story.
    d. delaying transport until law enforcement is present.

20. You are assessing your pediatric patient for possible shock. How should you perform the capillary refill test on your patient?
    a. Compress the soft tissue of the kneecap.
    b. Compress the tissue under the fingernail.
    c. Compress the tissue under the toenail.
    d. Compress the tissue of the forehead.

21. Trauma in children
    a. is the leading cause of death from age 12 to 20 years.
    b. is caused primarily by bicycle-related accidents.
    c. results in death within the first hour in 10 percent of all cases.
    d. is most commonly caused by blunt trauma.

22. Which of the following mechanisms of injury would require transporting to a Level 1 Pediatric Trauma Center, if one is available?
    a. Motor vehicle crash in which another occupant is killed
    b. Pedestrian struck at 5 mph
    c. Restrained occupant of a vehicle traveling 10 mph
    d. Fall from 5 feet onto concrete

23. Which of the following is the potential danger associated with excessive air in the stomach (gastric insufflations), which may occur as a result of positive-pressure ventilation?
    a. Interference with diaphragm movement and lung inflation
    b. Gastric rupture due to excessive air in the stomach
    c. Nausea and projectile vomiting
    d. Gastric regurgitation if placed into the semi-Fowler position

24. Which statement is correct relating to trauma in infants and children?
    a. The most common cause of hypoxia is the tongue obstructing the airway.
    b. Hypoperfusion is typically a sign of a closed head injury.
    c. Infants' and children's ribs are less pliable than adults' ribs.
    d. The capillary refill test is the most reliable assessment finding for shock.

25. Infant and child burn patients are at more risk of hypothermia and _____ , in part because of their greater skin surface in relation to body mass.
    a. respiratory compromise
    b. fluid loss
    c. fever
    d. scarring

26. Which statement is most correct regarding child abuse?
    a. Physical abuse is the provision of inadequate attention.
    b. Neglect is when an improper action causes an injury.
    c. The abused child will seldom exhibit fear when questioned about the injury.
    d. In many cases the child will be the victim of both abuse and neglect.

27. You suspect child abuse by a local caregiver. Which of the following best describes how you should proceed?
    a. Question neighbors about your suspicions, and flag your prehospital-care report by writing "suspected child abuse" on it.
    b. Refuse to leave the scene until the police arrive to investigate the caregivers.
    c. Record your objective observations, follow local reporting protocols, and maintain total confidentiality.
    d. Record all details of your observation, confront the caregiver, and contact the local child protective service agency.

28. A tube that is placed into the stomach for children who require long-term feeding is called a
    a. central line.
    b. shunt line.
    c. gastrostomy tube.
    d. nasogastric tube.

29. In children with tracheostomy tubes, the airway can be easily cleared of mucus by suctioning the tube with a suction catheter that is
    a. one-fourth the diameter of the tube.
    b. half the diameter of the tube.
    c. the same diameter as the tube.
    d. twice the size of the tube.

30. You are preparing to assess your pediatric patient by using the Pediatric Assessment Triangle (PAT). Which of the following best describes the PAT?
    a. It can be performed from across the room prior to patient contact.
    b. It is performed during the ongoing assessment of the patient.
    c. It is composed of appearance, work of breathing, and blood pressure.
    d. It requires specific knowledge of anatomy of the pediatric patient.

31. You are assessing your pediatric patient and suspect she may be experiencing cardiac compromise. You know the pediatric patient primarily compensates for cardiac compromise by
    a. dilating blood vessels.
    b. increasing the strength of contractions.
    c. changing the heart rate.
    d. increasing the respiratory rate.

32. While assessing your pediatric patient you know that the capillary refill test
    a. by itself is a good indicator of the perfusion status.
    b. should be performed by pressing the nailbeds.
    c. is a good indicator of the hydration status.
    d. indicates the status and effort of breathing.

33. Your pediatric patient presents with signs of shortness of breath but is still maintaining adequate respiratory depth and rate. This patient is considered to be in
    a. respiratory arrest.
    b. decompensated respiratory distress.
    c. early respiratory distress.
    d. impending apneic distress.

34. You are treating a pediatric patient for shortness of breath when you note that the tidal volume has become inadequate. You should
    a. apply oxygen with a nonrebreather mask.
    b. continue your treatment; this is not uncommon.
    c. decrease the oxygen; your patient is hyperventilating.
    d. immediately ventilate with a bag-valve mask with oxygen.

35. While treating your child patient, you notice that the wheezing has resolved without the use of medication. This often indicates
    a. the child has worsened and is no longer moving adequate air to create wheezes.
    b. the child compensatory response has been initiated and the wheezes are relieved.
    c. the hypoxic drive has increased the respiratory effectiveness and has relieved the wheezes.
    d. the bronchioles are contricting, lessening the restrictions in the airway.

36. You arrive on the scene, and the parents of a small child rush to meet you and hand you a limp, unresponsive 2-year-old patient. The parents state he choked on a hot dog, then became unresponsive. After you open the airway using the head-tilt/chin-lift, you should next
    a. open the mouth and look for a foreign body in the oropharynx.
    b. perform a blind finger sweep of the mouth.
    c. perform two back slaps while in the supine position.
    d. position the patient in a Fowler position and attempt to ventilate.

CASE STUDY

You are dispatched to a women's shelter for "baby not breathing." Upon arrival, the patient's mother reports that her 5-month-old male infant has had a cold and has been fussy for the past 2 days. Today, the child had episodes of coughing that "made him vomit." About 10 minutes ago he appeared to briefly stop breathing, and she called 9-1-1. The infant is lying quietly in his mother's arms. He is awake but lethargic with decreased muscle tone. Eyes appear "glassy." Airway is patent with very rapid, shallow, grunting respirations at 60 per minute. Skin is pale, very warm, and dry. The brachial pulse is strong and regular at 90 per minute. The anterior fontanel appears to be sunken. Capillary refill is greater than 2 seconds. There are no obvious injuries or signs of trauma.

1. The infant is exhibiting signs of
   a. decompensated respiratory failure.
   b. gastric distension and distress.
   c. early respiratory distress.
   d. progressive dehydration syndrome.

2. What is the most appropriate immediate treatment for the infant?
   a. Provide oxygen at 15 lpm and administer oral fluids.
   b. Provide oxygen at 15 lpm and immediate transport.
   c. Provide oral fluids in small amounts and rapid transport.
   d. Provide immediate positive-pressure ventilation with oxygen and transport.

During the SAMPLE history, the mother reports that the patient was born 7 weeks prematurely but has been doing fine. The patient is taking no medications and has no known allergies. She says that she fed him about 3 hours ago, but he has vomited several times since then. He has not had a wet diaper since this morning. She starts to cry and says it's her fault that the baby is so sick, but she couldn't afford to take him to the doctor when he "caught his cold."

3. In addition to the problem identified above, the infant is most likely suffering from
   a. dehydration.
   b. fever.
   c. seizure.
   d. flu.

ENRICHMENT

1. Croup
   a. is a bacterial infection of the upper airway.
   b. has a rapid onset of symptoms accompanied by a high fever.
   c. produces stridor on inhalation with a harsh "seal bark".
   d. patients should be administered dry oxygen.

2. Epiglottitis
   a. is a viral infection that causes swelling of the epiglottis.
   b. most commonly affects 5- to 10-year-olds.
   c. causes drooling and the patient sits up and leans forward.
   d. if left untreated has a 10 percent mortality rate.

3. Asthma
   a. occurs when the bronchioles dilate.
   b. is common in children without allergies.
   c. sufferers will assume a "tripod" position.
   d. attacks are not generally regarded as serious.

4. A severe attack of asthma that cannot be managed with medication is known as
   a. acute asthma.
   b. chronic asthma.
   c. pernicious asthma.
   d. status asthmaticus.

5. A condition that affects children less than 1 year of age and is caused when the small bronchi in the lungs become inflamed by a viral infection is called
   a. asthma.
   b. croup.
   c. bronchiolitis.
   d. chronic lung disease.

6. Chest compressions in children may be necessary if the heart rate drops below _____ with poor perfusion.
   a. 90/min
   b. 80/min
   c. 70/min
   d. 60/min

7. An infection of the brain and spinal cord by a virus or bacteria is called
   a. meningitis.
   b. bronchiolitis.
   c. croup.
   d. epiglottitis.

8. Place an X or a check mark next to each item below that is one of the *Six* categories that are assessed in the Pediatric Trauma Score (PTS).
   _____ a. Size/weight

   _____ b. Airway

   _____ c. Chest movement

   _____ d. Systolic blood pressure

   _____ e. Body temperature

   _____ f. Central nervous system

   _____ g. Fontanel status

   _____ h. Wounds

   _____ i. Suspicion of fractures

9. If the Pediatric Trauma Score is _____ or lower, rapidly transport the child to a Pediatric Trauma Center, if one is available.
    a. +8
    b. +9
    c. +10
    d. +11

10. When immobilizing an infant or child in a car seat
    a. use sandbags to immobilize the head.
    b. tape under the chin and around the seat.
    c. tape across the upper lip and around the seat.
    d. avoid the use of towels, blankets, or pads.

SCENARIO 23: **DOCUMENTATION EXERCISE**

Read the following scenario, and think about how you would document this call if you were the EMT who responded to the scene. Then answer the multiple-choice questions and fill in the sample prehospital-care report, basing your documentation on information from the scenario.

It is 11:30 PM on a cold winter evening. You and your partner have just finished cleaning the jump kit following a call for a vehicle versus a pedestrian when the station alarm sounds. "Unit 2, respond to 879 Venice Way for a child that has fallen; cross street, Edgewood Drive. Time out 2330 hours." You quickly return the contents to the jump kit and head to the rescue vehicle. Your partner, John, acknowledges the call and advises dispatch that you are responding.

You arrive at an upper-class residential area and quickly locate the home. It is a large three-story house. A man is standing out in the front yard waving you down. You pull into a circular driveway, step out of the vehicle with your BSI precautions in place, and are immediately met by the man. He quickly says, "Thank goodness you're here! It's my son. He fell and hit his head. He's not moving at all. You've got to hurry, please!" You reply, "Sir, my name is Rebecca, and this is John. We are EMTs, and we're here to help you and your son. What is your name, sir?" He says, "It's Ed River." As you remove the jump kit, oxygen, the pediatric immobilization device, and other equipment, you ask, "Mr. River, how old is your son?" He replies as you are walking toward the front door, "He just turned 18 months old." You continue your questioning. "How did he fall, and from how high did he fall?" As the father opens the front door, he says, "The only thing we can figure out is that he fell from the second-story area. I think he must have climbed over the railing and fell to the first floor. I found him on the hallway floor. He hasn't moved at all. You asked about how high he fell. I think it must be at least 15 feet, because we have really high ceilings on the first floor."

You ask dispatch to respond ALS, and they advise that the ALS unit is about 6 minutes away. You enter the front door and see a small boy lying on his right side. You estimate his weight at about 30 pounds. The mother is softly crying and holding the child's hand. When your eyes meet, you can see that she is terrified. As you move toward the child, you look up and observe the upper living area from which it is assumed that the child fell. As Mr. River had said, it is at least 15 feet up. The child's respirations appear to be adequate with no abnormal respiratory sounds present. John sets down the jump kit and immobilization device and places a nonrebreather mask on the child, adjusting the flow to 15 lpm. The child does not move. His eyes are closed and remain closed. He has a large laceration on the right frontal area of his head. The mother is holding pressure on the wound, and the bleeding appears to be controlled.

John quickly cuts the clothing from the boy and positions the pediatric immobilization device next to him. He holds manual stabilization of the cervical spine while you roll the child onto the immobilization device. The child is secured to the immobilization device with a cervical collar in place. You check for a pain response and observe an extension response to pain. Both arms and legs move. You size and place an oropharyngeal airway, and a gag reflex is not triggered.

You check the brachial pulse and find it strong and regular. The skin is warm, and the skin color is good. The capillary refill is less than 2 seconds. You perform a rapid trauma assessment while John takes the vital signs. You observe the laceration on the child's forehead. The child's pupils are unequal: the right pupil is fixed and dilated, and the left eye responds slowly to light. The eyes are deviated to the right. The ears and nose are clear of blood and fluid. On palpation of the skull, you feel a depressed area over the right parietal region. No obvious deformities of the neck are noted, and the trachea is in the midline. The breath sounds are clear and equal bilaterally. You note a probable closed fracture of the right forearm. No other physical findings are observed.

John completes the vital signs and tells you, "His breathing is 24 per minute and appears to be of normal depth. His pulse is 130 per minute and strong and regular. His pupils are unchanged from your as-sessment. The blood pressure is 96/48; his skin color is good; the radial and brachial pulses are strong. The capillary refill time is less than 2 seconds. The SpO_2 is 96 percent. You obtain a SAMPLE history from the father. He tells you that his son has no allergies, takes no medications, has no prior medical history, and last ate about 30 minutes ago.

You hear a knock at the door and see Paramedic Beck walk into the house. You give the paramedic a quick patient report and help place the patient into the ALS ambulance.

1. Rebecca requested ALS when the child's father told her that the child fell from a height of about 15 feet. She knew that any fall of at least _____ feet is a mechanism of injury that requires transport of the pediatric patient to a Level 1 Pediatric Trauma Center.
   a. 5
   b. 10
   c. 12
   d. 15

2. The average range for the pulse in this 18-month-old patient is expected to be
   a. 80–140 per minute.
   b. 80–130 per minute.
   c. 80–120 per minute.
   d. 70–110 per minute.

3. When providing spinal immobilization for this patient
   a. a spinal immobilization collar should not be applied.
   b. check for pulses, motor function, and sensation before and after immobilization.
   c. place padding under the head to account for the large occiput.
   d. secure the head to the immobilization device before the torso.

4. The child in this case could be more accurately referred to as a/an
   a. neonate.
   b. infant.
   c. toddler.
   d. preschooler.

5. The child in this case would be assigned a Pediatric Trauma Score of
   a. +5
   b. +7
   c. +9
   d. +12

EMERGENCY TRIP SHEET

TRIP #	
MEDIC #	
BEGIN MILES	
END MILES	
CODE___/___	PAGE___/___
UNITS ON SCENE	

	BILLING USE ONLY
DAY	
DATE	
RECEIVED	
DISPATCHED	
EN-ROUTE	
ON SCENE	
TO HOSPITAL	
AT HOSPITAL	
IN-SERVICE	

NAME   SEX M F DOB ___/___/___

ADDRESS   RACE

CITY   STATE   ZIP

PHONE (   )   -   PCP DR.

RESPONDED FROM   CITY

TAKEN FROM   ZIP

DESTINATION   REASON

SSN   -   -   MEDICARE #   MEDICAID #

INSURANCE CO   INSURANCE #   GROUP #

RESPONSIBLE PARTY   ADDRESS

CITY   STATE   ZIP   PHONE (   )   -

EMPLOYER

CREW	CERT	STATE #

TIME	ON SCENE (1)	ON SCENE (2)	ON SCENE (3)	EN-ROUTE (1)	EN-ROUTE (2)	AT DESTINATION
BP						
PULSE						
RESP						
EKG						

IV THERAPY
SUCCESSFUL Y N # OF ATTEMPTS ___
ANGIO SIZE _____ga.
SITE _____
TOTAL FLUID INFUSED _____ c
BLOOD DRAW Y N INITIALS

INTUBATION INFORMATION
SUCCESSFUL Y N # OF ATTEMPTS ___
TUBE SIZE _____ mm
TIME _____ INITIALS ___

MEDICAL HISTORY

CONDITION CODES				

MEDICATIONS

TREATMENTS

TIME	TREATMENT	DOSE	ROUTE	IN

ALLERGIES

C/C

EVENTS LEADING TO C/C

ASSESSMENT

TREATMENT

GCS | E___ V___ M___ TOTAL =

GCS | E___ V___ M___ TOTAL =

HOSPITAL CONTACTED

CPR BEGUN BY   B   P   TIME BEGUN

EMS SIGNATURE

AED USED   Y   N   BY:

RESUSCITATION TERMINATED - TIME

(   ) OSHA REGULATIONS FOLLOW

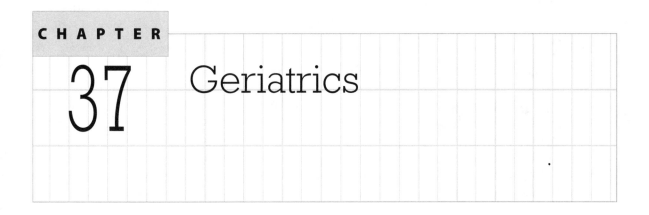

CHAPTER 37 Geriatrics

OBJECTIVES

Numbered objectives are from the United States Department of Transportation EMT-Basic National Standard Curriculum. Asterisked objectives, if any, pertain to material that is supplemental to the DOT curriculum.

Cognitive

* Discuss at least four factors that contribute to the geriatric patient being at a higher risk for medical emergencies.
* Discuss the general physiological changes in the body systems of the geriatric patient that are due to the normal aging process.
* Discuss special considerations for assessing the geriatric patient suffering from a medical or traumatic emergency.
* Outline the special considerations for obtaining an accurate medical history from a geriatric patient.
* List the emergency care steps and considerations for the geriatric patient suffering either a medical or a traumatic emergency.
* Discuss positioning, immobilization, and packaging of the elderly trauma patient with consideration of physical deformity.
* Recite and explain common disease processes that cause generalized complaints in the elderly.

KEY IDEAS

This chapter focuses on the assessment of the geriatric patient, one who is over the age of 65. Since this is the fastest growing segment of the population in the United States, and because the majority of EMS calls involve geriatric patients, it is important to understand the characteristics of this age group and how to tailor your assessment to their special needs. Key concepts include:

■ The elderly are at greater risk for nearly all types of injuries and illness.

■ Due to physiological changes caused by aging, the geriatric patient will present problems with different signs and symptoms than you would expect to find if your patient were younger.

■ Geriatric patients often have one or more coexisting long-term conditions or health problems that can mask or change the presentation of their current emergency problem.

TERMS AND CONCEPTS

1. Write the number of the correct term next to each definition.
    1. Arteriosclerosis
    2. Cardiac hypertrophy
    3. Chronic
    4. Dementia
    5. Kyphosis
    6. Osteoporosis
    7. Silent heart attack
    8. Syncope

    _____ a. Heart attack that does not cause chest pain

    _____ b. Condition resulting in the malfunctioning of normal cerebral processes

    _____ c. Long term, progressing gradually

    _____ d. Abnormal curvature of the spine

    _____ e. Disease process that causes the loss of elasticity in the vascular walls

    _____ f. Disease characterized by an abnormal loss of bone minerals

    _____ g. A brief period of unconsciousness due to lack of blood flow to the brain

    _____ h. Thickening of the cardiac walls without an increase in the size of the chamber

CONTENT REVIEW

1. Which of the following statements related to aging is accurate?
    a. Changes in body physiology associated with aging typically begin at about age 50.
    b. The trend is that people are not living as long with chronic disease.
    c. The aging body has fewer reserves with which to combat diseases and traumatic injuries.
    d. Illness is an inevitable part of aging.

2. Cardiovascular system changes associated with aging include
    a. increased arterial elasticity that speeds reaction to stimulation.
    b. a conduction system that carefully maintains heart rate and rhythm.
    c. increased cardiac output due to cardiac hypertrophy.
    d. increased blood pressure due to increased vascular resistance.

3. Aging causes a generalized deterioration of the respiratory system. This is characterized by decreased flexibility of the rib cage, alveolar degeneration, decreased elasticity of the lung tissue, and
    a. increased resistance to infection.
    b. blunted sensitivity to hypoxia.
    c. increased gas exchange through diffusion.
    d. enhanced cough and gag reflex.

4. Which of the following is the most significant musculoskeletal change associated with aging?
    a. Arthritis
    b. Kyphosis
    c. Fibrosis
    d. Osteoporosis

5. Slowing of reflexes commonly seen in the elderly is due to
   a. degeneration of nerve cells.
   b. increased muscle elasticity.
   c. increased impulse transmission.
   d. increased brain mass and weight.

6. Aging of the gastrointestinal system contributes to a variety of medical conditions as well as
   a. enhanced drug absorption.
   b. increased peristalsis.
   c. malnutrition.
   d. obesity.

7. Which statement best describes changes related to the renal system in the elderly as compared to other age groups?
   a. The kidneys become larger in size and weight.
   b. An increase in nephrons in the elderly allows for more blood to be filtered.
   c. It is more common for the elderly to suffer from drug toxicity if they take too much medication.
   d. Elderly patients' renal systems are more resistant to failure during acute illness or injury.

8. Which statement is most correct related to the scene size-up phase of an emergency call involving an elderly patient?
   a. Always wear an N-95 or a HEPA mask when treating a nursing-home patient with a cough.
   b. Elderly patients' diminished sensitivity to temperature changes means cold- or heat-related emergencies are less common for these patients.
   c. When you enter a nursing home, focus only on the patient you have been called to treat.
   d. Elderly patients are unlikely to suffer a medical and a traumatic problem at the same time.

9. Signs of dehydration in the elderly include
   a. eyes appear to bulge in the orbits.
   b. mucous membranes appear cyanotic.
   c. lips appear swollen.
   d. tongue appears furrowed.

10. Geriatric patients as a group
   a. deteriorate less quickly than other age groups.
   b. are more sensitive to pain than other age groups.
   c. suffer depression less than other age groups.
   d. abuse alcohol more than other age groups.

11. Which statement related to the initial assessment or management of the geriatric patient is correct?
   a. A sudden onset of altered mental status is common and is called dementia.
   b. A narrowed, more rigid esophagus means a reduced incidence of choking on food.
   c. You should never attempt to perform a jaw-thrust maneuver in an elderly patient.
   d. A resting respiratory rate of greater than 20 per minute is normal.

12. You are treating a 75-year-old woman with an altered mental status and no history of trauma. She should be transported
   a. in a Fowler's position.
   b. lying on her side to protect her airway.
   c. immobilized on a long spine board after applying a cervical collar.
   d. wearing a cervical collar but placed in a position of comfort.

13. You are treating a 78-year-old who fell from a ladder onto his concrete patio and is complaining of back and neck pain. Because of his severe kyphosis, he should be transported
    a. in whatever position is most comfortable.
    b. fully immobilized on a long spine board, wearing a rigid cervical collar.
    c. on a long spine board, using blankets to fill the void from the curvature of the spine.
    d. lying on his left side to prevent aspiration of stomach contents.

14. Due to depressed pain perception, geriatric patients may have a "silent heart attack." Rather than experiencing chest discomfort, they may more commonly complain of
    a. lower abdominal pain.
    b. lower back pain.
    c. weakness and fatigue.
    d. tingling in the fingers.

15. Congestive heart failure commonly occurs in older patients because the heart no longer pumps effectively and blood begins to "back up" into the lungs or peripheral vessels. Results may include fatigue and difficulty breathing. Treatment includes administering oxygen and expediting transport
    a. immobilized to a long spine board.
    b. in a Fowler's position (sitting up).
    c. lying on the side to prevent aspiration.
    d. supine on the stretcher.

16. Your 80-year-old patient suffers from chronic obstructive pulmonary disease (COPD). She is alert and complains of increasing difficulty breathing over the past few days. She denies having any pain. Emergency care for your patient would include administering oxygen by nonrebreather mask and
    a. assisting her in taking nitroglycerin.
    b. assisting her ventilations with positive pressure.
    c. transporting her in a Fowler's position if tolerated.
    d. assisting her in using a metered-dose inhaler.

17. You are treating a 77-year-old patient, who is complaining of a sudden onset of difficulty breathing and chest pain that is localized and does not radiate. He is slightly cyanotic. His breathing is labored at 16 per minute. He has a history of heart problems and recently had surgery. Your first priority in emergency treatment is
    a. administering oxygen by nonrebreather mask.
    b. administering positive-pressure ventilation.
    c. having him sit up with pillows behind his back.
    d. placing him in a lateral recumbent position.

18. After you perform the emergency treatment in item 17, your patient's respiratory rate decreases to 8 per minute. Your most accurate conclusion would be that
    a. your treatment has caused his condition to improve, and no further treatment is required.
    b. your treatment has caused his condition to deteriorate, and you will contact medical direction for advice.
    c. his condition is deteriorating because he is unable to sustain the labor of breathing, and you need to provide positive-pressure ventilation.
    d. his condition is improving because these spells come and go spontaneously.

19. An altered mental status in the geriatric patient is
    a. usually a difficult condition to manage.
    b. generally caused by senility.
    c. most often accompanied by a headache.
    d. most often due to hypotension.

20. For each item in the following list, write Y (yes) or N (no) to indicate if it is a common cause of altered mental status in the elderly.

    _____ a. Decreased blood-glucose level

    _____ b. HIV and HIV-related complexes

    _____ c. Hypothermia or hyperthermia

    _____ d. Respiratory disorders and hypoxia

    _____ e. Medical or traumatic head injury

    _____ f. Infection

21. Key treatment of a cerebrovascular accident (CVA, or stroke) includes
    a. aggressive oxygenation and ventilation.
    b. complete immobilization of the head and neck.
    c. rapid transport to the medical receiving facility with delayed assessment en route.
    d. administering fluids to maintain hydration and perfusion.

22. Which statement is correct related to drug toxicity in the elderly patient?
    a. Younger patients are more at risk for drug toxicity than older patients.
    b. Younger patients buy more prescription drugs than older patients.
    c. Treatment for drug toxicity is based on treating the drug's effects.
    d. You should leave over-the-counter and prescription drugs at the patient's home.

23. You are treating your elderly patient from a nursing facility. As you gather a history from the nurse, she states that the patient has a medical history of "cardiac hypertrophy." You know this to be
    a. a thickening of the cardiac walls without any increase in atrial or ventricular chambers, which decreases stroke volume.
    b. a thinning (reduction) of the heart walls increasing the atrial or ventricular chambers, thus increasing stroke volume.
    c. a deterioration in the conduction system of the heart, resulting in the inability of the heart to initiate and transmit a normal impulse.
    d. a systemic increase in the conduction system of the heart, resulting in the ability of the heart to adapt to increased load and demand on the heart.

24. A drop in the systolic blood pressure and an elevation of the heart rate when the elderly patient goes from a lying to a standing position is known as
    a. Trendelenburg hypotension.
    b. supine hypotension.
    c. hemostatic hypotension.
    d. orthostatic hypotension.

25. Which of the following factors contributes to the development of environmental emergencies among the elderly?
    a. Aging enhances the body's ability to control temperature.
    b. Limitations on mobility allow the elderly to maintain body warmth.
    c. Medications the elderly take have little impact on ability to control temperature.
    d. Situational factors, such as fixed income, lead to environmental emergencies.

26. Number the list below in the proper order from 1 to 5 to provide emergency care to an elderly patient who is suffering from hypothermia.

    _____ Remove wet clothing.

    _____ Remove the patient from the environment.

    _____ Protect the airway.

    _____ Wrap the patient in a dry blanket.

    _____ Maintain normal breathing and circulation.

27. In the elderly patient, which of the following receptors become less sensitive in detecting hypoxia or carbon dioxide levels in the blood?
    a. Baroreceptors
    b. Chemoreceptors
    c. Oxygen receptors
    d. Kodiak receptors

28. The characteristic curvature of the spine that is caused by narrowing of the vertebral disks in the elderly patient is known as
    a. lumbarosis.
    b. spineosis.
    c. curveosis.
    d. kyphosis.

CASE STUDY

It is early one Sunday afternoon, and the emergency services are relaxing by watching the Buccaneers play the Saints. The Buccaneers have just scored a touchdown when you are dispatched to an 88-year-old woman, Mrs. Walter, who has suffered a fall. As you enter the house, Mrs. Walter's daughter tells you that her mother had pneumonia 3 months ago but has been doing well since then. You note no hazards nor find any obstacles to extrication. You find your patient seated on the couch holding her right arm very carefully across her chest. When you introduce yourself and your partner, Mrs. Walter apologizes for bothering you on a Sunday afternoon. She goes on to say that she lost her balance and fell while coming down a flight of stairs. You find Mrs. Walter to be alert and oriented. Her airway is patent, and her breathing is regular at 16 per minute with good air exchange. Core and peripheral pulses are strong and regular at 78 per minute. Her skin is slightly pale and moist but warm to the touch. Your partner auscultates her blood pressure at 168/98 in her left arm. Mrs. Walter complains that her right shoulder is very painful where she hit the wall as she fell. You note that there is an obvious deformity near her shoulder and that her right arm seems to droop at an unnatural angle, even though she is supporting it with her left hand.

1. Which statement best describes how you should next proceed with Mrs. Walter's care?
   a. Establish and maintain stabilization of the head and neck.
   b. Provide positive-pressure ventilation.
   c. Apply a splint to the injured arm.
   d. Contact adult protective services.

2. Which of the vital-sign findings is of concern related to Mrs. Walter's condition?
   a. Pulse
   b. Respirations
   c. Skin color and condition
   d. Blood pressure

PEDIATRICS AND GERIATRICS: CHAPTERS 36–37

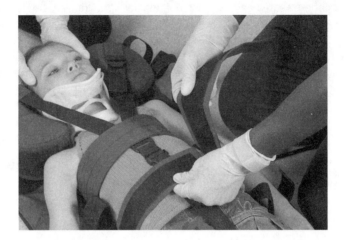

Calls to emergencies involving infants and children are among the most stressful for many EMTs, partly because they are relatively infrequent, partly because many EMTs are not familiar with children, partly because the emotions and reactions of the parents or other caregivers adds to the stress of the event, and partly because the plight of a sick or an injured child can be heartrending.

Q   **What are the similarities between emergencies involving infants and children and those involving adults?**

A   Infants and children have many of the same medical and trauma problems as adults. They bleed, suffer shock, develop allergies, get stung by insects, and swallow poisonous substances, just as adults do. Most treatments are the same as those for adults.

Q   **What are the important differences between adults and infants or children as they may affect emergency care?**

A   Some important anatomical differences were discussed in the Airway module. Children have smaller mouths and noses, relatively larger tongues, softer airway and chest structures, and larger heads that require padding under the shoulders to keep the airway aligned. All of these factors require special alertness to possible airway occlusion.

Q   **Isn't it hard to communicate with children and their parents?**

A   It helps to know something about the way children develop. You can also use common sense. You can't ask a baby how he feels, but you can note whether he is alert and crying vigorously or, instead, is lying lethargically and looking ill. Involving the parents or other caregivers can help to keep the adults calm. They can provide information about what is normal for this child and can comfort the child by holding him.

Q   **What is the chief concern involving infants or children?**

A   *Respiration.* In fact, the primary goal in treating any infant or child is the anticipation and recognition of respiratory problems. With children, respiratory difficulties can rapidly lead to respiratory failure and death.

Q **What are the signs of respiratory distress in the infant or child?**

A Be especially alert for signs of *early* respiratory distress, including a higher-than-normal breathing rate; nasal flaring; retractions of the tissues and muscles above, below, and over the rib cage; audible breathing such as stridor, wheezing, or grunting; or "seesaw" breathing (effort of inspiration draws chest in, forces abdomen out). From early respiratory distress, the child may deteriorate into decompensated respiratory failure (a respiratory rate over 60 per minute, poor tidal volume, cyanosis, decreased muscle tone, poor peripheral perfusion, and altered mental status), and finally to respiratory arrest (respirations less than 10 per minute or absent, unresponsiveness, slow, or absent heart rate, weak or absent peripheral pulses).

Q **What is the emergency care for respiratory distress in the infant or child?**

A If the child is in early respiratory distress and breathing is adequate, provide oxygen and immediate transport. If the child is deteriorating into decompensated respiratory failure or respiratory arrest, establish and maintain a patent airway, suction fluids, and provide positive-pressure ventilation with supplemental oxygen. If distress is mild, the child may prefer to sit up. If the child is very ill or unresponsive (without suspected spinal injury), place her on her side to aid drainage from the mouth. If spinal injury is suspected, immobilize her in a supine position with padding beneath the shoulders as needed to keep the airway aligned. Transport without delay.

Q **What are the special concerns regarding trauma in infants and children?**

A A child's relatively larger, heavier head will propel the head forward in a crash so that head injuries are common. The child's less-developed ribs, chest, and abdominal walls mean that they may more easily sustain internal injuries without broken ribs or other observable signs of injury. If you observe signs of possible child abuse or neglect, treat the child's injuries as you would ordinarily. Do not confront the caregivers, but report your suspicions to the proper authorities according to your state laws or local protocols.

38 Ambulance Operations

OBJECTIVES

Numbered objectives are from the United States Department of Transportation EMT-Basic National Standard Curriculum. Asterisked objectives, if any, pertain to material that is supplemental to the DOT curriculum.

Cognitive

7-1.1 Discuss the medical and nonmedical equipment needed to respond to a call.

7-1.2 List the phases of an ambulance call.

7-1.3 Describe the general provisions of state laws relating to the operation of the ambulance and privileges in any or all of the following categories:
- Speed
- Warning lights
- Sirens
- Right-of-way
- Parking
- Turning

7-1.4 List contributing factors to unsafe driving conditions.

7-1.5 Describe the considerations that should be given to:
- Request for escorts
- Following an escort vehicle
- Intersections

7-1.6 Discuss "due regard for safety of all others" while operating an emergency vehicle.

7.1-7 State what information is essential in order to respond to a call.

7-1.8 Discuss various situations that may affect response to a call.

7-1.9 Differentiate between the various methods of moving a patient to the unit based on injury or illness.

7-1.10 Apply the components of the essential patient information in a written report.

7-1.11 Summarize the importance of preparing the unit for the next response.

7-1.12 Identify what is essential for completion of a call.

7-1.13 Distinguish among the terms cleansing, disinfection, high-level disinfection, and sterilization.

7-1.14 Describe how to clean or disinfect items following patient care.

KEY IDEAS

As an EMT, you have the responsibility of getting safely to the scene of an emergency and transporting your patients safely to medical care. This chapter focuses on the safe and effective operation of an ambulance. It also provides information on how to prepare yourself, your equipment, your medical supplies, and your vehicle for the emergency call.

- Operation of an emergency vehicle gives you certain privileges; however, at no time is it justified to operate an ambulance in a manner that endangers or jeopardizes anyone else.

- The EMT that fails to exercise due regard for the safety of others incurs personal liability for any consequences that may result from that disregard.

- Operation of an ambulance requires your familiarity and compliance with agency guidelines or procedures and state and local laws and regulations governing all aspects of emergency vehicle operation.

- Practice roadway-safety procedures by not trusting oncoming traffic, not turning your back to approaching traffic, positioning the first arriving vehicle to create a barrier, wearing highly visible vests, turning off headlights at night that may blind oncoming traffic, using other emergency vehicles to slow and redirect traffic, using other warning signs and measures to slow traffic (including traffic cones), and assigning a person to monitor oncoming traffic.

- The major phases of an ambulance call include daily prerun vehicle and equipment preparation, dispatch, en route to the scene, at the scene, en route to the receiving facility, at the receiving facility, en route to the station or response area, and post-run.

- Infection-control procedures play a crucial role in preparing your unit and yourself to return to service.

- If your EMS agency interacts with or provides aeromedical emergency service, you must be familiar with landing-zone safety considerations and must always comply with them when performing your job.

CONTENT REVIEW

1. A "privilege" associated with the operation of an emergency vehicle is
   a. driving the posted speed limit.
   b. stopping at red lights.
   c. parking properly.
   d. passing in a no-passing zone.

2. Which of the following demonstrates a failure to exercise "due regard for the safety of others"?
   a. You are en route to the scene of an emergency and cautiously move through a red light, slowing down as you enter the intersection.
   b. En route to an emergency scene, you drive the wrong way down a one-way street without using any warning devices.
   c. You park your vehicle over the crest of a hill on a busy highway, post flares, and direct traffic around your location.
   d. You exceed the speed limit in accordance with state and local regulations while responding to the scene of an emergency.

3. To be a good emergency-vehicle operator, the EMT should
   a. always travel as fast as possible.
   b. hold the steering wheel at the 9 o'clock and 12 o'clock positions.
   c. always travel the shortest route to the emergency scene.
   d. brake into a curve and gradually accelerate when going out.

4. Which of the following *best* describes the appropriate use of escorts?
   a. Since the use of escorts will decrease your response time to the scene of an emergency, they should always be used.
   b. The use of escorts significantly minimizes the dangers associated with emergency driving; they should always be used.
   c. The use of escorts doubles the hazards associated with emergency driving and should only be used as a last resort.
   d. The use of escorts doubles the hazards associated with emergency driving and should never be used.

5. When using a siren
   a. pull directly behind a car and blast your siren.
   b. it is safe to assume that drivers are aware of you.
   c. operators tend to increase their speed by 30 mph.
   d. it creates emotional stress for you and the patient.

6. During your daily inspection of the ambulance, you note that the brakes appear to be unsafe. You discuss this with your supervisor, who tells you to drive the vehicle anyway. You should
   a. document the incident and drive the vehicle.
   b. document the incident and drive the vehicle with extra care.
   c. document the incident and respectfully refuse to operate the vehicle.
   d. documentation is not required; drive the vehicle as requested.

7. Mark an X or check mark to indicate which of the following is information that should be provided by dispatch.
   _____ a. Location of the call
   _____ b. Patient's physician's name
   _____ c. Nature of the call
   _____ d. Name, location, and callback number of the caller
   _____ e. Patient's insurance provider
   _____ f. Location of the patient at the scene
   _____ g. Number of patients and severity of the problem
   _____ h. Patient's height and weight

8. En route to the scene, it is a good practice to do which of the following?
   a. Determine and clarify the responsibilities of each team member.
   b. Prealert medical direction of the nature of the call.
   c. Drive as fast as possible to reduce response time.
   d. Check on fuel levels to ensure you have enough for the return trip.

9. An incomplete list of the major phases of an ambulance call appears below. Fill in the blanks with the omitted phases.

   1. Daily prerun vehicle and equipment preparation
   2. Dispatch
   3. En route to the scene
   4. _____
   5. En route to the receiving facility
   6. _____
   7. _____

10. At the scene of a collision, if no other vehicles are on-scene, the EMT should park the ambulance
    a. in such a way as to provide a safety zone.
    b. as close to the patient as possible.
    c. on the opposite side of the roadway.
    d. only where directed by law enforcement.

11. Stay a minimum of _____ feet from wreckage or a burning vehicle and _____ feet from hazardous materials spills.
    a. 2,000; 100
    b. 100; 2,000
    c. 200; 1,000
    d. 1,000; 200

12. Upon arrival at the emergency scene
    a. determine the responsibilities of team members.
    b. rapidly move all patients to the ambulance.
    c. carefully observe the complete incident as you approach.
    d. always leave your headlights on to alert oncoming traffic.

13. En route to the receiving facility, conduct an ongoing assessment at least every _____ minutes for a stable patient and every _____ minutes for an unstable patient.
    a. 5/15
    b. 10/10
    c. 15/5
    d. 20/1

14. Allowing family or friends in the patient compartment during transport to the hospital
    a. may be helpful if the patient is a child.
    b. is prohibited by most states' EMS statutes.
    c. is helpful if the family or friend is emotionally distressed.
    d. is prohibited by federal EMS statutes.

15. A complete oral report should be given to emergency-department personnel at the patient's bedside in order to
    a. ensure proper continuity of care.
    b. expedite the patient's admission into the hospital.
    c. reassess the patient's condition and interventions.
    d. reassure the patient.

16. The written prehospital-care report
    a. is never given to the patient.
    b. may substitute for all other hospital reports.
    c. is not necessary if you have given an oral report.
    d. should be left at the emergency department.

17. A post-run activity is
    a. changing a soiled uniform.
    b. washing your hands.
    c. providing an oral report to hospital personnel.
    d. leaving a copy of the prehospital-care report at the hospital.

18. A substance or process that kills all microorganisms is called
    a. a low-level disinfectant.
    b. an intermediate-level disinfectant.
    c. a high-level disinfectant.
    d. sterilization.

19. An intermediate-level disinfectant solution for surfaces that come into contact with intact skin is made by using a _____: _____ solution of household bleach to water.
    a. 1:10
    b. 1:20
    c. 1:50
    d. 1:100

20. Write the number of the correct level of disinfection or sterilization with the surface or equipment for which it is appropriate.
    1. Low-level disinfection
    2. Intermediate-level disinfection
    3. High-level disinfection
    4. Sterilization

    _____ a. Reusable instruments that made contact with mucous membranes

    _____ b. Environmental surfaces with no visible contamination and no suspected TB

    _____ c. Instruments that are used invasively

    _____ d. Surfaces that come in contact with intact skin

21. Appropriate guidelines for setting up a helicopter landing zone include
    a. putting a fifth warning device on the upwind side.
    b. designating a 75 × 75-foot area for a nighttime landing zone.
    c. keeping spectators at least 100 feet away.
    d. designating a 50 × 50-foot area for a daytime landing zone.

ENRICHMENT

1. National Association of Emergency Medical Technicians (NAEMT) guidelines for ensuring operational safety and security measures require
   a. security briefings at the end of each shift.
   b. decreased involvement of EMS crews in development of security measures.
   c. never leaving EMS vehicles unattended with the keys in the ignition.
   d. reducing the tracking systems of EMS vehicles.

2. Night driving
   a. results in fewer fatal collisions than do daytime driving conditions.
   b. is more difficult for younger people as compared to older drivers.
   c. can be improved by staring directly at the high beams of oncoming cars.
   d. can be improved by the use of quartz-halogen headlights in EMS vehicles.

3. A technique for safe driving at night is to
   a. use the high beams when entering a curve.
   b. dim your headlights within 50 feet of an approaching driver.
   c. keep your eyes moving; avoid focusing on one object.
   d. flick high beams up and down to remind a driver to dim his bright lights.

4. When driving in bad weather, be aware that
   a. the roads are slipperiest at the end of a rainstorm.
   b. if hydroplaning begins, you should hold the wheel steady.
   c. stopping on ice requires three times the stopping distance to stop.
   d. hydroplaning can begin at speeds of 50 mph.

5. Carbon monoxide in ambulances
   a. is easy to detect due to its distinctive odor.
   b. occurs with greater outside air pressure.
   c. can be reduced by opening the rear windows.
   d. may be harmful in amounts over 1 part per million.

39 Gaining Access and Extrication

OBJECTIVES

Numbered objectives are from the United States Department of Transportation EMT-Basic National Standard Curriculum. Asterisked objectives, if any, pertain to material that is supplemental to the DOT curriculum.

Cognitive

7-2.1 Describe the purpose of extrication.
7-2.2 Discuss the role of the EMT-Basic in extrication.
7-2.3 Identify what equipment for personal safety is required for the EMT-Basic.
7-2.4 Define the fundamental components of extrication.
7-2.5 State the steps that should be taken to protect the patient during extrication.
7-2.6 Evaluate various methods of gaining access to the patient.
7-2.7 Distinguish between simple and complex access.

KEY IDEAS

Your primary role in a rescue situation is gaining access to the patient as quickly as can be safely accomplished in order to perform patient assessment and care. Your two major priorities are to keep yourself and your partner safe and to prevent further harm to the patient.

■ Proper protective clothing and equipment must be used at every incident in which hazards (such as shattered glass, sharp metal, flammable liquids, battery acid, and body fluids) are present.

■ If you are first to arrive at the scene, you may be responsible for scene size-up and scene stabilization until police, fire, and other rescue personnel arrive. The most frequent rescue situations are motor vehicle collisions. Related hazards include downed electrical lines and uncontrolled traffic.

■ After all hazards are addressed and the scene is secure, the vehicles involved must be properly stabilized by specially trained rescue personnel. A vehicle is considered stable when it is in a secured position and can no longer move, rock, or bounce.

■ Most emergency calls do not present access problems. However, when they do, it is best to call for rescuers who have had specialized training. Residential access includes locating the patient first and evaluating the need for a forced entry based on dispatch information, what you observe at the scene, and your conversation with the patient. In a motor vehicle collision, the access of choice is a door.

■ The role of the EMT in vehicle stabilization and patient extrication is that of patient care provider. Once specialized rescue personnel assure you that a vehicle is stabilized and the scene is safe, you may approach the patient to initiate care. Patient care always precedes removal from the vehicle unless delay would endanger the life of the patient, EMS personnel, or other rescuers.

■ After gaining access to a patient, provide the same care you would provide to any trauma patient. In addition, you are responsible for assisting the patient through the extrication process and preparing him mentally and physically for disentanglement from the wreckage. Be sure to stabilize and, if possible, immobilize the spine securely before you remove the patient from the vehicle by normal or rapid extrication procedures.

CONTENT REVIEW

1. When should you first begin to plan for access and extrication problems?
   a. When receiving dispatch information
   b. While en route to the incident
   c. While you are approaching the scene
   d. After effectively evaluating the scene

2. Which of the following will present the most frequent rescue problems for an EMT-Basic?
   a. Water-rescue incidents
   b. Motor vehicle collisions
   c. Partial or complete building collapse
   d. Work-site accidents

3. All ambulances should carry which of the following to assess the scene from a safe distance?
   a. An air-particle sniffer
   b. A cellular telephone
   c. Powerful binoculars
   d. Protective outerwear

4. Which of the following is the most appropriate equipment for personnel involved in the vehicle extrication process?
   a. Full protective turnout gear
   b. Work uniform with helmet
   c. Protective coveralls, helmet, and work gloves
   d. Safety helmet with safety shield

5. When dealing with electrical power lines, which of the following is correct?
   a. Downed lines are electrically alive only when arcing.
   b. Power lines that are not arcing are considered safe.
   c. Always assume downed lines are electrically alive.
   d. Remove power lines only when wearing rubber gloves.

6. In general, which of the following is the safest method of traffic control at a serious vehicle collision?
   a. Stop all traffic and turn it around.
   b. Stop all traffic and reroute it to different roads.
   c. Slowly guide the vehicles around the scene.
   d. Hold all traffic in place until the scene is cleared.

7. While working a vehicle collision, you notice a small sweater in the rear seat of one of the vehicles. What might this indicate?

8. A vehicle is stable when which of the following takes place?
   a. Cribbing has been placed front and rear.
   b. All four tires are on a flat surface.
   c. It can no longer move, rock, or bounce.
   d. The engine is off, and the parking brake is set.

9. The majority of electric current hazards associated with auto collisions can be most simply and quickly eliminated when someone
   a. disconnects the battery.
   b. pulls the main fuse.
   c. disables the coil wire.
   d. turns off the ignition.

10. Briefly explain what steps should be taken to provide patient access in a vehicle collision before turning off or disconnecting the vehicle's power.

11. If it is necessary to disconnect the car battery, cut or use a wrench to
    a. remove the negative battery cable first.
    b. disconnect the cable on the starter.
    c. disconnect the positive cable first.
    d. lift the battery out of the engine compartment.

12. You are preparing to gain access to your patient trapped in a vehicle. You determine that you will need to use tools and specialized equipment. This type of access is known as
    a. simple access.
    b. complex access.
    c. special access.
    d. pinned access.

13. Police are on the scene, and you are about to make forcible entry into a residence for a medical emergency. Which of the following is the quickest, easiest, and least costly method of forcible entry?
    a. Breaking a window
    b. Forcing a door open
    c. Cutting a door lock
    d. Calling a locksmith

14. The patient is pinned inside a vehicle involved in a collision. He is in the driver's seat, facing front. How should you approach him?
    a. From the left side
    b. From the right side
    c. From the front
    d. From directly behind

15. Your patient is pinned inside a vehicle involved in a collision. What is the best way to tell him to unlock the door?
    a. "Unlock the door, but please turn your body at the shoulders."
    b. "Turn your body at the shoulders, then try to unlock the door."
    c. "Try to unlock the door, but don't move your head or neck."
    d. "Without moving your head or neck, try to unlock the door."

16. When using a sharp tool like a screwdriver to break a vehicle window, the tool should be placed _____ of the window.
    a. against the direct center
    b. against the upper center
    c. against a lower corner
    d. against an upper corner

17. In which of the following situations would removal from the vehicle precede patient care?
    a. The patient is hysterical and tries to extricate himself.
    b. Delaying removal would endanger the patient or rescue personnel.
    c. The vehicle extrication will take over an hour.
    d. There is minor damage, and the patient can be extricated quickly.

18. To protect yourself, the patient, and other EMT from the glass and flying debris that commonly result from disentanglement operations, you should do which of the following?
    a. Cover the patient with your body.
    b. Direct the patient to move to the back seat.
    c. Share your personal protective equipment with those at the scene.
    d. Use blankets, a tarp, or a spine board.

19. To help reduce your patient's fears while being extricated, you should do which of the following?
    a. Reassure the patient that you are highly skilled.
    b. Explain the activities, noises, and movements.
    c. Try to have the patient think of pleasant thoughts.
    d. Explain that this is an everyday, routine occurrence.

20. The only exception to the rule that the spine must be stabilized and, if possible, immobilized before removing a patient from a vehicle is when
    a. the patient does not complain of pain or discomfort.
    b. the patient appears intoxicated and adamantly refuses treatment.
    c. the patient is in her last trimester of pregnancy.
    d. when another patient blocks access to a critically injured patient.

CASE STUDY

You and your partner are working overtime as a standby crew at a local polo match. The last chukker has been completed when you hear a loud screech followed by a terrible crash. You both look toward the highway and see a large luxury car wrapped around a utility pole. Joe quickly advises dispatch of the situation, that the match has ended, and that you will be responding. As you approach the scene, you notice an electrical line that is broken 80 feet from the pole and is lying across the hood of the car. A crowd of bystanders has begun to surround the scene. Joe radios dispatch, advises them of the utility line, and requests a priority response from the power company. A polo-grounds security guard tells you that his personnel have shut off the power. You can visualize the patient in the car; the middle-age man is trying to remove his seatbelt.

1. Which of the following is the correct way to secure this scene?
   a. Secure an area that is more than 80 feet in all directions. Do not approach the vehicle. Yell instructions to the patient and advise him to stay in the vehicle.
   b. Secure an area up to 75 feet in all directions in case the power is restored. Approach the vehicle, since the guard advised that the power is off, and begin to assess the patient.
   c. There is no reason to secure a perimeter since the power is off; however, you should advise bystanders to keep back so you can work.
   d. Ask bystanders to keep back at least 40 feet (half the distance from the pole). This will keep them clear of danger. Then yell to the patient to stay in the vehicle.

2. Until you are able to gain access, which of the following is the most appropriate way to keep this patient from moving his head and neck?
   a. Instruct the patient to place his hands on either side of his head and apply manual stabilization.
   b. Instruct the patient to close his eyes and try to block out what is happening around him.
   c. Tell the patient to focus and keep his attention on an object directly in front of him.
   d. Have the patient try to lie down across the front seat and remain absolutely still.

3. Briefly explain how you and your partner can decrease the fears that this patient may experience during the noise and confusion that often accompany disentanglement.

ENRICHMENT

1. You have responded to a motor vehicle crash. What is the first step to stabilizing an upright vehicle?
   a. Remove the door next to the patient.
   b. Immobilize the suspension.
   c. Disconnect the battery cable.
   d. Let the air out of the tires.

2. You are on the scene of a motor vehicle crash where a vehicle has come to rest on its side. The first step in stabilizing this vehicle is to
   a. immobilize the suspension by placing step chocks or blocks beneath the undercarriage.
   b. cut the "A" and "B" posts, then roll the roof downward toward the ground.
   c. place block cribbing or step chocks into the void below both tires near the ground.
   d. attach a pulling device from the undercarriage of the vehicle to an immovable object.

3. You are on the scene of a crash where a four-door, mid-size car has come to rest on its roof. Which of the following could lead to collapse of the car's roof?
   a. Use of high-pressure air bags
   b. Removing the battery cables
   c. Opening of a door
   d. Cribbing the voids

4. You are using the hydraulic spreaders to gain access to a patient in the front seat of a vehicle. You know that the front doors are most easily opened by prying at the latch site on the
   a. "A" post.
   b. "B" post.
   c. "C" post.
   d. "D" post.

5. Your patient is trapped inside a vehicle that is on its side. Access to the patient is best gained by
   a. opening the trunk or rear hatch.
   b. lifting the door on top of the car.
   c. cutting the roof off the car.
   d. removing the rear window.

40 Hazardous Materials Emergencies

OBJECTIVES

Numbered objectives are from the United States Department of Transportation EMT-Basic National Standard Curriculum. Asterisked objectives, if any, pertain to material that is supplemental to the DOT curriculum.

Cognitive

7-3.1 Explain the EMT-Basic role during a call involving hazardous materials.
7-3.2 Describe what the EMT-Basic should do if there is reason to believe that there is a hazard at the scene.
7-3.3 Describe the actions that an EMT-Basic should take to ensure bystander safety.
7-3.4 State the role the EMT-Basic should perform until appropriately trained personnel arrive at the scene of a hazardous materials situation.
7-3.5 Break down the steps to approaching a hazardous situation.
7-3.6 Discuss the various environmental hazards that affect EMS.
7-3.11 Describe basic concepts of incident management.
7-3.12 Explain the methods for preventing contamination of self, equipment, and facilities.

KEY IDEAS

Hazardous materials spills and incidents are increasing in frequency. The EMT's role in such emergencies is to recognize that a hazardous materials emergency exists and to secure the scene until trained rescuers arrive. This chapter reviews recognition and EMS management of hazardous materials emergencies. Personal safety of the EMT is emphasized.

■ The principle dangers from hazardous materials are toxicity, flammability, and reactivity.

■ The amount of injury caused by a hazardous material depends on the dose, concentration, route of exposure, and amount of time the patient is exposed.

■ The primary concerns in any hazardous-material emergency are rescuer safety, public safety, and patient safety.

■ The U.S. Department of Transportation's regulations require vehicles containing hazardous materials to be marked with specific hazard labels or placards and accompanied by shipping papers.

■ Resources for hazardous-materials identification and management include state and local agencies, state and local hazardous-materials teams, the U.S. Department of Transportation's *Hazardous Materials: Emergency Response Guidebook*, CHEMTREC (1-800-424-9300), CHEMTREL, Inc. (1-800-255-3924), and your regional poison-control center.

■ Avoid contact with any unidentified material, regardless of the level of protection offered by your clothing and equipment.

- The most essential part of hazardous-materials rescue is pre-incident planning. Plan for the worst possible scenario and tailor the plan to the individual community. As part of your plan, predesignate an incident-command officer, establish a clear chain of command and a system of communications, and predesignate receiving facilities.

- An early priority at the scene of any hazardous-materials emergency is to establish safety zones in which rescue operations may be carried out. These zones are the hot (exclusion) zone, the warm (contamination-reduction) zone, and the cold (support) zone.

- Do not enter the hazardous-materials area unless you are trained at least to the hazardous-materials technician level and are trained in the use of SCBA (self-contained breathing apparatus) and chemical protective clothing. If you have had no training, radio immediately for help. While you are waiting for help to arrive, protect yourself and bystanders by keeping uphill, upwind, upstream, and away from danger.

TERMS AND CONCEPTS

1. Write the number of the correct term next to each definition.
   1. Warm zone
   2. Cold zone
   3. Hazardous material
   4. Hot zone

   _____ a. Includes chemicals, wastes, and other dangerous products

   _____ b. Area adjacent to the warm zone in a hazardous-materials emergency; normal triage, treatment, and stabilization are performed here; also called support zone

   _____ c. Area where contamination is actually present; it generally is the area that is immediately adjacent to the accident site and where contamination can still occur; also called exclusion zone

   _____ d. Area that is established surrounding or immediately adjacent to the hot zone, the purpose of which is to prevent the spread of contamination; also called contamination-reduction zone

CONTENT REVIEW

1. Which of the following is the primary concern in any hazardous-materials emergency?
   a. Preservation of property
   b. Rescuer, public, and patient safety
   c. Rapid control and removal of the hazard
   d. Locating placards and shipping papers

2. What factors determine a patient's response to a hazardous-material exposure?
   a. Material, concentration, and exposure route
   b. Environment, exposure route, preexisting medical condition, and material
   c. Dose, concentration, route of exposure, and exposure time
   d. Environment, material, preexisting medical condition, and dose

3. A hazardous-materials warning placard required by the U.S. Department of Transportation is usually
   a. a circle with a triangle in the center.
   b. two concentric circles.
   c. a four-sided diamond shape.
   d. a triangle with the point down.

4. In the internationally recognized NFPA 704 Hazardous Material Identification System, a blue diamond indicates a
   a. health hazard.
   b. acid/alkali hazard.
   c. fire hazard.
   d. reactivity hazard.

5. An important resource available to rescuers 24 hours a day is a public-service division of the Chemical Manufacturer's Association. It is referred to as
   a. Chemical Transportation Emergency Center (CHEMTREC).
   b. Chemical Transportation Awareness Program (CHEMAWARE).
   c. Chemical Emergency Response Guide (CHEMERG).
   d. Chemical Manufacturer's Association Center (CHEMMAC).

6. Hazardous materials
   a. should be detected by relying on your senses.
   b. are always easily detectable.
   c. may create colored vapor clouds.
   d. spills need not be treated as dangerous.

7. The principal dangers hazardous materials present are
   a. toxicity, flammability, and solubility.
   b. toxicity, flammability, and reactivity.
   c. toxicity, flammability, and carcinogenic properties.
   d. tolubility, toxicity, and carcinogenic properties.

8. A concise print reference guide that lists more than a thousand hazardous materials, each with a four-digit UN identification number that is cross-referenced to complete emergency instructions, is called the
   a. *Emergency Response and HAZMAT Directory.*
   b. *Emergency Response Guidebook.*
   c. *American and International Guidebook.*
   d. *HAZMAT Response Guide.*

9. Which of the following is one of the four levels of training that OSHA and EPA have identified as necessary for dealing with hazardous-materials emergencies?
   a. Hazardous Materials Generalist
   b. EMR Awareness
   c. On-Scene Hazardous Materials Advisor
   d. Hazardous Materials Professional

10. Smoke from a hazardous-materials fire
    a. is transformed into a harmless state because of the intense temperatures of hazardous-materials fires.
    b. is transformed into a mildly toxic state because of the intense temperatures of hazardous-materials fires.
    c. threatens the immediate safety of victims and rescuers and threatens their long-term health.
    d. only threatens the immediate safety of victims and rescuers.

11. Before a hazardous-material emergency occurs
    a. two command officers should be appointed for all decision making.
    b. agencies should develop internal, confidential communications plans.
    c. predesignate the hospital receiving facilities that will be utilized.
    d. train and prepare for the most likely scenario that may occur.

12. Number the list below in the proper order from 1 to 3 to show the three general priorities in a hazardous-materials emergency, which never changes.

    _____ Decontaminate clothing, equipment, and the vehicle.

    _____ Protect the safety of all rescuers and victims.

    _____ Provide patient care.

13. Which statement best describes correct activities or actions in the hot zone?
    a. Bystanders are allowed only in the designated area of the hot zone.
    b. Smoking, eating, and drinking are allowed in some areas of the hot zone.
    c. At least three entry points into and out of the hot zone must be established.
    d. Rescue, initial decontamination, and treatment of life threats take place in the hot zone.

14. Prior to air transport of a contaminated patient, be sure to
    a. establish a landing zone within the hot zone.
    b. decontaminate the patient fully.
    c. contact the patient's family.
    d. contact the receiving facility.

15. If you have no training to handle a hazardous-materials emergency, radio immediately for help and
    a. keep downhill, downwind, downstream, and away from the danger.
    b. keep downhill, upwind, upstream, and away from the danger.
    c. keep uphill, upwind, upstream, and away from the danger.
    d. keep uphill, downwind, downstream, and away from the danger.

16. Failure to properly decontaminate equipment and the interior of the vehicle can result in
    a. mechanical failure.
    b. chronic chemical exposure.
    c. electronic equipment deterioration.
    d. damage to external surface areas.

CASE STUDY 1

You have responded to a call for an overturned tractor-trailer on a remote stretch of highway. From a distance, you observe green smoke escaping from the back of the trailer. A man, standing about 100 yards away, waves you down. You pull over and watch him walk up to you. The man is about 45 years old and looks well. He has a normal gait and does not appear to be injured. You ask him, "Why did you call the ambulance?" He says, "I don't know who called you. I called the police. Hey, I was alone, I fell asleep, I ran off the road. I bounced around inside the truck, and then I crawled out." While talking to the patient, you use your binoculars and spot a diamond-shaped panel on the back of the truck. You take out your *Emergency Response Guidebook* to look up the UN ID number and determine that the number refers to chlorine gas.

1. What is your next *best* action to take?
    a. Enter the truck cab and search for shipping papers.
    b. Approach from downwind to survey the scene.
    c. Enter the truck cab and search for additional victims.
    d. Quickly request additional assistance.

2. After taking the action above, what is your next *best* action?
    a. Call CHEMTREC for hazard-control information.
    b. Enter the trailer and begin decontamination procedures.
    c. Keep uphill, upwind, and protect yourself and the patient.
    d. Crack open the trailer doors to vent and prevent buildup of fumes.

CASE STUDY 2

You have responded to a hazardous-materials accident. The patient is being decontaminated. You arrive on-scene and report to the staging area. Shortly after, you are called to the cold zone to transport the patient.

1. You are accidentally splashed with contamination from an anxious and fatigued rescuer. Contamination can occur most easily in which of the following areas of your body?
    a. Lower legs and feet
    b. Lower arms and hands
    c. Under the arms and in the groin
    d. Back

2. How should you decontaminate yourself?
    a. Wash with green soap and plenty of running water, irrigating skin for at least 20 minutes.
    b. Use high-pressure hoses to wash and irrigate skin for at least 20 minutes.
    c. Use baking soda to neutralize the contaminant, then stand under running water for at least 20 minutes.
    d. Blot your skin with towels and dispose of the towels in a sealed biohazard container.

3. What precautions should be undertaken prior to transport of the decontaminated patient?
    a. Treat the patient's major and minor injuries in the hot zone before moving.
    b. Cover exposed areas of the vehicle with plastic sheeting.
    c. Transport the patient's clothing with the patient and leave it at the hospital.
    d. Transport with the patient any contaminated patient-care equipment used in the hot zone.

CASE STUDY 3

You have responded to a call for a man down at a local fertilizer distributor. You arrive on-scene and observe smoke billowing from the building. A bystander is preparing to enter the building to put the fire out with a garden hose.

1. What should you do?
   a. You should remove the bystander, evacuate the area, and contact dispatch.
   b. You, the bystander, and your partner should enter to put out the fire.
   c. You should contact dispatch while your partner puts out the fire.
   d. You should contact dispatch and remain near the building to direct firefighters.

ENRICHMENT

1. In a radiation accident the patient may suffer from
   a. contamination by radiation only.
   b. exposure to radiation only.
   c. both exposure to and contamination by radiation.
   d. immediate cardiac failure due to radiation exposure.

2. Which statement is most correct related to radiation accidents?
   a. Every EMT should quickly decontaminate all patients exposed to radiation.
   b. If a Radiation Safety Officer is not available, transport the patient wrapped in a sheet.
   c. The type of radioactive material involved is the most critical factor in how a radiation emergency will be managed.
   d. Alpha rays can be stopped by clothing.

3. This is caused by exposure to large amounts of radiation. It starts the day after the exposure and can last from a few days to 7 or 8 weeks.
   a. Radiation sickness
   b. Radiation injury
   c. Radiation syndrome
   d. Radiation poisoning

4. The Federal Nuclear Regulatory Commission recommends that an individual in an emergency situation not be exposed to more than a one-time whole-body dose of _____ roentgens.
   a. 10
   b. 15
   c. 20
   d. 25

5. This occurs when the patient has been exposed to a dangerous amount of internal radiation that results in a host of diseases, including cancer and anemia.
   a. Radiation sickness
   b. Radiation injury
   c. Radiation syndrome
   d. Radiation poisoning

SCENARIO 24: DOCUMENTATION EXERCISE

Read the following scenario, and think about how you would document this call if you were the EMT who responded to the scene. Then answer the multiple-choice questions and fill in the sample prehospital-care report, basing your documentation on information from the scenario.

It is 1:30 P.M. on an overcast Monday. You have just returned to the station after completing a patient transfer from a nursing home to the local hospital when the station alarm sounds. "Rescue 1, respond to 5243 Old Dixie Highway, the Jasper Refrigerated Storage Company, cross street, Highway 17 North, for a suspected ammonia exposure. Multiple patients may be involved. HAZMAT is responding. Rescue 2, 7, 5, and 10 are also responding. Report to the staging area in front of the Texaco Gas Station at Old Dixie and Western Avenue. Time out 1330 hours." You and your partner, Colleen, quickly make your way to the vehicle and advise dispatch you are responding.

You arrive at the staging area in about 10 minutes. You are met by the staging-area officer, who advises you that an ammonia leak occurred and that the HAZMAT crew is entering the building, looking for victims. Twenty minutes pass, and the staging officer advises you to respond to the storage company to transport a patient removed from the building. You respond to the storage company.

You arrive at an area the HAZMAT team has established as a triage area for patients that have been removed from the building. The triage officer tells you that the patient was exposed to ammonia gas and is experiencing mild respiratory distress. The patient is lying on the ground, and oxygen is being administered via a nonrebreather mask at 15 lpm. She is alert and looks at you as you approach. She appears to be about 25 years old and seems to be in minor distress. She appears to be breathing adequately with no abnormal respiratory sounds present. Her skin color looks good. You reach down and feel her pulse while you introduce yourself and your partner.

"Hi, my name is Tyrone, and this is Colleen. We are EMTs, and we're here to help you." Her pulse is strong and regular, and her skin is warm and dry. "What's your name?" She says, "My name is Jill Epson." You say, "How do you feel, Jill?" Jill says, "It is difficult to breathe at times. However, it's much better now than it was a few minutes ago."

You auscultate the patient's chest and find the breath sounds to be clear and equal bilaterally. The triage officer hands you a patient-care record that has Jill's vital signs and physical evaluation recorded. The vitals are that she is alert and oriented to person, place, and time; her respirations are 16 per minute and normal; her pulse is 90 per minute, strong and regular; her skin is warm and dry and normal color; her blood pressure is 130/76 and her SpO_2 is 98 percent. You place Jill on the stretcher, maintaining the oxygen flow, and place her in the ambulance. Colleen obtains a SAMPLE history while on the way to the hospital, takes a second set of vital signs, and completes a physical exam. The vital signs are stable, and no negative physical findings are observed. Jill tells Colleen that she was trapped in a back area of the building and inhaled only a small amount of ammonia gas. She complains of a sore throat and is having some slight difficulty breathing. She takes no medications, has no prior medical history, and last ate at noontime.

1. Command for this HAZMAT situation should be assumed by
   a. two command officers.
   b. one command officer.
   c. three command officers.
   d. no command is necessary.

2. The receiving facility to which the patient is being transported should be
   a. predesignated.
   b. a Level I trauma center.
   c. a burn center.
   d. a respiratory-care center.

3. Tyrone auscultated Jill's chest for the presence of
   a. pulmonary embolism.
   b. pneumothorax.
   c. pulmonary edema.
   d. cardiac dysrhythmia.

4. For HAZMAT responses, Tyrone and Colleen are most likely trained to the level of
   a. EMR Awareness.
   b. EMR Operations.
   c. Hazardous Materials Technician.
   d. Hazardous Materials Specialist.

5. The area where the ammonia contamination is present would be designated the
   a. hot zone.
   b. warm zone.
   c. contamination zone.
   d. control zone.

EMERGENCY TRIP SHEET

TRIP #
MEDIC #
BEGIN MILES
END MILES
CODE___/___ PAGE___/___
UNITS ON SCENE

BILLING USE ONLY				
DAY				
DATE				
RECEIVED				
DISPATCHED				
EN-ROUTE				
ON SCENE				
TO HOSPITAL				
AT HOSPITAL				
IN-SERVICE				
CREW		CERT	STATE #	

NAME   SEX M F DOB ___/___/___

ADDRESS   RACE

CITY   STATE   ZIP

PHONE (   )   -   PCP DR.

RESPONDED FROM   CITY

TAKEN FROM   ZIP

DESTINATION   REASON

SSN   -   -   MEDICARE #   MEDICAID #

INSURANCE CO   INSURANCE #   GROUP #

RESPONSIBLE PARTY   ADDRESS

CITY   STATE   ZIP   PHONE (   )   -

EMPLOYER

TIME	ON SCENE (1)	ON SCENE (2)	ON SCENE (3)	EN-ROUTE (1)	EN-ROUTE (2)	AT DESTINATION
BP						
PULSE						
RESP						
EKG						

IV THERAPY
SUCCESSFUL Y N # OF ATTEMPTS _____
ANGIO SIZE _____ga.
SITE _____
TOTAL FLUID INFUSED _____ cc
BLOOD DRAW Y N INITIALS

INTUBATION INFORMATION
SUCCESSFUL Y N # OF ATTEMPTS _____
TUBE SIZE _____ mm
TIME _____ INITIALS _____

MEDICAL HISTORY

CONDITION CODES				

MEDICATIONS

TREATMENTS

TIME	TREATMENT	DOSE	ROUTE	INIT

ALLERGIES

C/C

EVENTS LEADING TO C/C

ASSESSMENT

TREATMENT

GCS	E___ V___ M___ TOTAL =
GCS	E___ V___ M___ TOTAL =

HOSPITAL CONTACTED

CPR BEGUN BY   B   P   TIME BEGUN

EMS SIGNATURE

AED USED   Y   N   BY:

RESUSCITATION TERMINATED - TIME

(   ) OSHA REGULATIONS FOLLOWED

CHAPTER

41 Multiple-Casualty Incidents

OBJECTIVES

Numbered objectives are from the United States Department of Transportation EMT-Basic National Standard Curriculum. Asterisked objectives, if any, pertain to material that is supplemental to the DOT curriculum.

Cognitive

7-3.7 Describe the criteria for a multiple-casualty situation.
7-3.8 Evaluate the role of the EMT-Basic in the multiple-casualty situation.
7-3.9 Summarize the components of basic triage.
7-3.10 Define the role of the EMT-Basic in a disaster operation.
7-3.11 Describe the basic concepts of incident management.
7-3.13 Review the local mass-casualty incident plan.
  * Outline the ways to get help in a multiple-casualty incident.
  * Describe various approaches for reducing rescue personnel stress during a multiple-casualty incident or disaster.

KEY IDEAS

A multiple-casualty incident (MCI) can occur without warning at any time or place. This chapter reviews fundamental management techniques for MCIs, including the National Incident Management System (NIMS). Be sure to review your local community plans for specific MCI procedures and plans.

■ An MCI is an event that places excessive demands on personnel and equipment.

■ In any MCI, call for plenty of help as quickly as possible.

■ The National Incident Management System provides for flexibility and standardization in managing any disaster or MCI.

■ The incident command system (ICS) is effective because it consistently uses standardized, common terminology; adopts a manageable span of control; identifies clear objectives to be accomplished (incident action plans [IAPs]); utilizes an integrated communications system; and uses a system of accountability at all levels.

■ There is only one designated incident commander at the scene. He or she may appoint finance/administration, logistics, operations, and planning sections and chiefs as necessary. The section chiefs then establish units and unit leaders.

■ Large-scale multiple-casualty incidents may require establishing triage, treatment, transport, staging, and morgue units under the direction of an EMS branch director. The EMS branch director reports to the operations chief who reports to the incident commander.

- Triage is a system used for sorting patients to determine the order in which they will receive care. Primary triage is performed at the site of the incident immediately upon arrival of the first EMS crew. Secondary triage, or patient reassessment, is performed in the triage unit.

- Typically, there are four triage priority levels. Priority 1 (P-1/highest priority/red/immediate) are patients who require immediate care and transport; Priority 2 (P-2/second priority/yellow/delayed), delayed emergency care and transport; Priority 3 (P-3/lowest priority/green/minor), minor injuries and ambulatory patients; and Priority 4 (P-4/black/deceased), deceased or fatal injuries.

- Typical patient-identification systems use colors to signify priorities of care: highest = red, second = yellow, lowest = green, deceased = black.

- To reduce stress on yourself and other rescue personnel who are involved in an MCI, rest at regular intervals. Be aware of your exact assignment. Several workers should watch for signs of physical exhaustion and stress in other rescuers. Plenty of food and drinks should be provided, and workers should be encouraged to talk among themselves.

TERMS AND CONCEPTS

1. Write the number of the correct term next to each definition.

1.	Disaster	7.	Secondary triage
2.	Incident commander	8.	Staging unit
3.	Incident command system	9.	Supply unit
4.	Mobile command unit	10.	Transportation unit
5.	Multiple-casualty incident	11.	Treatment unit
6.	Primary triage	12.	Triage unit

_____ a. Monitors, inventories, and directs available ambulances to the treatment unit at the request of the transportation unit leader

_____ b. An event that places excessive demands on EMS personnel and equipment

_____ c. The person responsible for coordinating all aspects of the incident

_____ d. Unit responsible for prioritizing patients for emergency medical care and transport

_____ e. The headquarters for the incident manager; the EMS command post

_____ f. A sudden catastrophic event that overwhelms natural order and causes great loss of property and/or life

_____ g. Unit responsible for inventory and distribution of the medical materials and equipment necessary to render care

_____ h. Evaluation of patients that takes place immediately upon arrival of the first EMS crew to quickly categorize the severity of the patients' conditions and priority for treatment and transport

_____ i. Identifies the authority and responsibilities for activities occurring at a disaster or multiple-casualty incident.

_____ j. Unit responsible for collecting and treating patients in a centralized treatment area

_____ k. Reevaluation that occurs in the triage unit to categorize the severity of the patient's condition and priority for treatment and transport

_____ l. Unit that coordinates patient transportation with the triage unit leader and communicates with the hospitals involved

CONTENT REVIEW

1. Which system provides for a consistent approach to managing disasters by federal, state, or local responders to an incident?
   a. Federal Multiple Command System (FMCS)
   b. National Incident Management System (NIMS)
   c. International Single Command System (ISCS)
   d. Regional Disaster Command System (RDCS)

2. The incident commander is stationed in the
   a. incident command post.
   b. supply unit.
   c. transport unit.
   d. triage unit.

3. A child that is unresponsive to all stimuli or responds to pain with incomprehensible sounds or inappropriate movement (does not localize pain or has no purposeful flexion or extension) is tagged
   a. red.
   b. yellow.
   c. green.
   d. black.

4. Any patient who is able to walk at the scene of a multiple-casualty incident is initially tagged
   a. red.
   b. yellow.
   c. green.
   d. black.

5. You have responded to a bus crash with many victims. The scene is safe, and the bus is stable. Which best describes "primary triage" at this scene?
   a. Primary triage is conducted by the first-arriving EMS crew after removal of the patients from the bus.
   b. Primary triage is conducted by the first-arriving EMS crew inside the bus before moving the patients.
   c. Primary triage is conducted by the first-arriving EMS crew once patients are placed in the triage sector.
   d. Primary triage is conducted by the second-arriving EMS crew once patients are placed in the triage sector.

6. The primary goal of triage is to accomplish which of the following?
   a. Sorting of patients according to criticality
   b. Providing comprehensive treatment on each patient
   c. Performing a detailed physical exam on each patient
   d. Transporting all patients as rapidly as possible

7. Which of the following best describes secondary triage?
   a. Occurs as the patient is extricated from the hot zone and is designed to initially evaluate the patient's condition
   b. Occurs when the patient is within the actual incident site and is designed to evaluate the patient's condition
   c. Occurs during the transporting of the patient to the receiving facility and is designed to reevaluate the primary patient categorization
   d. Occurs as the patient is brought into the triage unit and is designed to reevaluate the initial patient categorization

8. In the START triage system, you should do which of the following?
   a. Check respirations only.
   b. Check respirations and perfusion only.
   c. Check mental status only.
   d. Check ability to walk, respirations, perfusion, and mental status.

9. When assessing the respirations of a patient utilizing the START triage system, you have opened a patient's airway but the patient is not breathing and has no respiratory effort. Your next immediate action should be to
   a. tag the patient as "red" and immediately move him to the treatment area.
   b. tag the patient as "black" and move on to the next patient.
   c. tag the patient as "yellow" and move on to the next patient.
   d. tag the patient as "red" and reposition the patient's airway.

10. Patients who are transported first in a four-level priority-triage system are which of the following?
    a. Priority 1 (red)
    b. Priority 2 (yellow)
    c. Priority 3 (green)
    d. Priority 4 (black)

11. In the START system, a patient with respirations greater than 30 per minute should be assigned to which of the following priorities?
    a. Priority 1 (red)
    b. Priority 2 (yellow)
    c. Priority 3 (green)
    d. Priority 4 (black)

12. A typical patient-tagging system uses colors to triage and identify patients. Red would be used to signify a
    a. high-priority patient.
    b. second-priority patient.
    c. third-priority patient.
    d. fourth-priority patient.

13. Patients should be organized in the treatment unit according to which of the following?
    a. Approximate age
    b. Order in which they were brought to the treatment area
    c. Kind of injury or condition
    d. Triage or priority level

14. Which of the following will help to reduce stress on rescuers during an MCI incident?
    a. Have rescuers work in 8- to-10-hour shifts and then perform less stressful tasks.
    b. Give a motivating talk to any rescuer who becomes hysterical.
    c. Provide plenty of nourishing food and drinks.
    d. Encourage rescue workers not to talk among themselves.

15. What age group is the JumpSTART pediatric triage system used for?
    a. Newborns to 5 years old
    b. Newborns to 8 years old
    c. One year to 8 years old
    d. For any patient that looks like a child

CASE STUDY

You have been dispatched to the scene of a bus–train collision. You are the senior EMT on the vehicle, and you are the closest responding unit to the scene. Your partner quickly pulls out the local "MCI Response Packet" and reviews the MCI plan. You arrive on-scene and observe a large commercial bus that has been struck by a train. The bus has been pushed approximately 50 yards from the crossing. There is extensive damage to the bus. There are many bystanders who are next to the bus waving at you to hurry. Several patients have been removed from the bus and are being treated by bystanders. A law-enforcement officer grabs you by the arm as you exit the vehicle and tells you, "You had better get some help out here! There are at least 40 people injured. There are victims lying all over the place. Tell them to hurry!"

1. What is your *best* first action to take?
    a. Establish a mobile command sector.
    b. Request additional help and assistance.
    c. Have the walking wounded patients walk to the treatment area.
    d. Triage all patients to determine the total number of injured patients.

2. During your primary triage, a child patient on-scene responds to pain by localizing it. The patient should be tagged
    a. red.
    b. yellow.
    c. green.
    d. black.

3. On this scene, the treatment unit
    a. leader radios the hospital that ambulances are en route.
    b. should be located close to the area where ambulances arrive.
    c. must not be marked in order to limit bystander traffic.
    d. is necessarily limited to only one location or area.

4. Utilizing the START triage system, perform the primary triage on the following adult patients from the bus–train collision. Tag each patient using the appropriate universally recognized categorization color: red, yellow, green, or black. (Red = immediate care and transport, priority 1; Yellow = delayed emergency care and transport, priority 2; Green = minor injuries and ambulatory patients, priority 3; Black = deceased or fatal injuries, priority 4)

_____ a. An ambulatory patient who has a large, bleeding leg wound

_____ b. A patient who is breathing about 12 times each minute, but does not follow simple commands

_____ c. A patient breathing 22 times each minute, who has a radial pulse, capillary refill less than 2 seconds, and squeezes your fingers on command

_____ d. A patient who is deeply unresponsive and bleeding from the ears

_____ e. A patient who has no obvious injuries and no respirations or respiratory effort after opening the airway

ENRICHMENT

1. Alerts for evacuation must be repeated often and with clarity to convince people that the disaster is really about to occur. Which of the following is likely to be considered part of the minimum information that must be contained in the evacuation alert message?
   a. Location where federal and state assistance will be available following the incident
   b. Safe routes to take out of the area
   c. The name of the local mayor or political official in charge
   d. Estimated time before the evacuated will be able to return to the area

2. During a disaster, the reactions of children depend on their age, individual disposition, family support, and community support. Which of the following groups is more likely to experience extreme aggression and stress that is severe enough to disrupt their lives?
   a. Infants
   b. Preschoolers
   c. Elementary-school-age children
   d. Preadolescents and adolescents

3. Which of the following is considered appropriate when dealing with the psychological impact of disasters?
   a. Giving assurances to your patients that are not true but are intended to help them deal with the problem
   b. Encouraging your patients to talk about the disaster and its long-term effects
   c. Delaying the reuniting of families as soon as possible to lessen the emotional stress
   d. Discouraging patients to do necessary chores to help them get over their problems

42 EMS Response to Weapons of Mass Destruction

OBJECTIVES

Numbered objectives are from the United States Department of Transportation EMT-Basic National Standard Curriculum. Asterisked objectives, if any, pertain to material that is supplemental to the DOT curriculum.

Cognitive

* Define weapons of mass destruction.
* Discuss the role of EMS, particularly the role of the EMT-Basic in response to a weapons-of-mass-destruction attack.
* Describe the primary, secondary, and tertiary effects of an explosive detonation.
* Describe the characteristics of and the signs and symptoms and emergency medical care for the following chemical agents: nerve agents, vesicants, cyanide, pulmonary agents, riot-control agents, and industrial chemicals.
* List the agents or specific findings for the following types of biological agents and emergency care for biological agents: pneumonia-like agents, encephalitis-like agents, biological toxins, and other biological agents.
* Discuss the types of radiation (X-ray and gamma, neutron, beta, and alpha), types of radiation exposure (primary and fallout), types of radiation injuries, assessment, and medical care for radiation injuries.
* Describe appropriate personal protection and patient decontamination for chemical, biological, and nuclear weapons exposure.

KEY IDEAS

This chapter focuses on EMS preparedness for response to terrorism involving weapons of mass destruction (WMD), including conventional weapons and explosives and incendiary devices, as well as chemical agents, biological agents, and nuclear weapons and radiation. Signs and symptoms (how to recognize a WMD attack) and appropriate emergency medical care are discussed for each category, as are personal protection and patient decontamination issues.

■ The goal of an EMS response to weapons of mass destruction (WMD) is to successfully manage patients affected by the attack.

■ The weapons of mass destruction include chemical, biological, radiological, nuclear, and explosive (CBRNE).

■ The general prehospital approach to an incident involving WMD is similar to that for any disaster involving multiple casualties. Various factors must be considered and planned for prior to the event, including provisions for supplies and equipment, medical direction, training for providers, response protocols, and issues of scene safety.

- Explosives and incendiary devices are, and will most likely remain, the WMD most commonly used by terrorists. Explosives and incendiary devices cause primary, secondary, and tertiary effects, inflicting damage on the lungs, abdomen, and ears and causing crush and shrapnel injuries.

- Chemical agents include nerve agents, vesicants, cyanide, pulmonary agents, riot-control agents, and industrial chemicals.

- Biological agents are classified as pneumonia-like agents, encephalitis-like agents, biological toxins, and other biological agents.

- Nuclear detonation results in three mechanisms of death and injury: radiation, blast injuries, and thermal burns.

- Many of the same principles that are applied to dealing with hazardous materials can be applied to a chemical, biological, or nuclear incident.

TERMS AND CONCEPTS

1. Write the number of the correct term next to each definition.
   1. Biological agents
   2. Nerve agents
   3. Persistence
   4. Vesicants
   5. Volatility
   6. Weapons of mass destruction

   _____ a. Agents that block the action of acetycholinesterase in the plasma of the blood, red blood cells, and nervous tissue

   _____ b. A characteristic of agents that do not evaporate quickly and tend to remain as a puddle for a long period of time

   _____ c. Chemical agents that most commonly result in damage to exposed skin, lungs, and eyes and that cause blisters, tissue burning, and tissue damage on contact

   _____ d. Agents that are made up of living organisms, or the toxins produced by the living organisms, used to cause disease in a target population

   _____ e. The tendency of a chemical agent to evaporate

   _____ f. Weapons intended to cause widespread and indiscriminate death and destruction

CONTENT REVIEW

1. Which of the following is correct regarding the appropriate prehospital response to an incident involving weapons of mass destruction (WMD)?
   a. Coordinated community preplanning for a WMD attack is necessary.
   b. A single EMS agency is likely to have enough equipment to handle a WMD attack.
   c. If a statewide disaster plan is in place, it will be both unnecessary and confusing for regional and local agencies to also develop their own disaster plans.
   d. The general approach is significantly different than that for any disaster involving multiple casualties.

2. Which are the most widely used weapons of mass destruction used by terrorists?
   a. Chemical agents
   b. Nuclear agents
   c. Biological agents
   d. Explosive and incendiary agents

3. Incendiary device(s)
   a. create similar injury patterns to conventional explosives.
   b. are difficult to improvise and manufacture.
   c. include napalm, thermite, and magnesium.
   d. burns are assessed in a vastly different manner from thermal burns.

4. The mnemonic SLUDGE is used to help remember the signs and symptoms associated with
   a. nerve agents.
   b. cyanide.
   c. vesicants.
   d. pulmonary agents.

5. Two drugs that are used to counteract the effects of nerve agents are
   a. epinephrine and calcium chloride.
   b. atropine and pralidoxime.
   c. calcium chloride and magnesium.
   d. epinephrine and magnesium.

6. These agents cause blisters, burning, and tissue damage on contact and were once called "blistering agents." They are called
   a. nerve agents.
   b. cyanide.
   c. vesicants.
   d. pulmonary agents.

7. A substance that disrupts the ability of the cell to use oxygen and leads to cellular hypoxia and eventually death is
   a. phosgene.
   b. cyanide.
   c. tularemia.
   d. ricin.

8. Phosgene, halogen compounds, and nitrogen–oxygen compounds are examples of
   a. nerve agents.
   b. cyanide.
   c. vesicants.
   d. pulmonary agents.

9. The management for exposure to riot-control agents should focus on
   a. administering activated charcoal.
   b. removing the patient from the environment.
   c. administering amyl nitrite or sodium nitrite.
   d. covering the eyes with moist dressings.

10. Biological agents that can be used as weapons of mass destruction are categorized into what four groups?
    a. Pneumonia-like agents, encephalitis-like agents, biological toxins, and other biological agents
    b. Biological agents, intestinal agents, viral agents, and bacterial agents
    c. Viral agents, bacterial agents, fungal agents, and other agents
    d. Anthrax agents, plague agents, tularemia agents, and other agents

11. Two common encephalitis-like agents are
    a. smallpox and Venezuelan equine encephalitis.
    b. botulinum and ricin.
    c. staphylococcus and botulinum.
    d. epsilon toxin and cholera.

12. The three primary mechanisms of death or injury associated with nuclear detonation are
    a. alpha radiation, beta radiation, and gamma radiation.
    b. radiation, blast, and thermal burns.
    c. neutron radiation, beta radiation, and alpha radiation.
    d. x-ray radiation, gamma radiation, and neutron radiation.

13. This type of radiation is the most penetrating type and can travel long distances. It is called
    a. gamma radiation.
    b. beta radiation.
    c. alpha radiation.
    d. delta radiation.

14. There are two types of radiation exposure associated with a nuclear explosion. After primary exposure, this is the second form of radiation exposure and contains radioactive dust and particles. It is called
    a. blast injury.
    b. fallout.
    c. shock wave.
    d. barotrauma.

15. A conventional explosive attached to radioactive materials is referred to as a
    a. radiological dispersal device.
    b. radioactive weapon.
    c. radioactive-conventional weapon.
    d. weapon of destruction.

CASE STUDY

It is 4:00 PM on a cold winter day. You are watching TV and relaxing at home when a newsbreak advises you that a nuclear device has just been detonated in a large city located about 60 miles from the town where you live. A mutual-aid call goes to surrounding emergency service personnel to respond to the disaster area. You pack your bags and quickly head to the EMS station for assignment. As you and a crew of ten of your fellow EMTs are heading to the disaster site, you try to remember the information you learned in your multiple-casualty and weapons-of-mass-destruction training.

1. You know that the mechanism that causes most deaths and injury associated with nuclear detonation is the
   a. blast and thermal burns.
   b. neutron and alpha radiation.
   c. radiation.
   d. fallout.

2. Which of the following is correct regarding blast injuries associated with nuclear detonation?
   a. The nuclear ignition produces a small contained-gas cloud.
   b. Shock-wave injuries are of a different nature from those caused by conventional weapons.
   c. The intensity of shock-wave injuries is greater the further the victim is from ground zero.
   d. The windblast is strong enough to cause structural collapse, crush injuries, and entrapment.

3. Your agency's personnel have all received specialized hazardous materials (HAZMAT) training. Therefore, your crew is prepared to act as an initial-response crew.
   a. The statement is true, because all the principles of a nuclear and a HAZMAT emergency are identical.
   b. The statement is true, because similar principles apply to dealing with a nuclear and a HAZMAT emergency.
   c. The statement is false, because the procedures for dealing with a nuclear emergency are very different from those for a HAZMAT emergency.
   d. The statement is false, because plenty of trained personnel should be available by the time you arrive on-scene.

OPERATIONS: CHAPTERS 38–42

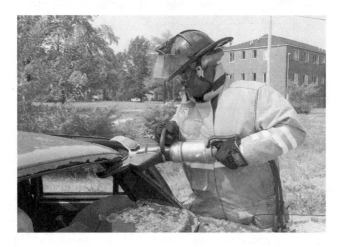

Previous modules have dealt with the assessment and emergency care of patients. In the operations module, you have been learning primarily about the daily nuts-and-bolts, nonmedical aspects of your job as an EMT, as well as approaches to some special situations such as gaining access and the management of hazardous-materials emergencies, multiple-casualty incidents, and weapons-of-mass-destruction attacks.

Q **What are the major aspects of ambulance operation?**

A For the EMT who will drive the ambulance, development of safe and effective driving skills and knowledge of the special laws regulating operation of emergency vehicles are essential. All members of the crew must participate in the necessary chores of making sure that the unit is operational, that the ambulance is fully supplied at all times, and that the unit is properly cleaned and disinfected before notifying dispatch that you are clear for the next call. Specific tasks must be performed during each of the eight phases of an ambulance call: prerun preparation, dispatch, en route to the scene, at the scene, en route to the receiving facility, at the receiving facility, en route to the station, and post-run.

Q **What is the primary role of the EMT during a rescue operation?**

A If you are not a trained member of a rescue crew, you must call for expert assistance and wait until they have secured the scene; for example, by stabilizing a collision vehicle. Your role as an EMT is to gain access to the patient or patients as quickly as can be safely accomplished in order to perform patient assessment and care, even as the rescue operation proceeds. Your major priorities at the rescue scene are to keep yourself and your partner safe and to prevent further harm to your patient.

Q **What is the role of the EMT at a hazardous-materials emergency?**

A The EMT is not required to deal with hazardous materials. You should be able to identify the possibility of a hazardous-materials accident from a safe distance, call for the assistance of a specialized hazardous-materials team, and protect yourself and bystanders by keeping uphill, upwind, upstream, and away from the danger. Patients will be removed from the accident site and decontaminated by those equipped to do so. However, even after decontamination, there may still be some contamination present on patients or equipment. Exercise caution and take measures to protect your equipment and vehicle from contamination. Prior to transport, cover all benches, floor, and other exposed areas of your unit with thick plastic sheeting secured with duct tape. Leave all contaminated clothing and equipment at the scene. Following the incident, wash your unit and equipment, your clothing, and yourself thoroughly following local procedures and policies. Seek medical help immediately if you develop symptoms of illness following a hazardous-materials incident.

Q   **What is the role of the EMT at a multiple-casualty incident?**

A   Emergency care at a multiple-casualty incident will be conducted according to a preset disaster response plan. Jurisdictions use an incident command system (ICS) as outlined in the National Incident Management System. In an ICS, the following sectors are usually established at the scene of the large-scale multiple-casualty incident: incident command unit, supply unit, triage unit, treatment unit, staging unit, and transportation unit. Patients are generally triaged under a four-level priority system. Patients are transported and treated by priority level (Priority 1 [red], Priority 2 [yellow], Priority 3 [green], and Priority 4 [deceased]). As an EMT arriving at a multiple-casualty scene, unless you are the first and senior EMT to arrive and must take initial command, you will be assigned to a unit and a task for which—ideally—you will have practiced and prepared in advance of the emergency.

Q   **What is the primary goal of EMS response to a weapons-of-mass-destruction attack?**

A   The primary goal of EMS response to a WMD attack is to successfully manage the patients affected by the attack. The general prehospital approach to an incident involving WMD is similar to that for any disaster involving hazardous materials and/or multiple casualties.

43 Advanced Airway Management

OBJECTIVES

Numbered objectives are from the United States Department of Transportation EMT-Basic National Standard Curriculum. Asterisked objectives, if any, pertain to material that is supplemental to the DOT curriculum.

Cognitive

8-1.1 Identify and describe the airway anatomy in the infant, child, and adult.
8-1.2 Differentiate between the anatomy in the infant, child, and adult.
8-1.3 Explain the pathophysiology of airway compromise.
8-1.4 Describe the proper use of airway adjuncts.
8-1.5 Review the use of oxygen therapy in airway management.
8-1.6 Describe the indications, contraindications, and techniques for insertion of nasal gastric tubes.
8-1.7 Describe how to perform Sellick's maneuver (cricoid pressure).
8-1.8 Describe the indications for advanced airway management.
8-1.9 List the equipment required for orotracheal intubation.
8-1.10 Describe the proper use of the curved blade for orotracheal intubation.
8-1.11 Describe the proper use of the straight blade for orotracheal intubation.
8-1.12 State the reasons for and proper use of the stylet in orotracheal intubation.
8-1.13 Describe the methods of choosing the appropriate size endotracheal tube in an adult patient.
8-1.14 State the formula for sizing the infant or child endotracheal tube.
8-1.15 List complications associated with advanced airway management.
8-1.16 Define the various alternative methods for sizing the infant and child endotracheal tube.
8-1.17 Describe the skill of orotracheal intubation in the adult patient.
8-1.18 Describe the skill of orotracheal intubation in the infant and child patient.
8-1.19 Describe the skill of confirming endotracheal tube placement in the adult, child, and infant patient.
8-1.20 State the consequence of and the need to recognize unintentional esophageal intubation.
8-1.21 Describe the skill of securing the endotracheal tube in the adult, child, and infant patient.

KEY IDEAS

In some situations, manual maneuvers and basic airway adjuncts are inadequate to maintain or even to establish an airway. In these situations, the use of advanced airway adjuncts is necessary. For this reason, some EMS jurisdictions and medical directors now require EMT to become proficient in advanced airway management skills. These skills are difficult to master and require a high degree of accuracy; performed correctly, however, they offer a real opportunity to save lives.

- It is important to know the anatomy of the upper airway, especially the landmark structures that differentiate the opening of the larynx from the opening of the esophagus, to avoid accidental insertion of the tracheal tube into the esophagus—a dangerous and possibly fatal error.

- It is important to understand how the right and left mainstem bronchi branch from the trachea at the level of the carina, the right mainstem bronchus, at a much lesser angle than the left. If the tracheal tube is advanced too far, it is likely to enter the right mainstem bronchus so that air is entering only the right lung, causing inadequate oxygenation.

- It is critical to master the techniques of confirming correct placement of the tracheal tube by watching for chest rise and fall and auscultating the lungs and the epigastrium.

- It is critical to understand differences in airway anatomy of infants and children as compared to adults. An infant's larger head will cause the supine infant's head to tilt forward, constricting the airway; padding must be placed under the infant's shoulders to keep the airway aligned. The infant's or young child's tongue is larger in proportion to the mouth and cannot only cause obstruction by falling back into the airway but can also interfere with visualization of anatomical structures during intubation. The infant and child airway is narrowest at the level of the cricoid cartilage, so that a tube that passes easily through the vocal cords may be too large to pass through the cricoid ring; tubes a half-size larger and smaller than the size you estimate must be available to deal with such problems. Infant and child airway structures are softer; pressure on the cricoid and overextension of the neck during intubation can constrict the airway. Airway structures are shorter in infants and children, making intubation of the mainstem bronchus more likely.

- Before advanced airway techniques are initiated, basic airway techniques including manual opening of the airway, hyperventilation of the patient, and oropharyngeal suctioning must be performed.

- Indications for the use of tracheal intubation include the following: the EMT is unable to ventilate the apneic patient with standard methods such as mouth-to-mask or bag-valve-mask ventilation; the patient cannot protect his own airway (is unresponsive to any stimulus or has no cough or gag reflex).

- Because the EMT must get very close to the patient's open mouth and contact with the patient's secretions, vomitus, and blood is unavoidable, body substance isolation including gloves, eye protection, and mask are essential during advanced airway procedures.

- The equipment used in tracheal intubation includes the laryngoscope (used to lift the epiglottis and provide a light source for visualization of the vocal cords and glottic opening); the tracheal tube; a stylet to stiffen the tube during insertion; a water-soluble lubricant; a 10-cc syringe to inflate the cuff at the distal end of the tube and create an airtight seal; a securing device to prevent the tube, once correctly positioned, from slipping inward or pulling outward; suctioning equipment, including a large-bore rigid catheter for clearing the oropharynx and a flexible French catheter for tracheal suctioning; towels or padding to raise the head or shoulders as needed for airway alignment; and a stethoscope for auscultation of the lungs and epigastrium to confirm tube placement. Special sizes of equipment must be used for infants and children. For best displacement of the tongue and visualization of the glottic opening, a straight blade is preferred in infants and children up to 8 years old; a curved blade could be used for children 8 years and older. Uncuffed tubes are used in children under 8 years old because the narrow cricoid ring seals the airway.

- Sellick's maneuver, also called cricoid pressure, is pressure applied over the cricoid cartilage to close off the esophagus (cutting off airflow into the stomach and helping to prevent vomiting of stomach contents) and to slightly move the glottic structures into a better position for visualization.

- Some of the more common complications of tracheal intubation include the following: hypertension (elevated blood pressure), tachycardia (increased heart rate), and arrhythmias (irregular heart rhythms); in infants and children and some adults, bradycardia (decreased heart rate) and hypotension (depressed blood pressure) may be seen; trauma to the lips, tongue, gums, teeth, and airway; inadequate oxygenation and hypoxia from prolonged (longer than 30 seconds) attempts at intubation during which the patient is receiving no oxygen; right mainstem bronchial intubation; misplacement of the tracheal tube in the esophagus; vomiting from stimulation of the gag reflex; deflation of the cuff, causing air leakage; laryngospasm caused by stimulation of the epiglottis or vocal cords; and accidental extubation or self-extubation if the patient becomes responsive enough to pull out the tube.

■ Nasogastric intubation (insertion of a flexible tube through the nose into the stomach) may be required in infants and children to relieve gastric distension that is preventing effective ventilation or when the patient is unresponsive and at risk of vomiting stomach contents.

■ Contraindications to use of the nasogastric (NG) tube are as follows: An NG tube should not be inserted into a patient who has suffered major facial, head, or spinal trauma. Consult medical direction about oral insertion in such patients. An NG tube should not be inserted into a patient suspected of suffering an airway disease, which can cause spasms or exacerbate swelling to the point of occluding the airway. An NG tube should not be inserted into a patient who has ingested some caustic substances or hydrocarbons. Consult medical direction.

■ Possible complications of nasogastric intubation include tracheal intubation; nasal trauma; stimulation of the gag reflex, causing vomiting; curling or kinking of the tube; perforation of the esophagus; and (rarely) passage of the tube into the cranium through a basilar skull fracture.

■ Orotracheal suctioning (suctioning of the trachea to the level of the carina, as differentiated from oropharyngeal suctioning of the mouth and pharynx) can be performed by inserting a soft catheter through the tracheal tube to remove heavy secretions that might block the airway. Possible complications include hypoxia (which can be prevented by aggressive hyperoxygenation of the patient before and after suctioning and applying suction for no more than 15 seconds at a time); cardiac arrhythmias or abnormal (fast or slow) heart rates resulting from stimulation of the airway or from hypoxia; coughing (which can increase pressure inside the skull and decrease blood flow to the brain, which is very dangerous in the case of head injury or stroke); damage to the mucosa caused by the catheter; and bronchospasm if the catheter is inserted beyond the carina into the bronchi.

MEDICAL TERMINOLOGY

Term	Prefix	Word Root Combining Form	Suffix	Definition
epiglottis (ep-uh-GLOT-is)	epi- (upon, over, above)	glottis (the sound-producing area of the larynx)		A small, leaf-shaped flap of tissue, located above the glottis, which covers the entrance of the larynx during swallowing
epistaxis (EP-uh-STAK-sis)	epi- (upon, over, above)		-staxis (dripping, trickling)	Medical term for a nosebleed
laryngoscope (luh-RINJ-uh-skope)	laryng/o- (larynx)	scope (watcher)		A device with a lighted distal end used to lift the epiglottis and permit visualization of the vocal cord
laryngoscopy (LAIR-inj-OS-kuh-pe)	laryng/o- (larynx)	scopy (viewing, examining)		A procedure of using a laryngoscope to visualize the glottic opening and vocal cords
nasogastric (NAY-zo-GAS-trik)		nas/o (nose); gastr (stomach)	-ic (pertaining to)	Pertaining to the nose and stomach; example: *nasogastric tube (NG)*, a specialized catheter that is inserted through the nose and esophagus into the stomach

Term	Prefix	Word Root Combining Form	Suffix	Definition
orotracheal (OR-o-TRAY-ke-ul)		or/o (mouth); -trache (trachea)	-al (pertaining to)	Pertaining to the mouth and trachea
pneumonia (nu-MO-nyuh)		pneumon (lung)	-ia (condition of)	Inflammation of the lungs caused by bacteria, viruses, or chemical irritants
pulmonectomy (PUL-mo-NEK-tuh-me)		pulmon/o (lung)	-ectomy (surgical excision)	Surgical excision of the lung or part of the lung; synonym: *pneumonectomy*
rhinostenosis (rye-no-stuh-NO-sis)		rhin/o (nose); sten (narrowing)	-osis (condition of)	Narrowing of the nasal passages
tracheal (TRAY-ke-ul)		trache (trachea)	-al (pertaining to)	Pertaining to the trachea
tracheitis (TRAY-ke-EYE-tis)		trache (trachea)	-itis (inflammation)	Inflammation of the trachea
tracheostomy (TRAY-ke-OS-tuh-me)		trache/o (trachea)	-stomy (opening)	Opening surgically created in the trachea

1. While reviewing your patient's chart at a local care facility, you note the patient has a history of tracheitis. You know that the word root *trache* refers to the trachea and the suffix *-itis* means
   a. pertaining to.
   b. inflammation.
   c. surgical excision.
   d. condition of.

2. Your patient has a medical history of rhinostenosis. You know that the suffix *-osis* means
   a. condition of.
   b. edema.
   c. dripping.
   d. bleeding.

3. The medical term *rhinostenosis* contains the word roots *rhino,* which means nose, and *sten,* which means
   a. within.
   b. swelling.
   c. enlargement.
   d. narrowing.

4. The medical term *orotracheal* contains the word root *oro.* You know that this translates as
   a. ears.
   b. neck.
   c. mouth.
   d. tongue.

5. When you read the medical term *laryngoscopy*, you recognize the suffix *-scopy*, which means
   a. tumor, cancer.
   b. instrument, equipment.
   c. viewing, examining.
   d. touching, feeling.

TERMS AND CONCEPTS

1. Write the correct term next to each definition.

   1. Carina
   2. Cricoid cartilage
   3. Cuneiform cartilage
   4. Epiglottis
   5. Extubation
   6. Glottic opening
   7. Laryngoscopy
   8. Murphy eye
   9. Thyroid cartilage
   10. Trachea
   11. Vallecula

   _____ a. The procedure of using a laryngoscope to lift the epiglottis to visualize the vocal cords and glottic opening

   _____ b. A tubular structure that extends from the lower portion of the larynx to the bronchi

   _____ c. The bulky shieldlike structure that forms the anterior surface of the larynx

   _____ d. The point of bifurcation at about the level of the fifth thoracic vertebra where the trachea splits into the right and left mainstem bronchi

   _____ e. The removal of a tube, such as a tracheal tube

   _____ f. The space between the vocal cords

   _____ g. Elongated cartilage attached to the posterior arytenoids

   _____ h. A firm and complete circular ring located below the thyroid cartilage and attached to the first ring of the trachea

   _____ i. A leaf-shaped cartilaginous structure that covers the opening of the larynx during swallowing

   _____ j. A depression located between the base of the tongue and the epiglottis

   _____ k. A small hole opposite the bevel at the distal end of a tracheal tube

1. Fill in each term, naming the epiglottis and nearby structures, on the appropriate line.

   Epiglottis
   Glossoepiglottic ligament
   Tongue
   Vallecula

   A _____
   B _____
   C _____
   D _____

   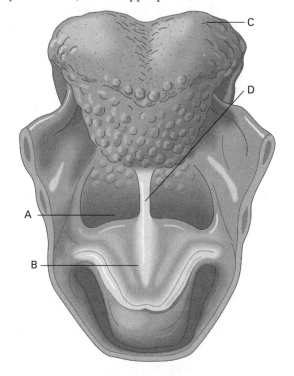

2. Fill in each term, naming the glottis and associated structures, on the appropriate line.

   Aryepiglottic fold
   Corniculate cartilage
   Cuneiform cartilage
   Epiglottis
   False vocal cords
   Glottis
   True vocal cords

   A _____
   B _____
   C _____
   D _____
   E _____
   F _____
   G _____

   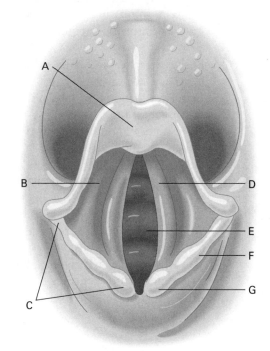

3. Which of the following explains why it is easier to misplace a tracheal tube into the right mainstem bronchus than into the left mainstem bronchus?
   a. The left bronchioles branch from the trachea at a greater angle than the right.
   b. The right bronchioles branch from the trachea at a greater angle than the left.
   c. The left mainstem bronchus branches from the trachea at a lesser angle.
   d. The right mainstem bronchus branches from the trachea at a lesser angle.

4. To keep the airway aligned and ensure airflow for the infant or small child, you should do which of the following?
   a. Place a small, folded towel under the shoulders.
   b. Place padding under the back of the head (occiput).
   c. Place a small, folded towel or padding under the feet.
   d. With patient lying prone, place padding under the head.

5. Which of the following airway sounds indicates that the tongue is occluding the upper airway?
   a. Wheezes
   b. Crackles
   c. Snoring (sonorous) sounds
   d. Rales

6. When you hear gurgling sounds during ventilations, which of the following is correct?
   a. Gurgling indicates that the patient has a stoma, and this is a normal sound.
   b. Gurgling indicates a narrowing of the airway, and a bronchodilator is needed.
   c. Gurgling indicates an obstructed airway, and immediate back slaps are needed.
   d. Gurgling indicates liquid in the airway, and immediate suction is needed.

7. Your patient requires tracheal intubation. Which of the following statements is correct pertaining to intubating your patient?
   a. Tracheal intubation requires manual maneuvers such as head-tilt/chin-lift to maintain the airway.
   b. Because tracheal intubation does not isolate the airway from the esophagus, aspiration may still occur.
   c. Better ventilations are achieved because the bag-valve mask is directly attached to the endotracheal tube.
   d. Deep suctioning must be achieved prior to endotracheal intubation because the suction catheter cannot be used.

8. For which of the following patients is tracheal intubation indicated?
   a. You are able to adequately ventilate your 22-year-old female apneic patient with standard methods.
   b. Your responsive patient presents with tachypnea and a poor tidal volume, indicating inadequate respirations.
   c. The unresponsive patient coughs when you attempt to place an oropharyngeal airway prior to attempting intubation.
   d. After inserting an OPA and ventilating the patient, you determine the patient cannot protect her own airway.

9. You have just intubated your patient. Which of the following describes secondary tracheal tube placement confirmation?
   a. Auscultation of the epigastrium
   b. Auscultation of the chest
   c. Direct visualization of tube placement
   d. Application of the end-tidal CO_2 detector

10. Which of the following is the most appropriate way to determine if a patient has lost the gag reflex?
   a. You are able to insert your index finger into the back of the throat without incident.
   b. You are able to insert an oropharyngeal airway without incident.
   c. You are able to insert a hard suction catheter without incident.
   d. You are able to insert the tracheal tube into the oropharynx without incident.

11. Which of the following body substance isolation devices may be used but is not required to be worn when performing tracheal intubation?
   a. Gloves
   b. Mask
   c. Eye protection
   d. Nonporous gown

12. Which of the following best describes the cricoid pressure used to bring the glottic opening into the best position for visualization by the intubator?
   a. Backward, upward, rightward pressure
   b. Anterior, inferior, lateral pressure
   c. Posterior, inferior, left-lateral pressure
   d. Backward, downward, leftward pressure

13. On the curved laryngoscope blade, the broad surface and tall flange are used to
   a. spread the teeth to keep the mouth open.
   b. lift the vallecula indirectly.
   c. lift the epiglottis directly.
   d. hold the tongue out of the way.

14. The curved laryngoscope blade lifts the epiglottis by
   a. pressing on the corniculate cartilage to lift the epiglottis indirectly.
   b. pressing on the glossoepiglottic ligament to lift the epiglottis indirectly.
   c. placing the tip under the epiglottis to lift it directly.
   d. displacing the aryepiglottic fold to lift the epiglottis directly.

15. If the laryngoscope light is not working or is not bright and white, briefly explain what should be checked to rectify the problem.

16. In an emergency, which size tracheal tube will fit either an adult male or an adult female?

    a. 7.0 mm i.d.

    b. 7.5 mm i.d.

    c. 8.0 mm i.d.

    d. 9.0 mm i.d.

17. Fill in each term, naming a part of the tracheal tube, on the appropriate line.

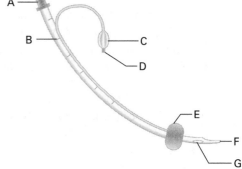

15 mm adapter	A _____
Bevel	B _____
Centimeter marker	C _____
Cuff	D _____
Inflation port	E _____
Murphy eye	F _____
Pilot balloon	G _____

18. What is the purpose of the Murphy eye on the tracheal tube?

    a. Permits airflow in the case of tube obstruction

    b. Permits easy access for suctioning the trachea

    c. Permits attachment of securing device

    d. Protects the stylet tip from injuring the trachea

19. Which of the following is true of a properly placed tracheal tube?

    a. Distal tip of tube is in the esophagus, midway between the carina and vocal cords.

    b. Distal tip of tube is in the trachea, midway between the carina and vocal cords.

    c. Proximal tip of tube is in the trachea, with distal tip extending past the carina.

    d. Proximal tip of tube is in the trachea, midway between the carina and vocal cords.

20. Which of the following is considered improper regarding the use of the stylet?

    a. Lubricate the stylet with a water-soluble lubricant.

    b. Place the stylet in the tube and bend into hockey-stick shape.

    c. Extend the tip of the stylet past the Murphy eye approximately 1 cm.

    d. Hold the tube securely with your hand when removing the stylet.

21. When checking a tracheal tube prior to insertion, you should inject _____ of air into the cuff to ensure that it is working properly.

    a. 5 cc

    b. 10 cc

    c. 15 cc

    d. 20 cc

22. The function of the distal cuff of the tracheal tube is to

    a. secure the tube and prevent dislodgement.

    b. indicate the amount of air within the tube.

    c. apply lateral pressure to the esophagus and prevent regurgitation.

    d. seal the trachea, preventing air from leaking around the tube.

23. Which best describes how to perform Sellick's maneuver on the patient you are preparing to intubate?

    a. Place the index finger and thumb of one hand on the anterior aspect of the throat just lateral to the midline of the cricoid cartilage; then apply pressure backward to close off the esophagus.

    b. Place the index fingers from both hands on the anterior aspect of the throat midline of the cricoid cartilage; then apply pressure backward to close off the esophagus.

    c. Place the index finger from one hand directly superior to the cricoid cartilage at the midline and apply firm pressure upward to close off the trachea.

    d. Place the index and thumb of one hand on the posterior aspect of the throat lateral to the midline of the epiglottis; apply downward pressure, closing off the trachea.

24. Which of the following is the correct sequence for inserting the laryngoscope?

    a. Hold scope in left hand, insert into left corner of mouth, sweep tongue to right.

    b. Hold scope in left hand, insert into right corner of mouth, sweep tongue to left.

    c. Hold scope in right hand, insert into left corner of mouth, sweep tongue to left.

    d. Hold scope in right hand, insert into right corner of mouth, sweep tongue to right.

25. You are preparing to intubate your unresponsive and apneic patient. Which of the following anatomical characteristics or landmarks identify the esophagus and not the glottic opening where the tracheal tube must pass for a successful intubation?

    a. Round opening

    b. Cartilaginous structures

    c. Vocal cords

    d. Oval sphincterous passageway

26. Briefly describe how to use primary and secondary techniques to confirm correct tracheal tube placement.

27. Which of the following are possible complications of tracheal intubation in an adult?

    1. Bradycardia

    2. Heart dysrhythmia

    3. Hypertension

    4. Hypotension

    5. Tachycardia

    a. 4 and 5

    b. 1, 2, and 4

    c. 2, 3, and 5

    d. 1, 2, 3, 4, and 5

28. For which of the following patients would intubation be inappropriate?

    a. Prolonged positive-pressure ventilation is required.

    b. The patient is responsive and in severe respiratory distress.

    c. The patient is apneic and in respiratory arrest.

    d. Bag-valve-mask and mouth-to-mask ventilations are inadequate.

29. Which of the following statements is incorrect regarding the straight laryngoscope blade?
    a. The straight blade is preferred in infants because it displaces the tongue better for visualization.
    b. The straight blade directly lifts the epiglottis, exposing the vocal cords.
    c. Straight blades come in sizes 0–4, sizes 0–2 usually being used for infants and children.
    d. The straight blade is placed into the vallecula to put pressure on the glossoepiglottic ligament to lift the epiglottis.

30. Which of the following is appropriate for selecting tracheal tube size in the infant and child?
    a. Refer to a sizing chart or commercially available resuscitation tape.
    b. Use this formula: tube size = (12 + patient's age in years) ÷2.
    c. Match the child's thumb with the outside diameter of the tube.
    d. Measure the outside diameter of the right nare.

31. You are assessing your patient and note fluid in the airway. Which of the following airway sounds indicates fluid in the airway?
    a. Gurgling
    b. Stridor
    c. Snoring (sonorous) sounds
    d. Crackles

32. For which of the following child patients is nasogastric intubation indicated?
    a. You are unable to provide positive-pressure ventilation due to gastric distention.
    b. The patient requires ventilation with a bag-valve mask and supplemental oxygen.
    c. The patient ingested a caustic poison and then became unresponsive and apneic.
    d. The patient is unresponsive to all stimulation, and his breathing is labored.

33. Briefly list the contraindications for nasogastric intubation in infants and children.

34. You have just inserted a tracheal tube in your patient and are preparing to confirm placement. Which of the following devices may provide inaccurate results in patients who are extremely obese, in late pregnancy, suffering status asthmaticus, or with large amounts of secretions?
    a. Colorimetric device
    b. Esophageal detector
    c. End-tidal CO_2 detector
    d. Electronic CO_2 device

35. Which of the following is the correct way to measure for a nasogastric tube?
    a. Measure from angle of jaw around the ear, extending downward until the distal end is past the xiphoid process.
    b. Measure from tip of nose around the ear, extending downward until the distal end is past the xiphoid process.
    c. Measure from corner of mouth around the ear, extending downward until the distal end is past the xiphoid process.
    d. None of these

36. Briefly explain the five possible complications of orotracheal suctioning.

37. Once the patient has been successfully intubated, it is necessary to continuously monitor the patient for deterioration that may result from a problem associated with the tracheal tube or ventilation device. Which common mnemonic can be used to help determine causes for deterioration in the patient's oxygenation or ventilation status?
   a. BURP
   b. DOPE
   c. SOAP
   d. COPD

38. You have just attempted to place an endotracheal tube into your patient's airway. Which of the following would indicate that the tracheal tube has been placed into the esophagus rather than the trachea?
   a. You hear air sounds entering the lungs.
   b. You do not hear air sounds over the epigastrium.
   c. The end-tidal carbon dioxide detector registers the presence of CO_2.
   d. The esophageal detector remains collapsed and does not reinflate.

39. You are preparing to suction your pediatric patient as you prepare to intubate. At what should the negative suction pressure be set?
   a. 40 to 80 mmHg
   b. 80 to 120 mmHg
   c. 120 to 160 mmHg
   d. 160 to 200 mmHg

40. Your system's medical director allows for the use of cuffed tracheal when intubating the child patient. You know which of the following formulas is correct when selecting the proper cuffed tracheal tube for the child patient?
   a. Cuffed tube size = 3 + (age in years ÷ 4)
   b. Cuffed tube size = 3 + (age in years ÷ 8)
   c. Cuffed tube size = 4 + (age in years ÷ 4)
   d. Cuffed tube size = 4 + (age in years ÷ 8)

CASE STUDY

It's a beautiful summer afternoon in the coastal community where you work. You and your partner, Jill, are relaxing at your EMS station when the radio alerting system sounds: "Unit 5, respond to a report of a boating accident at Inlet State Park. Park rangers are reporting a middle-age male not breathing." You and Jill request paramedic backup, but you anticipate that your unit will arrive before the backup. As you arrive on scene, you find a crowd surrounding the patient. Park rangers are performing rescue breathing with a pocket mask. One of the park rangers advises you that the patient fell out of the boat, and then the boat crashed onto the rocks. Jill reports that the patient has a strong pulse but is unresponsive to painful stimulus and apneic. You ask the park ranger to hold in-line stabilization of the patient's neck, since he fell from a moving boat.

1. Which of the following procedures should you immediately undertake for this patient?
   a. Measure a tracheal tube, prepare the laryngoscope, and visualize the glottic opening.
   b. Perform a jaw thrust, insert an oropharyngeal airway, and hyperoxygenate with a bag-valve mask.
   c. Have the park rangers continue artificial ventilation with the pocket mask until paramedic backup arrives.
   d. Describe the patient's condition to medical direction, and then proceed according to on-line orders.

2. Is advanced airway management indicated in this case? Briefly explain your answer.

While ventilating the patient, you note a gurgling sound in the upper airway. You inspect the oropharynx and find that it is full of seawater.

3. Which of the following is the most appropriate treatment for this condition?
   a. Turn the patient's head to the side to allow the seawater to drain.
   b. Do nothing; seawater will not injure the patient's oropharynx.
   c. Immediately suction the seawater with a rigid catheter.
   d. Immediately suction the seawater with a soft catheter.

At this point, you and Jill decide to initiate tracheal intubation. As you prepare the appropriate equipment, Jill is hyperventilating the patient.

4. Which of the following is the most appropriate rate at which to ventilate this patient?
   a. Ten to 12 breaths per minute for up to 1 minute prior to intubating
   b. Sixteen to 18 breaths per minute for at least 1 minute prior to intubating
   c. Twenty to 22 breaths per minute for at least 2 minutes prior to intubating
   d. Twenty-four or more breaths per minute for at least 1 minute prior to intubating

Jill ceases ventilations so that you can attempt to intubate the patient. You immediately initiate visualization of the patient's glottic opening. Jill silently counts to herself and will advise you when the patient needs to be ventilated again.

5. Briefly explain how you and Jill would work together to achieve maximum visualization of the glottic opening.

6. Jill will notify you that the patient needs to be ventilated after silently counting to _____ seconds.
   a. 15
   b. 30
   c. 45
   d. 60

After identifying the glottic opening and being careful not to lose sight of it, you watch as you guide the tracheal tube through the opening. You remove the laryngoscope from the patient's mouth and carefully remove the stylet from the tube. You then inflate the cuff. Jill attaches the bag-valve device to the tracheal tube and begins to ventilate so that you can confirm tube placement. The chest rises and falls during ventilations, and there are no gurgling sounds in the epigastrium. However, when you auscultate the lung fields, the left side is silent, but there are normal breath sounds on the right.

7. Approximately how far beyond the vocal cords should you place the proximal end of the cuff on this patient?
   a. One-half inch to 1 inch past the vocal cords
   b. One inch to 1½ inches past the vocal cords
   c. One-and-one-half inches to 2 inches past the vocal cords
   d. One-half inch to 2 inches past the vocal cords

8. Which of the following best describes the cause of the unequal lung sounds and the action that should be taken?
   a. The tube is past the carina and in the left mainstem bronchus. Deflate the cuff and pull back enough to restore lung sounds on the right side. When equal sounds are restored, reinflate the cuff.
   b. The tube is past the carina and in the right mainstem bronchus. Deflate the cuff and pull back enough to restore lung sounds on the left side. When equal sounds are restored, reinflate the cuff.
   c. The tube has not been properly secured in place and has been pulled out of the trachea. Hyperventilate the patient, reinsert the tube, secure in place, and reassess for correct placement.
   d. The tube has been misplaced in the esophagus. Remove the tube, hyperventilate the patient, insert the tube into the trachea, secure in place, and reassess for correct placement.

After correcting the problem with the unequal lung sounds, you place an end-tidal carbon dioxide detector on the tracheal tube. The paramedic backup team has arrived, and you proceed to give them a complete assessment and report. The senior paramedic, Lieutenant Wilson, assesses the lung sounds and advises that there is good chest rise and fall, no sounds are heard over the epigastrium, and breath sounds are present and equal in both lungs. The patient responds to treatment and is released from the hospital a few days later. You and Jill are justified in feeling that you have saved the man's life by performing basic and advanced airway-management procedures efficiently and correctly.

ENRICHMENT

1. Which statement is correct pertaining to the digital intubation technique?
   a. Direct visualization of the hypopharynx occurs when performing digital intubation.
   b. Digital intubation is the preferred method of intubating the alert trauma patient.
   c. The EMT lifts the epiglottis by inserting his fingers into the patient's mouth.
   d. Manipulation of the head or neck by the EMT is required when digitally intubating.

2. You are preparing to intubate your patient using the transillumination intubation technique. Which of the following statements is correct regarding this technique?
   a. A major problem with this technique is the inability to see the stylet light in bright ambient light.
   b. The use of this technique is contraindicated and dangerous when performed in the trauma patient.
   c. Placement is confirmed when the light appears lateral to the upper aspect of the thyroid cartilage.
   d. A light at the front of the neck that appears dim or hard to see indicates placement into the trachea.

3. For which of the following patients is the use of a pharyngeotracheal-lumen (PtL®) airway appropriate?
   a. A 10-year-old male drowning victim
   b. A 4-foot-11-inch female in cardiac arrest
   c. A 55-year-old unresponsive female who has a gag reflex
   d. A 17-year-old unresponsive smoke-inhalation patient

4. You are ventilating a deeply unresponsive patient with the esophageal-tracheal Combitube® airway when the patient regains responsiveness. You should
   a. reassure the patient by calmly explaining the procedure.
   b. immediately remove the ETC and prepare to suction the patient.
   c. apply firm cricoid pressure (Sellick's maneuver) to reduce spasms.
   d. deflate the cuff and pull back the ETC 2 centimeters and then reinflate.

5. You are preparing to use the laryngeal-mask airway (LMA) for a patient who is unresponsive and apneic. Which insertion method is correct for this device?
   a. Advance the LMA into the hypopharynx until resistance is met.
   b. Lift the epiglottis directly with the distal end, and advance into the trachea.
   c. Insert the LMA until the teeth or gums are positioned between the two black rings.
   d. Following the natural curvature of the oropharynx, advance until the teeth strap touches.

6. The process of monitoring the exhaled carbon dioxide in the body is known as
   a. carbonemetry.
   b. oxygenometry.
   c. capnometry.
   d. geometry.

7. The normal physiologic range for end-tidal CO_2 ($ETCO_2$) is
   a. 18–22 mmHg.
   b. 28–32 mmHg.
   c. 38–42 mmHg.
   d. 48–52 mmHg.

8. With which of the following tracheal-intubation devices would you feel the "bumps" of the tracheal rings prior to passing the tracheal tube?
   a. Bougie (Eschmann) tracheal-tube introducer
   b. Standard malleable stylet
   c. Transillumination (lighted stylet)
   d. Wisconsin straight-lighted blade

ADVANCED AIRWAY MANAGEMENT: CHAPTER 43

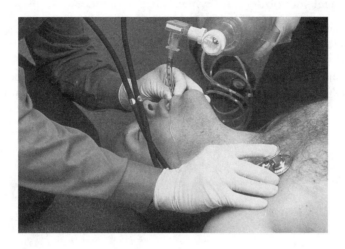

In the past, performance of advanced airway procedures was reserved for ALS personnel. However, it is the EMT who is usually first on the scene, and the ability of the EMT to perform advanced airway procedures before ALS assistance arrives may, in some situations, make the difference between life and death for the patient. For this reason, although advanced airway skills are difficult to master and maintain, some jurisdictions, at the discretion of the medical director, may now require that EMTs receive advanced airway-management training. If you are assigned to such a jurisdiction, this module will be required. If not, you may skip this module, or you may want to study it as additional background.

Q **At the discretion of the medical director, and if trained to perform them, what advanced airway procedures may be performed by EMTs?**

A Orotracheal intubation, nasogastric intubation in infants and children, and orotracheal suctioning.

Q **What is orotracheal intubation, and when is it performed?**

A Orotracheal intubation is the insertion of a tube through the mouth and along the oropharynx and larynx, directly into the trachea. (Because the tube goes into the trachea, it is called a tracheal tube.) The advantages of orotracheal intubation include isolation and complete control of the airway, to prevent aspiration of vomitus and other substances. Not every patient requires tracheal intubation. It should be attempted only after basic airway techniques (such as the head-tilt/chin-lift maneuver, suctioning, and insertion of an airway adjunct such as an oropharyngeal airway) and normal ventilation methods (such as mouth-to-mask or bag-valve-mask ventilation) have been attempted. Orotracheal intubation should then be attempted if ventilation by ordinary methods is ineffective and if the patient cannot protect his own airway (is unresponsive to any stimuli and has no gag or cough reflex). Extreme care must be taken to confirm that the tube is correctly placed in the trachea. Mistaken placement of the tube in the esophagus or advancement of the tube into the right mainstem bronchus can cause severe hypoxia and death.

Q **What is nasogastric intubation, and when is it performed?**

A Nasogastric intubation is performed by the EMT primarily to relieve gastric distention in infants and children. (It is far easier to mistakenly force air into the esophagus in an infant or a child than in an adult. If distention is severe, it will force the diaphragm upward against the lungs and prevent adequate ventilation.) A flexible tube is measured from the tip of the nose around the ear to below the xiphoid process. The lubricated tube is inserted through a nostril and into the esophagus. The tube is then attached to low suction to aspirate gastric contents. A nasogastric (NG) tube should not be inserted in a patient who has suffered major facial, head, or spinal trauma nor in a patient with suspected airway disease.

Q   **What is orotracheal suctioning, and when is it performed?**

A   Orotracheal suctioning is performed by inserting a soft suction catheter through an already-inserted tracheal tube to clear secretions. The tube can be advanced down the endotracheal tube to the level of the carina (the point where the right and left mainstem bronchi branch off from the trachea). There are two main indications for orotracheal suctioning: (1) obvious secretions in the endotracheal tube and (2) poor compliance or increased resistance when ventilating through the endotracheal tube, which may indicate a blockage in the tube. Because the patient cannot receive oxygen during orotracheal suctioning, aggressive hyperoxygenation before and after suctioning is required, and suction must be limited to 15 seconds or less in order to prevent hypoxia.

1. Which department of the United States government was charged with developing an Emergency Medical Services (EMS) system and upgrading prehospital emergency care?
   a. Department of Assessment Standards
   b. Department of Technical Assistance
   c. Department of Labor and Employment
   d. Department of Transportation (DOT)

2. The process of ensuring scene safety is *best* described by which of the following?
   a. Ensuring scene safety is accomplished upon arrival on-scene.
   b. Ensuring scene safety is dynamic and ongoing.
   c. Ensuring scene safety begins with patient contact.
   d. Ensuring scene safety is continued until patient contact.

3. You are dispatched to a rock climber injured on a very steep hillside. Knowing that you are not trained in this type of rescue, you should
   a. wait for a trained rescue crew.
   b. climb down to the patient.
   c. secure the patient with ropes.
   d. from below, climb up to the patient.

4. You are dispatched to a residence where all of the family members, including the dog, are experiencing similar signs of disorientation. What should you suspect?
   a. The dog has infected the family.
   b. The patients have the flu.
   c. The patients are suffering from the same virus.
   d. The environment is toxic.

5. The chief complaint is the patient's answer to the question
   a. "Where does it hurt?"
   b. "Why did you call EMS?"
   c. "What do you think is wrong with you?"
   d. "Can you point with one finger where the pain is?"

6. A life-threatening condition that is found during the initial assessment should be treated
   a. once the initial assessment is completed.
   b. once the patient priorities are established.
   c. immediately as it is found.
   d. after assessing the circulation.

7. Inadequate breathing should be suspected in an unresponsive adult patient with a respiratory rate of
   a. less than 12 or greater than 22 per minute.
   b. less than 10 or greater than 24 per minute.
   c. less than 10 or greater than 20 per minute.
   d. less than 4 or greater than 20 per minute.

8. The focused history and physical exam is performed to do which of the following?
   a. Identify any additional injuries or conditions that may also be life threatening.
   b. Rapidly make the initial identification of life-threatening conditions.
   c. Identify potential hazards that may be present on the scene.
   d. Rapidly identify the total number of patients ill or injured.

9. An unresponsive trauma patient with a midfacial fracture, unequal pupils, and abnormal posturing to painful stimulus requires
   a. rapid transport without spinal immobilization.
   b. hyperventilation at 20 breaths per minute with supplemental oxygen.
   c. placement of a nasopharyngeal airway and hyperventilation at 20 per minute.
   d. spinal immobilization and rapid transport only.

10. The "S" in the SAMPLE history represents
    a. Signs and symptoms
    b. Symptoms and severity
    c. Signs and setting
    d. Setting and scenario

11. The chest of the adult medical patient should be auscultated at which of the following?
    a. Third intercostal space at the midclavicular line and fifth intercostal space at the midaxillary line
    b. First intercostal space at the midclavicular line and sixth intercostal space at the midaxillary line
    c. Second intercostal space at the midclavicular line and fourth intercostal space at the midaxillary line
    d. Sixth intercostal space at the midclavicular line and sixth intercostal space at the midaxillary line

12. The detailed physical exam is
    a. always conducted on every patient.
    b. most often performed on-scene prior to transport on the critical patient.
    c. performed to rapidly identify life threats.
    d. performed following the focused history and physical exam and after life-threatening injuries are controlled.

13. A pupil that is large in size and not responding to light should be referred to as
    a. Dilated and glazed
    b. Fixed and dilated
    c. Fixed and constricted
    d. A consensual reflex

14. The purpose of the ongoing assessment is to do which of the following?
    a. Determine potential scene hazards and obstacles
    b. Determine patient changes and assess treatments
    c. Establish priorities of patient management
    d. Evaluate system effectiveness and benchmarks

15. Vital signs in the unstable patient should be reassessed every _____ minutes.
    a. 2
    b. 3
    c. 5
    d. 15

16. You are preparing to treat your patient with a particular drug. Which of the following should alert you to stop the therapy?
    a. A side effect
    b. A therapeutic effect
    c. An indication
    d. A contraindication

17. There are many different routes by which medications may be administered. Which of the following describes the correct route for administration of nitroglycerin spray?
    a. Oral
    b. Sublingual
    c. Inhalation
    d. Intramuscular

18. When you must lift a patient, you should do which of the following?
    a. Keep your back in an unlocked position
    b. Keep your back in a locked-in position
    c. Lean backward from the waist and bend knees
    d. Lean forward from the waist and lock knees

19. When pulling an object, you should keep the load
    a. between your shoulders and hips and close to your body.
    b. between your shoulders and waist and away from your body.
    c. above the shoulders and avoid bending at the waist if possible.
    d. below the waist and avoid bending at the waist when possible.

20. In which of the following circumstances should you perform an emergency move?
    a. The patient is unresponsive but is breathing and has a pulse.
    b. It is necessary to gain access to a patient who needs spinal immobilization.
    c. The patient is responsive but has an obvious head injury.
    d. It is necessary to gain access to other patients who display immediate life threats.

21. From the following, when would the use of a stair chair be inappropriate?
    a. The corridors and stairway are narrow.
    b. The patient has an injury to the chest.
    c. The patient weighs more than 200 pounds.
    d. The patient has an altered mental status.

22. To help take the weight of the fetus off the large blood vessels and nerves, a woman in advanced pregnancy should be placed in which position?
    a. On her left side
    b. Trendelenburg
    c. Supine
    d. Prone

23. Each 3-month period of the approximately 9-month pregnancy is referred to as a
    a. Trimester
    b. Trigeminal
    c. Stage
    d. Period

24. The third stage of labor is the period during which
    a. complete cervical dilation occurs.
    b. the placenta is expelled.
    c. the infant moves through the birth canal.
    d. the amniotic sac ruptures.

25. Which of the following is the organ that contains the developing infant?
    a. Perineum
    b. Cervix
    c. Placenta
    d. Uterus

26. Delivery of the infant can be expected within a few minutes if contractions are
    a. Six to 7 minutes apart and last from 15 to 20 seconds
    b. Four to 5 minutes apart and last from 15 to 25 seconds
    c. Three to 4 minutes apart and last from 20 to 25 seconds
    d. Two to 3 minutes apart and last from 60 to 90 seconds

27. When suctioning the newborn's airway during birth, which of the following should you do?
    a. Suction the nose first, then the mouth.
    b. Suction the mouth first, then the nose.
    c. Turn the head to the side to expel the contents.
    d. Suction either the nose or the mouth first.

28. A newborn infant has bluish skin discoloration of the extremities, adequate breathing, and a heart rate of 100 bpm. Which of the following is the *most* appropriate treatment?
    a. Begin CPR immediately and provide ventilations.
    b. Provide ventilations by bag-valve mask with supplemental oxygen.
    c. Provide free-flow oxygen by the "blow-by" method.
    d. Insert a nasogastric tube to decompress the stomach.

29. Which of the following describes a difference found in the infant or child's airway that is not found in the adult?
    a. The tongue is smaller and takes up less space in the pharynx.
    b. The nose and mouth are larger in the infant and child.
    c. The epiglottis is more U-shaped and can protrude into the pharynx.
    d. The trachea is wider, harder, and less flexible.

30. A "patent airway" is
    a. partially obstructed by foreign body.
    b. an airway that is open.
    c. also called an oropharyngeal airway.
    d. completely obstructed by the tongue.

31. You are preparing to use an oropharyngeal airway on your patient. You know that
    a. it is available in adult sizes only and contraindicated in the child.
    b. it passes through and extends below the larynx to hold the tongue in position.
    c. it can be used on partially responsive patients.
    d. it is rotated 180 degrees in the adult patient while inserting.

32. Which of the following is true about the nasopharyngeal airway?
    a. It is available in one adjustable size.
    b. It is more likely to stimulate vomiting than an oropharyngeal airway.
    c. It may injure the nasal mucosa.
    d. It must be inserted flange first with the bevel toward the septum.

33. The depth of a patient's breathing may also be referred to as which of the following?
    a. Chest ventilation
    b. Tidal volume
    c. Total volume
    d. Breathing capacity

34. Excessively rapid breathing is referred to as which of the following?
    a. Tachypnea
    b. Eupnea
    c. Dyspnea
    d. Bradypnea

35. Your patient's minute volume is inadequate. Which of the following should you use to correct this problem?
    a. Nonrebreather mask
    b. Bag-valve mask
    c. Nasal cannula
    d. Oxygen by blow-by

36. The preferred method for ventilation of a patient using the bag-valve-mask device requires that
    a. one EMT should ventilate the patient.
    b. the EMT who ventilates should be positioned at the patient's side.
    c. the EMT squeezing the bag should also hold the mask.
    d. two EMTs should ventilate the patient.

37. The flow-restricted, oxygen-powered ventilation device provides
    a. a flow rate of more than 50 lpm of 60 percent oxygen.
    b. easy operation, requiring little or no training.
    c. 100 percent oxygen with each ventilation.
    d. positive-pressure ventilation for the adult or child patient.

38. A full oxygen cylinder will generally read
    a. 1,000 PSI
    b. 1,500 PSI
    c. 1,750 PSI
    d. 2,000 PSI

39. The safe use of oxygen includes
    a. use of oil-based lubricants on the regulator.
    b. keeping cylinders secured when in transit.
    c. use of a valve that has been modified from another gas cylinder.
    d. storing cylinders below 200°F.

40. The preferred method for the delivery of oxygen in the prehospital setting is with which of the following?
    a. Nasal cannula
    b. Simple face mask
    c. Nonrebreather mask
    d. Partial rebreather mask

41. Which of the following signs and symptoms is most commonly associated with a patient who is suffering an altered mental status with a history of diabetes controlled by medication?
    a. Slow heart rate
    b. Combativeness
    c. Warm, dry skin
    d. Calmness

42. Before oral glucose may be administered, which of the following criteria must first be met, in addition to an on-line or off-line order from medical direction?
    a. Unresponsiveness, history of diabetes controlled by diet, ability to swallow
    b. Altered mental status, history of diabetes controlled by medication, ability to swallow
    c. Unresponsiveness, history of diabetes controlled by injections, present gag reflex
    d. Open airway, history of diabetes controlled by exercise, present gag reflex

43. When assessing pulse quality, the term "thready" refers to which of the following?
    a. Strong pulse
    b. Regular pulse
    c. Weak pulse
    d. Irregular pulse

44. To gather the most effective information during the history taking of your alert patient, you should
    a. ask open-ended questions.
    b. ask yes-or-no questions.
    c. question a family member.
    d. ask challenging questions.

45. Which of the following sets of vital signs is considered normal for a 42-year-old male?
    a. Pulse 82, blood pressure 154/72, breathing rate 28
    b. Pulse 112, blood pressure 146/92, breathing rate 18
    c. Pulse 78, blood pressure 142/68, breathing rate 12
    d. Pulse 48, blood pressure 122/54, breathing rate 10

46. Which of the following is a meeting that may precede a CISD (critical incident stress debriefing) to allow the rescuers to vent their emotions and get information before the larger group meeting?
    a. Defusing
    b. Critiquing
    c. Teaching
    d. Debriefing

47. Which of the following is the single most important way you can prevent the spread of infection?
   a. Wearing gloves
   b. Wearing a mask
   c. Hand washing
   d. Cleaning equipment

48. When might it be appropriate to apply a surgical mask to the patient?
   a. When blood may be splashed into the patient's face
   b. When you suspect an airborne infectious disease
   c. When the patient is suspected of having AIDS
   d. When transporting more than one patient at a time

49. Dark red blood that flows steadily from a wound usually indicates a severed or damaged
   a. Artery
   b. Vein
   c. Capillary
   d. Arteriole

50. Your patient has a large laceration to the forearm. After you have applied direct pressure and elevation, the wound continues to bleed profusely. You should
   a. compress the popliteal pressure point.
   b. compress the femoral pressure point.
   c. compress the brachial pressure point.
   d. compress the carotid pressure point.

51. Which of the following is a sign or symptom of shock?
   a. Constricted pupils
   b. Absent peripheral pulses
   c. Red, warm, dry skin
   d. Slow, deep breathing

52. A child from 1 to 3 years old is referred to as which of the following?
   a. A neonate
   b. An infant
   c. A toddler
   d. A preschooler

53. Which of the following is the primary goal in treating any infant or child patient?
   a. To recognize and treat respiratory problems
   b. To provide rapid transport to the medical facility
   c. To reduce pain and suffering
   d. To determine the cause of the illness or injury

54. Which of the following is an indication of respiratory arrest in the infant or child patient?
   a. Regular respirations
   b. Respiratory rate less than 10 per minute
   c. Hyperactive patient
   d. Strong peripheral pulses and an elevated heart rate

55. Which of the following is the *best* indication of a complete airway obstruction in the infant or child patient?
   a. Crying or talking
   b. Stridor upon inspiration
   c. Pale, cool, clammy skin
   d. Ineffective or absent cough

56. The normal ranges of respirations in the infant and the child are, respectively,
   a. 25–50 and 15–30
   b. 30–40 and 20–25
   c. 40–50 and 15–20
   d. 30–40 and 10–20

57. Which of the following is a sign of hypoperfusion in the infant or child patient?
   a. Warm, pink, dry skin
   b. Rapid, bounding pulse
   c. Capillary refill under 2 seconds
   d. Absence of tears when crying

58. SIDS (sudden infant death syndrome) has a peak incidence at around _____old.
   a. 2 weeks
   b. 1 month
   c. 4 months
   d. 1 year

59. Gastrostomy tubes in the child are used to provide
   a. long-term drainage of cerebrospinal fluid.
   b. long-term feeding directly to the stomach.
   c. long-term intravenous access.
   d. long-term airway access.

60. You are the primary triage officer on an MCI (multiple-casualty incident). The first patient you triage is not breathing. You take steps to open the airway, but the patient is still not breathing. You would tag this patient as
   a. Red/first priority
   b. Black/no priority
   c. Yellow/second priority
   d. Green/third priority

61. In triage tagging, which of the following injuries would indicate a yellow or priority-2 patient?
   a. Able to walk, minor injuries
   b. Respirations < 30/minute, obeys commands
   c. Respirations > 30/minute, unresponsive
   d. Does not obey commands/signs of shock

62. A patient is found in severe respiratory distress, sitting upright and leaning slightly forward, supporting himself with his arms. This position is called which of the following?
   a. Trendelenburg position
   b. Tripod position
   c. Distress position
   d. Trapezoid position

63. A cough that produces mucus is known as which of the following?
    a. Diminished cough
    b. Productive cough
    c. Paradoxical cough
    d. Wet cough

64. What is cyanosis?
    a. An early sign of hypoperfusion
    b. An early sign of breathing difficulty
    c. A late sign of breathing difficulty
    d. A late sign of altered mental status

65. An infant with cyanosis, an altered mental status, and a slow heart rate should be provided
    a. positive-pressure ventilation with supplemental oxygen.
    b. oxygen via simple face mask.
    c. oxygen via nonrebreather mask.
    d. oxygen via the "blow-by" method.

66. Which of the following is an "S" question in the OPQRST questions used to evaluate a patient with respiratory distress?
    a. "When did the difficulty in breathing start?"
    b. "Does lying flat make the breathing more difficult?"
    c. "How bad is this breathing difficulty on a scale of 1 to 10?"
    d. "What were you doing when the breathing difficulty started?"

67. A patient with difficulty in breathing is considered which of the following?
    a. A high-priority patient
    b. A low-priority patient
    c. A medium-priority patient
    d. A patient not assigned to a priority

68. A loose flap of skin and soft tissue that has been torn loose or pulled completely off is known as an
    a. Articulation
    b. Amputation
    c. Avulsion
    d. Abrasion

69. You are treating a patient who has an abdominal injury with exposed organs. Which treatment is most appropriate?
    a. Apply a sterile dressing moistened with saline, then an occlusive dressing.
    b. Apply an occlusive dressing, then sterile gauze moistened with saline.
    c. Apply a dry, sterile cotton dressing; then use direct pressure to help control bleeding.
    d. Apply a dry gauze dressing to control bleeding, then cover with an occlusive dressing.

70. Which of the following is the most appropriate way to transport an amputated body part?
    a. Place the body part in a plastic bag; label the bag; immediately place the bag on ice.
    b. Immediately immerse the body part in a bag of ice water; label the bag; transport.
    c. Wrap the body part in dry, sterile dressing; place in a plastic bag; label the bag; keep the part cool.
    d. Do not delay to wrap or label the part; transport the part immediately.

71. Which of the following is an early sign or symptom of neurological deficit that is commonly found in the patient suffering a stroke?
    a. Paralysis to both legs
    b. Bilateral numbness to hands
    c. Stiff neck
    d. Loss of vision in one eye

72. Which of the following is the *most* appropriate means of administering oxygen to the stroke patient who is unresponsive and breathing inadequately?
    a. Nasal cannula with a flow of 4–6 lpm
    b. Nonrebreather mask with a flow of 15 lpm
    c. Positive-pressure ventilation at 8 per minute
    d. Positive-pressure ventilation at 20 per minute

73. Implied consent applies to which of the following?
    a. The patient adamantly refuses treatment then becomes unresponsive.
    b. The patient is of legal age and able to make rational decisions.
    c. The parent or legal guardian has consented to treatment and transport.
    d. The patient consents orally or by a nod or an affirming gesture.

74. In a malpractice suit, injuries to the patient are deemed to be the direct result of negligence by the EMT. This is called
    a. Battery
    b. Damages
    c. Secondary negligence
    d. Proximate cause

75. Which chamber of the heart receives oxygen-rich blood from the lungs?
    a. Left ventricle
    b. Right ventricle
    c. Left atrium
    d. Right atrium

76. Which of the following is the most appropriate emergency medical treatment for a responsive patient suffering from a cardiac emergency?
    a. Administer oxygen at 10 lpm via nonrebreather mask and consider calling for ALS backup.
    b. Administer oxygen at 15 lpm via nonrebreather mask and consider calling for ALS backup.
    c. Administer oxygen at 10 lpm via nasal cannula and consider calling for ALS backup.
    d. Administer oxygen at 6 lpm via nasal cannula and consider calling for ALS backup.

77. You are preparing to administer nitroglycerin. Which of the following statements is correct regarding nitroglycerin?
    a. It constricts the coronary arteries, increasing the blood flow to the heart.
    b. A second dose can be administered 2 minutes after the first dose.
    c. The patient's systolic blood pressure must be above 100 mmHg.
    d. Nitroglycerin is indicated in patients suffering from a head injury.

78. When using the AED, the decision to transport the patient to the emergency facility should occur after which of the following conditions is met?
    a. A total of two shocks have been delivered by the AED.
    b. The AED has given a no-shock message.
    c. The patient regains a pulse and then slips back into cardiac arrest.
    d. The patient has been shocked four times and remains pulseless.

79. Which of the following statements is correct regarding the AED?
    a. After depressing the shock button, you should say, "Clear the patient."
    b. Before delivering shocks in the ambulance, stop and turn the motor off.
    c. The AED cannot be used on a patient who has an implanted pacemaker.
    d. Shocking a patient who has taken nitroglycerin sublingually is contraindicated.

80. You are treating an adult patient who has partial-thickness burns that encircle the right arm and cover the anterior trunk. What is the total BSA burned and the severity?
    a. 36 percent; critical burns
    b. 27 percent; critical burns
    c. 36 percent; moderate burns
    d. 27 percent; moderate burns

81. You are treating a patient with dry lime burns on both legs. Which of the following is the appropriate treatment?
    a. Remove clothing; do not attempt to brush the chemical off; flush for 20 minutes while transporting.
    b. Remove clothing; brush the chemical off; flush for 20 minutes while transporting.
    c. Brush the chemical off; remove clothing; flush for 20 minutes; then transport.
    d. Remove clothing; do not attempt to brush the chemical off; flush for 20 minutes; then transport.

82. When dealing with a patient suffering from a behavioral emergency, which of the following statements to the patient would be *most* appropriate?
    a. "You have nothing to worry about; everything will be better before long."
    b. "Trust me; things will be all right after we go to the hospital and see the doctor."
    c. "I'm sensitive to your problems, and I'm sure you can be cured."
    d. "Even with all of your problems, you seem to have people who care about you."

83. Which of the following restraints are considered humane and should be used when restraining a patient who may be a danger to you or himself?
    a. Metal police handcuffs
    b. Soft leather restraints
    c. Disposable flex cuffs
    d. Wide adhesive tape

84. When an error is made while writing the prehospital-care report, how should you correct the mistake?
    a. Use a commercially available correction fluid.
    b. Erase the mistake, then write over the error.
    c. Draw a single line through the error and initial it.
    d. Completely blacken out the mistake and initial it.

85. Your patient is adamantly refusing treatment and transport to a medical facility. The patient is also refusing to sign a refusal-of-care form. Which of the following should you do?
    a. Have the police respond to the scene, and force the patient to sign the form.
    b. Advise the patient that if the form is not signed, he will have to be transported.
    c. Have someone else sign the form, verifying that the patient refused to sign.
    d. If the patient refuses to sign the form, there is nothing you can do. Clear the scene.

86. According to the National Fire Protection Association (NFPA) 704 system, a diamond-shaped symbol identifies potentially dangerous cargo. Which color and number represent an extreme health hazard?
    a. Red diamond with the number 1 inside the triangle
    b. Red diamond with the number 4 inside the triangle
    c. Blue diamond with the number 1 inside the triangle
    d. Blue diamond with the number 4 inside the triangle

87. At a hazardous materials scene, the zone where contamination is actually present or that is immediately adjacent to the accident site and where contamination can still occur is the
    a. Safety zone
    b. Hot zone
    c. Warm zone
    d. Cold zone

88. While you are waiting for specially trained personnel to arrive to handle a hazardous-materials scene, you should protect yourself and bystanders by
    a. keeping downhill and upwind from the scene.
    b. keeping uphill and downwind from the scene.
    c. keeping downhill and downwind from the scene.
    d. keeping uphill and upwind from the scene.

89. Which of the following is a division of the nervous system that influences the activities of skeletal muscles and movements throughout the body?
    a. Automatic nervous system
    b. Voluntary nervous system
    c. Autonomic nervous system
    d. Involuntary nervous system

90. A spinal injury resulting from hanging would be caused by which of the following mechanisms of spine injury?
    a. Flexion
    b. Extension
    c. Lateral bending
    d. Distraction

91. Manual stabilization of the potentially spine-injured patient's neck should
    a. not be released until the cervical-spine immobilization collar is applied.
    b. be released if the patient complains of discomfort.
    c. not be released until the patient is completely immobilized to a backboard.
    d. be released if the patient's level of responsiveness deteriorates.

92. A patient who is walking around at a collision scene
    a. does not have a spinal injury.
    b. should not be immobilized.
    c. may have a spinal injury.
    d. should always be immobilized.

93. Paralysis to all four extremities is called which of the following?
    a. Quadriplegia
    b. Paraplegia
    c. Biplegia
    d. Hemiplegia

94. Your patient has ingested a poisonous plant and will only respond to painful stimuli. In which position should you place the patient?
    a. Lateral recumbent
    b. Supine
    c. Fowler's
    d. Trendelenburg

95. After administering activated charcoal to a 6-year-old patient who has ingested all of her mother's blood-pressure medicine, the patient vomits. You should now
    a. contact medical direction to authorize one repeat dose of 10 grams.
    b. contact medical direction to authorize one repeat dose of 25 grams.
    c. contact medical direction to authorize one repeat dose of 60 grams.
    d. not contact medical direction; repeating the dose is contraindicated.

96. When treating a patient who has inhaled a poisonous gas, your *first* treatment priority is to
    a. administer high-flow oxygen.
    b. place the patient on his side.
    c. start positive-pressure ventilation.
    d. move the patient out of the toxic environment.

97. Your patient has been involved in a farm accident. All conventional methods of shutting down the tractor have failed. Which of the following methods of shutting off the engine may be used but may cause engine damage?
    a. Pulling the air shut-off lever instead of using the key
    b. Discharging a 20-pound CO_2 extinguisher into the air intake
    c. Closing the fuel valve at the bottom of the fuel tank
    d. Clamping the fuel line by using a pair of Vise-Grip pliers

98. Which of the following best describes silo gas?
    a. Carbon dioxide, rotten-egg-like smell, lighter than air, can kill within hours
    b. Carbon monoxide, gasoline-like smell, lighter than air, can kill within minutes
    c. Methane gas, vodka-like odor, heavier than air, can kill within hours
    d. Red-brown to yellow-green in color, bleachlike odor, heavier than air, can kill within minutes

99. Which of the following terms means "toward the center of the body"?
    a. Superior
    b. Medial
    c. Dorsal
    d. Lateral

100. Which of the following terms refers to the center of each of the collarbones?
   a. Midclavicular
   b. Distal
   c. Midanterior
   d. Midaxillary

101. In this body position, the patient is lying on her back with her head elevated at a 45-degree to 60-degree angle.
   a. Supine position
   b. Lateral recumbent position
   c. Fowler's position
   d. Trendelenburg position

102. Which heart valve is located between the left atrium and the left ventricle?
   a. Mitral valve
   b. Aortic valve
   c. Pulmonary valve
   d. Tricuspid valve

103. Which organ is solid, is located in the left upper quadrant of the abdominal cavity, and aids in the filtration of blood?
   a. Gallbladder
   b. Spleen
   c. Ileum
   d. Duodenum

104. The five vertebrae that form the lower back and are located between the sacral and the thoracic spine form the
   a. Iliac spine
   b. Humeral spine
   c. Cervical spine
   d. Lumbar spine

105. When the amount of heat the body produces or gains exceeds the amount the body loses, the result is which of the following?
   a. Heat stroke
   b. Hyperthermia
   c. Heat cramps
   d. Hypothermia

106. Coma and severely depressed vital signs occur when the temperature reaches approximately what core body temperature?
   a. 70° F
   b. 79° F
   c. 89° F
   d. 90° F

107. Which of the following is an early finding of hypothermia?
   a. Decreased vital signs
   b. Decreased level of responsiveness
   c. Apathy
   d. Muscular shivering

108. A hyperthermic patient with moist, pale skin that is normal to cool in temperature should be
    a. placed in a bath filled with ice water.
    b. moved to a cool environment.
    c. placed in a supine position with the head elevated.
    d. given fluids if unresponsive.

109. A patient has been stung by a bee. Which of the following methods is the *best* way to remove the stinger?
    a. Use tweezers.
    b. Use your fingers.
    c. Use forceps.
    d. Gently scrape it.

110. You are treating a patient who has been struck in the head with a baseball bat. Which of the following is the correct way to treat bleeding that is coming from the patient's right ear? Cover the ear with a sterile gauze dressing and
    a. then apply a pressure dressing.
    b. then apply an occlusive dressing.
    c. do not try to stop the bleeding.
    d. then apply direct pressure by hand.

111. Your patient responds to painful stimuli by extending both arms down to his sides and extending his legs, then arching his back. Which of the following describes this response?
    a. Lowest level of purposeful response, known as flexion or decorticate posturing
    b. Indicates an upper-level brainstem injury, known as extension or decerebrate posturing
    c. Second-lowest level of nonpurposeful response, known as flexion or decorticate posturing
    d. Second-lowest level of purposeful response, known as extension or decerebrate posturing

112. Which of the following signs and symptoms best describes those that may be found in a patient who is suffering from an abdominal aortic aneurysm?
    a. Sudden onset of tearing pain felt in the chest and left arm; pale, cool skin
    b. Abdominal pain with pale skin above the chest and normal color below
    c. Constant, severe abdominal pain and a pulsating abdominal mass
    d. Sudden onset of intermittent abdominal pain that radiates to the neck

113. Which is the correct way of performing the physical assessment of a patient with acute abdominal pain?
    a. Have the patient first point to the area that is most painful; then palpate each quadrant, beginning with the area farthest from the pain.
    b. Palpate the lower two quadrants first; next, palpate the upper two quadrants; then have the patient point to the area that is most painful.
    c. Have the patient first point to the area that is most painful; palpate that area first, moving toward the less painful areas.
    d. Palpate all four quadrants to find the area that is most painful.

114. Which of the following is the main purpose for assessing the elderly patient's mental status?
    a. To determine the degree of senility
    b. To determine if circulation is adequate
    c. To determine if a stroke has occurred
    d. To determine the possible need for airway protection

Course Review Self-Test

115. Which of the following is correct regarding an altered mental status in an elderly patient?
    a. An altered mental status is not caused by a chronic condition such as Alzheimer's disease.
    b. An altered mental status never results from the use of drugs and medications.
    c. An altered mental status is normal and to be expected in an elderly patient.
    d. An altered mental status may be the result of the acute onset of an emergency such as a stroke.

116. Nearly one-third of all elderly victims of heart attack never experience pain. This is widely known as
    a. An atypical heart attack
    b. A painless heart attack
    c. A false heart attack
    d. A silent heart attack

117. Which of the following is the access route of choice to gain access to the passenger compartment of a car?
    a. Driver's window
    b. Passenger window
    c. Door
    d. Back window

118. Which of the following is a makeshift tool that can be used in an emergency to gain access through a car's window?
    a. The car's whip antenna
    b. The car's hubcap
    c. The car's seatbelt
    d. The car's rear door handle

119. In a vehicle collision, the up-and-over or the down-and-under pathway commonly occurs with which of the following?
    a. Lateral impact
    b. Rear-end impact
    c. Rollover
    d. Frontal impact

120. A "whiplash" injury is commonly caused by which of the following?
    a. Lateral impact
    b. Rear-end impact
    c. Rollover
    d. Frontal impact

121. Which of the following is the most common mechanism of injury?
    a. Motor vehicle collisions
    b. Motorcycle collisions
    c. Gunshot wounds
    d. Falls

122. Penetrating injuries are classified as which of the following?
    a. Hollow, solid, and mixed
    b. Open, closed, and mixed
    c. Low, medium, and high velocity
    d. Partial, complete, and closed

123. Which of the following is called "pathway expansion" and is caused by a pressure wave resulting from the kinetic energy of the bullet?
   a. Cavitation
   b. Profile
   c. Drag
   d. Trajectory

124. Which of the following are the three phases of an explosion that cause specific injury patterns?
   a. First, second, and third phase
   b. Initial, medial, and final phase
   c. Preliminary, general, and specific phase
   d. Primary, secondary, and tertiary phase

125. You are treating a patient with an injured forearm and no other apparent or suspected injuries. There is no distal pulse, and the extremity appears cyanotic. Which of the following is correct?
   a. Complete the initial assessment and transport immediately.
   b. Align the limb with gentle traction; stop only when the pulse returns.
   c. Transport immediately, align the limb, and stop only when the pulse returns.
   d. Align the limb with gentle traction; stop if pain or crepitus occurs.

126. Which of the following describes the correct way to immobilize long-bone injuries?
   a. Immobilize the joint above the injury.
   b. Immobilize the joint below the injury.
   c. Immobilize the joints above and below the injury.
   d. Immobilize the injured long bone only, not the joints.

127. Use of the traction splint is inappropriate in which of the following circumstances?
   a. When the pelvis has also been injured
   b. When the injury is within 3 inches of the hip
   c. When the injury is to the middle of the thigh
   d. When the injury is within 6 inches of the knee

128. After receiving an on-line order from medical direction, you should do which of the following?
   a. Tell medical direction that you have received the order.
   b. Repeat the order back to medical direction, word for word.
   c. Have medical direction repeat the order at least twice.
   d. Write the order on a notepad.

129. In radio terms, which of the following means "message received and understood"?
   a. Copy
   b. Over
   c. Clear
   d. Break

130. When trying to rescue a responsive patient who is struggling near the shore of a lake, which order of rescuing the patient is preferred?
1. Swim to the patient by using a flotation device.
2. Reach to the patient by holding out an object.
3. Throw a weighted polypropylene rope to the patient.
4. Row a boat to the patient if one is immediately available.
   a. 3, 2, 1, 4
   b. 2, 3, 4, 1
   c. 3, 2, 4, 1
   d. 2, 4, 3, 1

131. You are treating a suspected spine-injured patient who is still in the water. Which of the following is correct?
   a. If the patient is found face down, roll the patient over quickly and remove from the water, using any available resources.
   b. To prevent any movement of the head and neck, avoid rescue breathing until the patient is removed from the water.
   c. Slide a long backboard under the patient, secure the torso and legs, then place a cervical-spine immobilization collar.
   d. Place a cervical-spine immobilization collar, slide a long backboard under the patient, then secure the torso and legs.

132. When operating an emergency vehicle, you must exercise "due regard for the safety of others." Which statement is true regarding this concept?
   a. You will not be held responsible for your actions if your emergency lights and siren are operating.
   b. Even under the special laws that apply in cases of true emergency, you can be held liable if you do not exercise reasonable care for the safety of others.
   c. You will not be held responsible for your actions if you exceed the speed limit by no more than 10 miles per hour over the posted speed limit.
   d. You must slow down only at red lights, stop signs, or school crossings.

133. Using a police escort is
   a. appropriate in a dangerous neighborhood.
   b. appropriate when high-speed transport is required.
   c. appropriate in a high-traffic area.
   d. a last resort, usually not a good idea.

134. Which of the following is the first major phase of an ambulance call?
   a. Arrival at scene
   b. Dispatch
   c. Equipment preparation
   d. Post-run

135. A daytime landing area for a small helicopter requires an area of
   a. 30 × 30 feet
   b. 40 × 40 feet
   c. 50 × 50 feet
   d. 60 × 60 feet

136. The four corners of a helicopter landing area should be marked. Where should a fifth device be positioned?
    a. On the approach side of the landing area
    b. At the location of the patient
    c. On the upwind side of the landing area
    d. At the location of the ambulance

137. Which of the following, a chronic brain disorder, is the most common cause of seizures?
    a. Diabetes
    b. Stroke
    c. Head injury
    d. Epilepsy

138. Which of the following conditions is a dire medical emergency that requires aggressive airway management?
    a. Postictal state
    b. Status epilepticus
    c. Tonic-clonic seizure
    d. Grand mal seizure

139. Which of the following drugs is considered to be a central nervous system depressant?
    a. Alcohol
    b. Cocaine
    c. LSD
    d. Ephedrine

140. In which of the following overdose cases (in which the drug taken is known) would the talk-down technique *not* be appropriate?
    a. PCP
    b. LSD
    c. Heroin
    d. Cocaine

141. The patient with an eye injury should be asked to follow your finger as you move it left and right, up and down, in order to evaluate
    a. ability to focus on far object.
    b. ability to focus on near object.
    c. abnormal gaze.
    d. reactivity to light.

142. Removal of a foreign particle from the eye should not generally be attempted in the field. If required, you should attempt removal of a particle only if
    a. it is lodged on the conjunctiva.
    b. it is lodged on the globe.
    c. it is lodged on the cornea.
    d. it is lodged on the iris.

143. An injury to the globe of the eye should be treated with
    a. patches applied lightly to both eyes.
    b. a firm compress applied to both eyes.
    c. firm hand pressure to the globe of the injured eye.
    d. direct pressure to the globes of both eyes.

144. When a patient has suffered an injury to the face, which of the following *best* states the other areas or structures to which compromise or injury should be suspected?
    a. The airway, spine, and skull
    b. The airway and spine
    c. The spine and skull
    d. The airway and skull

145. Which of the following is the correct way to dress and bandage a bleeding neck wound?
    a. An occlusive dressing covered by a regular dressing and a circumferential bandage
    b. A bulky dressing covered by an occlusive dressing and a circumferential bandage
    c. An occlusive dressing covered by a regular dressing and direct pressure
    d. A regular dressing covered by an occlusive dressing and a self-adhesive bandage

146. When administering an epinephrine auto-injector to a patient who is experiencing a severe allergic reaction, which of the following is the correct injection site?
    a. Any of the large arm veins
    b. Right or left buttocks
    c. Lateral portion of the thigh
    d. Deltoid or shoulder muscle

147. Which of the following key categories of signs and symptoms specifically indicates a severe allergic reaction (anaphylaxis) and indicates immediate intervention and administration of epinephrine?
    a. Itchy, watery eyes with a slow heart rate
    b. Intense itching, increased blood pressure
    c. Respiratory or airway compromise and shock (hypoperfusion)
    d. Hives with a warm, tingling feeling to the hands

148. Your patient has been stabbed in the chest. You quickly expose the chest and find an open wound to the anterior chest. Which of the following is your correct *first* action?
    a. Perform a focused history and physical exam.
    b. Perform a rapid trauma assessment.
    c. Seal the wound with a nonocclusive dressing.
    d. Seal the wound with a gloved hand.

149. Which of the following is an *early* sign or symptom that indicates a complication associated with the sealed chest wound and a developing tension pneumothorax?
    a. A breathing rate that is faster than normal
    b. A heart rate that is slower than normal
    c. High blood pressure with a widening pulse pressure
    d. Tracheal deviation away from the injured side

150. You are treating a patient with an abdominal injury but no suspected spinal injury. Which of the following is the *best* position in which to place the patient?
    a. On the left side with the legs straight
    b. Supine with the legs flexed at the knees
    c. Fowler's position with the legs flexed
    d. Trendelenburg position with the legs straight

151. The mnemonic CBRNE is sometimes used to remember types of weapons of mass destruction. It stands for
    a. Chemical, biological, radiological, nuclear, explosive
    b. Concussion, biochemical, radiological, nitroglycerin, environmental
    c. Chemical, bacterial, radioactive, neurological, extractive
    d. Corrosive, biochemical, radio, nuclear, environmental

152. Many of the same principles that apply to hazardous-materials emergencies also apply to weapons-of-mass-destruction emergencies. Which of the following is one of these principles?
    a. All rescuers will be involved in decontamination of patients.
    b. Zones must be established to limit exposure to rescuers.
    c. Rescuers will not require specialized suits and breathing apparatus.
    d. Preplanning and coordination of agencies is not important or imperative.

OPTIONAL: ADVANCED AIRWAY MANAGEMENT

153. The most important indicator of proper tracheal tube placement is
    a. Auscultation of the epigastrium
    b. Auscultation of breath sounds
    c. Seeing the tip of the tube pass between the vocal cords
    d. Watching for chest rise and fall

154. In orotracheal intubation, where should the tube be inserted?
    a. Through the nose and into the esophagus
    b. Through the mouth and into the trachea
    c. Through the mouth and into the esophagus
    d. Through the nose and into the larynx

155. In orotracheal intubation, the epiglottis must be lifted in order to
    a. provide visualization of the vocal cords and glottic opening.
    b. prevent aspiration of blood, secretions, and vomitus.
    c. open the esophageal structures.
    d. move the tongue aside.

156. Which of the following is true regarding an orotracheal intubation?
    a. The straight blade is inserted into the vallecula to lift the epiglottis directly.
    b. The curved blade is fitted under the epiglottis to spread the glottic opening directly.
    c. The straight blade is inserted between the vocal cords to separate them directly.
    d. The curved blade is inserted into the vallecula to lift the epiglottis indirectly.

157. During Sellick's maneuver, where is pressure applied?
    a. To the stomach, to relieve gastric distention
    b. To the larynx, to prevent regurgitation and aspiration
    c. To the cricoid cartilage, to push the glottic structures into the visual field
    d. To the 10 cc syringe, to inflate the distal cuff

158. Endotracheal tubes in infants and children who are under 8 years old are typically
  a. uncuffed because the narrow cricoid ring seals the trachea.
  b. measured from the tip of the nose, around the ear, to the xiphoid process.
  c. not used because of the danger of severe gastric distention.
  d. one-half size larger than the diameter of the patient's thumb.

159. Which of the following is a contraindication for the insertion of a nasogastric tube in an infant or a child?
  a. You are unable to provide effective positive-pressure ventilation due to gastric distention.
  b. The patient is unresponsive and at risk of vomiting gastric contents.
  c. Ingested poisons need to be diluted.
  d. The patient has suffered major facial trauma.

160. Which of the following is true regarding orotracheal suctioning?
  a. A rigid catheter is used to suction the oropharynx.
  b. A soft catheter is used to suction to the level of the carina.
  c. A soft catheter is used to suction to the level of the larynx.
  d. A rigid catheter is used to suction to the level of the xiphoid process.

The number(s) following each answer refer to the textbook page(s) where the answer can be found or supported.

Chapter 1: Introduction to Emergency Medical Care

TERMS AND CONCEPTS

1. a. 4   b. 5   c. 1   d. 6   e. 3   f. 2   *(p. 2)*

CONTENT REVIEW

1. **b.** The other items are AEMT or Paramedic skills. *(p. 9)*
2. **a.** *Your* safety first and always; then other rescuers/bystanders safety. When the scene is secure, you may then provide care for the patient. *(p. 9)*
3. **c.** All the items listed are potential hazards. Be especially aware of the hazards from traffic at nighttime scenes. *(p. 9)*
4. **c.** The risk of being struck by traffic at nighttime scenes is reduced by wearing reflective clothing and providing adequate scene lighting. Being struck by traffic on nighttime scenes is a key threat to all on-scene personnel. All responders must take precautions to protect and ensure a visible and safe working area. It is never considered "just part of the job," and don't hold a lighted flare in your hand. *(p. 10)*
5. **b.** This will result in much discussion. The best answer, given the situation described, is to move or retreat to an area where you can observe the scene and await the arrival of law enforcement. You should not approach until law enforcement tells you the scene is safe. *(p. 10)*
6. **b.** Quality improvement *(p. 14)*
7. **b.** Disposable gloves, eye protection, mask, and gown are the most commonly used equipment worn to protect against infectious diseases. Disposable gloves and eye protection are the most commonly worn. If the potential for splash of body fluid exists, then the mask and cover gown would be added. Leather gloves, turnout gear, helmets or hard hats, and boots would be worn at an accident scene. Self-contained breathing apparatus is used mainly by hazardous materials teams when toxic fumes are present. *(p. 10)*
8. **b.** The medical director is responsible for clinical and patient-care aspects of the EMS system, including both on-line and off-line medical direction and involvement in educational programs and refresher courses. The medical director's primary responsibility is to develop and establish guidelines under which emergency service personnel function. *(p. 13)*
9. **b.** The EMT functions as a designated agent of the system medical director. *(p. 13)*
10. Be honest in your rankings. Ask a friend to rank you on these items; then compare the results. Nobody's perfect, but you must recognize your limitations so you can improve. *(pp. 12–13)*
11. **d.** Patient advocacy includes actions such as collecting patient valuables (if time permits), protecting patients from onlookers, and honoring the patient's requests (if possible). *(p. 11)*
12. **c.** Agencies commonly accessed by 9-1-1 include law enforcement, fire services, and EMS. *(p. 5)*

CASE STUDY

1. **d.** Law enforcement has the primary responsibility for traffic control. At this scene, the car was just over the crest of a hill. This could create a potential hazard to rescuers while working this scene. If law enforcement is not on-scene when you arrive, you (or others) will need to control traffic until they arrive.
2. **a.** The fire department has the primary responsibility for extrication and hazard control at this scene. The fire/rescue department, if properly trained, may need to secure downed power lines in emergency situations when the power company is not on-scene. Otherwise, the power company would deal with electrical hazards.
3. **b.** EMS/ambulance service has the primary responsibility for patient care and transport. In many areas, the fire service also provides EMS.
4. **d.** Do what you can, when you can, for the patient. Patient advocacy requires doing what is in the patient's best interest.
5. **a.** Prehospital care reports are the most commonly used instruments. Feedback from crews, patients, and family are other instruments that may be used but are not as common as the use of the prehospital care report.
6. **c.** The correct answer in this case is based on personal judgment. Traffic is certainly a hazard given that the accident occurred on a steep hill at night. The danger of fire is a possibility at any vehicle accident, and the vehicle could have been in an unstable position. Downed power lines in this case are the greatest potential threat because of the

nighttime conditions and the frequent difficulty in seeing downed lines.

Chapter 2: The Well-Being of the EMT

TERMS AND CONCEPTS

1. a. 1 b. 3 c. 2 d. 5 e. 4 *(p. 18)*

CONTENT REVIEW

1. **b.** The five emotional stages associated with
death and dying are denial, anger, bargain-
ing, depression, and acceptance. *(p. 20)*

2. **a.** A **b.** I **c.** I **d.** A (Talk to the unresponsive patient as if he is alert, because
many unresponsive patients are able to hear.
Family members, if cooperative and not preventing appropriate treatment, should be allowed to remain in the room during
resuscitation efforts. Never offer false reassurance. Try saying instead that you are
"doing everything possible." Listen to the
patient carefully, and deliver any messages to
family members.) *(pp. 20–21)*

3. **a.** Irritability, loss of appetite, and loss of interest in work are signs of stress. The others are
signs of normal adaptation responses.
(p. 23)

4. **a.** Defusing *(p. 25)*

5. **a.** "Pathogens" describe microorganisms that
spread disease. Viruses and bacteria are two
specific types of pathogens. *(p. 26)*

6. **a.** Handwashing *(p. 27)*

7. **c.** Before attempting any rescue situation involving specialized threats such as hazardous
materials, biological agents, high-angle rescue, or white-water rescue, specialized rescue
teams should be requested. *(p. 33)*

8. **a.** 5 **b.** 2 **c.** 3 **d.** 1 **e.** 4.   Identify hazards with binoculars and guidebook, await
scene control by hazmat team, put on necessary protective clothing, and then (and only
then) provide patient assessment and emergency care. *(p. 33)*

9. **a.** Call for police assistance before entering a
potentially violent scene. *(p. 34)*

10. **b.** Avoid disturbing a crime scene, but remember that your priority as an EMT is patient
care. *(p. 35)*

CASE STUDY

1. **d.** Acceptance. The patient has obviously accepted his death and is dealing rationally
with his very difficult situation.

2. **a.** The situation is considered a high-stress incident and may require CISD (critical incident
stress debriefing).

3. **d.** Police, communications, EMS, and emergency-department personnel are all involved
in the defusing. The patient's family should
not be involved.

4. **a.** I **b.** I **c.** I **d.** I (All choices are inappropriate. Don't mask the symptoms and re-
sults of stress by using alcohol or drugs.

Exercise should be encouraged along with
sharing events with coworkers and requesting
a slower-duty station rather than a busier station.)

ENRICHMENT

1. **d.** Hepatitis B may cause no signs or symptoms
at all. (If they do occur, they may include fatigue, nausea, abdominal pain, headache,
fever, and/or jaundice.) Hepatitis B is commonly transmitted by contact with a chronic
carrier's blood or body fluids. It is a serious
disease that may occur over months. The infection may be prevented by obtaining a vaccination. *(pp. 35–36)*

2. **c.** The best action to take, given the responses
provided, is to contact your supervisor for
specific instructions. The supervisor will implement your organization's exposure-control policy. *(p. 36)*

3. **c.** Tuberculosis is a highly infectious disease
spread by droplets from coughing and from
direct contact with sputum. This disease is
making a dramatic comeback. Researchers
are concerned because new drug-resistant
strains of tuberculosis are developing. Wearing a HEPA or N-95 respirator is recommended (not SCBA). *(p. 36)*

4. **c.** HEPA or N-95 respirators provide sufficient
respiratory protection. Surgical face masks
provide limited protection from tuberculosis.
A self-contained breathing apparatus is not
necessary. *(p. 37)*

5. **d.** AIDS is chiefly spread by sexual contact involving the exchange of semen or blood or
through contact with vaginal or cervical secretions, infected needles, infected blood or
blood products, or transmission between an
infected mother and her child. *(p. 37)*

6. **b.** AIDS is caused by a virus that destroys an infected individual's immune system. This disease process generally presents without signs
and symptoms. AIDS is more difficult than
hepatitis B to contract. *(p. 37)*

7. **b.** Hepatitis C is not prevented by a vaccine, is
the most common bloodborne infection in
the United States, is not easily transmitted,
and causes no symptoms in about 80 percent
of all cases. *(p. 36)*

8. **c.** The actions you can take to prevent exposure
are to leave the surgical mask on the patient
(if one is not in place you should place one
on the patient) to prevent droplet spread; to
look for signs of fever and respiratory symptoms for up to 10 days following contact
with the patient to avoid touching your eyes,
nose, or mouth with your gloved hands; and
by washing your hands after glove removal.
(pp. 37–38)

9. **a.** The severe signs and symptoms of West Nile
virus include high fever, headache and stiff
neck, confusion and disorientation, seizures,
muscle weakness, paralysis, and vision loss.
(p. 38)

10. **d** Multidrug-resistant organisms are commonly encountered during patient transport from hospital intensive care units, in burn units, and in long-term-care facilities. They are considered a significant threat to the EMT and are commonly transmitted by person-to-person contact. The organisms include methicillin/oxacillin-resistant *Staphylococcus aureus* (MRSA), vancomycin-resistant enterococci (VRE), penicillin-resistant *Streptococcus pneumoniae* (PRSP), and drug-resistant *Streptococcus pneumoniae* (DRSP). *(p. 38)*

Chapter 3: Medical, Legal, and Ethical Issues

TERMS AND CONCEPTS

1. **a.** 5 **b.** 4 **c.** 3 **d.** 1 **e.** 2 **f.** 6 **g.** 11 **h.** 7 **i.** 8 **j.** 10 **k.** 9 *(p. 41)*

CONTENT REVIEW

1. **c.** The EMT's scope of practice is defined by the National EMS Scope of Practice Model, by the National Standard Curriculum, and by state laws, regulations, and policies. A national EMS act does not exist. Just because an EMT has the knowledge to perform certain skills does not permit the EMT to utilize the skills on a patient. *(pp. 43–44)*
2. **d.** Battery *(p. 45)*
3. **c.** Good Samaritan law *(p. 44)*
4. **a.** Standard of care *(p. 43)*
5. **b.** The patient's expressed or implied consent *(pp. 45, 54)*
6. **a.** Implied consent (It is not minor consent, which must be given by a parent or guardian.) *(p. 45)*
7. **a.** To refuse care, a patient must be mentally competent and informed. He or she is not legally required to sign a release, although the EMT should attempt to get a signed and witnessed release for the legal protection of the EMT and the EMS system. *(p. 46)*
8. **b.** Pushing away or any other indication that care is not welcome—before or after care is begun—constitutes valid refusal if the patient is a competent adult. *(p. 46)*
9. **b.** Abandonment *(p. 50)*
10. **d.** Patient information may not be given to an off-duty EMT, your wife, or any other person without a legitimate need for the information. A health-care provider needs to know this information in order to continue medical care. *(p. 51)*
11. **b.** The duty to act refers to your obligation to provide care to the patient while you are on duty. Some states require EMTs to stop and render aid even when off duty. *(pp. 43–44)*
12. **c.** When you are not sure whether the patient can make a rational decision, you should consult medical oversight. *(pp. 46–49)*

13. **d.** A willful threat to a patient that can occur without actual touching is called assault. *(p. 50)*
14. **b.** The Health Insurance Portability and Accountability Act (HIPAA), as it relates to the EMT, includes limits on disclosure of patient information, training on specific policies, obtaining patient signatures, and the assignment of an EMS privacy officer. *(p. 51)*
15. **c.** The Consolidated Omnibus Budget and Reconciliation Act (COBRA) and the Emergency Medical Treatment and Active Labor Act (EMTALA) are both federal regulations designed to ensure public access to emergency care regardless of ability to pay. *(pp. 51–52)*

CASE STUDY 1

1. **b.** The most important concerns you should have relating to this patient's refusal of treatment is the patient's understanding of the possible consequences of his refusal. He appears to have a hearing problem that may impact his ability to completely understand the ramifications of his actions. The patient also seems to be mentally competent. You should also be concerned that the patient quickly signed the release without reading it. Do not let your partner influence what you know to be proper patient-care decisions.
2. **d.** The other choices should be pursued only when all efforts to persuade the patient have failed.

CASE STUDY 2

1. **a.** Y **b.** Y **c.** Y **d.** Y (This situation meets all four criteria for a successful negligence suit.)

Chapter 4: The Human Body

MEDICAL TERMINOLOGY

1. **a.** Nature
2. **c.** Between; *intervertebral* means "between the vertebrae."
3. **b.** Over, above
4. **a.** Study of
5. **d.** Skin; *subcutaneous* means "below the (dermis) skin."
6. **a.** perfusion **b.** my/o **c.** glottis **d.** vertebra **e.** hypo **f.** card/ium **g.** peri **h.** axil **i.** pleur **j.** inter

TERMS AND CONCEPTS

1. **a.** transverse line **b.** posterior **c.** prone **d.** superior **e.** normal anatomical position **f.** midaxillary **g.** inferior **h.** lateral **i.** anterior **j.** distal **k.** midline *(pp. 40, 68–70)*

CONTENT REVIEW

1. **c.** The patient's right *(p. 45)*
2. **a.** midline **b.** proximal **c.** distal **d.** medial **e.** lateral **f.** palmar **g.** plantar **h.** anterior **i.** posterior **j.** superior **k.** midaxillary **l.** inferior *(pp. 58–63)*

3. **a.** Bilateral refers to right and left; the femur is the thigh bone. *(p. 62)*
4. **a.** Posterior means "toward the back." *(p. 62)*
5. **c.** Lateral means "toward or on the side"; recumbent means "lying down." *(p. 62)*
6. **d.** Thoracic spine *(p. 64)*
7. **a.** Cervical spine (the neck) *(p. 64)*
8. **d.** Ball-and-socket joints *(p. 67)*
9. **c.** Voluntary muscles can be consciously controlled; involuntary muscle movements are automatic. *(p. 69)*
10. **b.** The unresponsive patient may not be able to protect his airway, partly because the epiglottis fails to close over the trachea. *(pp. 71–73)*
11. **b.** The thoracic cavity increases, creating lower pressure inside the chest than in the atmosphere, causing air to flow into the lungs. *(p. 73)*
12. **b.** The infant's or child's tongue takes up proportionately *more* space in the smaller mouth. *(p. 74)*
13. **d.** Use of accessory muscles (e.g., muscles of the neck, above the clavicles, below the ribs) to aid in breathing is a sign that normal breathing mechanisms are not functioning adequately. The other choices are signs of adequate breathing. *(pp. 75–76)*
14. **A.** cranium **B.** zygomatic bone **C.** maxilla **D.** cervical vertebra **E.** sternum **F.** xiphoid process **G.** iliac crest **H.** ilium **I.** pelvic girdle **J.** greater trochanter **K.** symphysis pubis **L.** frontal bone **M.** parietal bone **N.** occipital bone **O.** temporal bone **P.** mandible **Q.** clavicle **R.** scapula **S.** ribs **T.** humerus **U.** elbow **V.** ulna **W.** radius **X.** sacrum **Y.** coccyx **Z.** carpals **AA.** metacarpals **BB.** phalanges **CC.** femur **DD.** patella **EE.** tibia **FF.** fibula **GG.** tarsals **HH.** metatarsals **II.** calcaneus *(p. 66)*
15. **a.** Gas exchange takes place between capillaries and alveoli and between capillaries and the body's cells. *(pp. 73, 76)*
16. **d.** Atria, ventricles *(p. 76)*
17. **d.** The white blood cells *(p. 80)*
18. **c.** The carotid (in the neck) is a central pulse. The radial (wrist), brachial (upper arm), and tibial (ankle) are considered peripheral pulses (away from the center). *(p. 80)*
19. **d.** Perfusion ("hypo" in hypoperfusion means "low," so hypoperfusion is low, or inadequate, perfusion.) *(p. 81)*
20. **a.** Brain and spinal cord *(p. 83)*
21. **b.** Pituitary *(p. 85)*
22. **d.** Largest organ, protects against bacteria, regulates temperature *(p. 87)*
23. **d.** In the semi-Fowler's position, the patient is placed on his back with the torso elevated less than 45 degrees. In the Fowler's position, the patient is placed on his back with the torso elevated 45–60 degrees. *(p. 51, 98)*
24. **a.** Vasoconstriction, decreasing the diameter of the vessel, and vasodilation, increasing the diameter of the vessel, are controlled by smooth muscle within the vessels. Vasoconstriction will increase the resistance inside the vessel, making it harder for the blood to pass through, and will result in an increase in pressure. Whereas vasodilation will result in a decrease in the resistance inside the vessel, making it easier for the blood to flow through, and decreasing the pressure. *(p. 69)*
25. **d.** *Ventilation* defines the mechanical process of how air is moved in and out of the lungs. Ventilation is primarily based on changes in pressure inside the chest causing air to flow into or out of the lungs. *Respiration* refers to the process of moving oxygen and carbon dioxide across membranes in and out of the cells, capillaries, and alveoli. Thus, respiration deals with the actual gas exchange process. *Oxygenation* is a form of respiration where the oxygen molecule moves across a membrane from an area of high-oxygen concentration to an area of low-oxygen concentration. Cells are oxygenated when the oxygen moves out of the blood in the vessel and into the cell where it is used in metabolism. *(p. 71)*
26. **b.** The diaphragm contributes about 60–70 percent of the effort to breathe, whereas the intercostals muscles contribute the remaining 30–40 percent. *(p. 73)*
27. **c.** An apical pulse is felt on the left side of the chest over the left ventricle. The pulse being felt is from the mechanical contraction of the left ventricle. Since you are only feeling the mechanical contraction of the heart and not the pressure wave of blood, it does not provide an assessment of the effectiveness of the heart or blood volume. *(p. 80)*
28. **d.** About 97 percent of the oxygen carried in the blood is attached to the hemoglobin molecule, which is on the surface of the red blood cell. The remaining 3 percent, not enough to survive on alone, is dissolved in the blood. *(p. 81)*
29. **a.** The main source of energy comes from the cell metabolizing glucose (a simple sugar molecule). *(p. 82)*
30. **a.** *Alpha 1* causes the vessels to constrict (vasoconstriction) thus shunting blood to the core of the body. This causes the skin to become cool, pale, and diaphoretic. *Alpha 2* is thought to regulate the release of alpha 1. *Beta 1* has all of its effects on the heart. It will increase the heart rate, increase the force of contraction, and will speed up the electrical impulse traveling down the heart's conduction system. *Beta 2* will cause smooth muscle to dilate, especially in the bronchioles and in some vessels. *(p. 85)*

CASE STUDY

1. Supine is on the back (face up).
2. **a.** Large laceration to right midclavicular line (center of right clavicle) superior to (above) the right nipple (right = patient's right)

3. **a.** Deformity to the proximal (nearest the torso) end of the left (patient's left) humerus (upper arm bone)

4. **b.** Bilateral (to both legs) femoral region (area around and including the thigh bone) deformity with puncture wound to the left (patient's left) lateral thigh (toward the outside of the thigh, away from the body's midline, which runs between the legs) proximal to (nearer the torso in relation to) the patella (kneecap)

5. Trendelenburg position is supine with lower body elevated approximately 12 inches. (It is sometimes called "shock position," but its use for shock patients is controversial.)

ENRICHMENT

1. **a.** The pancreas is a solid organ located behind the stomach. The pancreas contains small areas of specialized tissue called the islets of Langerhans, which produce the hormones somatostatin, glucagon, and insulin. *(p. 85)*

2. **c.** The spleen is a solid organ located in the upper left quadrant of the abdomen. It helps to filtrate the blood and, because it contains a dense network of blood vessels, it serves as a reservoir of blood the body can use in an emergency such as hemorrhage. *(p. 86)*

3. **a.** Ureters carry the waste from the kidneys to the bladder. The urethra carries urine from the bladder out of the body; the duodenum is the first section of the small intestine that receives partly digested food from the stomach; the hepatic ducts receive bile from the right and left lobes of the liver. *(p. 89)*

Chapter 5: Baseline Vital Signs and History Taking

MEDICAL TERMINOLOGY

1. **a.** systol **b.** sphygm/o **c.** diastol **d.** tachy **e.** auscultat **f.** ic **g.** brady **h.** card **i.** cyan **j.** osis or ia

TERMS AND CONCEPTS

1. **a.** 5 **b.** 1 **c.** 3 **d.** 4 **e.** 7 **f.** 2 **g.** 6 **h.** 10 **i.** 8 **j.** 9 *(p. 121)*

CONTENT REVIEW

1. **c.** Skin *(p. 103)*
2. **c.** Counting the number of respirations in 30 seconds and multiplying by 2 *(pp. 104–105)*
3. **a.** Normal respirations are described. *(p. 105)*
4. **a.** In assessing the quality of a patient's breathing, the EMT determines the depth of respirations (how much air the patient is moving in and out) and how well it is moving (whether there are difficulties moving the air in and out). *(p. 105)*
5. **A.** carotid **B.** brachial **C.** radial **D.** femoral **E.** posterior tibial **F.** dorsalis pedis *(p. 105)*

6. **c.** Count the number of beats in 30 seconds and multiply by 2 *(p. 107)*
7. **b.** Brachial *(p. 106)*
8. **d.** 120–150 beats per minute is normal range for an infant. *(p. 106)*
9. **b.** Strong and regular at 60 beats per minute *(p. 107)*
10. **a.** Pale conjunctiva *(p. 108)*
11. **c.** To help assess skin color in dark-skinned people and infants and children, the palms of the hands and the soles of the feet should be checked, in addition to the nail beds, oral mucosa, and conjunctiva. *(p. 108)*
12. **c.** Relative skin temperature is assessed by using the back of your hand on the patient's skin. *(p. 108)*
13. **d.** Dry skin is normal. Wet or moist skin may indicate hypoperfusion. *(p. 109)*
14. **d.** The high limit for capillary refill in infants, children, and adult men is 2 seconds; for females it is 3 seconds; and for elderly patients it is 4 seconds. *(p. 109)*
15. **d.** Size, equality, and reactivity are assessed. *(p. 110)*
16. **b.** Arteries *(p. 111)*
17. **d.** If the pulse pressure (difference between the systolic and diastolic pressures) is less than 25 percent of the systolic pressure, it is considered a narrow pulse pressure. During auscultation of the blood pressure, the systolic pressure is recorded as the first distinct sound of two or more distinct beats. The diastolic pressure is recorded as the last sound heard. When using a sphygmomanometer and stethoscope, the blood pressure is always reported and expressed as an even number. *(pp. 111–113)*
18. **a.** 124/82 mmHg is considered normal. To estimate the systolic pressure in the adult female patient at rest who is less than 40 years of age, add the patient's age to 90. The normal range for the diastolic pressure is 60–90 mmHg. *(pp. 111–112)*
19. **c.** A sphygmomanometer and a stethoscope *(pp. 112–113)*
20. **a.** 6 **b.** 5 **c.** 2 **d.** 4 **e.** 3 **f.** 1 The correct sequence is as follows: **1.** Position the patient's arm. **2.** Palpate the radial pulse, inflate to 70 mmHg, and increase by 10 mmHg until the radial pulse is no longer palpable. Note the number and deflate the cuff. **3.** Place the stethoscope in your ears. **4.** Inflate the cuff 30 mmHg above the noted number. **5.** Deflate the cuff at 2 mmHg per second. **6.** Note the systolic and diastolic sounds. *(p. 113)*
21. **c.** In the stable patient, vital signs should be checked at least every 15 minutes. *(p. 119)*
22. **a.** A **b.** L **c.** S **d.** M **e.** P **f.** S **g.** A **h.** E **i.** S **j.** L **k.** M **l.** P *(pp. 119–120)*
23. **c.** Testing orthostatic vital signs are conducted by taking the patient's pulse and blood pressure in a supine and then in a standing position. An increase in the patient's pulse by 10–20 bpm and a decrease in the patient's

blood pressure by 10–20 mmHg is a positive finding and can indicate significant blood or fluid loss.   *(pp. 115–116)*

24. **a.** Pulse oximetry is a method of detecting hypoxia in patients and monitoring the effectiveness of airway and ventilation therapy. A reading of 97 percent does not eliminate the potential of hypoxemia in a patient. Other factors may be creating a false reading, such as in patients with hypoperfusion or hypothermia. Readings are commonly affected if the patient is wearing fingernail polish. *(pp. 116–119)*

CASE STUDY

1. **d.** Mr. Baker is in severe respiratory distress. His breathing rate is faster than normal at a rate of 26 breaths per minute, and his breathing quality is both labored (using accessory muscles) and noisy (audible wheezing and gurgling); in addition, his SpO_2 is 90 percent.

2. **d.** His skin is slightly cyanotic, cool, and moist. His bluish skin color indicates that he has inadequate oxygenation and poor perfusion. Cool, moist skin also indicates hypoperfusion.

3. **a.** His radial pulse is weak (thready) and irregular, which indicates that he is in shock (hypoperfusion). The rate of 50 beats per minute is slower than normal, which may also point to heart problems. An auscultated blood pressure at 80/50 mmHg also indicates hypoperfusion. Your impression is that his heart is not working very efficiently, and as a result his circulation is inadequate.

4. Signs and symptoms: Mr. Baker states that he can't breathe. Rapid, noisy (audible wheezing and gurgling), labored breathing. Skin is slightly cyanotic, cool, and moist. Weak, irregular pulse. Allergies: Mrs. Baker says that her husband has no allergies. Medications: Digoxin and Lasix taken daily, nitroglycerin as needed for angina. None today, according to wife. Pertinent past history: heart attack 5 years ago. Ate a bowl of soup at lunch; did not eat supper. Events leading to illness: shoveled snow this morning and since then has been increasingly short of breath but denied having chest pain.

5. **a.** Mr. Baker should have his vital signs reassessed every 5 minutes because he is an unstable patient, in severe respiratory distress, and showing signs of inadequate oxygenation and perfusion.

Chapter 6: Preparing to Lift and Move Patients

TERMS AND CONCEPTS

1. **a.** Body mechanics involves use of the most effective methods of gaining a mechanical advantage when lifting or moving; it also means use of lifting and moving techniques that help prevent injury. *(p. 125)*

2. **b.** In a power grip the palm and all fingers are in contact with the object, with all fingers bent at the same angle. *(p. 126)*

3. **c.** A power lift is done with feet apart, knees bent, back and abdominal muscles tightened, back straight, lifting force driven through feet and ankles, and the upper body rising before the hips. *(p. 128)*

CONTENT REVIEW

1. **a.** Reaching a great distance to lift a light object *(p. 129)*

2. **a.** Leg, hip, and gluteal muscles (avoid lifting with your back muscles; avoid reaching) *(p. 130)*

3. **b.** Keeping your shoulders, hips, and feet in vertical alignment *(p. 130)*

4. Flexibility training, cardiovascular conditioning, strength training, and nutrition. *(p. 125)*

5. **c.** Always try to lock the back. Lifting the upper body first reduces movement of the back. *(p. 127)*

6. **b.** Place the weaker leg slightly forward of the good leg *(p. 129)*

7. **a.** Leaning to the opposite side   *(p. 129)*

8. **d.** Use a spotter to direct and navigate *(pp. 139, 143)*

9. **c.** Twenty inches   *(p. 129)*

10. **b.** Push rather than pull; keep the load between hips and shoulder. *(p. 129)*

11. **a.** The patient that presents with neurological deficit should be carefully extricated from the vehicle; there were no other hazards in this case. All of the others should have been rapidly extricated from the vehicle to protect the patient and rescuers. The last patient stopped breathing and needed immediate treatment after rapidly extricating them from the vehicle. *(p. 132)*

CASE STUDY

1. **b.** Keep their backs locked and stay as close to the stretcher as possible, avoiding leaning

2. **c.** Lower the stretcher onto its wheels so the stretcher does part of the work, with the rescuers at the back pushing it along the boardwalk

3. All of these

4. **a.** The power lift is recommended for *all* patients, especially heavy patients.

Chapter 7: Airway Management, Ventilation, and Oxygen Therapy

MEDICAL TERMINOLOGY

1. **a.** Two, double
2. **c.** Dark blue
3. **b.** Surgical incision
4. **b.** Trachea
5. **d.** Opening

TERMS AND CONCEPTS

1. **a.** 3 **b.** 1 **c.** 18 **d.** 2 **e.** 5 **f.** 19 **g.** 22 **h.** 21 **i.** 20 **j.** 8 **k.** 16 **l.** 10 **m.** 13 **n.** 7 **o.** 6 **p.** 14 **q.** 15 **r.** 9 *(pp. 211–213)*

CONTENT REVIEW

1. **c.** In the infant and child the tongue takes up more space in the mouth and thus may occlude the airway. The nose and mouth are proportionately smaller in the infant and child. The cricoid cartilage is narrower and less rigid. The diaphragm and intercostal muscles do not effect the airway. *(p. 160)*
2. **A.** Mandible **B.** Thyroid cartilage **C.** Trachea **D.** Cricoid cartilage **E.** Nasal cavity **F.** Nasopharynx **G.** Soft palate **H.** Oropharynx **I.** Tongue **J.** Epiglottis **K.** Vocal cords **L.** Larynx **M.** Esophagus *(p. 155)*
3. **a.** The diaphragm also is responsible for approximately 60–70 percent of the effort involved in breathing. *(p. 157)*
4. **b.** The carina is the point at which the trachea splits and becomes the right and left mainstem bronchi. The bronchi continue to branch into the bronchioles and eventually into the alveoli. *(pp. 156, 211)*
5. **c.** Sweep the mouth with your *gloved* index finger. *(p. 164)*
6. To perform the head-tilt/chin-lift maneuver, place one hand on the patient's forehead, apply firm backward pressure, tilt the head backward, place the tips of the fingers of the other hand under the bone of the chin, and lift the chin. *(p. 164)*
7. **a.** Jaw-thrust maneuver *(p. 165)*
8. **d.** Neutral *(p. 165)*
9. **d.** All of these *(p. 167)*
10. **c.** Hard catheter *(p. 169)*
11. **c.** 15, 5 *(p. 169)*
12. **c.** Suction for 15 seconds, provide positive-pressure ventilation for 2 minutes, repeat *(p. 169)*
13. **c.** Measure from the level of the front teeth to the angle of the jaw. *(p. 171)*
14. **c.** The flange rests on the flare of the nostril. *(p. 171)*
15. **a.** Hypoxia is the medical term used to describe the insufficient oxygenation of the cells. Ventilation is the term used to describe the mechanical process of moving air into and out of the lungs. *(p. 179)*
16. In a patient who is breathing adequately, **a.** The rate will be within normal limits. **b.** The rhythm will be a regular pattern, with inhalations and exhalations about equal in length. **c.** The quality will include breath sounds that are equal and full bilaterally, with the chest rising and falling adequately and equally with each breath and no excessive accessory muscle use (children normally use abdominal muscles in breathing more than adults do). **d.** The depth, or tidal volume, will seem adequate as you feel and hear the breath with your ear next to the patient's mouth and nose and as you see the chest rise and fall adequately. *(p. 180)*
17. **c.** Cyanotic nail beds, skin, or mucous membranes are a late and severe sign of hypoxia. Restlessness, headache, and an altered mental status are all early signs of hypoxia; these are important to recognize so immediate treatment can be initiated to prevent severe hypoxia from developing. *(p. 159)*
18. Normal ranges are as follows: adult, 10–24; child, 15–30; infant, 25–50 respirations a minute. *(p. 159)*
19. **a.** Bilateral chest rise *(p. 177)*
20. **b.** The modified lateral (recovery) position should be used in the patient with an altered mental status in whom you do not suspect a spinal injury. Cricoid pressure is only indicated if you are ventilating the patient. A nonrebreather mask or oropharyngeal airway will not prevent aspiration. *(p. 167)*
21. **c.** Provide positive-pressure ventilation *(p. 176)*
22. **c.** It helps to reduce the regurgitation of the stomach contents into the lung tissue. Cricoid pressure is used only in the patient who is receiving positive-pressure ventilation. It is not tolerated by the responsive patient, even one with an altered mental status, and should not be performed unless the patient is being ventilated. *(p. 184)*
23. **b.** Exhaled oxygen contains about 16 percent oxygen, which is enough to oxygenate a patient with mouth-to-mouth or mouth-to-nose ventilation. *(p. 186)*
24. **b.** The rescuer must breathe into the mask; ventilations are not delivered automatically. *(p. 188)*
25. **a.** An adult should be ventilated every 5–6 seconds; an infant or child should be ventilated every 3–5 seconds. *(p. 188)*
26. **A.** Face mask **B.** Nonrebreathing patient valve **C.** Bag **D.** Intake valve/oxygen-reservoir valve **E.** Oxygen reservoir **F.** Oxygen-supply connecting tube *(p. 191)*
27. **c.** 21 percent (the same as atmospheric air) *(pp. 191, 201)*
28. **b.** It allows delivery of ventilations enriched from an oxygen source. *(p. 191)*
29. **c.** Establish in-line stabilization and perform a jaw-thrust maneuver, then ventilate. *(pp. 193–194)*
30. **d.** Improper use can cause severe damage to the lungs. *(p. 195)*
31. **a.** As soon as the chest begins to rise *(p. 195)*
32. **c.** Reevaluate the position of the head, chin, and mask seal *(p. 195)*

33. b. Consult with medical direction *(p. 196)*
34. b. Approximately 2,000 pounds per square inch *(p. 201)*
35. b. Petroleum jelly and some adhesive tapes *(p. 202)*
36. c. High-pressure regulator *(p. 203)*
37. c. Quickly open and shut the valve on the cylinder. *(pp. 202–203)*
38. b. Remove the mask from the patient's face, then turn off the oxygen. *(p. 205)*
39. d. 15 liters per minute (A lesser flow may not inflate the reservoir bag and may cause hypoxia.) *(p. 207)*
40. c. Have someone familiar with the child hold the mask close to the child's face. *(p. 208)*
41. a. When the patient will not tolerate a nonrebreather mask *(p. 208)*
42. a. 1–6 liters per minute *(p. 208)*
43. c. Nonrebreather mask *(p. 209)*
44. d. Leave them in the mouth for a better mask seal *(p. 201)*
45. d. Patients stricken by carbon monoxide poisoning may have an abnormally elevated SpO_2 reading, even though the patient is severely hypoxic. This inaccurate reading is due to the pulse oximeter's inability to distinguish between hemoglobin saturated with oxygen and hemoglobin saturated with carbon monoxide. The mass amounts of carbon dioxide attached to the hemoglobin will provide an erroneously high reading. This patient still needs high concentrations of oxygen. He is actually severely hypoxic. *(p. 204)*
46. b. The respiratory system responds primarily to changes in the carbon dioxide levels. Thus, it is said that healthy people breathe on a hypercarbic (high carbon dioxide) drive. When the carbon dioxide level decreases in the blood, the chemoreceptors sense this and send signals to the respiratory muscles to slow down the respiratory rate and depth, and the respirations return to normal. Oxygen is much less of a stimulus for changes in breathing in healthy people. *(pp. 158, 211)*
47. b. Oxygen. Because of the constant high carbon dioxide levels, the chemoreceptors are no longer really sensitive to the changes in carbon dioxide. The COPD patient's chemoreceptors must rely on the oxygen levels in the blood to regulate breathing. *(pp. 158, 211)*
48. c. You should immediately provide positive-pressure ventilations with the BVM that is attached to supplemental oxygen. Signs of inadequate breathing are tachypnea, bradypnea, or poor tidal volume. *(p. 176)*
49. d. *Never* place a patient in a prone position. Placing a patient in this position may reduce the effectiveness of ventilation by pushing the abdominal contents upward against the diaphragm, limiting its movement. This may lead to inadequate ventilation and severe hypoxia. *(p. 167)*
50. a. The vagus nerve may be stimulated, causing the patient to become bradycardic. *(p. 169)*

51. a. Respiratory rate and tidal volume *(p. 173)*
52. b. To increase the tidal volume (the amount of air breathed in and out) you should assist the patient's breaths by delivering a breath with the BVM each time the patient begins to breath in. There is no reason to increase the rate because the patient is breathing 12 times a minute. Increasing the tidal volume will help to reduce hypoxia. *(p. 173)*
53. c. This patient should receive ventilations at a rate of 8–10 breaths per minute because this patient is pulseless and CPR is initiated using the LMA. *(p. 188)*
54. d. You should immediately ventilate the newborn at a rate of 40–60 times each minute. *(p. 188)*
55. b. If the jaw thrust is ineffective in opening or maintaining an airway, use the head-tilt/chin-lift maneuver to ventilate the patient, even if the potential for a spine injury exists. Opening the airway and providing adequate ventilation is a priority in patients in cardiac arrest and takes precedence over other procedures. *(p. 190)*
56. a. The patient has a respiratory rate that is too fast (tachypnea), which leads to an inadequate tidal volume (hypopnea). You should initially assist the ventilation at the patient's rate by delivering the ventilation with each breath. Over the next 5–10 ventilations, slowly adjust the rate so that you are now ventilating every 5–6 seconds with one of the patient's breaths. Remember to reassure your patient. *(p. 198)*
57. c. You should select an infant or child mask for a good fit over the stoma. Suction should be limited to no more than 3–5 inches. Position the head in a neutral, comfortable position for the patient; position will not affect the airway in a stoma patient. Ventilations should be over 2 seconds; watch for chest rise. *(p. 199)*
58. b. Encourage the patient to cough to try to expel the object. Never perform a blind finger sweep. Do not try to reposition the head or administer abdominal thrusts. *(p. 201)*

CASE STUDY 1

1. Answers should include at least three of these indications: her position (upright, tripod position); that she is obviously anxious; her gasping breaths; her statement, "I can't breathe."
2. d. Nonrebreather mask at 15 liters per minute. Be prepared to assist ventilations with the bag-valve mask. (The Venturi and simple face masks are not recommended for prehospital use, and the nasal cannula should be used only if the patient will not tolerate the nonrebreather mask.)
3. a. Use a rigid catheter (with large bore), insert without suction, suction for 15 seconds (more time risks hypoxia).
4. c. Nasopharyngeal airway (responsive patient can't tolerate oral airway), bevel first (the other is upside down)

5. **b.** Continue to ventilate at a rate of 10–12 breaths each minute and suction as before. (She has a pulse, so CPR is not appropriate. Suctioning must be done so ventilations are effective. Check pulse often. If pulse becomes absent, begin CPR or defibrillation if available.)

CASE STUDY 2

1. **c.** In-line stabilization with jaw thrust. (This patient has a suspected spinal injury from the fall.)
2. **d.** Suction, using the rigid or hard catheter. (Turning the head may compromise the spine. Finger sweeps and soft French catheter are inadequate.)
3. **d.** Any or all of these could be the cause of the chest failing to rise with ventilations (as well as BVM failure or operator error).

Chapter 8: Scene Size-Up

TERMS AND CONCEPTS

1. **a.** T **b.** T **c.** M **d.** T **e.** M **f.** M (A medical condition is one brought on by illness or by substances or by environmental factors that affect the function of the body. Trauma is a physical injury or wound caused by external force or violence.) *(p. 231)*
2. **a.** 5 **b.** 1 **c.** 2 **d.** 4 **e.** 3 *(p. 237)*

CONTENT REVIEW

1. **a.** EMTs, patients, and bystanders *(p. 220)*
2. **d.** While receiving dispatch information *(p. 221)*
3. **c.** Protective gloves *(p. 220)*
4. **a.** Ask some bystanders to hold up a sheet *(p. 230)*
5. **d.** Call for additional resources *(pp. 220, 234)*
6. **a.** Consider all power lines to be energized until a power-company representative advises you they are not. *(p. 223)*
7. **b.** Notify your dispatcher and wait for a rescue crew *(pp. 224–225)*
8. **d.** Enter the scene only after it has been secured by police *(p. 226)*
9. **c.** Knock while standing off to the knob side *(p. 227)*
10. **a.** A large-caliber gunshot is considered a mechanism of injury, or what caused the injury. A laceration and a deformed and swollen wrist are both the result of a specific mechanism of injury. Hot and dry skin is considered a sign. *(p. 231)*

CASE STUDY 1

1. **d.** Stage your vehicle outside the scene, with no lights or siren, until scene safety is confirmed
2. **b.** Immediately call for additional transporting and ALS units
3. **c.** The patient is unresponsive. Don't touch the gun but notify the police. (The gun is not interfering with treatment, so there is no need to attempt to move it.)

4. **c.** Retreat temporarily until the police can give you support

CASE STUDY 2

1. Answers may include any three of the following: the address of the call gives a clue about whether this is or is not generally a safe neighborhood; "elderly" helps you to anticipate a geriatric patient; "cough for months" indicates a medical condition and alerts you to take BSI precautions; a husband calling about his wife may mean a relatively safe domestic environment; the fact that no one is presently answering the phone may indicate that the emergency is severe or that the caller is also ill.
2. **d.** Before entering the house, both EMTs should put on gloves, eye protection, and an N-95 or a HEPA respirator.
3. **a.** Because the patient presents signs of TB, you continue to wear the N-95 or HEPA respirator and advise the hospital of the precaution.

Chapter 9: Patient Assessment

MEDICAL TERMINOLOGY

1. **a.** pnea **b.** dys **c.** a **d.** icter **e.** ic **f.** quadri **g.** para **h.** hemi **i.** plegia

TERMS AND CONCEPTS

1. **a.** 13 **b.** 2 **c.** 7 **d.** 6 **e.** 4 **f.** 11 **g.** 12 **h.** 9 **i.** 10 **j.** 8 **k.** 1 **l.** 5 **m.** 3 *(p. 237)*

CONTENT REVIEW

1. **d.** The primary purpose of the patient assessment is to determine the illness or injury and to establish transport priorities. Comprehensive medical and trauma evaluations are not performed in the prehospital environment because such examinations may delay transport and result in increased patient morbidity and mortality. *(p. 242)*
2. **c.** The scene size-up and the initial assessment are the first two of the six components of patient assessment. *(pp. 241–242)*
3. **b.** Any of these techniques might be useful, but given the overt physical threats, the best course is to leave until the scene is controlled. *(p. 243)*
4. **b.** The patient has significant mechanisms of injury (hit by a car, laceration on forehead) for spine trauma. Bring the head to a neutral in-line position while maintaining in-line stabilization of the head and neck. The patient responds to questioning; therefore, his airway is assumed to be patent. *(p. 247)*
5. **c.** Until the patient is fully immobilized to a backboard *(p. 266)*
6. **c.** *Every* patient must receive an initial assessment. *(p. 242)*
7. **c.** The initial assessment is always performed in this sequence on all patients: Form a general impression, assess mental status, assess airway, assess breathing, assess circulation, establish patient priorities. *(p. 243)*
8. **a.** General impression *(p. 243)*

9. **d.** "Why did you call EMS today?" (or "What seems to be the problem today?") elicits the patient's own statement without suggesting an answer. *(p. 245)*

10. **d.** The patient is not alert but does respond to a verbal stimulus, a subtle yet important difference. *(p. 248)*

11. **c.** This patient responds to a verbal stimulus. Patients a and b respond only to a painful stimulus. Patient d is completely unresponsive. *(pp. 247–250)*

12. **b.** Appropriate methods of eliciting a pain response in an unresponsive patient include the use of central (trapezius pinch, supraorbital pressure, sternal rub, armpit pinch) or peripheral (nail-bed pressure; pinching the web between the thumb and index finger; pinching the finger, toe, hand, or foot) stimuli. *(p. 249)*

13. **a.** If the patient is talking to you, he is moving air in and out. Observing the speaking pattern also helps in assessing breathing status. *(p. 251)*

14. **b.** Relaxation of upper-airway muscles. The tongue and other soft tissues tend to fall back and cover the opening to the trachea. *(p. 251)*

15. **b.** Snoring respirations—use a head-tilt/chin-lift or jaw-thrust maneuver. If gurgling respirations are noted, quickly suction the airway. For snoring respirations use a head-tilt/chin-lift or jaw-thrust maneuver. For crowing respirations or stridor, avoid inserting anything in the airway, which could result in dangerous spasm of the airway. *(p. 251)*

16. **b.** Indications of a life-threatening breathing problem in an adult patient are cyanosis and deteriorating mental status. *(pp. 253–254)*

17. **c.** Positive-pressure ventilation can be delivered by bag-valve mask device, by mouth-to-mask, or by a flow-restricted, oxygen-powered ventilation device. The other devices listed are used to deliver oxygen passively to patients who are breathing adequately. *(p. 254)*

18. **c.** In a cold environment the vessels in the skin constrict to decrease the blood flow to the skin. In a hot environment the vessels in the skin dilate, causing the blood to be shunted to the skin. The alpha properties of circulating epinephrine cause the vessels in the skin to constrict (shunting blood away from the skin) and are responsible for stimulation of the sweat glands. Epinephrine (adrenalin) is released as a protective mechanism by the body during shock or hypoperfusion. Anemic patients take longer to become cyanotic when hypoxic. *(pp. 257–258)*

19. **b.** When assessing the pulse in the initial assessment, determination of the exact pulse rate is not required. It is important to determine if it is present or not, the approximate heart rate (fast, normal, or slow), and the regularity and strength of the pulse. *(p. 255)*

20. **c.** A peripheral (radial, brachial, or femoral) or central (carotid) pulse will not be felt if the systolic blood pressure is less than 60 mmHg. *(p. 256)*

21. **b.** The nail beds. Problems associated with environmental temperature, medical illnesses, and smoking can affect the color of the nail beds. *(p. 257)*

22. **a.** Cyanotic skin indicates reduced tissue oxygenation. Red skin may indicate anaphylaxis, vasogenic shock, or poisoning. Yellow skin may result from liver failure. Pale or mottled skin may result from a decrease in perfusion, such as might occur from blood loss. *(pp. 257–258)*

23. **d.** Cool, clammy skin is one of the major signs of shock (hypoperfusion). *(p. 258)*

24. **b.** Greater than 2 seconds (Two seconds can be counted by saying "One one-thousand, two one-thousand" or the words "capillary refill.") *(p. 258)*

25. All require rapid assessment and transport except 3 and 5. *(p. 261)*

26. **b.** Properly performed, the rapid trauma assessment takes only moments and should always be completed before moving the patient to the stretcher. *(p. 287)*

27. All are considered significant mechanisms of injury except 2 and 4. *(p. 265)*

28. **c.** Significant mechanisms of injury for an infant or child include a fall from a height greater than 10 feet, a vehicle collision at a medium speed, a bicycle collision, and a vehicle collision where the child was unrestrained. *(p. 265)*

29. **b.** For a trauma patient with significant mechanism of injury, altered mental status, suspected multiple injuries, or critical findings in the initial assessment, perform the focused history and physical exam in this sequence: rapid trauma assessment, baseline vital signs, SAMPLE history. *(p. 264)*

30. **d.** For a trauma patient with no significant mechanism of injury and no multiple injuries and who is alert and oriented, perform the focused history and physical exam in this sequence: focused trauma assessment, baseline vital signs, SAMPLE history. *(p. 264)*

31. **b.** The patient's Glasgow Coma Scale is 5 (eye opening = 1, verbal response = 1, motor response = flexion 3, total = 5). Immediately establish an airway and hyperventilate (at 20 pm in the adult), using positive-pressure ventilation, when possible head injury with signs of brain herniation is present (abnormal posturing, fixed or unequal pupils). *(pp. 267, 274)*

32. **a.** A patient with a Glasgow Coma Score of less than 8 has a severe alteration in brain function. It is an important finding if a patient with a potential head injury is unresponsive, then regains responsiveness for a short time, and then begins to exhibit a deteriorating mental status report. Time is the first orien-

tation to be lost in an altered mental status, and self is the last. *(p. 267)*

33. Deformities, contusions, abrasions, punctures/penetrations, burns, tenderness, lacerations, swelling *(pp. 268–270)*

34. **d.** The use of your sense of smell is missing from this list. *(p. 270)*

35. **c.** In assessing the neck, in addition to the "DCAP-BTLS" criteria, the EMT should inspect for jugular vein distention, tracheal deviation or tracheal tugging, subcutaneous emphysema, and posterior cervical muscle spasms. *(p. 277)*

36. **c.** Determine the presence and equality of breath sounds by auscultating the right and left chest at the apex and base of the lungs. *(p. 280)*

37. **a.** When assessing the abdomen during the rapid trauma assessment, the EMT should palpate for tenderness, distention, and rigidity. *(p. 281)*

38. **a.** The EMT should not palpate the pelvis when the patient complains of pain in the pelvic region or has obvious pelvic deformity. The other choices are not contraindications to palpating the pelvis. *(p. 282)*

39. **a.** "PMS" refers to indicators that circulation and nerve function to the extremities are intact: pulses, motor function, and sensation. *(p. 282)*

40. **a.** Log roll the patient while maintaining in-line stabilization. *(p. 283)*

41. **c.** Apply the CSIC (cervical spine immobilization collar) after the neck has been assessed. (You can't fully assess the neck with a collar on, although most have holes on the anterior surface to allow later inspection.) Remember that the CSIC does not fully immobilize the head and neck; therefore, manual in-line stabilization must continue to be maintained after CSIC is in place until the patient is fully immobilized to the long spine board. *(pp. 272, 278)*

42. **d.** Vital signs should be reassessed every 5 minutes in an unstable patient (every 15 minutes in a stable patient). This applies to both trauma and medical patients. *(pp. 285, 299, 302, 304)*

43. Signs and symptoms, allergies, medications, pertinent past history, last oral intake, events leading to the incident *(pp. 286–287)*

44. **c.** If there is a suspicion of other injuries, always perform a head-to-toe rapid trauma assessment. *(p. 290)*

45. **d.** The focused history and physical exam in the responsive medical patient should be performed in this sequence: SAMPLE history, focused medical assessment (focused on the area of the patient's complaint), vital signs. *(p. 292)*

46. **b.** The focused history and physical exam in the unresponsive medical patient should be performed in this sequence: rapid medical assessment (head to toe), vital signs, SAMPLE history. *(p. 292)*

47. **d.** In the rapid medical assessment, palpate the abdomen for tenderness, rigidity, distention, and pulsating masses. *(p. 297)*

48. **a.** When assessing the extremities during the rapid medical assessment, be sure to check around the hands, feet, and ankles for peripheral edema or swelling. *(p. 298)*

49. **a.** The vital signs are respiration, pulse, skin, pupils, blood pressure, and in many EMS systems pulse oximetery. *(p. 299)*

50. Onset, provocation, quality, radiation, severity, time *(pp. 302–303)*

51. **c.** The recovery position permits fluids to drain from the mouth of the unresponsive patient and helps prevent airway blockage or aspiration. Placing the patient on his left side ensures that he will be facing the EMT who is riding with him in the back of the ambulance. *(pp. 300–301)*

52. **b.** Gather both prescription and over-the-counter medications to bring to the hospital with the patient. Both will be important clues for hospital personnel. *(p. 301)*

53. **c.** If the patient doesn't have a specific complaint on which you can focus the physical exam, perform a head-to-toe rapid assessment. *(p. 303)*

54. **b.** If a patient is one who required a head-to-toe rapid assessment, he is also a candidate to receive a head-to-toe detailed assessment if time and the patient's condition permit. *(p. 305)*

55. **d.** It is important to determine the last oral intake when testing a patient's blood glucose level. A fasting blood glucose in the diabetic patient may be 120–140 mg/Dl. If an unresponsive medical patient requires ventilation, put him in a supine position. Pain is typically produced by ischemia, inflammation, infection, and obstruction. *(pp. 299, 300, 301)*

CASE STUDY 1

1. **c.** The patient is exhibiting signs of brain herniation. Hyperventilate at a rate of 20 ventilations per minute while maintaining in-line stabilization.

2. **a.** Rapid trauma assessment and, if possible, detailed physical exam

3. **c.** The presence of a pulse indicates that the patient has a blood pressure of *at least* 60 mmHg.

CASE STUDY 2

1. **a.** Y **b.** Y **c.** Y **d.** Y **e.** Y (All are clues to an airway problem in this patient.)

2. **c.** Head-tilt/chin-lift

3. **a.** In all patients, the EMT must assess the adequacy of both the respiratory rate and the tidal volume in order to determine if the patient is moving enough air per minute to sustain life. Either an inadequate respiratory rate or an inadequate tidal volume will require administration of positive-pressure ventilation.

4. **c.** Rapid medical assessment

5. a. 3 (eye opening = 1, verbal response = 1, motor response = 1, total = 3)

CASE STUDY 3

1. b. Suggest a task for the girlfriend.
2. c. Apply direct pressure, then a pressure dressing.
3. c. Focused trauma assessment (focused on the injury), vitals, SAMPLE history

CASE STUDY 4

1. b. SAMPLE history, including OPQRST questions to get a full description of the pain
2. d. Ask an open-ended question.
3. a. A focused medical assessment
4. b. The patient is responsive and has adequate breathing, so CPR and positive-pressure ventilation are obviously inappropriate. The patient did not refuse treatment but gave consent by saying, "As long as you're here, you may as well check me out." If he had refused, you would have tried to persuade him to accept treatment and transport.

CASE STUDY 5

1. b. Capillary refill should be checked in a child.
2. b. His symptoms are too generalized to permit a focused assessment.
3. b. The patient displays classic signs of shock (hypoperfusion), including a weak, rapid pulse and pale, cool, and clammy skin. A child with these signs is likely to deteriorate quickly. He is a high priority for rapid transport.
4. b. Oxygen by nonrebreather mask

Chapter 10: Communication

TERMS AND CONCEPTS

1. **a.** 3 **b.** 1 **c.** 4 **d.** 2 **e.** 5 *(p. 341)*

CONTENT REVIEW

1. d. The base station generally uses a high output of between 80 and 150 watts of transmission power, should be located in a high area to improve signal transmission, should be located in close proximity to the hospital that serves as the medical command center, and serves as a dispatch and coordination area that is in contact with other system elements. *(p. 331)*
2. a. Allow communications over a wide area *(p. 332)*
3. d. Cellular telephones within an EMS system usually have excellent sound quality, may become overwhelmed during disaster situations, are usually easily maintained, and are cost efficient and often improve communication privacy. *(p. 332)*
4. b. License base stations *(p. 333)*
5. b. Radio use must be brief, efficient, and professional, *not* as if talking on the telephone. Always listen for other radio traffic before transmitting, and use the "echo method" by

repeating information when receiving orders or information. *(pp. 333–334)*
6. c. Provide instructions about what to do until help arrives. *(p. 335)*
7. 1. Announce arrival on-scene. **2.** Announce departure from scene and ETA. **3.** Announce arrival at hospital. **4.** Announce you are clear and available for another call. **5.** Announce arrival back at base *(p. 335)*
8. d. The patient's mental status and, additionally, baseline vital signs, pertinent physical exam findings, description of care provided, the patient's response to the treatment provided, and the estimated time of arrival *(pp. 335–336)*
9. b. Repeat instructions back word for word *(pp. 335–336)*
10. a. Question the order *(p. 336)*
11. c. It is not necessary to obtain permission from police and fire personnel before beginning patient care. Obtain information while going to or at the side of the patient, and always ask for information about what happened and what care has been given. *(p. 337)*
12. a. See if a companion or a bystander can interpret; talking loudly and slowly does not help if the person doesn't understand English, although talking slowly might help if the person has limited English. *(p. 338)*

CASE STUDY

1. Report on arrival at the scene: "Unit 3 to Dispatch. We are on the scene at the playground at 1031 Bruce Road. Over."
2. Report en route to the hospital: "Washington Memorial, this is Green County BLS Unit 3 en route to you with an ETA of 12 minutes. We have a 3-year-old male with a 1-inch laceration to his chin due to a fall on the playground. He is alert and oriented. Mother reports no allergies. His vital signs are blood pressure 80/68 mmHg, pulse strong at 80, respirations 28 and of good quality with an SpO_2 of 96 percent on room air. His skin is flushed, warm, and moist. Capillary refill is less than 2 seconds. Pupils are normal. The wound has been dressed and bandaged. The bleeding is controlled. Patient reports injury 'hurts bad.' Over."
3. Report to the hospital personnel when transferring care: "This is Mikey Smith. He has a 1-inch laceration to his chin. Mrs. Smith reports that he has no allergies. We applied a dressing and a bandage. The bleeding is controlled. Current vitals: blood pressure is 80/68 mmHg, pulse 80, respirations 28, skin normal, pupils normal, SpO_2 of 96 percent on room air."

ENRICHMENT

1. a. Radio codes provide clear, concise information that shortens radio airtime. These codes are not regulated by the FCC and are generally not understood by the patient. *(p. 339)*
2. d. Ten-Codes, as well as other codes, have recently been abandoned by many EMS agencies in favor of the use of standard English.

Ten-Codes are published by the Association of Public-Safety Communications Officials (APCO), primarily for use by dispatch, although they are also sometimes used by other EMS personnel. *(p. 339)*

3. **c.** 2032 hours represents 8:32 PM. (Hours from 1:00 AM to noon = 0100 to 1200 hours; hours from 1:00 PM to midnight = 1300 to 2400 hours. To arrive at the military time representing 8:32 PM, add 832 to 1200 hours.) *(p. 339)*

Chapter 11: Documentation

TERMS AND CONCEPTS

1. **a.** 4 **b.** 2 **c.** 1 **d.** 3 *(p. 359)*

CONTENT REVIEW

1. **c.** To ensure the continuity of patient care *(p. 343)*

2. **a.** The documentation provided in the prehospital-care report (PCR) typically becomes a part of the patient's permanent medical record, is of great benefit in a lawsuit brought against the EMT, is frequently created in an electronic form, and is commonly used for preparation of bills and for submission to insurance companies. *(p. 344)*

3. **b.** The use of accurate and synchronous clocks is critical for proper EMS documentation of both dispatch needs and medical information needs. *(p. 348)*

4. **b.** Pertinent information about the scene (include only objective and pertinent subjective information) *(pp. 348–349)*

5. **c.** The patient denies back and neck pain. (These are symptoms that would be expected in this kind of accident, so the denial is a pertinent negative.) *(p. 349)*

6. **b.** At least two sets of vital signs should be obtained. Be sure to document the time taken and the patient's position when taken. *(p. 348)*

7. **b.** Patient information must not be given out to friends, reporters, or others who are merely curious. *(p. 350)*

8. **a.** When dealing with a patient that has refused treatment, document your explanation of possible consequences of failing to accept care, and have the patient sign the form acknowledging refusal of treatment. Discuss the situation with medical direction, complete as much of the assessment as the patient will permit, ensure that the patient is not under the influence of drugs or alcohol. Documentation of the call is generally more involved and frequently will be more difficult to document. The issue of patient competency is a primary concern of the EMT. *(p. 350)*

9. **a.** Objective information is measurable or verifiable in some way. A sign is an objective observation. A symptom is a subjective observation based on the individual's perception. A symptom a patient denies having is a pertinent negative. *(p. 348)*

10. **c.** Draw a single line through the incorrect entry and initial it. *(pp. 351–352)*

11. **a.** Triage tags *(p. 352)*

12. **a.** Additional special documentation by the EMT is required for suspected abuse of a child or an elderly patient, possible exposures to communicable diseases, and for injury to a member of the EMS crew. *(p. 352)*

13. **c.** Next of kin (usually the immediate family) is not included in the DOT minimum data set and does not usually appear on PCR forms. *(pp. 347–348)*

14. **a.** QID (four times a day) **b.** x (times) **c.** a (before) **d.** Pt (patient) **e.** Rx (prescription) **f.** q (every) **g.** Tx (treatment) **h.** c (with) **i.** STAT (immediately) **j.** s (without) **k.** PO (orally, by mouth) **l.** TID (three times a day) *(pp. 354–357)*

CASE STUDY

1. Patient-care report narrative section for this call: Fifty-year-old male complains that his right ankle is "a little sore" after slipping on a wet floor approximately one-half hour ago. Patient found to be alert and oriented, having no apparent difficulty breathing, and in no apparent distress. No signs of bleeding. Pulse is strong and regular. Skin is pink, warm, and dry. Focused physical exam reveals right ankle is markedly swollen, discolored, and very tender to gentle palpation. Pedal pulse is present. Good motion and sensation in injured extremity. Foot is slightly pale but warm to touch. Denies any other injuries. Vital signs: BP 138/78 mmHg, pulse 68, respirations 18 and adequate, PaO_2 on room air is 96 percent. Pupils normal. No allergies or medications. Patient denies any medical problems. Last meal (soup and a sandwich) about one-half hour earlier. States he felt fine all day but slipped on some water on the floor and twisted his ankle. Patient advised ankle should be splinted for transport to the hospital for evaluation and X-rays. Patient refuses, stating that his wife is already en route to take him to the doctor. Advised against weight bearing on injured ankle until evaluated by doctor. Encouraged to call 9-1-1 should any problems arise. B. Jones, EMT

2. **a.** The patient should review the patient-care report (PCR) and sign a refusal of treatment form. Be prepared to answer any questions that the patient may have.

3. **a.** You must not share any information pertaining to this patient with the safety officer. You should briefly and politely explain that legally you cannot discuss this case with him. Even giving what might seem like general information may be a violation of the patient's rights.

ENRICHMENT

1. **d.** The mnemonics SOAP, CHART, and CHEATED all help to organize information

on the prehospital-care report (PCR). Regarding response a., the mnemonic for the level of responsiveness is AVPU.
(*pp. 352–353*)

2. **d.** The "A" in the mnemonics SOAP, CHART, and CHEATED stands for "assessment" in each case, representing the assessment portion of information gathering.
(*pp. 352–353*)

Chapter 12: General Pharmacology

TERMS AND CONCEPTS

1. a. 2 b. 1 c. 3 d. 9 e. 6 f. 10 g. 8 h. 7 i. 5 j. 4 k. 11   (*p. 375*)

CONTENT REVIEW

1. **c.** Identified in local protocols   (*p. 364*)
2. **b.** Carried on the unit or prescribed for the patient   (*p. 364*)
3. **a.** Epinephrine   (*pp. 365–366*)
4. **c.** Ask a family member to retrieve the medication. (Never ask a patient to retrieve his medication. This activity could aggravate his condition.)   (*p. 365*)
5. **a.** The brand name is also known as the trade name.   (*p. 366*)
6. **b.** Isoetharine is also known by the trade name Bronkosol®.   (*p. 367*)
7. **b.** The trade name of salmeterol (generic name) is Serevent®.   (*p. 367*)
8. **d.** The sublingual route   (*p. 366*)
9. **a.** Shaken (The solids in a suspension will settle to the bottom.)   (*p. 367*)
10. **b.** Contraindications   (*p. 370*)
11. **a.** The six essential items of information are indications, contraindications, dose, administration, actions, and side effects.(*p. 369*)
12. **b.** Epinephrine is given by injection with a spring-loaded auto-injector. (Be careful to avoid a needle stick.)   (*p. 367*)
13. The correct sequence is 7, 1, 2, 4, 6, 3, 5. The correct sequence for administering a medication is: **1.** Obtain an order from medical direction. **2.** Ensure selection of the proper medication. **3.** Verify the patient's prescription. **4.** Check the expiration date. **5.** Check for discoloration or impurities. **6.** Verify the form, route, and dose. **7.** Document medication administration.   (*pp. 370–372*)
14. **a.** Package inserts, *AMA Drug Evaluation,* and the *Physician's Desk Reference* are common sources of medication information.   (*p. 373*)
15. Oxygen (*p. 367, Table 12-1*)
16. Oral glucose (*p. 367, Table 12-1*)
17. Altered mental status with diabetic history (*p. 367, Table 12-1*)
18. Poisoning, overdose (*p. 000, Table 12-1*)
19. Chest pain (*p. 367, Table 12-1*)
20. Nitroglycerin spray (*p. 367, Table 12-1*)
21. Chest pain (*p. 367, Table 12-1*)
22. Adrenalin® (*p. 367, Table 12-1*)
23. Proventil®, Ventolin® (*p. 367, Table 12-1*)
24. Alupent®, Metaprel® (*p. 367, Table 12-1*)

25. Breathing difficulty associated with respiratory conditions (*p. 367, Table 12-1*)
26. Isoetharine (*p. 367, Table 12-1*)
27. Breathing difficulty associated with respiratory conditions (*p. 367, Table 12-1*)
28. Serevent® (*p. 367, Table 12-1*)
29. Bitolterol   (*p. 367, Table 12-1*)
30. Breathing difficulty associated with respiratory conditions (*p. 367, Table 12-1*)
31. Xoponex (*p. 367, Table 12-1*)
32. Maxair   (*p. 367, Table 12-1*)
33. Breathing difficulty associated with respiratory conditions (*p. 367, Table 12-1*)
34. Brethaire   (*p. 367*)
35. Bayer, Ecotrin, Empirin, Acriptin, Bufferin, Buffex (*p. 367, Table 12-1*)
36. Patient experiencing chest pain or chest discomfort suggestive of an acute coronary syndrome (*p. 367, Table 12-1*)

CASE STUDY

1. **c.** Never administer medication unless prescribed to the patient and/or you are ordered to do so by medical direction.
2. **b.** False. The medications should not be administered to a patient who has an altered mental status.
3. **c.** Chest pain or chest discomfort suggestive of an acute coronary syndrome

Chapter 13: Respiratory Emergencies

MEDICAL TERMINOLOGY

1. **b.** Breathing
2. **d.** Fast
3. **a.** No, not, without, lack of
4. **d.** Bad, difficult, painful
5. **b.** Absence of breathing; respiratory arrest

TERMS AND CONCEPTS

1. a. 2 b. 7 c. 3 d. 6 e. 9 f. 1 g. 5 h. 8 i. 4 j. 10 (*p. 377*)
2. Apnea and respiratory arrest   (*p. 378*)

CONTENT REVIEW

1. **d.** A patient who is having difficulty breathing but has an adequate tidal volume and respiratory rate is in respiratory distress. Because the tidal volume and respiratory rate are still adequate, the patient is compensating and is in need of supplemental oxygen via a nonrebreather mask at 15 lpm.   (*p. 379*)
2. **c.** Hypoxia will cause the patient to become agitated and aggressive. Hypercarbia will cause the patient to become confused.   (*p. 381*)
3. **b.** Pale, cool, clammy skin is an early sign of hypoxia in the patient. Cyanosis is a clear but late sign of hypoxia.   (*p. 381*)
4. **a.** Severe respiratory distress   (*p. 380*)
5. **a.** Speaking a couple of words between breaths (*p. 409*)
6. **d.** Patient will be confused and disoriented. (*p. 381*)

7. **a.** Crowing, gurgling, snoring, and stridor all indicate a possible partial obstruction from secretions, blood, vomitus, or a foreign body. Clear the airway with suction, manual maneuvers, and airway adjuncts as needed. *(pp. 381, 395)*

8. **b.** May be in an acute state of hypoxia *(p. 381)*

9. **a.** Immediately begin positive-pressure ventilation. (A respiratory rate of 14 is below the normal respiratory range for children of 15–30 breaths per minute.) *(p. 397)*

10. **c.** Apply oxygen by nonrebreather mask at 15 lpm. *(p. 382)*

11. **d.** This patient is presenting with obvious signs of imminent respiratory failure and should be immediately treated with positive-pressure ventilation. *(p. 381)*

12. **a.** Following the initial assessment *(pp. 393, 401)*

13. **a.** A patient complaining of respiratory difficulty who is breathing 20 times a minute with adequate tidal volume should be placed on a nonrebreather mask at 15 liters per minute. Patients b, c, and d should all receive immediate positive-pressure ventilations. Simply put, any patient whose breathing is too fast (tachypnea) or too slow (bradypnea) or who has a poor tidal volume (amount of air moved in and out of the lungs, shallow breathing) in any combination must receive positive-pressure ventilations immediately. *(p. 407)*

14. **c.** The patient is working so hard to breathe that the tissues are being pulled inward. *(pp. 381, 384)*

15. **b.** Impending respiratory failure. Immediate and aggressive treatment is required. *(p. 385)*

16. **c.** Paradoxical motion (can cause ineffective ventilation) *(p. 387)*

17. **c.** When in doubt, provide positive-pressure ventilation with supplemental oxygen. Delays can permit rapid deterioration and adversely affect the patient's outcome. *(p. 387)*

18. **b.** A pulse oximeter reading (SpO_2) of less than 90 percent is a significant indication of severe hypoxia. *(pp. 385, 404)*

19. **1.** Provide oxygen first. **2.** Assess vital signs, which may reveal signs of severe respiratory distress such as elevated pulse or blood pressure. **3.** Pursue administration of a prescribed MDI, if the patient has one, to alleviate symptoms. **4.** Complete the focused history and physical exam. **5.** Place the patient in a position of comfort (most patients will find breathing is easiest in a sitting position) and transport to the hospital. *(p. 387)*

20. **a.** If your patient presents with a sudden onset of shortness of breath with decreased breath sounds to one side of the chest with no evidence of trauma, you should suspect a possible spontaneous pneumothorax. *(p. 407)*

21. **b.** Don't delay transport. Perform the ongoing assessment en route. *(p. 387)*

22. **b.** After the medication has been delivered, encourage the patient to try to hold his or her breath as long as possible. The canister should be shaken for 30 seconds prior to administration. The patient must inhale while the canister is depressed. Since the medication will be aimed into the mouth, the patient must breath through the mouth, not the nose, to take the medication into the lungs. *(p. 388)*

23. **a.** Use of accessory muscles, retractions during inspiration, grunting, tachypnea, tachycardia, nasal flaring, grunting, prolonged exhalation, frequent coughing, cyanosis in the extremities, and anxiety are signs of respiratory difficulty. A sore or hoarse throat is not a sign of respiratory difficulty. *(p. 394)*

24. **a.** See-saw or rocky breathing is a sign of respiratory failure. Loss of muscle tone or a limp appearance is associated with respiratory failure in infants and children. *(p. 394)*

25. **c.** Immediately initiate positive-pressure ventilation and transport. This is a dire emergency *(p. 394)*

26. **c.** Position of comfort to reduce the work of breathing and maintain an open airway *(p. 395)*

27. **b.** The child usually sits straight up, juts the neck out, and drools. Do not perform foreign body airway obstruction maneuvers if epiglottitis or other disease is suspected. These may seriously aggravate the condition. Foreign body maneuvers should be performed only if there is clear evidence that the child is choking and has not seemed to be ill. *(p. 395)*

28. **d.** Croup *(p. 395)*

29. **a.** Active exhalation requires the patient to use energy to exhale and force air from the lungs, leading to faster muscle fatigue and early respiratory failure. *(p. 384)*

30. **d.** Kussmaul's sign describes the distension of the jugular veins during inhalation and their return to normal during exhalation. This is an indication of a severely increased pressure in the chest or around the heart. *(p. 384)*

31. **b.** An extremely fast respiratory rate (tachypnea) will not allow enough time for the lungs to fill adequately. This will lead to an inadequate tidal volume and inadequate breathing. *(p. 402)*

32. **c.** Subcutaneous emphysema is an indication of an air leak in the chest or neck. Subcutaneous emphysema can be felt much easier than it can be seen on inspection. Due to gravity, the air will travel upward toward the neck and head in the patient who is in a seated position. *(p. 384)*

33. **a.** You should ventilate at 10–12 times per minute, imposing your ventilation over the patient's spontaneous breathing. *(p. 404)*

34. **d.** Beta 2 metered-dose inhalers also have Beta 1. The Beta 2 MDI has some Beta I properties, which is a side effect or a nondesired ef-

fect that will increase the heart rate. (p. 387)

CASE STUDY

1. **b.** Breathing is adequate, although respiration rate is at the high end of the normal range. However, patient is experiencing breathing difficulty and so should receive high-flow oxygen.
2. **a.** Provocation (what provokes the illness; what makes it better or worse)
3. **b.** The body attempts to make up for inadequate oxygenation. (Asthmatic attacks are usually sporadic with no symptoms between attacks; the range of normal respiration rates is the same for all adults; Albuterol should reduce a rapid breathing rate by improving oxygenation.)
4. **c.** Beta agonist, which relaxes the smooth muscle and dilates the airway
5. The indications for administration of an MDI are as follows: (1) the patient exhibits signs and symptoms of breathing difficulty; (2) the patient has a physician-prescribed metered-dose inhaler; and (3) approval has been given by medical direction to administer the medication.
6. **b.** Consult medication to consider re-administering
7. **d.** Fowlers or semi-Fowlers (sitting up with back straight or at a slightly reclining angle). This is usually the "position of comfort" for the patient, permitting the greatest ease of breathing.

ENRICHMENT

1. **b.** Pulmonary embolism is caused by an obstruction of blood flow in the pulmonary arteries caused by an occlusion. The reduction in blood flow leads to hypoxia.   (p. 404)
2. **a.** A spontaneous pneumothorax is a sudden rupture of the portion of the visceral lining of the lung, causing a partial collapse. This condition occurs without any type of penetrating or blunt trauma as its cause.   (p. 407)
3. **a.** Wheezing is best described as a high-pitched, musical whistling sound heard on inhalation and exhalation. Wheezing is an indication of swelling and constriction of the inner lining of the bronchioles.   (pp. 385–386)
4. **b.** The patient diagnosed with emphysema will often appear to have a barrel chest with an otherwise thin physique. These patients are more often males. The disease is characterized by the destruction of the alveolar walls and distention of the alveolar sacs.   (pp. 386, 396)
5. **d.** The patient in acute pulmonary edema should be kept in an upright sitting position and transported without delay. Laying the patient flat in a supine position could exacerbate the condition, increasing fluid buildup and difficulty with breathing.   (p. 406)

DOCUMENTATION EXERCISE

1. **b.** The patient's age does not play a role in whether a patient must be ventilated with positive-pressure ventilation. The decision to ventilate is based strictly on the patient's ability to breathe adequately or not. Mrs. Springer had obvious signs of respiratory failure, such as decreased air movement and increasing respiratory rate. She also displayed several signs of hypoxia, such as decreased mental status, cyanosis, and an abnormally low SpO_2 reading.
2. **a.** The bluish-gray color of the skin and mucous membranes is known as cyanosis. Cyanosis is a good indication of hypoxia and the need for immediate intervention.
3. **d.** The bubbly, crackling sound produced with inhalation is associated with the alveoli and terminal bronchioles' popping open with each inhalation. Crackles, also called rales, are associated with fluid in the lungs and may indicate pulmonary edema or pneumonia.
4. **b.** P—provocation, or what makes the symptoms worse. Lying flat made Mrs. Springer's breathing worse. Sitting upright on the edge of the bed improved her breathing.

Chapter 14: Cardiac Emergencies

MEDICAL TERMINOLOGY

1. **a.** per (through) **b.** atri (atrium) **c.** fus (pour) **d.** arter (artery) **e.** ion (process) **f.** ary (pertaining to) **g.** ven (vein) **h.** ventriculus (small cavity) **i.** infarct (necrosis of an area) **j.** myo (muscle) **k.** card (heart).

TERMS AND CONCEPTS

1. **a.** 2 **b.** 7 **c.** 9 **d.** 6 **e.** 10 **f.** 8 **g.** 4 **h.** 5 **i.** 1   (p. 462)
2. **a.** 2 **b.** 4 **c.** 3 **d.** 1   (pp. 438–440)

CONTENT REVIEW

1. **A.** Pulmonary artery **B.** Lung capillaries **C.** Pulmonary vein **D.** Veins **E.** Venules **F.** Bronchi **G.** Alveoli **H.** Arteries **I.** Arterioles **J.** Body capillaries   (pp. 415–416)
2. **b.** The heart (pumps the blood); the blood vessels (carry the blood); the blood (the fluid within the system)   (p. 415)
3. **c.** Hypoperfusion resulting from nervous-system interference creates a vascular system that is too large for the amount of available blood.   (p. 420)
4. **b.** Assess airway, breathing, circulation, skin   (p. 422)
5. **c.** Administer oxygen at 15 lpm by nonrebreather mask.   (p. 422)
6. **c.** Severity   (pp. 423–424)
7. **d.** A silent heart attack   (p. 425)
8. **a.** Sublingual   (p. 431)
9. **d.** The patient has a suspected head injury. Other contraindications include the following: the patient's baseline systolic blood pressure is below 90 mmHg systolic or the systolic blood pressure has decreased greater than 30 mmHg from the baseline; the heart rate is less than 50 beats per minute (bpm) or

greater than 100 bpm; the patient is an infant or a child; three doses have already been taken by the patient; or the patient has recently taken tadalafil (Cialis), vardenafil (Levitra), or sildenafil (Viagra).   *(pp. 431, 433, 434)*

10. b. The EMT's assessment and care is the same, no matter what the cause of the patient's chest discomfort or pain. (The EMT should not spend time trying to diagnose the cause of chest discomfort or pain. Administer oxygen; administer aspirin if allowed by local protocol; reassure the patient; consult medical direction regarding administering physician-prescribed nitroglycerin and requesting ALS backup; initiate early transport. Be alert for the occurrence of cardiac arrest, and should this occur, be prepared to perform defibrillation and CPR as appropriate.)   *(p. 426)*

11. a. Because of the potential for serious side effects, you should not administer nitroglycerin to a patient who is taking Viagra (sildenafil), tadalafil (Cialis), or vardenafil (Levitra). You should contact medical direction for specific orders.   *(pp. 427, 433)*

12. a. The requirements for placement of the AED are patients who are older than 1 year of age (for patients 1–8 years of age, a dose-attenuator system is preferred, but the adult AED may be applied) in cardiac arrest (no breathing, no pulse, and unresponsive to verbal or pain stimuli). The AED is not intended for cardiac arrest resulting from trauma.   *(p. 440)*

13. d. Respiratory compromise is a primary cause of death in infants and children.   *(p. 440)*

14. a. The components of the chain that are *most critical* to patient survival from cardiac arrest are high-quality cardiac compressions and early defibrillation.   *(p. 435)*

15. c. Defibrillation   *(p. 435)*

16. c. Ventricular fibrillation is the most common initial rhythm in sudden cardiac arrest.   *(pp. 438, 454)*

17. c. The AED, not the operator, administers the defibrillation.   *(p. 437)*

18. d. Survival from ventricular fibrillation, sudden cardiac arrest decreases by 7–10 percent for each 1-minute delay to patient defibrillation.   *(p. 435)*

19. d The AED is contraindicated in patients less than 1 year of age.   *(p. 440)*

20. c. There are three positions for electrode-pad placement. In the anteriolateral position, the sternum pad [−] is placed on the right upper border of the sternum; the top edge should be just below the clavicle. The apex pad [+] should be placed over the left lower ribs at the anterior axillary line (below and to the left of the nipple). In the anterior-posterior position, the sternum pad [−] is placed on either the upper left or right posterior thorax, and the apex pad [+] is placed over the left lower ribs at the anterior axillary line (below and to the left of the nipple). In the biaxillary position, the sternum pad [−] is placed on the right lower lateral thorax, and the apex pad [+] is placed over the left lower lateral thorax.   *(pp. 442–445)*

21. a. 6, 3, 1, 2, 5, 4, 7 (BSI and initial assessment; CPR and prepare AED; turn on power; attach cables and pads; begin narrative; stop CPR, clear, press button to begin analysis; clear patient and press button to deliver shock if indicated.   *(pp. 442–446)*

22. b. Stop the vehicle and turn off the motor during analysis. Deliver two (or three) shocks if required.   *(p. 446)*

23. d. Battery failure   *(p. 448)*

24. b. Refresher training and practice is recommended every 90 days, or 3 months.   *(p. 451)*

25. d. Contact with water, metal, and nitroglycerin patches are all safety hazards during AED operation.   *(p. 447)*

CASE STUDY 1

1. c. Nonrebreather mask at 15 lpm

2. b. Mr. Hansen is experiencing cardiac compromise and early transport is necessary

3. a. Reassure him that this is a common side effect of nitroglycerin and the headache pain should pass

4. b. Continue to evaluate him and to update the receiving facility (ongoing assessment)

CASE STUDY 2

1. b. Stop CPR, perform an initial assessment, and verify the absence of pulse/breathing.

2. b. Resume CPR and prepare the AED for operation.

3. d. After any "no shock" message, check the pulse and breathing and, if no pulse, resume CPR for 2 minutes (5 cycles of 30:2 compressions to ventilations), then initiate reanalysis.

CASE STUDY 3

1. c. If the downtime is less than 4–5 minutes or the arrest is witnessed, deliver a shock quickly. Attach the defibrillation pads, turn on the AED, and initiate the rhythm analysis.

2. d. If you are working alone, leave the patient briefly to call for help from EMS. You may also leave the patient to call EMS if the AED gives a "no shock" message, you detect a pulse, you have delivered two (or three) shocks, or other help arrives.

3. b. If the pulse returns, immediately check the breathing. Continued positive-pressure ventilation may be required for a time after the heartbeat has returned.

CASE STUDY 4

1. c. If, before ALS arrives, the patient regains a pulse, or you have given a total of two (or three shocks), or if the AED has given three consecutive "no shock" messages, transport. Do not wait for ALS arrival.

ENRICHMENT

1. **d.** The primary contributing factor to the development of coronary disease is the development of atherosclerosis. Atherosclerosis results in a reduction in the coronary arteries' internal diameter, a buildup of fatty plaque, and an inability of the coronary vessels to dilate. *(pp. 421, 451)*

2. **b.** Factors that affect the signs and symptoms and severity of acute coronary syndrome include the site of the occlusion, the artery occluded, how much blood the coronary artery supplies to the heart, the size or portion of the heart muscle not being supplied with oxygenated blood, and the length of time the artery has been occluded. *(p. 451)*

3. **b.** Collateral circulation develops in an attempt to move blood to areas that are lacking blood flow due to the occlusion. *(p. 451)*

4. **d.** Angina pectoris is a symptom of inadequate blood supply to the heart muscle. *(p. 452)*

5. **c.** The typical signs and symptoms of angina pectoris include steady discomfort in the chest, pain that rarely lasts longer than 15 minutes, nausea or vomiting, and a complaint of indigestion. *(p. 452)*

6. **a.** Appropriate emergency medical care for angina pectoris includes administering a patient's prescribed nitroglycerin, establishing an open airway and providing oxygen at 15 lpm, applying the pulse oximeter upon patient contact, and administering 160–325 mg of aspirin, if local protocol permits. *(p. 454)*

7. **b.** An acute myocardial infarction is infrequently the result of a coronary spasm, is commonly known as a heart attack, and involves heart-muscle death in about 20 minutes following occlusion. Myocardial infarction is defined as the death of heart muscle. *(pp. 453–454)*

8. **d.** In the patient suffering from acute myocardial infarction, ventricular fibrillation is the most common cause of cardiac arrest and usually occurs within the first hour following the onset of symptoms. Thrombolytic drugs will dissolve the clot and restore blood flow to the heart, preventing further damage, but they will not reverse damage that has already occurred, which is why early administration of these drugs is so important. Ischemic heart tissue can cause dysrhythmias. *(p. 454)*

9. The filled-in chart should appear as shown below and on the following page. *(pp. 341, 343–345)*

Sign/Symptoms	Acute Angina Pectoris	Myocardial Infarction	Heart Failure
Steady discomfort usually located in the center of the chest but may be more diffuse throughout the front of the chest	X	X	
Chest discomfort radiating to the jaw, arms, shoulders, or back	X	X	
Nausea or vomiting	X	X	
Severe dyspnea		X	
Cyanosis		XX	
Anxiety	X	XX	
Dyspnea	X	XX	
Signs and symptoms of pulmonary edema			X
Complaint of indigestion pain	X	X	
Distended neck veins—JVD (late sign)			X
Sense of impending doom		X	
Distended and soft, spongy abdomen			X
Tachypnea			X
Diaphoresis	X	X	X
Discomfort usually described as pressure; tightness; or aching, crushing, or heavy feeling	X	X	
Edema in the ankles, feet, and hands			X
Lightheadedness or dizziness		X	X
Fatigue on any exertion			X
Crackles and possibly wheezes on auscultation of the chest			X

Sign/Symptoms	Acute Angina Pectoris	Myocardial Infarction	Heart Failure
Tachycardia			X
Weakness		X	X
Upright position with legs, feet, arms, and hands dangling			X
Decreased SpO$_2$ (oxygen saturation) reading			X

10. **d.** Heart failure is categorized as right-sided or left-sided failure and can be caused by a valve disorder, hypertension, pulmonary embolism, and certain drugs. Right-sided heart failure frequently results in peripheral or dependent edema or swelling. Heart failure results when the heart no longer has the ability to adequately eject blood from the ventricle. (*pp. 453–455*)

11. **d.** Management of the heart-failure patient with pulmonary edema is similar to the treatment of the patient with an acute myocardial infarction. Treatment infrequently results in the development of a pneumothorax from positive-pressure ventilation treatment, although this may certainly occur. Treatment is not complicated by a common medication that heart-failure patients take, diuretics or "water pills." Drastic improvement following positive-pressure ventilation is possible. (*pp. 454–456*)

12. **b.** Depolarization is the stage when the heart muscle changes from positive to negative and causes the heart muscle to contract. Repolarization is the second stage, in which the electrical charges return to a positive charge and cause relaxation of the heart muscle. (*p. 457*)

13. **c.** The QRS complex is the second wave form and represents the depolarization or contraction of the ventricles. (*p. 457*)

14. **a.** The T wave is the third wave form in the normal ECG and represents the repolarization or relaxation of the ventricles (b is represented by the P wave, c by the QRS complex). (Repolarization of the atria is overshadowed by the QRS complex and so is not visible on the normal ECG.) (*p. 457*)

15. **b.** The PR interval is calculated from the beginning of the P wave to the beginning of the QRS complex. The PR interval represents the time it takes the heart's electrical impulse to travel from the atria to the ventricles. (*p. 457*)

DOCUMENTATION EXERCISE 2

1. **b.** Mr. Chambless is most likely suffering from an acute myocardial infarction. He is suffering from severe chest discomfort (9 or 10 in severity), pain in the center of his chest that radiates down the left arm that has been ongoing for at least 1 H hours.

2. **c.** The timing (over one-half hour in duration) and location of discomfort (mid-sternal) suggests an AMI.

3. **c.** Mr. Chambless's clenched fist positioned over the center of his chest is called Levine's sign.

4. **c.** The use of the AED on Mr. Chambless is inappropriate unless he becomes pulseless and breathless.

5. **c.** OPQRST method: onset, provocative/palliative, quality, radiation, severity, and timing.

DOCUMENTATION EXERCISE 3

1. **b.** Ventricular tachycardia (V-Tach) with a rate greater than 180 beats per minute will usually make the AED respond with a shock-advise message. However, some patients in V-Tach remain responsive. Since they are responsive, they are not appropriate candidates for defibrillation. (The rhythm detected by the AED after the first shock was ventricular fibrillation, or V-Fib.)

2. **d.** The AED is a very sensitive instrument and can sense spontaneous patient movement, movement of the patient by others, and engine vibrations. This movement can make the AED report inaccurately. Therefore, you should ensure that no one is touching the patient during this time, and if the patient is in the back of a moving ambulance, you should pull over, stop, and shut off the vehicle engine to gain an accurate message. Another reason to clear the patient is that anyone in contact during shock delivery may be injured.

3. **a.** According to the American Heart Association, the links in the Chain of Survival are early access, early CPR, early defibrillation, and early advanced life support.

Chapter 15: Altered Mental Status and Diabetic Emergencies

MEDICAL TERMINOLOGY

1. **d.** Sugar
2. **a.** Blood condition
3. **a.** Many, much, excessive
4. **b.** Urine
5. **c.** To eat, engulf

TERMS AND CONCEPTS

1. a. 4 b. 6 c. 2 d. 1 e. 5 f. 3   *(p. 464)*

CONTENT REVIEW

1. **d.** When the patient suffers from an altered mental status, this is an indication that the central nervous system has been affected. *(pp. 465–466)*

2. **c.** Stroke is considered a frequent medical cause of altered mental status. *(pp. 467–468)*

3. **d.** Blood-glucose meters or glucometers analyze glucose levels in the blood by obtaining a drop of capillary blood. The glucometers, widely used in EMS, are cost-effective, compact, and very portable. They measure blood glucose levels in milligrams per deciliter (mg/dl). Glucometers are widely used by diabetics because they are accurate and simple to use. *(pp. 471–472)*

4. **c.** A medical illness (An altered mental status may be caused by either traumatic injury or a medical illness, but a patient in bed with no evident mechanism of injury is likely to be suffering from a medical illness.) *(p. 468)*

5. **d.** Hyperglycemia can be defined as a blood-glucose level greater than 120mg/dl. Hypoglycemia (low blood-glucose level) is typically less than 60 mg/dl with signs and symptoms of hypoglycemia or less than 50 mg/dl without signs and symptoms of hypoglycemia. A normal BGL range is 80–120 mg/dl. *(p. 472)*

6. **b.** Flexion or extension posturing is commonly associated with trauma. The others are signs commonly associated with nontrauma or medical illness. *(p. 467)*

7. **a.** Ensure an open airway, provide high-flow oxygen by nonrebreather mask, place him in a lateral recumbent position, and transport. This is the recommended care for a patient with an altered mental status and no known history of diabetes controlled by medication. (Do not administer oral glucose unless the patient meets all three criteria for this medication: altered mental status, history of diabetes controlled by medication, and ability to swallow.) *(p. 487)*

8. **a.** Diabetes Type II is usually controlled by diet. Only in severe cases must insulin be administered. *(p. 482)*

9. **d.** When the blood-glucose level is decreasing, epinephrine (adrenalin) is released. This will produce the tachycardia, diaphoresis, and pale, cool skin typically seen in the hypoglycemic patient. Any of these may be true of the diabetic patient. *(p. 483)*

10. **d.** Your patient has a history of diabetes; asking whether the patient's family has a history of cancer will not likely help you assess this patient. You should ask, Did the patient take his medication the day of the episode? Did the patient eat (or skip any) regular meals on this day? Did the patient vomit after eating a meal on that day? Did the patient do any unusual exercise or physical activity on that day? *(p. 470)*

11. **c.** A diabetic emergency with signs and symptoms that mimic a stroke is a frequent occurrence in elderly patients. *(p. 474)*

12. **a.** A medical identification device indicating the patient has diabetes. *(p. 470)*

13. **b.** Determine if the patient can swallow. (Never give anything orally to a patient whose mental status is altered severely enough that he cannot swallow or protect his airway.) *(p. 474)*

14. **b.** Improvement after administration of oral glucose may happen quickly or may take 20 minutes or more. However, also be prepared for further deterioration of the patient's condition, and continually monitor the airway and breathing. Never insert anything in the mouth of a seizing patient. If oral glucose was administered with a tongue depressor and the patient seizes, immediately remove the tongue depressor. *(p. 474)*

15. **b.** Glucagon is a hormone that stimulates the breakdown of glycogen and allows the release of glucose molecules back into the blood. Glucagon does not contain sugar. *(p. 480)*

16. **d.** If a patient presents with signs of dehydration, check the blood-glucose level. Diabetic patients with high blood-glucose levels will have a tendency to lose large amounts of body water through excessive urination. *(p. 482)*

17. **a.** An altered mental status in the diabetic ketoacidosis patient is not from a lack of glucose to the brain but from dehydration and acidosis affecting the brain cells and causing dysfunction. *(p. 485)*

CASE STUDY

1. Probably a rapid onset if it occurred during jogging, anxious, speaks with inappropriate words, medical identification bracelet (insulin-dependent diabetic), episode follows a period of physical exercise, tachycardia (heart rate 104), skin cool and moist.

2. **b.** Nonrebreather mask at 15 lpm (Her breathing is adequate, so positive-pressure ventilation is not necessary at this time.)

3. **a.** The blood pressure is not one of the criteria for the administration of oral glucose. The three criteria for administration of oral glucose are as follows: (1) The patient must have an altered mental status: (2) The patient must have a history of diabetes controlled by medication: (3) The patient must be able to swallow.

4. In some jurisdictions, off-line medical direction allows the EMT Basic to administer oral glucose without direct consultation with medical direction, on the basis of standing orders or protocols. Some jurisdictions require on-line medical direction for the administration of oral glucose: approval given by radio or phone.

ENRICHMENT

1. b. Converting other noncarbohydrate substances into glucose is done by the hormone glucagon, not insulin. The other three choices are the main functions of insulin. *(p. 480)*

2. a. Glucagon's major role in the body is to raise and maintain the blood-glucose level. Glucagon converts liver glycogen and other substances into glucose to raise and maintain the blood-glucose level until the next meal. *(p. 480)*

3. b. In an elevated hyperglycemic state (above a BGL of 225 mg/dl), there is a large amount of glucose spilled into the urine from the kidneys. Glucose, a large molecule, draws water with it into the urine, resulting in the three Ps. *(p. 482)*

4. a. Type I diabetes mellitus patients most often have to administer insulin injections because their pancreas does not produce insulin. Typically, these patients are younger in age when diagnosed, most often under 40. They are usually lean from weight loss and are more likely to suffer from DKA and hypoglycemia. *(p. 482)*

5. d. The cells begin to burn fat for energy because glucose has collected in the blood. The BGLs are typically greater than 350 mg/dl, and signs of DKA usually do not occur for several days. Electrolytes in the body become unbalanced. *(pp. 482–484)*

6. c. Coma is a very late sign of DKA. All of the others are fairly early signs. *(pp. 484, 485, 486)*

7. c. The cells of the brain are not able to use proteins or fats for energy. Brain cells can only use glucose as fuel and will quickly suffer, shut down, and eventually die without it. *(p. 487)*

DOCUMENTATION EXERCISE

1. d. If the patient took his insulin and then forgot to eat, this would lead you to suspect the patient is hypoglycemic (low blood-glucose level). If the patient ate but did not take his insulin, you would suspect a hyperglycemic state (high blood-glucose level).

2. a. Acetone breath forms when the body has a buildup of ketones, which can be smelled in the patient suffering from diabetic ketoacidosis (DKA). The acetone smell may be mistaken for the smell of alcohol, but this patient is not intoxicated. Syrup of ipecac is not appropriate in this situation. DKA develops slowly, so unresponsiveness is probably not immediately impending.

3. c. Lowering the hand and warming the fingertips encourage better blood flow and produce a better blood sample.

4. d. Because the BGL is below 60 with signs and symptoms of hypoglycemia, this patient is considered to be hypoglycemic. A BGL of less than 50 without signs and symptoms of hypoglycemia is considered to be hypo-

glycemic. The normal range for a blood-glucose level is between 80 mg/dl and 120 mg/dl.

5. b. This patient met all three criteria before receiving the oral-glucose treatment (altered mental status, history of diabetes controlled by medication, ability to swallow). If your patient does not meet all of these criteria, oral glucose must not be given.

Chapter 16: Stroke

MEDICAL TERMINOLOGY

1. d. To speak
2. b. Bad, difficult, painful
3. d. Hardening
4. a. Half
5. b. Paralysis, stroke

TERMS AND CONCEPTS

1. a. 4 **b.** 2 **c.** 1 **d.** 3 *(p. 491)*

CONTENT REVIEW

1. a. Slurred speech *(p. 492)*

2. a. A stroke (which is a nontraumatic, or medical, brain injury) may result from any disruption of blood flow to the brain; for example, from a rupture to or blockage of a blood vessel in the brain. *(p. 494, with further explanation in the Enrichment section on pp. 502, 504)*

3. b. Chronic hypertension *(p. 493)*

4. b. Brain attack. An ischemic stroke is very similar to a heart attack. It has the same general cause (inadequate delivery of oxygenated blood because of a blood-vessel blockage) and the same level of seriousness as a heart attack. *(p. 493)*

5. c. Hypotension is a rare finding in the stroke patient. *(p. 501)*

6. b. An embolic stroke is another type of ischemic stroke that results from a piece of plaque or other material that breaks off from inside a vessel or within the heart and travels into the brain circulation until it becomes lodged in a cerebral vessel, cutting off distal circulation to brain tissue. *(p. 509)*

7. a. Weakness or paralysis affecting one side of the body *(p. 500)*

8. a. Administer positive-pressure ventilation with supplemental oxygen. *(pp. 501, 504)*

9. c. Lateral recumbent position (This will allow secretions to drain from the patient's mouth and help prevent aspiration when the patient cannot protect his airway. If the patient is responsive, place him in a supine position with head and chest elevated.) *(pp. 495, 501)*

10. d. One arm drifts downward *(p. 497)*

11. d. Perform an ongoing assessment every 5 minutes, paying close attention to airway, breathing, circulation, and mental status. *(p. 502)*

12. a. Elderly patients with a history of heart disease *(p. 494)*

13. **a.** Approximately one-third of those who suffer a transient ischemic attack (TIA) will go on to have a stroke. *(p. 495)*

14. **b.** Repeating a phrase with wrong or slurred words strongly suggests a stroke. *(pp. 496–497, 499)*

15. **d.** The elderly patient who has signs and symptoms of a stroke may, instead, be a diabetic who is suffering hypoglycemia. This patient may be a candidate for administration of oral glucose. The history of diabetes will also be important information for the hospital staff. *(pp. 497, 499)*

16. **d.** Time of onset is crucial information that must be relayed to the receiving hospital because clot-dissolving drugs can only be administered within 3 hours of the onset of the stroke. *(pp. 499, 500)*

17. **c.** Clot-dissolving drugs may be able to be given by the emergency department. *(p. 493)*

CASE STUDY

1. **a.** Place her on oxygen at 15 lpm by nonrebreather mask.

2. The victim of a nontraumatic brain injury may be suffering paralysis of the throat muscles, which will cause her to be unable to protect her airway, even if the airway is open. Vomiting is also a frequent consequence of a nontraumatic brain injury. Suctioning may be required to remove secretions or vomitus that the patient might aspirate.

3. **b.** Administer positive pressure ventilation at 10–12 ventilations per minute for the adult patient and 12–20 for the infant or child with the highest possible concentration of supplemental oxygen. (Extra oxygen can help prevent further deterioration of the injured brain. Since the patient is unresponsive with inadequate breathing, she cannot breathe on her own through a nonrebreather mask; positive-pressure ventilation is required to force the oxygen into her lungs.)

ENRICHMENT

1. **b.** Ischemic stroke is the type of stroke that occurs when a blood clot or other foreign matter blocks a cerebral artery. *(p. 502)*

2. **a.** Hemorrhagic stroke is the type of stroke that occurs from bleeding within the brain caused by a ruptured cerebral blood vessel. *(p. 502)*

3. **d.** Severe headache is a very common symptom of the hemorrhagic stroke. Onset is usually sudden with a rapid deterioration in mental status. Seizures and stiff neck are also common in this type of stroke. *(p. 503)*

DOCUMENTATION EXERCISE

1. **d.** This is a significant finding according to the Cincinnati Prehospital Stroke Scale. The patient not only slurred his words but used the wrong words. His apparent frustration can be caused by knowing what he wanted to say but being unable to do so.

2. **a.** A diabetic emergency can present with symptoms similar to those of a stroke. A normal blood-glucose level will help to rule out a diabetic emergency.

3. **a.** A stroke patient who can protect his airway should be placed with head elevated 15–30 degrees. If the patient's condition worsens so that he cannot protect his airway, he should be placed in the left lateral recumbent position. Also note that Cory has prepared the suction unit and BVM in anticipation that the patient may deteriorate.

4. **b.** Severe headache, sudden onset of symptoms, and history of hypertension treated by medication are all common indicators of hemorrhagic stroke. Seizures and stiff neck are also common with this type of stroke.

5. **c.** Establishing time of onset is crucial in order for hospital personnel to decide if clot-dissolving drugs can be administered. Although this patient has indications of suffering a hemorrhagic stroke, for which clot-dissolving drugs cannot be used, this decision must be made by hospital personnel. Our job is to gather appropriate information that can help hospital personnel with the decision process.

Chapter 17: Seizures and Syncope

TERMS AND CONCEPTS

1. **a.** 1 **b.** 5 **c.** 4 **d.** 2 **e.** 6 **f.** 7 **g.** 3 *(p. 510)*

CONTENT REVIEW

1. **a.** A head injury may cause a seizure in patients. *(pp. 510, 512)*

2. **a.** Aura—sensory perception that warns a patient a seizure is about to occur, sometimes described as a sensation that rises from the stomach toward the chest. Tonic phase—loss of responsiveness, followed by muscle contraction and rigidity. Hypertonic phase—extreme muscular rigidity with hyperextension of the back. Clonic phase—convulsions; jerky muscle activity. Postictal phase—recovery phase; confusion or disorientation to complete unresponsiveness, exhaustion, possible headache and weakness. *(p. 516)*

3. **d.** Postictal *(pp. 516–517)*

4. **a.** You should suspect a patient's seizure is triggered by a hypoglycemic state if the blood-glucose level is below 60 mg/dl. *(p. 515)*

5. **b.** Move objects away; guide the patient's movements. (Never place anything in the patient's mouth; it could break and cause airway obstruction. Do not attempt to restrain the patient, as this could cause injury.) *(p. 517)*

6. **c.** Following a generalized seizure, paralysis to one area or one side of the body may occur that may last up to 24 hours. This is known as Todd's paralysis and may indicate a space-occupying problem in the brain that is causing the seizure. *(p. 515)*

7. **b.** Positive-pressure ventilation and immediate transport are required for the status epilepticus patient.   *(p. 513)*
8. **c.** High fever   *(p. 522)*
9. **c.** The patient who has regained responsiveness between seizures (This patient still should be transported for evaluation at a medical facility but is not a high priority for immediate transport.)   *(p. 517)*
10. **b.** A typical fainting or syncopal episode is usually preceded by the patient's exhibiting yawning, diaphoresis, or nausea, or complaining of dizziness.   *(p. 517)*
11. **d.** The nasopharyngeal airway is soft and can be inserted when the teeth are clenched. A rigid oropharyngeal airway could break the teeth or be bitten off, risking airway obstruction.   *(pp. 513, 517)*
12. **b.** Lateral recumbent. The lateral recumbent position permits secretions to drain from the mouth and helps protect the airway and prevent aspiration. *(p. 517)*
13. **b.** The skin of a syncope patient is usually pale and moist.   *(p. 519)*

CASE STUDY

1. **a.** Guide body movements and move obstacles   *(p. 522)*
2. **d.** Positive-pressure ventilation with a nasopharyngeal airway in place and rapid transport (If Karl is in status epilepticus, positive-pressure ventilation is required. A nasopharyngeal airway cannot be bitten off as an oropharyngeal airway can.)   *(p. 513)*
3. The blood could have come from an injury from a fall or other mechanism; however, it often results when a seizing patient bites the tongue or cheek. Treat by suctioning.   *(pp. 512–513)*
4. **c.** Postictal   *(pp. 513, 514)*
5. **d.** Now that Karl is responsive, and since no head or spinal injury is suspected, place in a lateral recumbent position and administer oxygen by nonrebreather mask at 15 lpm.   *(p. 517)*

ENRICHMENT

1. **d.** The generalized seizure involves both hemispheres of the brain and usually renders the patient unconscious.   *(p. 521)*
2. **a.** The simple partial seizure, also known as a focal motor seizure or Jacksonian motor seizure, produces jerky muscle activity in one specific area.   *(p. 521)*
3. **d.** A febrile seizure is caused by a high fever (*febrile* means "feverish") and is most common in children between the ages of 6 months and 6 years.   *(p. 522)*

DOCUMENTATION EXERCISE

1. **b.** The grand mal or generalized tonic-clonic seizure usually presents with whole-body tonic-clonic movement. It is the most common type of epileptic seizure.
2. **b.** An aura is an odd sensation such as a sound, visual disturbance, smell, or taste that often precedes a generalized tonic-clonic seizure and warns the patient that a seizure is about to occur.
3. **c.** Status epilepticus is defined as a seizure that lasts longer than 10 minutes or seizures that occur consecutively without a period of responsiveness between the seizures. This is a dire emergency and requires immediate airway management and transport.
4. **a.** The postictal state is also known as the recovery stage, during which the patient may appear extremely tired, sleepy, weak, and disoriented. This stage may last 5–30 minutes or several hours. Supplemental oxygen should be administered during this stage.
5. **c.** Seizures may be caused by hyperglycemia or hypoglycemia. The glucometer will help to determine if the patient's blood-glucose level is too high, too low, or normal, as in this patient. Hypoxia can trigger seizures; the pulse oximeter is used to determine if the patient is hypoxic. Eclampsia is a complication of pregnancy. While seizures may occur with severe allergic reactions, a glucometer would not determine if there has been an allergic reaction.

Chapter 18: Allergic Reaction

TERMS AND CONCEPTS

1. **a.** 10 **b.** 2 **c.** 7 **d.** 5 **e.** 8 **f.** 4 **g.** 1 **h.** 9 **i.** 6 **j.** 3

CONTENT REVIEW

1. **a.** M **b.** S **c.** S **d.** M **e.** S **f.** S   *(p. 534, Table 18-3)*
2. **c.** Medications   *(p. 529)*
3. **c.** Allergens may enter the body by injection, ingestion, inhalation, or contact.   *(p. 529)*
4. **d.** The first time an antigen is introduced into the body chemical mediators are released and cause bronchoconstriction, *increased* capillary membrane permeability, and *vasodilation*. The treatment is the same as for anaphylaxis, and the patient will not have had a previous exposure.   *(pp. 528–529)*
5. **a.** Stridor or crowing indicates significant swelling to the upper airway, requiring positive-pressure ventilation.   *(p. 530)*
6. **a.** Deactivate the pop-off valve or cover it with your thumb in order to achieve adequate pressure to force air past swollen airway structures.   *(p. 530)*
7. **c.** Hives and itching are the hallmark signs of an allergic reaction.   *(p. 531)*
8. **d.** 20 minutes   *(p. 531)*
9. **b.** Respiratory compromise and/or shock must be present for an allergic reaction to be severe enough to be considered anaphylaxis. (Respiratory compromise is characterized by partial or complete airway occlusion, breathing difficulties, wheezing. Shock [hypoperfusion] may be indicated by absent or weak pulses, rapid heartbeat, decreased blood pres-

sure, and deteriorating mental status.) *(p. 533)*

10. a. Never underestimate the severity of an allergic reaction. Because death can occur within minutes, immediate intervention is imperative. Do not mistake anaphylaxis for conditions with similar signs and symptoms such as hyperventilation, anxiety attacks, alcohol intoxication, and hypoglycemia. *(p. 533)*

11. b. Common substances that cause anaphylactoid reaction include radiopaque contrast media, nonsteroidal anti-inflammatory drugs (NSAIDs), aspirin, opiates, and thiamine. *(p. 529, Table 18-1)*

12. b. Histamine release results in bronchoconstriction, vasodilation, and increased capillary membrane permeability. *(p. 527)*

13. d. Anaphylaxis is a major medical condition with a high mortality rate. It causes blood vessels to dilate, which decreases the blood pressure to dangerously low levels. It affects the entire body from the release of histamine by the immune system. Positive-pressure ventilation of the patient may be difficult due to severe bronchoconstriction and swelling of the airway. *(pp. 533, 534, 543, 536, 537)*

14. c. Signs and symptoms of severe allergic reaction including respiratory distress and/or shock (hypotension). *(pp. 536, 542)*

15. d. The upper airway is also likely to be swollen. *(p. 533)*

CASE STUDY

1. d. Although she looks well and is not having difficulty breathing, the patient's skin is flushed, she feels a "lump" in her throat, and her stomach "feels upset"— all early signs of anaphylaxis.

2. d. Airway and breathing compromise and poor perfusion

3. d. Excessive mucus in the lower airways

4. b. If the anaphylactic reaction is continuing to develop, coughing and hoarseness may occur along with other signs and symptoms.

DOCUMENTATION EXERCISE

1. a. Hives and itching are the hallmark signs of an allergic reaction.

2. a. Bronchoconstriction and swelling in the lower airway cause breathing difficulty and possible hypoxia.

3. c. The auto-injector is administered at the midpoint of the lateral thigh.

4. b. Headache and nausea are among the common side effects of epinephrine. Headache may also be a symptom of allergic reaction, but since Mr. Kendrick has had an injection of epinephrine, a recurrence of allergic symptoms is not likely.

5. d. The epinephrine may be administered directly through the patient's clothing, if necessary.

Chapter 19: Poisoning Emergencies

TERMS AND CONCEPTS

1. a. 5 (or 6) b. 3 c. 1 d. 2 e. 6 f. 4

CONTENT REVIEW

1. d. More than 1 million poisonings occur each year in the United States. Most poisoning emergencies result from accidental exposure and involve young children. Toxicology is the study of toxins, antidotes, and the effects of toxins on the body. Poisoning is commonly defined as an exposure to a substance other than a drug or medication. *(p. 548)*

2. c. Request assistance from a trained hazmat team. *(p. 558)*

3. c. A likely indicator of poisoning is chewed-up plants near a child patient. *(p. 552)*

4. c. While all of these things might eventually be done at the scene of a poisoning emergency, the medical priority is to maintain the patient's airway. *(p. 564, Figure 19-12A)*

5. c. Poisons may cause airway and breathing compromise as a result of alteration of mental status, respiratory depression, and direct damage to the airway tissues. *(p. 558)*

6. d. The most common inhaled poisons include carbon monoxide and carbon dioxide from industrial sites, sewers, and wells. Inhaled poisons cause thousands of deaths each year, not millions, and occur most often as a result of fires. Long exposure times to inhaled poisons are associated with poor, not good, survival rates. *(p. 555)*

7. c. Inhaled poisoning as a result of "huffing" paint. *(p. 555)*

8. a. Y b. Y c. N d. Y e. N f. N *(p. 553)*

9. b. Prevent further injury by rinsing the substance from his mouth and lips. Be careful when rinsing the mouth that the patient does not swallow the liquid. *(p. 554)*

10. c. Activated charcoal inhibits the absorption of poisons. *(p. 554)*

11. a. Activated charcoal is indicated for ingested poisons, when ordered by medical direction. *(p. 554)*

12. b. Activated charcoal is indicated for a 3-year-old who is responsive and crying after ingesting an unknown medication. (Crying indicates an open airway and a responsive patient.) The other choices are incorrect because activated charcoal administration is contraindicated by an altered mental status or for ingestion of caustics such as bleach. *(p. 555)*

13. c. The usual adult dosage of activated charcoal is 30–100 grams (1g/kg of body weight). *(p. 556)*

14. c. Actidose is a brand name for activated charcoal. *(p. 556)*

15. **b.** Activated charcoal is contraindicated in ethanol, ammonia, and food poisoning. (*p. 556*)
16. **a.** Blackened stool (Common side effects of activated charcoal include blackened stool, nausea, and vomiting. Other side effects are rare.) (*p. 557*)
17. **c.** Fire-related incidents (*p. 555*)
18. **b.** Difficulty breathing (*p. 558*)
19. **b.** An appropriate action in the management of toxic inhalation is to remove the patient to fresh air as soon as possible. This should be done by properly trained and equipped rescuers. (*p. 558*)
20. **a.** Prevent exposure to yourself from any poisons that may be absorbed through the skin. Wear protective gloves and ensure that the patient is properly decontaminated prior to transport. Chemical burns to the eye should be irrigated. Clothing and jewelry should be removed if contaminated. Dry powder should be brushed away. (Contact medical direction to see if this action should be followed by flushing.) (*p. 561*)

CASE STUDY

1. **a.** If you are not wearing a self-contained breathing apparatus or have not been properly trained for a hazardous material rescue, withdraw and request assistance. If you are properly trained and equipped, remove Mr. Johnson from the workshop and into fresh air as quickly as possible.
2. **a.** When Mr. Johnson is removed from the area, spinal immobilization should be maintained; an airway ensured; breathing checked; positive-pressure ventilation provided, if needed; and tight clothing loosened.
3. **a.** Y **b.** Y **c.** Y **d.** Y **e.** Y. All the actions are appropriate. A rapid trauma and/or medical assessment may be indicated. A complete physical exam should be completed to determine if any traumatic injuries are present.
4. **a.** Mr. Johnson requires an ongoing assessment every 5 minutes during transport to the hospital.

ENRICHMENT

1. **d.** Food poisoning does not commonly result in death, is increasing in incidence from prior years in the United States, is often caused by tainted seafood, and is difficult to detect because the signs and symptoms vary greatly. (*p. 556*)
2. **c.** Carbon monoxide poisoning is caused by an odorless gas that is difficult to detect. It decreases the amount of oxygen carried on the hemoglobin, which inhibits the ability of body cells to utilize oxygen. It causes thousands of deaths each year in the United States. (*pp. 556–557*)
3. **b.** Carbon monoxide poisoning should be suspected if flulike symptoms are shared by people in the same environment. The other

choices are not associated with carbon monoxide poisoning. (*p. 567*)
4. **d.** Cyanide can enter the body through inhalation, absorption, injection, or ingestion. It is found in many household products, including rodent poisons and silver polish, and in cherry and apricot pits. Inhalation can occur in fires where plastics, silk, and synthetic carpets are burning. (*pp. 567–568*)
5. **d.** The smell of bitter almonds is most closely associated with cyanide poisoning. (*p. 567*)
6. **c.** Strong acids have an extremely low pH; if ingested, they will cause the most severe burns in the stomach, producing severe and immediate abdominal pain. They will typically burn for only 1–2 minutes. (*p. 568*)
7. **c.** Alkalis have a high pH, will produce burns that are deeper than acid burns, will typically burn for minutes to hours after contact, and if ingested will likely injure the stomach tissue. (*p. 568*)
8. **b.** Hydrocarbon poisoning frequently involves children; toxicity is dependent upon the viscosity of the substance; activated charcoal is ineffective in treatment; and examples of products include kerosene, naphtha, turpentine, and mineral oil. (*p. 569*)
9. **d.** Methanol is also known as wood alcohol. It is commonly found in Sterno, paint removers, and windshield washer fluid. Poisoning can occur by ingestion, inhalation, or absorption. Ingestion will produce large amounts of acid in the body. (*p. 569*)
10. **b.** Isopropanol acts as a respiratory depressant. It is also known as isopropyl alcohol or rubbing alcohol, and poisoning occurs most frequently by ingestion. Isopropanol is found in cosmetics, degreasers, disinfectants, and solvents. (*p. 570*)
11. **a.** Ethylene glycol is commonly found in detergents, radiator antifreeze, and windshield de-icers. Poisoning occurs frequently in children due to its sweet taste. Poisoning occurs in three distinct stages, and activated charcoal may be recommended for treatment. (*pp. 570–571*)
12. **d.** About 75 percent of all Americans are allergic to urushiol, the poisonous element in poison ivy. For a reaction to occur, contact with poison ivy need not occur directly. Poison sumac is found mostly in the Southeast and West. Stinging nettle, crown of thorns, and buttercup can cause mild to severe dermatitis. (*p. 571*)
13. **c.** Poison-control centers are staffed and available for service 24 hours a day, 7 days a week; are able to provide information on any poisons; provide follow-up telephone calls to patients to monitor progress; and should routinely be consulted by the EMT when poisoning is suspected. Prior to providing treatment, be sure to contact medical direction for approval of treatment. (*p. 571*)

DOCUMENTATION EXERCISE

1. **c.** The blood pressure is not generally assessed in children less than 3 years of age. Better determinants of adequate perfusion in this age group are mental status, pulse, and skin temperature and color.

2. **a.** Activated charcoal acts to prevent absorption of the poison.

3. **b.** There is no one best answer to this question. Mrs. Wilson was clearly upset. By giving Mrs. Wilson a task it relieves her of her anxiety and calms the situation. Children at Jimmy's age most commonly will react to strangers and will not want to have the parent leave the room. In this case a good rapport was established and the mother could be of assistance in treating Jimmy and gathering information.

Chapter 20: Drug and Alcohol Emergencies

TERMS AND CONCEPTS

1. **a.** 5 **b.** 1 **c.** 3. **d.** 4 **e.** 2   *(p. 593)*

CONTENT REVIEW

1. **b.** The goals at the scene of a drug or an alcohol emergency are the identification and treatment of potential life threats, such as airway or breathing compromise. Treatment should never be delayed to identify the substance. *(p. 577)*

2. **a.** Three potential dangers at any drug or alcohol emergency scene are infectious disease, violent behavior, and weapons. *(p. 557)*

3. **b.** Transport the pill bottles to the emergency department with the patient. *(p. 557)*

4. **b.** Drug and alcohol emergencies may mimic many different medical and traumatic disorders, not just a few. These scenes are frequently the site of violent acts and physical abuse. Every scene demands the routine use of body substance isolation techniques. *(p. 557)*

5. **d.** Of the choices provided, the best answer is to ask bystanders about any events that may have precipitated the episode. *(p. 581)*

6. **a.** N **b.** Y **c.** N **d.** Y **e.** Y **f.** Y **g.** N **h.** N *(p. 580, Figure 20-2)*

7. **c.** Scene size-up and patient history *(p. 577)*

8. The emergency-care steps for the disoriented patient who reports overdose (or, in general, for any drug or alcohol emergency patient) are (1) establish and maintain a patent airway; (2) administer oxygen at 15 lpm by nonrebreather mask or positive-pressure ventilation with supplemental oxygen; (3) maintain body temperature; (4) if protocol permits, assess the blood-glucose level; (5) transport. *(p. 582)*

9. **a.** Hallucinogenic substances often produce a psychological emergency that may present as intense anxiety or paranoia ("bad trip"), depression, disorientation, or an inability to differentiate fantasy from reality. They may also present with tachycardia, dilated pupils, motor disturbances, and flushed face. PCP may cause paralysis, violence, rage, and status epilepticus. *(p. 578, Table 20-1)*

10. **b.** Touch can be comforting, but invading the drug- or alcohol-abuse patient's "personal space" can trigger a violent response. Always establish rapport, and obtain the patient's permission before touching him. *(p. 583)*

11. **a.** You should first "talk down" the patient and calm before transporting. Elements of the talk-down technique for the potentially violent patient who is suffering a "bad trip" include (1) Making the patient feel welcome; remaining relaxed and sympathetic. (2) Identifying yourself clearly and establishing rapport before touching the patient. (3) Reassuring the patient that his condition is caused by the drug and will not last forever. (4) Helping the patient verbalize what is happening to him. (5) Making simple statements to help orient the patient to time and place; encouraging him to feel more secure by helping him identify where he is and what is happening. (6) Forewarning the patient about what he may experience as the drug wears off. (7) Transporting the patient after he has been calmed. *(p. 583)*

12. **b.** Central-nervous-system-stimulant drugs typically cause dilated pupils, while narcotics cause pinpoint pupils. *(pp. 581–582)*

13. **c.** Bradycardia, hypotension; inadequate breathing rates and volume; cool, clammy skin; constricted pupils; and nausea are most commonly associated with narcotics. *(pp. 581–582)*

CASE STUDY

1. **b.** The first priority is to make sure the airway is clear while simultaneously assessing the breathing.

2. **c.** Activated charcoal would not be indicated for this patient because of the patient's altered mental status.

3. **b.** The patient is a priority transport and requires careful assessment of the patient's respiratory status, a complete physical exam, vital signs, an ongoing assessment every 5 minutes, and transport of a sample of the vomitus, pill bottles and the wine bottle to the hospital.

ENRICHMENT

1. **b.** The physically dependent drug user experiences a strong need to use the drug repeatedly, considers the drug constantly, and will experience severe physiological consequences of drug withdrawal. Tolerance of the drug may develop, in which larger and larger doses are needed. *(p. 587)*

2. **d.** Common signs and symptoms of drug withdrawal include nausea, abdominal cramping, tremors, anxiety, agitation, confusion, hallu-

cinations, and elevated heart rate and blood pressure. *(p. 587)*

3. **b.** A chronic brain syndrome resulting from the toxic effects of alcohol on the central nervous system combined with malnutrition is called Wernicke–Korsakoff syndrome. *(p. 588)*

4. **c.** The alcoholic syndrome consists of a combination of problem drinking and true addiction to alcohol. *(p. 587)*

5. **d.** Withdrawal syndrome occurs when the alcoholic's alcohol level falls below the amount usually ingested. The more the alcoholic was drinking, the more severe the syndrome will be. *(pp. 588–589)*

6. **d.** Stage 1 of alcohol withdrawal occurs within about 8 hours and is characterized by nausea, insomnia, sweating, and tremors. Stage 2 begins within 8–72 hours and is characterized by worsening of Stage 1 symptoms and hallucinations. Stage 3 occurs within 48 hours and is characterized by major seizures. Stage 4 is characterized by delirium tremens. *(p. 589)*

7. **b.** Delirium tremens is the last stage of alcohol withdrawal and is a life-threatening condition with a mortality rate between 5–15 percent. *(p. 589)*

8. **b.** Phencyclidine (PCP) is cheap to make and produces horrible psychological effects that can last for years. It is known by multiple names, such as angel dust, killer weed, supergrass, crystal cyclone, and many others. *(p. 589)*

9. **d.** Cocaine is now the drug most commonly involved in emergency-department visits. Its use in the United States has increased significantly. Cocaine may be inhaled through the nose, injected into the veins and muscles, or smoked (crack or free based). The treatment is generally the same as for PCP use. *(p. 589)*

10. **c.** The first priority of care for a patient under the influence of PCP is to protect the safety of yourself and your response crew. This is also true of cocaine. *(p. 591)*

11. **d.** Poisons intentionally inhaled commonly contain the chemical agent toluene, decrease the movement of oxygen across the alveolar membrane, have a more rapid onset of symptoms than injected poisons, and accumulate in the regions of the brain responsible for feelings of pleasure. *(p. 591)*

12. **c.** Methamphetamine is a stimulant; its use is increasing among teenagers; it is commonly called crystal meth; and it is used by ingestion, inhalation (snorting), and injection. *(p. 592)*

DOCUMENTATION EXERCISE

1. **b.** The signs or symptoms of potential LSD use that Ed was exhibiting include motor disturbances (shaking hands), dilated pupils, and hallucinations (hearing voices).

2. **c.** The technique Bonnie used is called the talk-down technique. It is appropriate for patients who have used hallucinogens or marijuana. This technique can help you reduce the patient's anxiety, panic, depression, or confusion.

3. **a.** The talk-down technique should not be used if the patient has taken PCP (phencyclidine). PCP causes paralysis, violence, and rage. The talk-down technique would not be useful for managing these patients and would likely further agitate them.

4. **a.** Y **b.** Y **c.** Y **d.** Y **e.** Y **f.** Y. Bonnie accomplished each step with her patient.

5. **a.** Personal safety is of utmost importance. If one is uncomfortable entering a scene or a scene becomes unsafe, evacuate the area and request law enforcement.

Chapter 21: Acute Abdominal Pain

TERMS AND CONCEPTS

1. **a.** 10 **b.** 4 **c.** 6 **d.** 8 **e.** 2 **f.** 3 **g.** 1 **h.** 12 **i.** 5 **j.** 7 **k.** 9 **l.** 11 *(p. 612)*

2. **a.** 10 **b.** 2 **c.** 8 **d.** 5 **e.** 6 **f.** 3 **g.** 9 **h.** 7 **i.** 4 **j.** 1 *(pp. 596–597)*

CONTENT REVIEW

1. **A.** Diaphragm **B.** Umbilicus **C.** Right upper quadrant (RUQ) **D.** Right lower quadrant (RLQ) **E.** Left upper quadrant (LUQ) **F.** Left lower quadrant (LLQ) *(p. 597)*

2. **A.** Hypogastric Region **B.** Umbilical Region **C.** Epigastric Region **D.** Right Iliac Region **E.** Right Lumbar Region **F.** Right Hypochondriac Region **G.** Left Hypochondriac Region **H.** Left Lumbar Region **I.** Left Iliac Region *(p. 597)*

3. **b.** The parietal (somatic) nerve fiber stimulation produces a sharp, intense, constant pain that can be pinpointed. The parietal nerve is associated with inflammation of the peritoneal lining of the abdomen. The visceral nerve produces an intermittent, generalized, dull, aching pain that is caused by ischemia, inflammation, or mechanical obstruction of the affecting organ. The phrenic nerve arises from the cervical roots down to the thorax to control breathing. The optic nerve is located behind the eye. *(pp. 599–600)*

4. **a.** Acute abdominal pain, acute abdomen, or acute abdominal distress *(p. 598)*

5. **b.** Consider the patient with abdominal pain to have a life-threatening condition until proven otherwise. *(p. 601)*

6. **d.** The position with knees drawn up is called a guarded position and is typically assumed by a patient with abdominal pain. *(p. 601)*

7. **a.** A criterion for priority transport of the acute abdomen patient is *any* of the following: (1) poor general appearance, (2) unresponsive, (3) responsive but not following commands, (4) shock (hypoperfusion), and (5) severe pain. *(p. 602)*

8. d. Certain types of bleeding do have a distinct smell that can sometimes be identified as you arrive at the patient's side. Patients with abdominal pain are likely to faint, usually in the bathroom. You should look for mechanisms of injury to rule out trauma as the cause of the abdominal pain. Bloody vomitus is not always present in the acute-abdomen patient. *(p. 605)*

9. a. Have the patient point to the area of the pain and palpate this quadrant last. *(pp. 599–600)*

10. c. Bloody vomitus or blood in the stool is the most likely sign associated with acute abdomen. *(p. 606)*

11. d. Never give anything by mouth (which can be vomited and aspirated) to an acute-abdomen patient. A supine position with legs flat is usually not comfortable for the acute-abdomen patient. Ongoing assessment should be performed every 5 minutes for the unstable patient. You should palpate the painful area last. *(p. 606)*

12. a. Cholecystitis, which is inflammation of the gall bladder. The other choices are not associated with acute abdomen. *(p. 609)*

13. a. Peritonitis. A modified Markle test that elicits a positive response indicates the patient may be suffering from peritonitis. *(p. 600)*

14. d. A narrowing pulse pressure (the difference between the systolic and diastolic blood pressure) with an increased heart rate and pale, cool, and diaphoretic skin is a sign of internal bleeding in the abdomen. *(p. 605)*

CASE STUDY

1. d. Remember the indicators of a serious medical emergency. This patient is displaying a poor general impression, a diminished mental status (slow to respond to questions, does not look at you when you enter), signs of hypoperfusion (rapid, weak pulse; cool, clammy skin; diminished mental status; nausea), and the patient is in severe pain.

2. c. Ask her to point with one finger to the area that is the most painful. Start with the area that is least painful. Palpate each abdominal quadrant of the abdomen, the most painful quadrant last.

3. a. Emesis (vomitus) should be saved for possible testing at the hospital.

4. c. This patient is an unstable patient who requires careful monitoring. Ongoing assessment should be performed at least every 5 minutes.

DOCUMENTATION EXERCISE

1. d. Severe "ripping or tearing" abdominal pain radiating to the back, inequality of femoral pulses, and a pulsating mass are all findings associated with an abdominal aortic aneurysm (AAA).

2. d. An aortic aneurysm can result in obstruction of blood flow to the femoral arteries, which

can yield complete or partial obstruction of blood flow.

3. d. Careful palpation was important in this case as deep or rough palpation could have ruptured the aneurysm.

4. a. Abdominal aortic aneurysm occurs in 20 percent of men over 50 years of age.

Chapter 22: Environmental Emergencies

TERMS AND CONCEPTS

1. 1. a. 1 **b.** 5 **c.** 2 **d.** 7 **e.** 10 **f.** 4 **g.** 13 **h.** 3 **i.** 11 **j.** 14 **k.** 6 **l.** 8 **m.** 9 **n.** 12 *(pp. 649–650)*

CONTENT REVIEW

1. d. The five basic mechanisms by which the body loses heat are radiation, convection, conduction, evaporation, and respiration. Which mechanism commonly leads to the greatest heat loss? Radiation: It accounts for 55–65 percent of heat loss. *(p. 617)*

2. b. Generalized hypothermia (also called generalized cold emergency) and local cold injury *(p. 619)*

3. a. Factors that may place a patient at greatest risk for developing generalized hypothermia include a cold environment, age (very old and very young), medical conditions (recent surgery, head injury, burns, generalized infections), and drugs and alcohol. *(p. 619)*

4. a. 4 **b.** 5 **c.** 1 **d.** 3 **e.** 2. The correct sequence is (1) Shivering, (2) Apathy and decreased muscle function, (3) Decreased level of responsiveness, (4) Decreased vital signs, (5) Death. *(p. 622, Figure 22-5)*

5. a. Emergency care for generalized hypothermia includes quickly but carefully removing the patient from the cold environment, administering warmed and humidified oxygen by nonrebreather mask at 15 lpm (or positive-pressure ventilation if required), and rewarming the patient as quickly and safely as possible. Do not allow the patient to exert himself in any way (including walking about). A quick clinical check of the patient's temperature is accomplished by the EMT's placing her hand on the patient's abdomen. Follow local protocols for specific guidelines. *(p. 627)*

6. b. Appropriate techniques for active rewarming include avoiding rewarming the unresponsive patient or a patient who is not responding appropriately. The body temperature should not be increased by more than 1°F per hour. Never immerse the patient in a hot tub of water or place in a hot shower. Heat is first applied to the torso rather than the extremities. *(pp. 627–628)*

7. a. 10 minutes (Make sure you familiarize yourself with normal spring, summer, and fall river, lake, and—if nearby—ocean temperatures in your area. Body temperatures can drop rapidly in what you *think* is relatively warm water.) *(p. 620)*

8. **d.** Guidelines for the emergency medical care of the patient with immersion hypothermia includes lifting the patient from the water in a horizontal position, asking the patient to make as little effort as possible to stay afloat until you reach him, removing the patient's wet clothing carefully and gently. Treatment is similar to generalized hypothermia management. *(p. 628)*

9. **b.** The stages of local cold injury are early (superficial) and late (deep). *(p. 622)*

10. **d.** Appropriate management of local cold injuries includes not rubbing or massaging the affected skin, not removing clothing that is frozen to the skin, avoiding the initiation of thawing if refreezing is possible, and carefully removing clothing and jewelry. *(p. 629)*

11. **d.** Guidelines for the rapid rewarming of local cold injuries includes maintaining the water temperature between 100°F and 110°F and dressing the area with a sterile, dry dressing. Rewarming is reserved for those with a delayed transport time with no chance of refreezing of tissue. The tissue should be kept in warm water until it is soft and skin color and sensation return to the affected part. *(p. 629)*

12. **b.** Hyperthermia *(p. 630)*

13. **a.** Factors that increase an individual's reaction to a heat-related injury include heart disease and various medical disorders such as kidney disease, cardiovascular disease, Parkinson's disease, thyroid disease, skin diseases, and dehydration. Hot temperatures, strenuous activity, extremes of age, and certain drugs and medications are additional predisposing factors. *(p. 634)*

14. **d.** Hot skin—either moist or dry—signals a dire medical emergency in a patient who has been exposed to heat. (In early stages of hyperthermia, the skin will be cool to the touch. If the skin is hot, hyperthermia is in an advanced and life-threatening stage. In about half the cases, the patient with hot skin will still be sweating. In the remainder of cases, sweat mechanisms will have shut down.) *(p. 637)*

15. **c.** When cooling a heat-emergency patient with hot skin, moist or dry, cooling takes priority over all other emergency-care procedures *except* management of the patient's airway, breathing, and circulation. One cooling method will generally not be effective to cool the patient; multiple methods are required. Be prepared to manage seizures and to prevent aspiration, and place cold packs in the patient's groin, at each side of the neck, in the armpits, and behind each knee to cool the large surface blood vessels. *(p. 637)*

16. **b.** If the patient is unresponsive (or has an altered mental status) or is vomiting, do not give fluids orally. *(p. 637)*

17. **d.** Most often the only time a hyperthermic patient with moist, pale skin that is normal to cool in temperature needs transport is if the patient is unresponsive or has an altered mental status, is vomiting or nauseated and will not drink fluids, has a history of medical problems, the body core temperature is above 101°F, or the patient's temperature is continuously rising. *(p. 637)*

18. **c.** The first step for any heat-emergency patient with cool or hot skin is to move the patient to a cool place such as the back of an air-conditioned ambulance or at least out of the sun and into the shade. *(p. 637)*

19. **c.** A rapid increase or decrease in the pulse with a decline in the patient's mental status is a grave finding. *(p. 638)*

20. **b.** Snake bites are uncommon and result in a small number of fatalities each year. Exercise special caution during the scene size-up to protect yourself from a bite or sting. Complications associated with airway and breathing difficulties occur infrequently but do occur. Most insect bites result in minor reactions, not major anaphylactic reactions. *(p. 638)*

21. **d.** Urban hypothermia occurs in individuals who live outdoors and are unable to escape the cold environment and in the elderly who attempt to reduce their home-heating bills. It is not limited to northern climates during the winter months and can occur in indoor temperatures of between 70 and 72°F. It occurs in individuals with a predisposition, disability, illness, or medication usage that renders them more susceptible to hypothermia. *(p. 620)*

CASE STUDY 1

1. **b.** Remove as much clothing as possible as quickly as possible.

2. **c.** Begin to cool the patient by one or a combination of the following methods: pour tepid water over the patient's body, place cold packs on the patient's groin, side of the neck, armpits, and behind each knee; wrap the patient in a wet sheet; fan the patient; keep the skin wet.

3. **d.** The use of cold water should be avoided in this patient because it may produce vasoconstriction and shivering.

CASE STUDY 2

1. **b.** Avoid the application of heat packs or cold packs and prevent the patient from moving about. The area should be washed with a mild agent or strong soap solution.

2. **a.** Lower the injection site slightly below the level of the heart and watch closely for signs of anaphylaxis. Cutting and suctioning of the site is not recommended. Epinephrine would not be administered unless the patient had a current prescription for the epinephrine, the patient was showing signs and symptoms of anaphylaxis, and you have authorization from

medical direction to administer the medication.

3. d. The patient must be observed closely for signs of developing anaphylaxis. These signs include respiratory distress, hives, and hypotension; all are signs of anaphylaxis.

CASE STUDY 3

1. c. Take longer than normal to assess the pulse in a hypothermia patient; the pulse may be present but extremely slow.
2. b. This patient is unresponsive, so passive (not active) rewarming should be utilized. Seek medical direction and follow local protocols.
3. d. Handle the patient gently. Keep the patient supine to improve blood flow to the brain. Ventilation of the patient is indicated at a normal rate; unnecessary hyperventilation can cause cardiac complications.

CASE STUDY 4

1. c. The signs and symptoms of early or superficial local cold injury include blanching of the skin, loss of feeling or sensation, continued softness of the skin in the injured area, and tingling sensation during any rewarming. Swelling and blisters would indicate later or deep cold injury.
2. a. Appropriate treatment for this patient includes removal of wet or restrictive clothing, not massaging the area, administering oxygen at 15 lpm, and splinting the area.
3. b. You must prevent the occurrence of refreezing of the tissue. Significant tissue loss can occur if the tissue is subjected to refreezing. All the other items are true except for using a moist, sterile dressing. Use a dry, sterile dressing.

ENRICHMENT

1. c. Lightning-strike injuries result in about 1,000–5,000 deaths per year, occur most frequently on Sundays, occur mostly in recreation and work-related situations, and typically involve one victim rather than multiple victims. *(p. 643)*
2. a. Lightning-strike patients are considered both medical and trauma patients, should be routinely spinal immobilized, are infrequently struck while talking on the telephone (2.4 percent of strikes), and can commonly suffer damage to the body's air-containing cavities. *(pp. 643–645)*
3. b. Dislocations and fractures associated with lightning strikes result from the thunder "blast wave," which results in a propelling or throwing of the patient, and strong muscular contractions. *(pp. 643–645)*
4. b. Coral snakes and pit vipers contribute to most snakebites in the United States today. The pit vipers include rattlesnakes, copperheads, and water moccasins. *(pp. 643–645)*
5. b. The signs and symptoms of a pit-viper bite are immediate and are gauged by how much poison was injected. The patient's size and weight are also factors. *(pp. 645–646)*

6. a. P b. P c. N d. N e. N f. P *(p. 645)*
7. a. The black widow spider has a shiny black body, thin legs, and a crimson red hourglass marking on its abdomen. *(p. 646)*
8. a. General signs and symptoms of a black widow spider bite include severe muscle spasms in the shoulders, back, chest, and abdomen. *(p. 646)*
9. c. The brown recluse spider bite is a serious medical condition and can result in severe tissue damage and necrosis at the site of the bite. *(pp. 646–647)*
10. a. Venom of aquatic organisms is destroyed by the application of heat. *(p. 647)*
11. d. Myxedema coma may make a person more susceptible to becoming hypothermic, occurs late in the progression of hypothyroidism, occurs in only about 0.1 percent of all hypothyroidism patients, and is precipitated by exposure to cold, a recent illness, or infection and trauma. *(pp. 642–643)*

DOCUMENTATION EXERCISE

1. c. Mrs. Holland is most likely suffering from heat stroke, which has a mortality rate that ranges from 20 to 80 percent.
2. a. The cooling of Mrs. Holland was appropriately performed.
3. d. A combination of factors allowed Roger to make the decision that Mrs. Holland was a priority transport. The hot air temperature with high humidity; headache; and flushed, hot, and dry skin all played a factor in Roger's decision. However, the presence of hot, dry skin, when combined with the other factors, is most important.
4. a. Roger and Katy did not provide any cool water for Mrs. Holland to drink. It is contraindicated due to Mrs. Holland's nausea and altered level of consciousness.
5. b. An air temperature of 95°F and a relative humidity of 75 percent represent a severe danger on the heat-and-humidity risk scale.

Chapter 23: Drowning and Diving Emergencies

TERMS AND CONCEPTS

1. a. 4 b. 3 c. 1 d. 2 *(p. 667)*

CONTENT REVIEW

1. b. Death from drowning is often associated with the use of alcohol. Drowning does not occur only in deep water, and the incidence would be reduced by use of personal flotation devices and supervision at swimming pools. *(p. 653)*
2. b. The two major age groups that are at most risk of death from drowning are children less than 5 years of age and teenagers. The third most common group is the elderly. *(p. 653)*
3. c. A drowning in which the victim does not aspirate water into the lungs is referred to as a dry drowning. *(p. 653)*

4. b. A patient with an altered mental status and a persistent cough would be considered symptomatic.   *(p. 658)*

5. c. Abdominal thrusts or the Heimlich maneuver should be used on drowning victims only if a foreign body airway obstruction is suspected.   *(pp. 653, 660)*

6. c. Rescue attempts near shore should be tried in this safest-to-riskiest sequence: Reach (by holding out an object), throw (something that floats), row (get a boat), go (wade or swim). Wade or swim only if you meet *all* of the following criteria: You are a good swimmer, you are specially trained in water rescue, you are wearing a personal flotation device, you are accompanied by other rescuers.   *(p. 655)*

7. a. An unresponsive patient found in shallow water should be suspected of having a spinal injury. (The other choices are also possible, but spinal injury should be your primary suspicion.)   *(pp. 653, 657, 666)*

8. c. Attempt resuscitation with full efforts. (Young patients submerged in cold water (<41°F) for 30 minutes or longer have been resuscitated.) Some experts advise resuscitation for every drowning patient regardless of water temperature. Resuscitation efforts should always be performed in an "all-or-none" manner. Resuscitate the patient fully or don't resuscitate the patient. So-called "show codes" or "slow codes" are not appropriate.   *(pp. 654, 657)*

9. d. Differences between salt-water and fresh-water drowning play no role in the goals and techniques of resuscitation. Approximately the same amount of surfactant is washed out in either case, and they result in the same incidence of respiratory distress.   *(p. 654)*

10. c. Mammalian diving reflex   *(pp. 654–657)*

CASE STUDY 1

1. d. Let's hope you didn't have to think much about this one! Begin resuscitation at once!

2. b. All the clues to possible spinal injury are present. You found the patient at the shallow end of the pool. The patient has a laceration on her forehead. These are signs that she may have dived into the pool and struck her head. Observed bleeding is minor. Checking for gastric distention may be necessary if positive-pressure ventilations are noted to be ineffective. This patient is not breathing on her own, so oxygen by nonrebreather mask is not appropriate.

3. d. Gastric distention occurs when the stomach fills with water (during submersion) or air (during artificial ventilation). The air or water in the stomach may put enough pressure on the diaphragm and lungs to interfere with the ability to ventilate the patient. If the patient is immobilized, roll the immobilized patient on her side and, with suction equipment immediately available (because the patient is likely to regurgitate stomach

contents), gently press on the epigastric region to relieve the distention. Suction the mouth and nose and then resume ventilation efforts. If the patient is not yet immobilized, roll her on her left side with manual stabilization of her spine and perform the procedures described above.

CASE STUDY 2

1. d. Complications from near-drowning can occur up to 72 hours after the incident. Even though this patient looks well now, he must be transported for evaluation by a physician.

2. b. Administer oxygen, monitor carefully, and transport on his left side to allow drainage in case he vomits.

3. b. This patient would be placed in the symptomatic category.

ENRICHMENT

1. c. Scuba-diving emergencies are increasing in incidence along with the popularity of the sport. They do not occur only near oceans; a diver can be far away from the ocean by airplane before symptoms occur. Scuba divers can drown. Scuba emergencies may be managed by the EMT as well as the paramedic.   *(p. 650)*

2. a. Boyle's law states that at a constant temperature the volume of a gas is inversely related to the pressure.   *(p. 662)*

3. a. Decompression sickness results from bubbles formed by the expansion of nitrogen in the blood. These can act as emboli and block circulation but do not reduce oxyhemoglobin loading. Decompression sickness is exacerbated by high altitudes and is more likely to occur in cold water than in warm water.   *(p. 664)*

4. c. The joint where the pain associated with decompression sickness is most commonly experienced is the shoulder, beginning as a mild pain and gradually increasing.   *(p. 664)*

5. The chart showing signs and symptoms associated with the three categories of decompression sickness should be filled out as follows.   *(pp. 664–665)*

Sign or Symptom	Type 1 DCS	Type 2 DCS	AGE
Pain in joints or tendons	X	X	X
Low back pain		X	
Skin rash, itching	X	X	X
Altered mental status		X	
Substernal burning sensation on inhalation		X	
Dyspnea		X	X
Headache, visual disturbance		X	X
Bloody sputum		X	X
Nausea and vomiting		X	X

6. b. The "squeeze" or barotrauma occurs during either ascent or descent as air pressure in body cavities becomes too great and damages tissues in these cavities. Rapidity of ascent exacerbates decompression sickness rather than barotrauma. Hypertension is not related to barotraumas. *(p. 665)*

DOCUMENTATION EXERCISE

1. c. Treatment and management should be focused on drowning, hypothermia, and traumatic injuries.

2. a. Laryngeal spasm occurs in 10–20 percent of cases and results in what is called a dry drowning.

3. d. The cold water could trigger the mammalian diving reflex, which results in laryngeal spasms, inhibition of breathing, slowing of the heart rate, and blood-vessel constriction.

4. a. Appropriate management of immersion hypothermia includes careful removal of wet clothing, the use of blankets, and moving the patient to a warm environment.

5. c. Deaths due to complications from immersion up to 72 hours after the immersion occur in 15 percent of immersion cases.

Chapter 24: Behavioral Emergencies

TERMS AND CONCEPTS

1. **a.** 7 **b.** 1 **c.** 9 **d.** 4 **e.** 2 **f.** 3 **g.** 8 **h.** 6 **i.** 5 *(p. 686)*

CONTENT REVIEW

1. a. N **b.** Y **c.** N **d.** Y **e.** N **f.** Y **g.** Y *(p. 671)*

2. a. A panic attack often presents with an overwhelming fear that is accompanied by rapid breathing. Patients often hyperventilate (breathe too deeply), which causes physical symptoms such as dizziness, tingling around the mouth and fingers, spasms of the hands and feet (carpal–pedal spasms), tremors, irregular heartbeat, palpitations (rapid or intense heartbeat), diarrhea, and sometimes feelings of choking, smothering, or shortness of breath. *(p. 671)*

3. c. Deep feelings of sadness and worthlessness accompanied by fatigue, loss of appetite, and a sense of hopelessness may be due to depression. *(p. 672)*

4. b. Schizophrenia is the term that is given to a group of mental disorders that present with bizarre delusions, hallucinations, and social withdrawal. *(p. 672)*

5. a. Y **b.** N **c.** Y **d.** Y **e.** Y **f.** N **g.** Y **h.** Y *(p. 673)*

6. d. When dealing with behavioral emergencies, it is important to understand that all individuals are susceptible to emotional injury, but each person has a greater ability to cope with crisis than he may believe. All individuals are affected, in some way, by disaster or injury. An emotional injury is just as real as a physical injury. *(p. 673)*

7. a. Careful and complete documentation is your best protection against legal problems. *(p. 683)*

8. b. Never attempt restraint until you have sufficient help and an appropriate plan. (Effective teamwork is more important than strength. Use only the minimal amount of force needed. Metal cuffs should not be used. Act quickly; surprise is a key element.) *(p. 680)*

9. c. The first priority in dealing with a behavioral emergency is to protect yourself and others from harm. Safety is of the utmost importance. *(p. 675)*

10. Only d, e, f, and h should be marked. Appropriate treatment for a behavioral emergency includes not making quick movements, not playing along with visual or auditory disturbances, letting the patient decide if he wants to involve family or friends, and not leaving the patient alone. The other choices are not appropriate treatments for a behavioral emergency. *(p. 674)*

CASE STUDY

1. d. Your first action should be to scan the scene for potential hazards.

2. a. You should always maintain eye contact and speak calmly. Never play along with visual or auditory disturbances or leave the patient alone. Always be truthful.

3. c. Your partner should keep you in his line of sight, be alert that the patient may become violent, try to obtain additional information, and try to disperse bystanders.

4. En route to the hospital, you should explain what you're going to do and seek his permission, then obtain baseline vital signs and complete your focused assessment. Continue talking quietly with Jim, and answer his questions honestly but do not create false expectations.

DOCUMENTATION EXERCISE

1. c. When managing a patient who has made a suicide attempt, the EMT's primary concern is to manage any injuries or medical conditions related to the suicide attempt.

2. a. Yes, Mrs. Raunecker was at great risk for following through on her suicide threat. She had numerous risk factors, including the recent death of her husband, loss of a job, depression, and previous suicide threats.

3. a. In questioning Mrs. Raunecker, Ted avoided the use of yes or no questions. Instead, he used open-ended questions, which allowed Mrs. Raunecker to freely express her feelings.

4. d. The interview with Mrs. Raunecker should have been conducted in a quiet surrounding with limited people present.

5. c. The search of Mrs. Raunecker's home was appropriate, given the circumstances.

Chapter 25: Obstetric and Gynecological Emergencies

TERMS AND CONCEPTS

1. a. 3 b. 8 c. 5 d. 7 e. 1 f. 4 g. 6 h. 2
   (pp. 721–722)

CONTENT REVIEW

1. c. Vagina (p. 690)
2. a. Uterine contractions that expel the fetus and placenta are generally referred to as labor. (p. 690)
3. c. The placental stage is the last stage. The three stages of labor are dilation, expulsion, and placental. Dilation occurs as the contractions begin and ends when the cervix becomes fully dilated. Expulsion ends with the delivery of the infant. The placental stage ends with the passage of the placenta (afterbirth). (p. 690)
4. c. *Gravida* refers to the number of pregnancies, while *para* refers to the number of births. The Roman numeral that follows each reports the numbers of events. *Primagravida* refers to a woman who is pregnant for the first time. *Primapara* refers to a woman who has given birth for the first time. (p. 693)
5. a. Altered mental status and seizures are both indications of a predelivery emergency. Other indications may include abdominal pain, nausea, vomiting, vaginal bleeding, weakness, dizziness, excessive swelling of the face and extremities, abdominal trauma, and shock. (p. 694)
6. a. Supine hypotensive syndrome is caused by the pressure of the combined weight of the enlarged uterus and fetus pressing on the inferior vena cava. The pressure may cause inadequate venous blood return to the heart and a drop in cardiac output, which may result in hypotension. (p. 694)
7. c. Transporting the patient on her side will minimize compression of the vena cava and improve her cardiac output. (p. 694)
8. d. Avoid packing the vagina, elevate the patient's feet 8 inches, and administer oxygen at 15 lpm. Provide general management for shock. (p. 695)
9. d. Care of this patient should include minimizing noise, light, and movement to prevent seizures. Administer oxygen at 15 lpm by nonrebreather mask. If necessary, provide positive-pressure ventilation and transport her on her side (to prevent supine hypotensive syndrome). (p. 695)
10. a. Contractions that occur every 2 minutes and last 60–90 seconds are a sign of imminent delivery. Other signs include crowning, patient feeling the infant's head in the birth canal, strong urge to push down, and the patient's abdomen being very hard. (pp. 690–691)
11. (1) Support the bony part of the infant's skull and exert gentle pressure against the perineum as the head delivers. Determine the position of the umbilical cord. (2) Suction the infant's mouth and nose. Support the body as it delivers, then again suction the mouth and nose. Dry and wrap the infant. (3) Keep the infant level with the vagina. Have your partner assume care of the infant. When the pulsations cease, clamp, tie, and cut the umbilical cord. (4) Observe for the delivery of the placenta. As it delivers, grasp it gently and rotate. Place in a plastic bag for transport to the hospital. (5) Place sanitary pad at the vaginal opening. Record the time of delivery and transport. Keep mother and infant warm en route. (pp. 700–703)
12. b. Emergency care for the patient with excessive post-delivery bleeding should include the administration of oxygen and firm massage of the uterus. If the mother appears to be in shock (hypoperfusion), transport immediately and initiate uterine massage en route. (p. 703)
13. d. Signs of abnormal delivery include any fetal presentation other than the normal crowning of the head, abnormal color or smell of the amniotic fluid, labor before 38 weeks of pregnancy, and recurrence of contractions after the first infant is born (indicates multiple births). (p. 703)
14. a. Management of a breech delivery includes positioning the mother in a supine head-down position to delay movement of the fetus into the birth canal, administering oxygen at 15 lpm, and transporting rapidly to the hospital. (p. 704)
15. d. Prolapsed cord. This is a true emergency. (pp. 703–704)
16. b. Insert a gloved hand into the vagina to relieve pressure on the cord. The mother should be transported immediately in a knee–chest position or Trendelenburg position. (pp. 703–704)
17. c. Meconium staining of the amniotic fluid should be managed by suctioning first the mouth and then the nose before the infant takes a first breath. It is critical to clear the airway before the infant begins to breathe to prevent aspiration of the meconium into the lungs. (p. 706)
18. d. In addition to the usual care for a newborn, care of the premature infant requires vigilant attention to prevent heat loss or contamination. Suctioning should be done very gently, and oxygen should be administered using a "blow-by" technique. (p. 706)
19. a. The APGAR score ranges from 0 to 10 and is a method to assess the newborn's overall condition at 1 minute and 5 minutes after delivery. Components of the APGAR assessment include appearance, pulse, grimace, activity, and respirations. (pp. 706–710)
20. c. The signs of a severely depressed newborn include a respiratory rate of over 60 per minute, an APGAR score of less than 4, a cyanotic body, and a heart rate over 180 per minute or under 100 per minute. (p. 710)

21. b. Emergency care for a newborn with shallow, gasping respirations and a heart rate that is less than 100 beats per minute should include assisting ventilations with a bag-valve mask and reassessing in 30 seconds. If there is no improvement, continue ventilations and again reassess in 30 seconds. *(p. 711)*

22. c. After taking appropriate BSI precautions and completing the initial assessment of the sexual assault victim, your focused history and physical exam should include tactfully questioning the patient about other potential injuries. Do not examine the genitalia of a sexual assault victim unless there is profuse or life-threatening bleeding. Clothing or other items should be bagged separately. Be sure to follow local protocols for evidence preservation. *(pp. 713–714)*

23. b. The APGAR score is initially performed at 60 seconds after birth and 5 minutes following birth. *(p. 706)*

24. a. Braxton–Hicks contractions are false labor contractions and are irregular. Interval times vary and the duration and intensity vary. *(p. 719)*

CASE STUDY

1. a. Initial management of this patient should first include immediately assisting respirations with a bag-valve mask with oxygen attached at 15 lpm.

2. b. This patient is critically injured and requires aggressive resuscitation. The management of supine hypotensive syndrome is of a secondary nature. However, if managed in this patient, it would be managed by placing a blanket or pillow under one side of the spine board. This relieves pressure on the inferior vena cava during transport.

3. a. CPR should be started immediately and continued throughout transport and until the fetus is surgically delivered at the hospital. Vigorous resuscitation of the mother to save the fetus is acceptable and appropriate.

ENRICHMENT

1. c. A placenta previa is associated with an abnormal implantation of the placenta over or near the cervical opening (os). The three types of placenta previa are total, partial, and marginal. *(p. 715)*

2. d. Multiparity (more than two deliveries), rapid succession of pregnancies, greater than 35 years of age, previous placenta previa, history of early vaginal bleeding, and bleeding following intercourse are all predisposing factors for placenta previa. *(p. 716)*

3. c. The hallmark sign is third-trimester painless vaginal bleeding of any color. *(p. 716)*

4. b. Abruptio placenta results from rupture of blood vessels under the placenta and subsequent separation from the uterine wall. It may be either a complete or a partial separation. *(p. 716)*

5. d. Predisposing factors for an abruptio placenta include hypertension, use of cocaine and other drugs, preeclampsia, multiparity, previous abruption, smoking, a short umbilical cord, premature rupture of the amniotic sac, and diabetes mellitus. *(p. 716)*

6. a. Constant abdominal pain associated with vaginal bleeding is the hallmark sign of abruptio placenta. *(p. 716)*

7. d. Preeclampsia chiefly affects women who have a history of diabetes, heart disease, kidney problems, or hypertension. It affects about 1 in 20 women and occurs most frequently in women in their 20 in the last trimester of pregnancy. *(p. 717)*

8. b. Preeclampsia is chiefly characterized by hypertension and swelling of the extremities. Blood pressure is usually greater than 140/90. *(p. 717)*

9. d. Ectopic pregnancy is the leading cause of maternal death in the first trimester of pregnancy. *(p. 718)*

10. c. Predisposing factors for development of an ectopic pregnancy include previous ectopic pregnancies, pelvic inflammatory disease, adhesions from surgery, and tubal surgery. *(p. 719)*

11. b. Signs and symptoms of ectopic pregnancy include a dull, ache-type pain that is poorly localized, then becomes a sudden, sharp or "knifelike" abdominal pain. Other signs and symptoms include vaginal bleeding; lower abdominal pain that radiates to one or both shoulders; tender, bloated abdomen; decreased blood pressure; a bluish discoloration around the umbilicus (if the rupture occurred hours earlier); and an urge to defecate. *(p. 719)*

DOCUMENTATION EXERCISE

1. d. Make sure no bleeding is taking place. A small amount of bleeding may be life threatening to a newborn. Ensure that the clamps are preventing any bleeding from taking place.

2. b. Crowning and Mary's need to bear down and push are classic indicators that birth is imminent.

3. d. The 1-minute APGAR score is 9. *(To check the score, see pages 706–710)*

4. d. The 5-minute APGAR score is 10. *(To check the score, see pages 706–710)*

5. d. 500 ml of bleeding is considered within normal limits. (The measurements ml and cc are approximately synonymous.)

Chapter 26: Mechanisms of Injury: Kinetics of Trauma

TERMS AND CONCEPTS

1. a. 1 **b.** 7 **c.** 4 **d.** 6 **e.** 3 **f.** 8 **g.** 5 **h.** 2   *(p. 745)*

CONTENT REVIEW

1. d. Mass and velocity   *(p. 727)*

2. **c.** Velocity is the most significant factor. (Review the formula for calculating kinetic energy. Notice that if you double the mass, you double the amount of kinetic energy. However, if you double the speed, the kinetic energy produced is four times as great.) *(p. 728)*

3. **d.** Acceleration (Deceleration is the rate at which a body in motion decreases its speed.) *(p. 728)*

4. **c.** The typical vehicular collision involves three impacts: the vehicle collision (it strikes an object), the body collision (it strikes the inside of the vehicle), and the organ collision (they strike the inside surface of the body). *(p. 729)*

5. **b.** Falls account for over half of all trauma incidents. *(p. 730)*

6. **a.** Vehicular collisions account for over one-third of all deaths due to trauma. *(p. 730)*

7. **c.** The group that is most likely to suffer injury from air-bag deployment are short adults, older adults, and infants and children less than 12 years of age. *(p. 737)*

8. **a.** In a motor vehicle collision, the "up and over" and "down and under" pathways are examples of injury patterns associated with a frontal impact. *(p. 730)*

9. **c.** When a passenger's head strikes the car windshield, the glass may crack in a typical "spider web" pattern. This is the term frequently used to describe the crack pattern caused by a vehicle occupant's head striking the windshield. (*p. 733*)

10. **b.** A rear-end impact *(p. 734)*

11. **c.** A lateral impact *(p. 734)*

12. **a.** Injuries due to rotational or rollover impact can create multiple-system injury and possible ejection if the patient was unrestrained *(p. 735*

13. **c.** Children turn toward the vehicle; adults turn away. *(p. 736)*

14. **b.** Femur, chest, abdomen, and head (Because a child is small and has a low center of gravity, he is likely to be struck high on the body, then thrown in front of the vehicle and run over.) *(p. 736)*

15. **d.** In a collision, a seatbelt worn too low can cause hip dislocations or fractures, not lower-leg fractures. Properly applied lap belts and shoulder straps don't prevent lateral head movement and air bags don't work well in multiple-collision events. A deployed airbag should be lifted from the steering wheel so the steering wheel can be checked for deformity. *(pp. 736–737)*

16. **d.** Leg burns are the most likely injury from the list provided. "Laying the bike down" is an evasive action meant to prevent ejection or separation of a motorcycle rider from his bike. Abrasions and burns are most likely, although a wide variety of injuries is possible. *(p. 738)*

17. **c.** 15, 10 *(p. 739)*

18. **b.** Three times his height *(p. 739)*

19. **a.** Between the nipple line and the waist *(p. 741)*

20. **b.** Blasts and explosions *(p. 741)*

CASE STUDY 1

1. **c.** An occupant of the same car was killed. Significant forces are involved in this accident. After the initial assessment, immobilize the patient and begin a rapid trauma assessment.

2. **b.** Along with high speed and death of another vehicle occupant, altered mental status is one of the factors that call for a high suspicion of significant mechanism of injury. You need to assess her mental status and monitor it carefully.

CASE STUDY 2

1. **d.** Knowing how the patient struck the ground will help you determine how the energy dissipated and what potential injuries resulted. The severity of trauma depends on the distance of the fall, the type of surface, and the body part that impacted first.

2. **b.** In a feet-first fall with knees locked, energy will travel all the way up the skeleton. When the patient is thrown forward, it may also cause a Colles' fracture, a fracture of the wrist that occurs when the patient tries to break his fall.

CASE STUDY 3

1. **c.** The patient with a penetrating injury between the nipple and waist requires evaluation for both a potential abdominal and chest injury. Lung tissue is relatively tolerant of cavitation caused by projectiles, a pneumothorax is a common result of injury to the chest, and the presence of rib fracture is highly likely in this patient.

2. **a.** It is critical to look for an exit wound and treat it if there is one. Obviously, the wound should not be probed, and nothing should be poured into the wound. Provide oxygen by nonrebreather mask, inspect for a sucking chest wound, and quickly seal the wound.

Chapter 27: Bleeding and Shock

MEDICAL TERMINOLOGY

1. **b.** Dripping, leaking
2. **a.** Blood
3. **d.** Tension
4. **b.** Contraction
5. **d.** Vessel

TERMS AND CONCEPTS

1. *Shock (hypoperfusion)* is the insufficient supply of oxygen and other nutrients to the body's cells, which results from inadequate circulation of blood. *(p. 748)*

2. The medical term for a nosebleed is *epistaxis*. *(p. 757)*

3. By compressing an artery at a *pressure point*, arterial blood flow can be reduced in an extremity. *(p. 753)*

CONTENT REVIEW

1. d. The circulatory system provides the human body with nutrients and blood. *(p. 766)*

2. d. The three main components of the circulatory system are the heart, the vessels, and the blood. *(p. 748)*

3. b. Adequate kidney function is not necessary to maintain tissue perfusion at the capillary level. Adequate blood volume, heart pumping, and vessel size are necessary to maintain perfusion. In addition to these, an intact respiratory system is also necessary. *(p. 748)*

4. c. The vital organs that are particularly sensitive to decreased perfusion and that play a major role in attempting to reverse shock are the heart, brain, lungs, and kidneys. *(p 748)*

5. a. 2 **b.** 3 **c.** 1 *(p. 749)*

6. a. Severe external bleeding should be controlled only after (or simultaneously with) ensuring an airway and breathing. *(p. 751)*

7. c. The first step in controlling severe bleeding is to apply direct pressure, then to elevate the extremity and apply ice or a cold pack. (Tourniquet or sling and swathe are inappropriate for this kind of injury. Compressing an artery at a pressure point may be necessary if direct pressure and elevation have not completely controlled major bleeding in an extremity.) *(p. 754)*

8. a. A vessel that is cut across (perpendicular to) the vessel will have a tendency to retract and clot off. A cut along the length of the vessel will have a tendency to open wider when it contracts. *(p. 749)*

9. a. Brachial pressure point **b.** Femoral pressure point *(p. 754)*

10. b. Tourniquets are used only as a last resort to control bleeding of an amputated extremity when all other methods have failed. *(p. 755)*

11. c. If the breathing is adequate, you should provide oxygen via nonrebreather mask at 15 lpm. If the breathing is inadequate, you should immediately provide positive-pressure ventilation with a BVM and supplemental oxygen. *(p. 758)*

12. Mechanisms of injury that can cause internal bleeding include falls, motor vehicle collisions, pedestrian impacts, blast injuries, and penetrating injuries. *(p. 758)*

13. c. Nothing should be given to the patient by mouth. *(p. 759)*

14. d. Shock (hypoperfusion) should be suspected in any patient who has suffered or may have suffered trauma. *(p. 760)*

15. a. Low blood pressure is a late sign of shock. *(pp. 761, 768)*

16. Shock (hypoperfusion) generally progresses in the following sequence: (1) Blood loss causes rapid heart rate and weak pulse. (2) Blood vessels constrict in extremities to conserve blood, causing cold, clammy skin. (3) Low oxygen levels to breathing-control centers of the brain make respirations rapid and shallow; nervous system reaction results in profuse sweating.

(4) Vasoconstriction fails, and blood pressure drops. (5) Leaking capillaries cause loss of vital blood plasma; unresponsiveness and death may result. *(Figure 27-13, p. 768)*

17. a. The sympathetic nervous system causes the peripheral blood vessels to constrict and shunt the blood to the vital organs. *(p. 758)*

18. Emergency care of shock includes the following: Take all BSI precautions. Maintain an open airway, and administer oxygen. Control any external bleeding. Apply and inflate the PASG when appropriate and as directed by local protocols and if approved by medical direction. Position the patient according to local protocol. Splint suspected bone or joint injuries. Cover the patient with a blanket to prevent loss of body heat. Transport immediately. *(pp. 766–767)*

19. d. If a tourniquet applied to an extremity does not completely stop arterial blood flow, the arterial blood will continue to flow into the extremity, but the venous blood will not be able to flow out. This will build up the arterial and venous pressure in the wound and increase the amount of bleeding. *(p. 756)*

20. b. The brain stimulates the adrenal glands to secrete epinephrine and norepinephrine, which has alpha and will cause the vessels to constrict, creating the pale appearance and cool sensation. It also stimulates the sweat glands, causing the clammy or diaphoretic presentation. The intent of alpha is to constrict the vessels and increase the systemic vascular resistance in an attempt to raise the blood pressure. *(p. 758)*

21. d. As the systolic blood pressure drops from the decrease in blood volume, the systemic vasoconstriction causes the diastolic blood pressure to be maintained or to increase, creating a narrow pulse pressure. *(pp. 759, 768)*

22. a. Medications such as Coumadin (warfarin) and other anticoagulant drugs, aspirin, ibuprofen, and other nonsteroidal anti-inflammatory drugs (NSAIDs). Other factors that may interfere with the clotting process and may lead to an increase in the rate of bleeding are as follows: Movement can disrupt the clotting process. A low body temperature may make the clotting process slower; therefore, it is very important to keep your patient warm. Intravenous fluids may increase the blood pressure, thereby breaking clots free, or the water or properties in the fluid may interfere with the clotting. *(p. 759)*

23. a. Infants and children will compensate for blood loss for a longer period of time than do adults; then they will deteriorate more rapidly once they begin to decompensate. *(p. 763)*

CASE STUDY

1. a. If you have not already done so, take BSI precautions because blood is spurting. Include eye protection and a mask as well as gloves. Place a sterile gauze over the large wound and apply fingertip pressure to the site. Due to the number of lacerations, have your partner apply a sterile pressure dressing to both hands and the other arm. Both extremities should be elevated above the level of the heart to slow the blood flow and aid in clotting. Since this patient has both venous and arterial bleeding, this is a potentially life-threatening situation.

2. c. His increasing agitation may be an early sign of shock. You should assess for other signs of shock, begin administration of oxygen via nonrebreather mask at 15 lpm, and then expedite transport.

3. b. You should place a new sterile bandage over the blood-soaked bandage. Removing the old bandage may remove blood clots and increase the bleeding.

ENRICHMENT

1. d. In compensatory shock, the blood pressure remains normal. The patient in compensatory shock may present with narrow pulse pressure, weaker pulse, slightly pale and cool skin, anxiety, and a slightly elevated heart rate. *(p. 768)*

2. d. A drop in the systolic blood pressure (the top number, or while the heart is contracting) is the main indicator of decompensated or progressive shock. *(p. 768)*

3. a. Unresponsiveness is a sign of late decompensated or progressive shock. Mottled skin and an absent peripheral pulse are other indicators. An elevated body temperature is not associated with shock. *(p. 769)*

4. b. The patient in irreversible shock may bleed from all orifices or may begin to leak blood from previous controlled wounds. *(p. 769)*

5. b. Vasogenic shock is a result of injury to the spine or head, resulting in a loss of control over the vascular system and dilated blood vessels. The volume of blood has not changed, but the container (vessels) has enlarged due to loss of muscle tone inside the vessel through dilation. This causes pooling of the blood in the periphery, away from the vital organs, and lowering of the blood pressure. *(p. 766)*

DOCUMENTATION EXERCISE

1. c. Venous bleeding is dark red and steadily flowing.

2. a. Arterial bleeding is bright red and spurting.

3. d. This patient has sustained a stab wound to the right lower flank. A distended abdomen with discoloration around the umbilicus indicates significant blood loss into the abdominal cavity. A major organ may have been penetrated, causing severe internal bleeding.

4. b. In a severe state of hypoperfusion, the body shunts blood from the extremities to the core by constricting peripheral blood vessels, making it hard or impossible to find a peripheral pulse.

5. c. A late sign of decompensated shock is loss of peripheral pulses. Other signs are tachycardia (abnormally fast heart rate), tachypnea (abnormally fast breathing rate), narrowing pulse pressure, unresponsiveness, and a significant drop in blood pressure.

6. d. If direct pressure to the wound on the right thigh fails to control bleeding, you should immediately apply firm, direct pressure to the right femoral pressure point. This will reduce the blood flow to the extremity.

Chapter 28: Soft Tissue Injuries

MEDICAL TERMINOLOGY

1. c. Away from

2. a. To pull

3. a. Skin

4. d. Blood

5. b. Skin

TERMS AND CONCEPTS

1. a. 8 **b.** 6 **c.** 5 **d.** 1 **e.** 10 **f.** 2 **g.** 4 **h.** 7 **i.** 9 **j.** 3 *(p. 796)*

CONTENT REVIEW

1. d. Epidermis, dermis, subcutaneous layer *(p. 774)*

2. b. 1, 2, 4. Aids in the elimination of water and various salts. Serves as a receptor organ. Protects the body from the environment. The white blood cells are produced by bone marrow. *(p. 774)*

3. b. An amputation is an open injury. Contusions and hematomas are closed injuries. A crush injury may be either open or closed. *(pp. 774–776)*

4. b. The hemostatic dressing has fibrinogen and thrombin on the surface of the dressing, which promotes clotting and stops bleeding when applied to wounds. *(p. 787)*

5. c. Take BSI precautions before approaching any patient. Assess the airway, breathing, and circulation. Assure open airway and adequate breathing. Treat for shock, if necessary. Then splint painful, swollen, or deformed extremities. *(pp. 776–780)*

6. d. Occlusive *(p. 782)*

7. b. On three sides only to allow air to escape as the patient exhales *(p. 782)*

8. c. Severe bleeding is usually associated with a jagged- or crushing-type amputation. If the amputation involves a clean cut through the vessels and soft tissue, there may not be severe bleeding. *(p. 778)*

9. a. 2, 4, 3, 1. Manually secure the object. Expose the wound area. Control bleeding. Use a bulky dressing to help stabilize the object. (An impaled object should never be removed in the field, unless it is through the cheek or impaled in the neck and is obstructing air flow through the trachea.) *(p. 783)*

10. **a.** Never directly immerse the part in water or in sterile saline, since this may cause tissue damage to the amputated part. *(p. 784)*
11. **a.** Occlusive dressings will help to prevent air from entering the wound and the bloodstream or tissue. *(p. 785)*
12. To apply a pressure dressing: (a) Cover the wound with several sterile gauze dressings. (b) Apply gloved-hand pressure until bleeding is controlled. (c) Bandage firmly to create enough pressure to maintain control of bleeding. Check distal pulses to be sure the bandage is not too tight. (d) If blood soaks through, apply additional dressings and bandage over the original ones. *(pp. 787–788)*
13. **c.** Distal pulses, motor function, and sensory function. (Bandages should be snug, not tight. To be sure the bandage is not interfering with circulation, always check distal pulses and motor and sensory function before and after bandage application.) *(p. 787)*
14. **a.** Sterile, moist gauze and then an occlusive dressing. (Avoid absorbent materials that could adhere to organs.) *(p. 783)*
15. **c.** It reduces the tension on the abdominal muscles and will make the patient more comfortable. *(p. 783)*

CASE STUDY 1
1. **c.** Venous bleeding (The bleeding from the patient's neck is dark red and flows steadily. If it were a combination of venous and arterial, you would expect some spurting from the wound.)
2. **a.** For a large open neck wound, place your gloved hand over the wound, then an occlusive dressing, and finally a pressure dressing.

CASE STUDY 2
1. **b.** With any penetrating chest injury, also suspect a spinal injury.
2. **d.** Given the number of shots fired, and in any case of a shooting, you need to look for additional entry and exit wounds.

ENRICHMENT
1. **c.** The most dangerous bites are those that occur over a vascular area, which can cause major bleeding and serious infections. *(p. 789)*
2. **d.** Breaking the jar may cause a severe laceration and bleeding. All the other answers are appropriate treatments. *(p. 789)*

DOCUMENTATION EXERCISE
1. **c.** The laceration occurred on the right side of the neck and produced dark red blood that flowed steadily. This would likely be from an affected jugular vein in the carotid area. If an artery had been affected, it would likely produce bright red blood that would spurt with each contraction of the heart.
2. **a.** The gloved hand will help prevent air from being sucked into the vein and carried to the heart, which can be lethal. Bleeding control

and prevention of an air embolism are major goals when treating this type of injury.
3. **d.** After applying your gloved hand over the wound to control the bleeding, you should apply an occlusive dressing. This dressing should extend beyond all the wound edges and be taped on all four sides. After you have applied the occlusive dressing, you should next apply a regular dressing. Apply only enough pressure to control the bleeding. A circumferential pressure dressing may compress the major blood vessels in the neck.
4. **b.** If blood has soaked through the original pressure dressing, indicating that the severe bleeding has continued, you should remove all of the original bandages and then apply direct fingertip pressure. After the bleeding is controlled, apply a dressing and bandage the wound.
5. **c.** You should immediately wrap the amputated part in sterile gauze. Keep the part dry by placing the part in a plastic bag and keep cool by placing the bag on ice.

Chapter 29: Burn Emergencies

TERMS AND CONCEPTS
1. **a.** 5 **b.** 3 **c.** 2 **d.** 1 **e.** 6 **f.** 4 *(p. 817)*

CONTENT REVIEW
1. Functions of the skin include (1) providing a barrier against infection, (2) providing protection from harmful agents in the environment and injury, (3) aiding in the regulation of body temperature, (4) sensation transmission (hot, cold, pain, touch), (5) aiding in elimination of some body wastes, (6) containing fluids necessary to the functioning of other organs and systems. *(p. 798)*
2. **a.** Body surface area *(p. 803)*
3. **a.** Superficial (first-degree) burn *(p. 799)*
4. **b.** The patient who has sustained a deep partial-thickness burn will present with red and blanched white skin. Other signs and symptoms may include thick-walled blisters that often rupture. The patient can still feel pressure at the site. There is poor capillary refill to the burn site. All of the other answers in this question are signs and symptoms of superficial partial-thickness burn. *(p. 800)*
5. **b.** Partial-thickness (second-degree) burn *(p. 800)*
6. **c.** Burns to the face are considered critical because of the potential for respiratory compromise or injury to the eyes. *(p. 801)*
7. **d.** A fourth-degree burn is often caused by electrical injuries and extends completely through the epidermis and dermis and deep into the muscles, blood vessels, and nerves. *(p. 799)*
8. **b.** In a child, partial-thickness burns of 10–20 percent BSA are considered moderate. *(p. 804)*

9. **c.** Children under age 5 and adults over age 55 have less tolerance for burn injuries. Because of relatively larger skin surfaces (in relation to body mass), children have the potential for greater fluid loss. Older adults have prolonged and possibly impaired healing processes. *(p. 803)*

10. Emergency care for burn injuries includes: (a) Remove patient from source of burn, and stop the burning process. (b) Assess airway, breathing, and mental status. (c) Classify the severity of the burn, and transport immediately if critical. (d) Cover the burned area with a dry, sterile dressing (if greater than 10 percent BSA). (e) Keep patient warm and treat other injuries as needed. (f) Transport to the appropriate facility. *(pp. 806–807)*

11. **a.** The rule of nines is not applied to superficial burns. The rule of nines is applied to superficial partial-thickness burns, deep partial-thickness burns, and full-thickness burns. *(p. 803)*

12. **b.** Separate burned fingers or toes with dry, sterile dressings to prevent adherence of burned areas. *(p. 809)*

13. **c.** Always apply a dry, sterile dressing to *both* eyes because the eyes move simultaneously, and if the patient moves the unburned eye, the burned eye will move, too. (Reassure the patient and keep him informed about what is going on.) *(p. 810)*

14. **b.** Dry chemicals should be brushed off before flushing with water. *(p. 810)*

15. **d.** A contact burn occurs from contact with a hot object like the exhaust pipe of a vehicle. A flame burn occurs when there is contact with an open flame. A flash burn is a type of flame burn that usually results from a flammable gas or liquid that quickly ignites. Hot gases may also cause upper-airway burns when inhaled. *(p. 805)*

16. **c.** In electrical burns, all tissue between entry and exit wounds is suspect for injury. *(p. 805)*

CASE STUDY

1. **b.** Cut around the area. Do not attempt to remove the adhered portion, since this may cause further damage to the soft tissues.

2. **c.** Singed nasal hair may be an indication of a compromised airway. Provide oxygen via nonrebreather mask at 15 lpm. If breathing becomes inadequate, use positive-pressure ventilations. (The child's loud crying indicates that breathing is still adequate.)

3. **c.** Using the rule of nines, approximately 14 percent of the child's body surface area is affected by the burn. Any partial-thickness burn affecting from 10 to 20 percent of the body surface area should be considered moderate in a child. It is considered critical because the foot is involved.

4. **b.** Use sterile, dry dressings on the burn, and keep the patient warm. (Remember that the heat-regulation function of burned skin is impaired.)

ENRICHMENT

1. **b.** Burns increase the capillary permeability, which leads to fluid leaking from the cells into the area between the cells, causing an extreme loss in fluid. This loss of fluid can lead to a decreased blood flow to the kidneys, which can cause a buildup of wastes in the blood. *(p. 814)*

2. **d.** Gastrointestinal dysfunction may be caused by decreased, not increased, blood flow to that system. Leakage of fluid from body cells will cause severe edema. Circumferential burns to the chest can prevent the chest from expanding fully. Scarring from burns can cause long-term muscle wasting and joint dysfunction *(p. 816)*

DOCUMENTATION EXERCISE

1. **d.** A scald occurs when the patient comes in contact with a hot liquid. The more viscous the liquid the more severe the burn because of increased contact time. Smothering the flames while the pan was on the stove with a lid or fire extinguisher could have prevented this burn.

2. **b.** The deep partial-thickness burn (second-degree) is characterized by thick-walled blisters of which some may have ruptured, red with blanched white patches, and poor capillary refill to the burn site. The patient can still feel pressure at the site.

3. **c.** This patient's burns included the anterior trunk, 18 percent; bilateral anterior legs, 18 percent (9 percent for the anterior portion of each leg); and genitalia area, 1 percent, for a total of 37 percent BSA.

4. **a.** This patient's burns are considered critical because they comprise over 20 percent deep partial-thickness burns. This patient's burns are 37 percent deep partial-thickness burns; she should be treated rapidly and transported without delay to an appropriate facility.

5. **b.** A dry, sterile, particle-free dressing should be used on this burn. A wet or moist dressing may cause the patient to become hypothermic. You must not apply creams. Do not apply dressings that are not particle free. Cotton or paper-type dressings may contaminate the burned area with particles and complicate the treatment and healing process.

Chapter 30: Musculoskeletal Injuries

TERMS AND CONCEPTS

1. **a.** 6 **b.** 1 **c.** 3 **d.** 2 **e.** 5 **f.** 4 *(p. 824)*

CONTENT REVIEW

1. **b.** Produces platelets (This is a function of the circulatory system.) *(p. 820)*

2. The six basic components of the skeletal system are (1) skull, (2) spinal column, (3) thorax,

(4) pelvis, (5) lower extremities, and (6) upper extremities. *(p. 821)*

3. **c.** Direct, indirect, and twisting *(p. 822)*

4. **d.** Pulselessness and cyanosis *(p. 822)*

5. **d.** A fracture to the femur or pelvis is considered a critical injury and must be managed to both immobilize the bones and reduce the associated bleeding. *(p. 822)*

6. The additional steps should be performed in the following order of priority: (1) Immobilize the patient to a spine board. (2) Initiate transport. (3) Perform further management of the life-threatening injuries and ongoing assessments every 5 minutes. (4) Splint the injured extremity. *(pp. 823, 824)*

7. **b.** An open injury *(p. 826)*

8. Signs and symptoms of bone and joint injury include deformity or angulation, pain and tenderness, grating or crepitus, swelling, disfigurement, severe weakness and loss of function, bruising, exposed bone ends, and joint locked into position. *(p. 824)*

9. **c.** A fracture to the femur bleeds heavily. Application of a traction splint will help to pull the bone in line and reduce the diameter of the thigh. This allows less blood to collect, thereby indirectly putting pressure on the bleeding bones. *(p. 832)*

10. **c.** When in doubt, splint! Pain, swelling, and deformity are signs and symptoms of a possible fracture. *(p. 831)*

11. **c.** Check distal pulses, motor function, and sensation before and after splinting and during the ongoing assessment. *(p. 837)*

12. **a.** The joints above and below the injury site *(pp. 824, 828)*

13. **a.** The PASG performs two functions: It stabilizes the fracture, and it decreases the compartment in which the pelvis can bleed. *(p. 837)*

14. **b.** Make one attempt at aligning the extremity. (Follow local protocol.) If pain, resistance, or crepitus increase, stop. *(p. 831)*

15. **b.** Never intentionally replace protruding bones or push them back below the skin. *(p. 831)*

16. **d.** The improvised splint should be padded so that the inner surfaces are not in contact with the skin. It should also be light in weight, firm, and rigid; long enough to extend past the joints above and below the site; and as wide as the thickest part of the injured limb. *(p. 832)*

17. **b.** Shoulder injury (The sling supports the arm, and the swathe holds it against the side of the chest.) *(p. 833)*

18. **d.** The position of function for a hand is fingers curled as if holding a ball. A roll of bandage in the hand can support this position. *(p. 834)*

19. **c.** Use a traction splint if the thigh is painful, swollen, or deformed. You do not have to be certain the femur has actually been fractured. However, do not apply a traction splint if there is injury to the hip, pelvis, or knee or within 1–2 inches of the knee because the

traction could aggravate these injuries. *(p. 836)*

20. **c.** It pulls on the thigh and realigns the broken femur. This helps relieve pain and reduces movement of the broken bone ends. *(p. 836)*

21. **b.** If the foot or ankle is injured, having the patient push down and pull back with the great (big) toe will give you the same results as if the entire foot was tested. *(p. 834)*

22. **d.** The pneumatic antishock garment (PASG) is an effective device that can be used to splint the pelvis and decrease the compartment size to reduce bleeding. Another splint used for the suspected pelvic fracture is a folded-sheet improvised pelvic wrap. There are also commercially produced devices used to splint the pelvis in the same manner as the pelvic wrap. *(p. 837)*

23. **a.** If the pressure in the space around the capillaries exceeds the pressure needed to perfuse the tissues, the blood flow is cut off, and the cells become hypoxic, leading to compartment syndrome. *(p. 837)*

CASE STUDY 1

1. **b.** Remember, check pulses, motor function, and sensation before and after splinting. (Apply a sling and swathe after checking PMS.)

2. **c.** Sensation is intact if the patient can tell you, without looking, which finger or toe you are touching.

3. **b.** The energy from the impact of this patient's hand with the ground travels up the arm and causes an injury to the collarbone (clavicle). This is a classic example of an injury caused by indirect force.

CASE STUDY 2

1. **c.** Do not release traction until after the splint has been applied.

2. **a.** Assess the pedal or posterior tibial pulse for a lower extremity, and assess the radial pulse for an upper extremity.

CASE STUDY 3

1. **a.** Paresthesia, or tingling, may indicate some loss of sensation.

2. **b.** The position of function is with the foot bent at the normal angle to the leg, not pushed downward or upward toward the shin or otherwise manipulated into an unnatural position.

3. **c.** If the injury involves a lower extremity, motor function is intact if the patient can tighten the kneecap and move the foot up and down as if pumping a gas pedal.

DOCUMENTATION EXERCISE

1. **d.** Crepitus is the sound or feeling of broken fragments of bone grinding against each other. Atelectasis is the condition in which the lungs are collapsed or airless. Eupnea describes good or normal breathing. Kyphosis

is the exaggerated curvature or "humpback" appearance of the thoracic spine.

2. a. Reducing the diameter of the thigh will allow less blood to accumulate, thereby indirectly putting pressure on the bleeding bone ends.

3. b. If your patient is unresponsive or becomes unresponsive, you should apply traction until the injured leg length is the same as the uninjured leg.

4. d. You should never elevate the extremity if you suspect a spinal injury. Because of the significant mechanism of injury, you should suspect a possible spinal injury. Applying ice packs will help reduce swelling. Although this was an open fracture, the bone ends have slipped back under the skin before you applied traction. Pulling manual traction while your partner readies the splint is appropriate.

5. d. You should evaluate the PMS distal to the injury every 15 minutes to ensure that the splint is not impairing circulation to the extremity.

Chapter 31: Injuries to the Head

TERMS AND CONCEPTS

1. a. 8 **b.** 1 **c.** 10 **d.** 2 **e.** 11 **f.** 3 **g.** 4 **h.** 7 **i.** 9 **j.** 6 **k.** 5 **l.** 12 *(p. 866)*

CONTENT REVIEW

1. a. Injury to the brain that results from shearing, tearing, and stretching of nerve fibers is called diffuse axonal injury. *(pp. 851, 859)*

2. c. The single most important sign in cases of suspected head injury is a decreasing mental status. *(p. 853)*

3. c. A tool that uses numerical values to carefully monitor a patient's level of consciousness is the Glasgow Coma Scale. *(p. 854)*

4. b. Jaw-thrust maneuver (This maneuver is performed without tilting the patient's head, which might aggravate a potential spine injury.) *(p. 851)*

5. d. The lowest level on the AVPU scale is unresponsiveness; that is, the patient does not respond to any stimulus, indicating the most serious injury. *(p. 854)*

6. c. Immediate transport and monitoring *(p. 854)*

7. d. A flexion response or decorticate posturing indicates an upper-brainstem injury, considered a nonpurposeful response, results in flexing of arms across the chest and extension of the legs and sometimes arching of the back. *(p. 854)*

8. c. When managing a patient with a suspected head injury, oxygenation and ventilation are of critical importance because any alteration in oxygenation or ventilation can make a head injury worse. It is critical to determine a baseline mental status so that subsequent comparisons can be accurately made. Any patient who lost consciousness, even if only for a brief period of time, requires evaluation at a hospital. A lowered SpO_2 can be a sign of a variety of disorders that interfere with oxygenation, not just a head injury. *(p. 854)*

9. a, c, and e. Cushing reflex is a triad of three signs that may signal increasing intracranial pressure. The systolic BP may significantly increase, the pulse rate may slow (bradycardia), and the respiratory pattern may be altered (normal, irregular, decreased, or absent). *(p. 857)*

10. d. Emergency care of a patient with a serious head injury should include hyperventilation at 20 per minute, avoidance of direct pressure on the skull, critical attention to airway and breathing status, and anticipation of potential seizure activity. *(p. 859)*

CASE STUDY 1

1. c. This patient is exhibiting Cushing's reflex, a sign of severe head injury.

2. b. The reflex described in question 1, Cushing's reflex, consists of a "triad" of signs. These three signs are an increasing blood pressure, slowing pulse, and alteration in respirations.

3. c. This patient would be best managed by ventilation at a rate of 20 per minute.

CASE STUDY 2

1. b. The bruising around Mrs. McDonald's eyes is a late sign of skull fracture called raccoon sign.

2. a. The bruising over the mastoid area is also a late sign of skull fracture. It is called Battle's sign.

3. Only a, b, d, e, f, g, and i should be marked. Treatments that should be provided for Mrs. McDonald include manual in-line stabilization, cervical spine immobilization device, oropharyngeal airway, oxygen at 15 lpm, ventilation at 20 per minute, immobilization to a spine board, and ongoing evaluation of mental status. The head-tilt/chin-lift is not appropriate for a potential head injury (use a jaw thrust); do not pack anything into the ear or nose to stop fluid flow (place a loose dressing over the area), and do not place pressure on a skull deformity.

ENRICHMENT

1. The chart showing signs and symptoms associated with the four types of brain injury should be filled out as shown on p. 468. *(pp. 859–864)*

Sign or Symptom	Concussion	Contusion	Subdural Hematoma	Epidural Hematoma
Momentary confusion	X	X		
Abnormal respiratory pattern			X	X
Retrograde and anterograde amnesia	X	X		
Loss of responsiveness followed by a return of responsiveness and then rapid deterioration				X
Weakness or paralysis on one side of the body			X	
Dilation of one pupil			X	
Fixed and dilated pupil				X
Posturing (withdrawal or flexion)				X
Repeated questioning about what happened	X			
Increasing blood pressure			X	X
Decreasing pulse rate			X	X
Seizures			X	X
Cushing's reflex				X
Vomiting	X	X	X	X

2. a. A mild form of diffuse axonal injury that presents with an altered mental status and progressively improves is called a concussion. *(p. 859)*

3. b. A contusion of the brain is usually caused by one of two types of injuries: coup–contrecoup and acceleration/deceleration. *(p. 861)*

4. d. This brain injury is typically the result of low-pressure venous bleeding above the tissue of the brain. It is called a subdural hematoma. *(p. 861)*

5. d. Subdural hematoma is the most common type of head injury. It occurs in 33 percent of all severe head injuries, is more common in patients older than 60, and is more likely in patients with abnormally long blood-clotting times. *(p. 863)*

DOCUMENTATION EXERCISE

1. c. Rolling the patient quickly on his side to suction his airway was an important and critical action to take. Whenever potential obstructions to the airway are noted, they must be removed rapidly.

2. a. This patient is most likely suffering from a high-level brainstem injury, as characterized by the flexion (decorticate) posturing that occurred following the application of pain.

3. d. This patient should be ventilated at a rate of 20 per minute.

4. a. This patient is likely suffering from hypoperfusion from bleeding in a body cavity, as indicated by the abrasion and distention to the patient's abdomen, skin temperature, rapid pulse rate, and weak radial pulse.

5. c. The patient's fractured ankle did not require immediate immobilization. Straps and padding could have been used to stabilize the ankle so long as the action would not delay transport to a hospital.

Chapter 32: Injuries to the Spine

TERMS AND CONCEPTS

1. a. 4 **b.** 3 **c.** 1 **d.** 2 *(p. 915–916)*

2. A. Cervical spine (first seven vertebrae, which form the neck); **B.** Thoracic spine (the next 12 vertebrae, which form the upper back); **C.** Lumbar spine (the next five vertebrae, which form the lower back); **D.** Sacral spine or sacrum (the next five vertebrae, which are fused together to form the rigid part of the back side of the pelvis); **E.** Coccyx (the four fused vertebrae that form the lower end of the spine) *(p. 870)*

CONTENT REVIEW

1. All should be marked except for d and g. Mechanisms of injury or types of emergency scenes that should alert you to the possibility of spinal injury include electrical injuries; blunt trauma; falls; motorcycle crashes; gunshot wounds to the head, neck, chest, abdomen, back, or pelvis; hangings; diving accidents; or any unresponsive trauma patient. Heart attacks and asthmatic attacks are medical emergencies, unless they also involve a fall or other mechanism of injury. *(p. 871)*

2. b. Maintain a high index of suspicion for spinal injury (regardless of the lack of obvious trauma). *(p. 873)*

3. d. Distraction is the mechanism of spinal injury that occurs when the vertebrae and spinal cord are stretched or pulled apart, as in a hanging. *(p. 871)*

4. c. Priapism (a persistent erection of the penis), if present (in male patients), is a classic sign of cervical-spine injury. Diaphragmatic breathing is associated with a cervical-spine injury. Never ask a suspected spinal injury patient to move about for any reason. Obvious deformity of the spine upon palpation is an uncommon finding. *(p. 877)*

5. d. When assessing for pulse, motor function, and sensory function in the patient with a spine injury, bilaterally check the radial and pedal pulses for presence, strength, and equality. Motor function is assessed in the upper and lower extremities. Upper: flex arms (C6), extend arms (C7), fingers spread

(T1), arm push (C7). Lower: push (S1 and S2), pull (L5). Sensory function is tested in each extremity for both pain and light touch. *(pp. 874–878)*

6. c. In manual spinal stabilization, the patient's nose is aligned with the navel, with the head neither flexed nor extended. *(p. 881)*

7. d. Two rescuers are needed to apply a cervical-spine immobilization collar, one to stabilize the neck manually while the other applies the device. Never use a soft collar; it permits too much movement. The collar by itself does not immobilize the patient. An improperly sized collar can cause more harm to the patient and further aggravate a potential spine injury. *(pp. 885–886)*

8. The chart showing techniques appropriate to immobilizing particular patients should be filled out as shown below. *(pp. 893–894)*

Patient type	Standing immobilization technique	Rapid extrication	Apply vest-type immobilization device	Immobilize to backboard
Standing patient	X			
Seated patient with critical injuries		X		X
Seated patient with no critical injuries			X	X
Supine or prone patient				X

9. b, c, d, and f should be marked. Appropriate management techniques for a patient with a spine injury include always immobilizing if in doubt about a spinal injury, establishing manual in-line stabilization as soon as possible, immobilizing the head in the position found if the patient complains of severe neck or spine pain or the head does not easily move, and recording and documenting the pulses and motor and sensory function in all extremities following immobilization. *(pp. 881–883)*

10. c. The log-roll technique is ideally performed using four rescuers; however, this is not always possible. Padding of all voids between the patient and the board should be performed to avoid extra movement. The cervical-spine immobilization collar should be placed before moving the patient onto the board. Immobilize the patient's torso to the board before the head. *(pp. 881–883)*

11. (1) Establish and maintain in-line manual stabilization. (2) Apply a cervical spine immobilization collar. (3) Log roll the patient onto the long spine board. (4) Place pads in the spaces between the patient and the board. (5.) Immobilize the patient's torso to the board with straps. (6) Immobilize the patient's head to the board. (7) Secure the patient's legs to the board. *(pp. 881–883)*

12. b. Immobilize the patient from a standing position while maintaining alignment. *(p. 893)*

13. d. A noncritical seated patient with a possible spine injury should have a cervical-spine immobilization collar and a short spinal immobilization device applied and then be transferred to a long spine board. The torso should be secured before the head is secured. *(pp. 893–898)*

14. c. Rapid extrication is indicated if the patient's condition is critical, the patient is on a scene that not safe, or the patient is blocking access to a critical patient. *(p. 902)*

15. a. Safe and effective rapid extrication requires constant cervical-spine stabilization. *(pp. 902–903)*

16. a. Removal of a helmet should generally not be attempted if the helmet fits well. Removal is obviously required if the patient is having breathing difficulties or is in cardiac arrest. Helmet removal can be adequately performed with two rescuers working carefully, and removal is not limited to any specific helmet type. *(pp. 904–905)*

17. a. Removing the helmet while leaving the shoulder pads in place may aggravate the injury by hyperextending the neck. *(p. 907)*

18. (1) Apply manual in-line stabilization. (2) Assess for life-threatening injuries or other reasons for removal from car seat. (3) Support the head in a neutral position, using towel rolls and tape. (4) Determine if padding is required between infant's body and seat. (5) Transport in the normal seated position after securing car seat to ambulance seat. *(p. 910)*

CASE STUDY

1. **b.** When immobilizing this patient, prevention of both lateral movement and movement up and down on the board is required. Pad the voids under the head and torso of this patient. A vest-type device is not required, and the EMT should not pad behind the cervical-spine immobilization collar.
2. **d.** Manual in-line stabilization can be released only after the head has been properly immobilized to the long spine board.
3. **b.** A minimum of three straps should be used to ensure proper immobilization.

ENRICHMENT

1. **a.** Spinal shock usually results from injury high in the cervical-spine region. *(p. 911)*
2. **b.** Findings associated with neurogenic shock include flushed, dry skin and a pulse rate of 60–100 per minute. *(p. 911)*
3. **a.** Neurogenic shock results in a relative hypovolemia; the same amount of blood is present within a dilated vascular space. The vascular dilation results from the loss of nervous system control. *(p. 911)*

DOCUMENTATION EXERCISE

1. **d.** The injury sustained by Wardell is most likely the result of lateral bending from the car being struck in the passenger side door.
2. **c.** Improper management and stabilization of Wardell's injury could produce three major complications of spinal injury: inadequate breathing effort, paralysis, and inadequate circulation.
3. **b.** The presence of numbness and tingling in Wardell's arm is a significant positive finding for a potential spinal injury.
4. **c.** Following immobilization with the short spinal immobilization device, Wardell should be placed on the long spine board. Don and Carly should reevaluate for pulse, motor, and sensory function following immobilization to the long spine board.
5. **d.** When securing Wardell to the long spine board, straps should be positioned, at a minimum, at the chest, hips, and above the knees.

Chapter 33: Eye, Face, and Neck Injuries

TERMS AND CONCEPTS

1. **a.** 3 **b.** 1 **c.** 9 **d.** 7 **e.** 8 **f.** 4 **g.** 2 **h.** 6 **i.** 5 *(pp. 918, 919)*
2. Labels on the left of the drawing, top to bottom: cornea, conjunctiva, pupil, aqueous humor. Labels in the center, top to bottom: iris, lens, vitreous humor. Labels on the right, top to bottom: retina, sclera. *(p. 919)*

CONTENT REVIEW

1. **c.** When conducting the focused history and physical exam on a patient with an eye injury, check the lids for bruising, swelling, and laceration; the pupils for equality and reactivity to light; and eye movement in all planes of motion (up, down, right, and left). *(p. 922)*
2. **b.** Stabilize the head and neck of the patient with facial trauma before doing anything else. *(p. 921)*
3. **d.** Suspect significant damage to the eye if there is unusual sensitivity to light. Also suspect significant damage if the patient has loss of vision that does not improve with blinking, loses part of the field of vision, has severe pain in the eye, or has double vision. *(p. 922)*
4. **d.** Every patient with an eye injury must be transported (in a supine position) for evaluation by a physician. *(pp. 925–929)*
5. **a.** Attempt to remove foreign objects from the conjunctiva only. All the rest should be removed by a physician. *(p. 923)*
6. **d.** Appropriate management of a lacerated eyelid includes preserving any avulsed skin and transporting with the patient. Cover the eye with a moist, sterile dressing, avoid the application of direct pressure, and cover the uninjured eye as well as the injured eye. *(pp. 925, 929)*
7. **b.** A patient with double vision, a marked decrease in vision, and loss of sensation above the eyebrow, over the cheek, or in the upper lip is most likely suffering from an orbital fracture. *(p. 924)*
8. **a.** Begin treatment of a chemical burn to the eye immediately during the initial assessment. Further delay will increase the injury. *(p. 926)*
9. **d.** Flush for at least 20 minutes. Remember to remove contact lenses, which can trap chemicals *(p. 926)*
10. **c.** Place the patient with an impaled or extruded eye injury in a supine position with the head immobilized. *(pp. 926, 927)*
11. **c.** They can be clearly seen by using a penlight. Contact lenses are frequently worn by people who also wear glasses. They may be worn in one eye only. Contact lenses should be removed in chemical burns of the eyes. *(p. 927)*
12. **a.** Pinch the soft lens between your thumb and index finger, allowing air to get underneath it. (If the lens has dehydrated, run sterile saline across the eye surface, slide the lens off the cornea, and pinch it up.) A suction cup device can be used for hard contacts. *(p. 927)*
13. **a.** When a patient with a painful, deformed, and swollen jaw has dentures that are still intact and in place, the dentures should be left in place. This provides proper alignment of the jaw when treating the injury. *(p. 930)*
14. **a.** Cover the exposed nerves and tendons with a moist, sterile dressing. Any other type of

dressing may dry out the nerves and tissues. (p. 935)

15. **b.** Rinse an avulsed tooth with saline to remove debris. Never scrub. Transport the tooth in a cup of saline or wrapped in gauze soaked in sterile saline. (p. 931)

16. **c.** Push or pull it out in the same direction in which it entered. (If not removed, it could fall into the mouth and obstruct the airway.) (p. 931)

17. **c.** Tape it to the outside of the mouth and monitor closely. (Don't insert your fingers; the patient may bite you, and you need your hands for other procedures. Don't have the patient hold the dressing; he may forget or lose responsiveness and let the dressing fall into the airway.) (p. 933)

18. **b.** Apply cold compresses to reduce the swelling, and then transport. (p. 933)

19. **d.** Clear or bloody fluid draining from the ear may indicate a skull fracture. Place a loose, clean dressing across opening to absorb the fluids. Do not exert any pressure. (pp. 933, 934)

20. **c.** To manage a severed blood vessel of the neck, *never* apply pressure to both sides of the neck at the same time; use an occlusive dressing secured with a figure-eight wrap, and position the patient on his left side, head down, for transport. (p. 937)

21. **b.** Hyphema is a condition where blood collects in the anterior portion of the eye. (p. 925)

22. **c.** Your initial management priorities for injuries to the mid-face or jaw are to establish manual spinal stabilization, ensure a patent airway, support breathing as necessary, and control life-threatening bleeding. (pp. 931, 932)

CASE STUDY

1. Yes, paramedic backup should be considered; the patient may need advanced airway procedures.

2. **d.** This is a high-priority patient. Transport immediately, and provide emergency care. Meet the paramedics en route.

3. **a.** Immediately begin flushing the eyes with saline. At the same time, place a gloved hand over the neck wound to control bleeding and administer high-flow oxygen.

DOCUMENTATION EXERCISE

1. **d.** When assessing Richard's pupils, Ali should carefully check the pupil in the right eye and then cover both eyes.

2. **b.** The figure-eight bandage, used to hold the occlusive dressing in place, is secured by placing the bandage over the dressing, across one shoulder, across the back, under the opposite armpit, and anchored at the shoulder.

3. **b.** Richard's complaints about numbness over his left eye and double vision just after the injury are most likely the result of an injury to the orbit.

4. **d.** Ali should have applied an occlusive dressing to the neck injury to prevent air from being sucked into the wound.

5. **d.** Richard's neck injury is a serious injury and must be carefully observed for swelling and airway compromise.

Chapter 34: Chest, Abdomen, and Genitalia Injuries

MEDICAL TERMINOLOGY

1. **b.** Spitting
2. **d.** Good, normal
3. **a.** Chest
4. **d.** Straight, breathing
5. **b.** New opening

TERMS AND CONCEPTS

1. **a.** 2 **b.** 4 **c.** 1 **d.** 3 **e.** 5 (p. 969)

CONTENT REVIEW

1. Chest cavity: aorta, heart, lungs, superior vena cava, trachea. Abdominal cavity: intestines, liver, spleen, stomach, urinary bladder. (p. 942)

2. **a.** The parietal pleura is the outermost layer of the pleura and lines the chest cavity. (p. 943)

3. **b.** Jugular vein distention that occurs during inhalation may be a sign of a tension pneumothorax or pericardial tamponade. The increased intrapulmonary pressure created during an inhalation prevents the emptying of the inferior and superior vena cava and results in jugular vein distention during inhalation. (p. 948)

4. **c.** As the pleural space expands, the lung collapses. (p. 943)

5. **d.** A central or sternal flail segment may result from ribs being separated from the cartilage on both sides of the sternum. (p. 945)

6. **a.** Initial assessment (Chest injury is potentially life-threatening.) (p. 947)

7. **b.** It is an attempt to reduce pain. (Shallow, rapid breathing can be inadequate and can easily lead to hypoxia.) (p. 947)

8. **c.** Gravity pulls fluids and other heavier matter downward, forcing air to flow upward. (p. 948)

9. **b.** When assessing for tracheal deviation, palpate the trachea immediately above the suprasternal notch. Palpation will reveal tracheal deviation before you will be able to visually notice deviation. (p. 948)

10. **c.** By providing positive-pressure ventilation, air is forced into the lungs, overriding the need for the patient's chest to create a negative pressure to draw the air into the lungs. You can effectively manage a flail segment through positive-pressure ventilations. (pp. 948, 962)

11. **c.** In tension pneumothorax, breath sounds will be absent on the injured side and decreased on the uninjured side. (The air on the injured side forces the mediastinum to shift,

compressing the cavity on the uninjured side, interfering with inflation of the lung on the uninjured side.) *(pp. 945, 949)*

12. **b.** Covering the wound with a gloved hand during the initial assessment, then applying an occlusive dressing taped on three or four sides are appropriate treatments. However, never assume that a corner of the occlusive dressing will not need to be lifted. If signs of respiratory distress develop, indicating development of a tension pneumothorax, a corner of the dressing should be lifted to allow air to escape and relieve the pressure. (Even a dressing taped on only three sides may become sucked into the wound and prevent air from escaping.) *(pp. 950–951)*

13. **b.** The hollow organs include the stomach, gallbladder, urinary bladder, and intestines. The liver, spleen, pancreas, and kidneys are solid organs. *(p. 953)*

14. **a.** The major complication associated with the laceration, or tearing, of a solid organ is major bleeding. Remember that a solid organ may bleed into the capsule that surrounds it for some time before the capsule ruptures and allows the blood to spill into the abdominal cavity. *(p. 953)*

15. **c.** Mechanism of injury (Because signs and symptoms may be subtle, the other choices are less reliable indicators.) *(p. 955)*

16. **d.** Start palpating farthest from the pain. *(p. 958)*

17. **c.** Supine, legs flexed at knees *(p. 959)*

18. **c.** An appropriate dressing for an abdominal evisceration is a sterile dressing soaked in saline or sterile water, then covered with an occlusive dressing. *(p. 959)*

19. **d.** The best care for any amputated part is to wrap it in a saline-moistened, sterile dressing; put it in a plastic bag; and place the bag on a cold pack or ice that has been wrapped in a towel. (Placing directly on ice may cause tissues to freeze.) Label the bag and transport the part with the patient. *(p. 960)*

20. **a.** Apply direct pressure with a moistened sterile compress such as a sanitary pad. *(p. 960)*

CASE STUDY

1. **c.** Immediately seal the open chest wound with a gloved hand. Any delay will worsen the patient's condition.

2. **c.** Only an occlusive dressing on an open chest wound needs to have an open side to allow air to escape from the chest cavity with breathing. Use a moist, sterile dressing covered with an occlusive dressing sealed on all sides with tape, cravats, or bandages.

3. **d.** Lift the corner of the occlusive dressing on the chest wound to release air that is potentially trapped and building up in the chest cavity.

ENRICHMENT

1. **a.** Pulmonary contusion, or bruised lung, is a serious condition usually caused by blunt trauma to the chest. Bleeding occurs in and around the alveoli and interstitial space, greatly decreasing the exchange of oxygen and carbon dioxide, leading to hypoxia. *(p. 962)*

2. **d.** Pericardial tamponade may result from blood filling the sac that surrounds the heart. Since the sac cannot expand, the result is compression of the heart muscle, resulting in the narrowing pulse pressure (the difference between the systolic and diastolic pressures). *(p. 967)*

3. **c.** Never completely wrap the chest or apply a swathe snugly. This may hamper normal respiration. Apply a sling and swathe and position the arm over the injured site; have the patient hold a pillow firmly over the injured site or allow the patient to guard the injury by placing his arm tightly over the injury site. *(p. 967)*

DOCUMENTATION EXERCISE

1. **b.** A flail segment is indicated by paradoxical movement.

2. **a.** Treat an abdominal evisceration by applying a saline-soaked sterile dressing first, then covering the dressing with an occlusive dressing or plastic wrap. Aluminum foil should not be used because it may lacerate the protruding organs. Never use absorbent cotton or other material that may cling to the organs.

3. **d.** This patient has a suspected spinal injury and has been placed on a backboard. You should not flex the legs if you suspect a spinal injury. You can initially splint the unstable chest with your gloved hand in the inward position. A pillow under the arm can help to stabilize the chest segment. Positive-pressure ventilations will continue to splint the chest segment by providing internal positive pressure.

4. **c.** You should suspect a pneumothorax if resistance develops to positive-pressure ventilations. You should ensure the airway is open by positioning the patient. Other signs that this patient may have developed a tension pneumothorax are that the breathing becomes more labored with severe tachypnea, there is slight cyanosis around his lips, and he has an SpO_2 of 84 percent.

5. **a.** A flail segment occurs when two or more consecutive ribs have been fractured in two or more places.

Chapter 35: Agricultural and Industrial Emergencies

CONTENT REVIEW

1. Hazards at the scene of an agricultural or industrial accident include toxic gases, chemicals, unstable equipment, fall hazards, and livestock. *(p. 974)*

2. **b.** The best approach to a tractor accident is to have at least two rescue teams at the scene—one to handle the potential fire hazard and one to provide patient extrication and treatment. *(p. 972)*

3. **c.** Never attempt rescue alone or without a lifeline at scenes involving agricultural storage areas. *(p. 978)*

4. **a.** If your patient was exposed to chemicals or manure, remove all clothing and flush the patient with copious amounts of water before transport. Be sure you are wearing appropriate protective clothing and equipment. Never use bleach or alcohol to flush a patient. Assessing for potential hazards should have been done during your initial scene survey. *(p. 974)*

5. **a.** Preserve all avulsed body parts, however mangled their appearance, and transport them with the patient, if possible. Do not delay the patient's transport if the body part is still entangled; have another unit disentangle the part and transport as soon as possible. *(p. 974)*

6. **a.** If you cannot free the patient by cutting the trapped clothing, you must remove the power takeoff (PTO) shaft from the equipment. It may be necessary to transport the patient to the hospital with the attached PTO shaft. Never use the self-reversing feature as this may cause more damage to the patient or rescuers. Do not release stored energy, and do not release pressure in the hydraulic hoses without specialized training. *(p. 977)*

7. **a.** 4 **b.** 5 **c.** 2 **d.** 1 **e.** 3 *(p. 975)*

8. **c.** Turning off the ignition switch may not shut off the engine of many types of equipment. Appropriate ways to stabilize agricultural equipment include blocking or chocking the vehicle, tying it to another vehicle, and setting the parking brake. When the equipment is stabilized, attempt to shut it down. *(p. 976)*

9. **a.** If the patient's life is threatened and other attempts to shut down the engine have failed, you should discharge a fire extinguisher into the air intake. (Note that this can cause extensive damage to the engine.) *(p. 976)*

10. **b.** Assume that a patient who has been buried in a grain tank is hypothermic. For that reason, always assume a patient is alive, even if he has been trapped for a long period of time. *(pp. 978–979)*

11. **d.** A corn or fresh-cut-grass odor is a common smell and not one of a silo gas. Signs of silo gas include bleachlike odor; yellowish or reddish vapor; red, yellow, or brown stains on surfaces touched by the gas; dead birds or insects near the silo; signs of illness in nearby livestock. *(p. 979)*

12. **c.** Never enter a livestock building or livestock area until all the animals have been secured. *(p. 980)*

13. **b.** Never assume the machine is locked and secured; verify it is safe before entering the danger area. Other guidelines for an industrial rescue include the following: check with the staff to determine potential hazards; if the patient is in a confined space or has been exposed to chemicals, wait for specialized hazardous material personnel for rescue and decontamination. *(p. 981)*

14. **d.** A wrap point is an aggressive component that moves in a circular motion. An example of a wrap point would be the PTO shaft of a tractor. *(p. 975)*

15. **b.** Do not attempt to stop or move machinery that you are not familiar with. Instruct a person who knows how to operate the machinery what needs to be done, such as shutting down the engine or motor. *(pp. 976, 977)*

CASE STUDY

1. **a.** Administer oxygen by nonrebreather mask at 15 lpm. Apply dressings as needed to control bleeding. Further assess the situation, and evaluate the need for additional assistance. You might consider having Mr. Wilson help you, depending on his emotional status.

2. **d.** Do not remove the impaled tine. It probably is controlling hemorrhage, so it should be stabilized with dressings in the position found to minimize movement and transported with the patient.

3. **b.** Continue manual in-line spinal stabilization and oxygen therapy. Stabilize the tine while Mr. Wilson removes the bolts holding it in place. Once that is done, have the forklift moved out of the way. Perform standing backboard procedures and immobilize John to the board.

Chapter 36: Infants and Children

TERMS AND CONCEPTS

1. **a.** Neonate, period of time from birth to discharge from the hospital: has total dependence on others; birth defects and unintentional injuries are common emergencies; no special assessment challenges. **b.** Infant, 0–1 year: recognizes the caregiver's face and voice; older infants are stressed by separation; start assessment from a distance and allow caregiver to hold infant for exam; frightened by initial stimulation around face, so begin exam with heart and lungs and end with the head. **c.** Toddler, 1–3 years: "do not like . . ." stage, so limit touch, avoid separation, limit clothing removal or involve caregiver; fear of pain/needles but

comforted by security objects; try toe-to-head exam. **d.** Preschooler, 3–6 years: concrete thinkers and literal interpreters, so explain simply and slowly before any action is taken; modest and resistant to attempts to unclothe, so involve caregiver; fear of pain, blood, and permanent injury but comforted by security objects; believe illness or injury is their fault and view it as punishment; allow them to see and "check out" equipment first; be sensitive, since stress may cause bladder or bowel accidents. **e.** School age, 6–12 years: cooperative and curious; usually have some understanding of EMS system; maturity levels are highly individualized; honesty very important, so seek their cooperation; modesty and body-image issues are common, so explanations are critical; fear of blood, pain, death, and permanent injury. **f.** Adolescent, 12–18 years: have concrete and abstract thinking skills, but believe nothing bad can happen to them; respect their privacy; obtain history when alone; peer influence strong; body conscious; may overreact. *(pp. 988–989)*

CONTENT REVIEW

1. **b.** Involve the caregivers if you can; it helps to calm them and acknowledges them as "experts" for this child. *(p. 988)*
2. **d.** Newborns and infants are obligate nose breathers; infants have proportionally larger tongues than adults as compared to the size of the mouth, which leaves little room for airway swelling; the smallest level of the airway in the child is at the level of the cricoid cartilage. The epiglottis is much higher in the airway than in the adult. *(p. 991)*
3. **c.** Hypothermia *(p. 993)*
4. **b.** Metabolic rates (Infants and children use oxygen from the bloodstream faster, making respiratory difficulties more dangerous.) *(p. 993)*
5. **c.** Respiratory system problems *(p. 996)*
6. **b.** The signs of early respiratory distress include an increase in the respiratory rate above normal; nasal flaring; intercostal, subclavicular, and subcostal retractions; neck muscle use; audible breathing noises; and "see-saw" respirations. *(p. 1038)*
7. **c.** Decompensated respiratory failure (Provide positive-pressure ventilation with supplemental oxygen and prompt transport.) *(p. 997)*
8. **c.** Respiratory arrest (Treat the patient aggressively with oxygenation and positive-pressure ventilation. Transport immediately.) *(p. 998)*
9. **b.** Normal respiration ranges from 25–30/min in an infant, and 15–30/min in a child. Measure the respiratory rate by counting the respirations for a full minute. Children generally breathe faster than adults. *(p. 1001)*
10. **c.** When assessing breath sounds in an infant or child, auscultate in the midaxillary line on the lateral chest. This is necessary since breath sounds are typically transmitted easily

from one side of the child's chest wall to the other. *(p. 1002)*
11. **b.** Urinary output *(p. 1002)*
12. (1) Support in prone head-down position. (2) Deliver five sharp back slaps. (3) Transfer to supine position and deliver five chest thrusts using two fingertips. (4) Look in mouth, sweep out visible object. (5) Attempt to ventilate; if unsuccessful, repeat sequence. *(p. 1014)*
13. **d.** Seizures in infants and children are caused by any condition that would produce seizures in adults. Seizures are high among children up to age 2. Seizures are caused by fever in about 5 percent of cases, and they can result in loss of bladder and bowel control. *(p. 1016)*
14. **b.** Status epilepticus occurs when a seizure lasts for longer than 10 minutes without a recovery period. This is a true emergency. Provide positive-pressure ventilation with supplemental oxygen. *(p. 1020)*
15. **d.** Management of the infant or child with a fever includes suctioning of secretions, if needed, for no longer than 5–10 seconds and, if there are seizures, the removal of clothing and sponging with tepid water. Don't use alcohol, ice, or cold water to cool the child. The EMT is not authorized to administer an antipyretic medication. *(pp. 1022–1023)*
16. **d.** Shock or hypoperfusion in children is uncommon because their blood vessels are able to constrict efficiently; it can occur in newborn children due to loss of body heat and an immature thermoregulatory system. Cardiac arrest in infants and children, when it does occur, is generally due to respiratory compromise. Shock in the pediatric patient occurs faster and is more serious than in adults. *(pp. 1023–1024)*
17. **a.** Management of an infant or child in shock includes keeping the patient warm, performing an ongoing assessment every 5 minutes, administering oxygen at 15 lpm via nonrebreather mask or blow-by (if breathing is adequate), and providing positive-pressure ventilation with supplemental oxygen at 20/min (if breathing is inadequate). *(p. 1025)*
18. **c.** Sudden infant death syndrome (SIDS) is also known as crib death or cot death, and it is the leading cause of death in infants 1 month to 1 year of age. Its occurrence cannot be predicted, and it cannot be diagnosed easily in the field. *(p. 1026)*
19. **b.** Management of SIDS should include immediate resuscitation efforts unless rigor mortis is present. Don't provide false reassurances to the family. Allow the caregivers to talk and tell their story. Transport immediately. *(p. 1027)*
20. **a.** Assess for capillary refill by compressing the soft tissue of the kneecap or forearm. Do not use distal portions of extremities. It must be used as only one of several indicators when

assessing the perfusion status. It alone can't provide a conclusion of poor perfusion. *(p. 995, 1002)*

21. **d.** Trauma in children is most commonly caused by blunt trauma. Trauma in children ages 1–14 is the leading cause of death. It is caused primarily by automobile-related deaths. It results in death within the first hour in 50 percent of all cases. *(p. 1028)*

22. **a.** Mechanisms requiring transport to a Level 1 Pediatric Trauma Center, if one is available, would include a motor vehicle crash in which the occupant is ejected from the vehicle or another occupant is killed or a pedestrian being struck at 10 mph or greater or thrown or dragged under or being run over by a vehicle. Other criteria include a fall from a height of 10 feet or more (not 5 feet) and an unrestrained occupant at speeds of 20 mph or greater. *(p. 1031)*

23. **a.** Interference with diaphragm movement and lung inflation may compromise respiratory effort. *(p. 1029)*

24. **a.** The most common cause of hypoxia is the tongue obstructing the airway. Hypoperfusion is typically not a sign of a closed head injury; infants and children have ribs that are more pliable than adults; capillary-refill test is not a reliable assessment of shock in and of itself. *(p. 1029)*

25. **b.** Fluid loss *(p. 1030)*

26. **d.** In many cases the child will be the victim of both abuse and neglect. Physical abuse is an improper action that causes an injury. Neglect is the provision of inadequate attention. The abused child will frequently exhibit fear when questioned about the injury. *(pp. 1030–1031)*

27. **c.** Objectively record your observations, follow local reporting protocols, and maintain total confidentiality. *(p. 1030)*

28. **c.** A tube that is placed into the stomach for children who require long-term feeding is called a gastrostomy tube. *(p. 1037)*

29. **b.** A suction catheter that is half the diameter of the tube *(p. 1035)*

30. **a.** The PAT can be performed from across the room before you actually make physical contact. This tool is especially useful because the necessary assessment information can be gathered during the general impression. The triangle is composed of three sides: appearance, work of breathing, and circulation. *(p. 996)*

31. **c.** The pediatric patient's cardiac compensation is primarily through changes in the heart rate. The pediatric patient does not have the ability to compensate by increasing the strength of cardiac contraction. *(p. 993)*

32. **c.** Capillary refill is a better indicator of the hydration status of the patient. It must be used as only one of several indicators when assessing the perfusion status. It alone can't provide a conclusion of poor perfusion. Assess for capillary refill by compressing the soft tis-

sue of the kneecap or forearm. Do not use distal portions of extremities. *(p. 995)*

33. **c.** If your pediatric patient is still maintaining an adequate respiratory depth and rate, the patient is said to be in early respiratory distress, otherwise known as "compensated respiratory distress." *(p. 997)*

34. **d.** If at any time the respiratory rate or tidal volume becomes inadequate, this is an indication that the patient has progressed from compensated respiratory distress to decompensated respiratory failure. This patient requires immediate ventilation with a bag-valve mask device or other acceptable ventilation device and supplemental oxygen. *(p. 997)*

35. **a.** When treating a patient that has wheezes and then the wheezing resolves without the use of medication, you should suspect the patient has become worse. If the wheezes are no longer heard, this may indicate the lack of adequate air movement. *(p. 1040)*

36. **a.** You should first open the airway and inspect the airway for the hot dog. *(pp. 998, 1015)*

CASE STUDY

1. **a.** The infant is exhibiting signs of decompensated respiratory failure.

2. **d.** The most appropriate immediate treatment for the infant is to provide positive-pressure ventilation with oxygen at 15 lpm and rapidly transport to the hospital.

3. **a.** In addition to the problem identified above, the infant is most likely suffering from dehydration. This is exhibited by the history of vomiting, no urinary output for the past few hours, a depressed fontanel, delayed capillary refill, and other physical findings of hypoperfusion and shock.

ENRICHMENT

1. **c.** Croup produces stridor on inhalation, with a harsh "seal bark." It results from a viral infection and has a slow onset of symptoms. Administer humidified oxygen. *(p. 1038)*

2. **c.** Epiglottitis is a bacterial infection that causes swelling of the epiglottis and most commonly affects 3- to 7-year-olds. It causes drooling, and the patient sits up and leans forward. If left untreated, it has a 50 percent mortality rate. *(pp. 1038–1039)*

3. **c.** Asthma occurs when the bronchioles constrict. It is common in children with allergies. Victims will assume a "tripod" position. All attacks must be regarded as serious. *(p. 1039)*

4. **d.** A severe attack of asthma that cannot be managed with medication is known as status asthmaticus. *(p. 1041)*

5. **c.** A condition that affects children less than 1 year of age and is caused when the small bronchi in the lungs become inflamed by a viral infection is called bronchiolitis. *(p. 1041)*

6. d. Chest compressions in children may be necessary if the heart rate drops below 60/min. *(p. 1041)*

7. a. An infection of the brain and spinal cord by a virus or bacteria is called meningitis. *(p. 1041)*

8. Only a, b, d, f, h, and i should be marked. The six categories of the Pediatric Trauma Score are size/weight, airway, systolic blood pressure, central nervous system, wounds, and suspicion of fractures. *(p. 1042)*

9. a. If the Pediatric Trauma Score is +8 or lower, rapidly transport the child to a pediatric trauma center, if one is available. *(p. 1042)*

10. c. Tape across the forehead and across the upper lip and around the seat. When immobilizing an infant or child in a car seat, never use sandbags to immobilize the head. Use towels or blankets to pad any voids that may be present. *(p. 1042)*

DOCUMENTATION EXERCISE

1. b. Any fall of at least 10 feet is a mechanism of injury that requires transport of the pediatric patient to a Level 1 Pediatric Trauma Center.

2. b. The average range for the pulse in this 18-month-old patient is 80–130 per minute.

3. b. When providing spinal immobilization for this patient, a spinal immobilization collar should be used. A quick check for pulses, motor, and sensory response should be performed prior to and after the patient is immobilized. Place padding under the shoulders to account for the large occiput, and secure the torso to the immobilization device before securing the head.

4. c. The patient in this case can be accurately referred to as a toddler. A neonate is the period of time from birth to discharge from the hospital, an infant from 1 to 12 months, a toddler from 1 to 3 years of age, a preschooler from 3 to 6 years of age.

5. a. The child in this case would be assigned a pediatric trauma score of +5. The Pediatric Trauma Score ranges from −6 to +12. The following score is assigned to this patient: Size/weight +1 (between 10 and 20 kg [22–40 lbs]). Airway +1 (constant observation required to maintain the patient's position or open airway; also if supplemental oxygen is needed). Systolic blood pressure +2 (pulse palpable at the wrist). Central nervous system −1 (comatose and unresponsive). Wounds +1 (minor wounds, including abrasions and lacerations). Suspicion of fracture +1 (simple closed fracture).

Chapter 37: Geriatrics

TERMS AND CONCEPTS

1. a. 7 b. 4 c. 3 d. 5 e. 1 f. 6 g. 8 h. 2 *(p. 1072)*

CONTENT REVIEW

1. c. Changes in body physiology typically begin at age 30; people are living longer with chronic diseases; and illness is not an inevitable part of aging. However, the aging body does have fewer reserves to combat the diseases and traumas that do occur. *(p. 1050)*

2. d. Cardiovascular system changes associated with aging include decreased arterial elasticity that speeds reaction to stimulation, degeneration of the conduction system that causes changes in rate or rhythm, decreased cardiac output due to cardiac hypertrophy, and an increased blood pressure due to increased vascular resistance. *(p. 1052)*

3. b. Blunted sensitivity to hypoxia *(pp. 1052, 1053)*

4. d. Osteoporosis *(p. 1053)*

5. a. Degeneration of nerve cells *(p. 1053)*

6. c. Malnutrition *(p. 1053)*

7. c. The kidneys become smaller in size, and there is a corresponding decrease in nephrons. The elderly patient's renal system is less resistant to failure during an acute illness or injury. The elderly more commonly suffer from drug toxicity when they take too much medication. *(p. 1053)*

8. a. You should always wear an N-95 or HEPA respirator when you are in contact with a potential tuberculosis patient. Elderly patients are more, not less, commonly the victims of heat- or cold-related emergencies. In a nursing home or other facility with multiple residents, be aware that a number of them may suffer from the same problem as your original patient, such as environmental temperature problems or toxic inhalation. It is not unlikely that an elderly patient will suffer from trauma and a medical problem at the same time, for example when a fainting spell causes a fall that results in injury. *(p. 1056)*

9. d. Signs of dehydration in the elderly include eyes that appear sunken in the orbits, membranes of the eyes and mouth that appear dry, and a tongue that appears furrowed. *(p. 1059)*

10. d. As a group, the elderly abuse alcohol *more* than other age groups. They deteriorate *more* quickly, are *less* sensitive to pain, and suffer *more* depression. *(pp. 1060–1061)*

11. d. A sudden onset of an altered mental status cannot be attributed to dementia. Dementia is a chronic condition with a slow rather than an acute onset. Reduced reflexes may cause a higher incidence of choking. Cervical arthritis may make the head-tilt/chin-lift maneuver difficult, so a jaw thrust may provide a better airway. A resting respiratory rate of greater than 20 per minute, fast in a younger patient, may be normal for the elderly patient. *(p. 1058)*

12. **b.** Lying on her side (the best way to protect the airway in a patient with an altered mental status) *(p. 1062)*

13. **c.** Immobilized with blankets (to accommodate his spinal curvature) *(p. 1062)*

14. **c.** Weakness and fatigue are common presentations of a silent heart attack in an elderly patient, as are trouble breathing, aching shoulders, and indigestion. The other choices are not common heart-attack presentations. *(p. 1063)*

15. **b.** Fowler's position (sitting up) (usually helps support breathing in the CHF patient) *(p. 1064)*

16. **c.** Fowler's position (sitting up) (usually helps support breathing in the COPD patient) *(p. 1066)*

17. **a.** Administering oxygen by nonrebreather mask (Mr. Herbert's sudden onset of breathing difficulty and pain that does not radiate may indicate a pulmonary embolism, not a heart attack with pain that usually radiates.) *(p. 1065)*

18. **c.** An elderly patient can easily become fatigued from labored breathing and lose the ability to sustain it. In this case, provide positive-pressure ventilation to sustain respiration and expedite transport. *(p. 1065)*

19. **a.** An altered mental status in a geriatric patient is usually difficult to manage. The other choices are not true. *(p. 1066)*

20. **a.** Y **b.** N **c.** Y **d.** Y **e.** Y **f.** Y (Other causes of altered mental status include decreased blood volume, effects of medications, dementia, heart rhythm disturbances, and heart attack.) *(p. 1067)*

21. **a.** A stroke patient requires aggressive oxygenation to prevent further deterioration of brain tissue. *(p. 1067)*

22. **c.** Older patients are more at risk for drug toxicity than younger patients, and older patients buy the greatest number of prescriptions. All medications that the patient is taking, including over-the-counter medications, should be taken to the hospital with the patient. Treatment of the drug-toxicity patient is based on treating the drug's effects. *(p. 1068)*

23. **a.** Cardiac hypertrophy is a thickening of the cardiac walls without any increase in atrial or ventricular chambers, which decreases stroke volume. *(p. 1051)*

24. **d.** Orthostatic hypotension is a drop in the systolic blood pressure and an elevation of the heart rate when the elderly patient goes from a lying to a standing position. *(p. 1052)*

25. **d.** Factors that contribute to the development of environmental emergencies among the elderly include situational factors, such as an inability to afford adequate heating or cooling. Aging, limitations on movement, and medications may all decrease the ability to regulate body temperature. *(p. 1070)*

26. (1) Protect the airway. (2) Maintain normal breathing and circulation. (3) Remove the patient from the environment. (4) Remove wet clothing. (5) Wrap the patient in a dry blanket. *(p. 1070)*

27. **b.** Chemoreceptors become less sensitive in detecting hypoxia or carbon dioxide levels in the blood. *(p. 1052)*

28. **d.** Kyphosis is a curvature of the spine that is caused by narrowing of the vertebral disks in the elderly patient. *(p. 1053)*

CASE STUDY

1. **a.** Establish and maintain stabilization of the head and neck. The patient fell down a flight of stairs. A significant mechanism of injury exists for a potential cervical-spine injury. She does not have symptoms that indicate a need for positive-pressure ventilation. Splinting and a call to adult protective services, if warranted, can take place later.

2. **c.** Mrs. Walter's skin is cool and pale, which may indicate circulatory compromise and possible hypoperfusion. She must be carefully observed and vitals repeated frequently until a trend can be established. Her pulse, respirations, and blood pressure are all within normal limits.

Chapter 38: Ambulance Operations

CONTENT REVIEW

1. **d.** A "privilege" associated with the operation of an emergency vehicle is passing in a no-passing zone. Other privileges include exceeding the posted speed limit, driving the wrong way down a one-way street, turning in any direction at an intersection, parking anywhere, leaving the ambulance standing in the middle of a street or intersection, and going through red lights or red flashing signals. You must avoid endangering life and property by driving with a due regard for the safety of others; otherwise, you are individually and personally responsible for any liabilities that result. *(p. 1078)*

2. **b.** Driving the wrong way down a one-way street without using any warning devices is obviously disregarding the safety of others. *(p. 1078)*

3. **d.** To be a good emergency vehicle operator the EMT should try to travel the posted speed limit when possible, hold the steering wheel at the 9 o'clock and 3 o'clock positions, travel routes that will ensure the quickest and safest response (it may not be the shortest route), brake into a curve and then gradually accelerate when going out of the curve. *(pp. 1078–1079)*

4. **c.** The use of escorts doubles the hazards associated with emergency driving; they should only be used as a last resort. *(pp. 1079–1080)*

5. **d.** When using a siren, never pull directly behind a car and blast your siren; always assume

that other drivers are unaware of you. Operators tend to increase their speed by about 15 mph when the siren is in operation. The siren creates emotional stress for you, your partner, and the patient. *(p. 1081)*

6. **c.** Legally, you may be within your rights to refuse to use a vehicle that you have reason to believe is unsafe. You may be legally liable for damage caused by a malfunctioning vehicle. Respectfully refuse to operate the vehicle. *(p. 1084)*

7. Only a, c, d, f, and g should be marked. The dispatcher should provide the following information: location of the call; nature of the call; name, location, and callback number of the caller; location of the patient at the scene; the number of patients; and the severity of the problem. *(p. 1084)*

8. **a.** Determine and clarify the responsibilities of each team member. *(p. 1085)*

9. The missing phases of the ambulance call are as follows: at the scene, at the receiving facility, and en route to the station. *(p. 1082)*

10. **a.** Position the ambulance to provide a safety zone. *(p. 1085)*

11. **b.** Stay a minimum of 100 feet from wreckage or a burning vehicle and 2,000 feet from hazardous materials spills. *(p. 1085)*

12. **c.** Prior to arrival at the emergency scene, determine the responsibilities of team members. Upon arrival at the emergency scene, carefully observe the complete incident as you approach, turn your headlights off (unless used to illuminate the scene) so that they don't blind oncoming drivers' vision, and rapidly move unstable patients to the ambulance. *(p. 1085)*

13. **c.** Every 15 minutes for a stable patient, every 5 minutes for an unstable patient *(p. 1087)*

14. **a.** Allowing family or friends in the patient compartment during transport to the hospital may be helpful if the patient is a child. It is not prohibited by state EMS statutes; a federal EMS statute does not exist; and it may be helpful if the patient's family or friend is emotionally stable. Ensure that companions use safety restraints while accompanying the patient. *(p. 1087)*

15. **a.** Ensure proper continuity of care *(p. 1090)*

16. **d.** It should be left at the emergency department. (Some EMS systems also may require you to leave a copy with the patient.) *(p. 1090)*

17. **a.** Appropriate post-run activities include changing a soiled uniform, completing an inventory of equipment and supplies, leaving the run report at the hospital before departing (and giving a copy to the patient if local protocol requires it), filling the fuel tank if necessary, and cleaning and disinfecting the ambulance after each call and at the end of the shift. Washing your hands and providing oral and written reports to hospital staff are performed while at the hospital. *(pp. 1090–1092)*

18. **d.** A process that kills all microorganisms is sterilization. *(p. 1092)*

19. **a.** 1:10 solution of household bleach and water *(p. 1092)*

20. **a.** 3 **b.** 1 **c.** 4 **d.** 2 *(p. 1092)*

21. **a.** Guidelines for setting up a landing zone include placement of a fifth warning device on the upwind side, establishment of a 100 × 100-foot area for a nighttime landing zone, keeping spectators at least 200 feet away, and establishment of a 60 × 60-foot area (small helicopter) for a daytime landing zone. Be sure to refer to your local aeromedical landing-zone guidelines for proper landing procedures. *(pp. 1093–1094)*

ENRICHMENT

1. **c.** National Association of Emergency Medical Technicians (NAEMT) guidelines for ensuring operational safety and security measures require security briefings at the beginning of each shift (or information sheets, postings, or supervisor briefings), increased involvement of EMS crews in the development of security measures, never leaving EMS vehicles unattended with the keys in the ignition, and increasing tracking systems of EMS vehicles. *(pp. 1094–1095)*

2. **d.** Nighttime driving conditions result in two and a half times more fatal collisions than do daytime driving conditions. It is more difficult for older drivers as compared to younger drivers and is improved by not staring directly at the high beams of oncoming cars. Night driving is improved by the use of quartz-halogen headlights. *(p. 1096–1097)*

3. **c.** Techniques for safe driving at night include not using your high beams when entering a curve, dimming your headlights within 500 feet of an approaching driver, keeping your eyes moving and avoiding focusing on one object, and not flicking high beams up and down to remind a driver to dim his bright lights. *(pp. 1096–1097)*

4. **b.** When driving in bad weather, the roads are slipperiest at the start of a rainstorm. If hydroplaning begins, hold the wheel steady, release the accelerator, and gently pump the brake. Stopping on ice requires five times the stopping distance. Hydroplaning can begin at speeds of 35 mph. *(pp. 1097–1098)*

5. **b.** Carbon monoxide in ambulances is difficult to detect due to its being odorless, colorless, and tasteless. It occurs with greater outside air pressure, can be reduced by keeping the rear windows closed, and may be harmful in amounts over 10 parts per million. *(p. 1098)*

Chapter 39: Gaining Access and Extrication

CONTENT REVIEW

1. **a.** When receiving dispatch information *(p. 1106)*
2. **b.** Motor vehicle collisions *(p. 1107)*
3. **c.** Binoculars can help you assess the scene from a safe distance. *(p. 1103)*
4. **a.** Full protective turnout gear (This includes coat, bunker pants, steel-toed boots, helmet with ear flaps and wide brim and a face shield, eye protection, and heavy leather gloves over disposable gloves.) *(p. 1103)*
5. **c.** *Always* assume downed power lines are alive. (Call the electric-service company for assistance.) *(p. 1104)*
6. **b.** Stop all traffic and reroute it to different roads. (Remember, however, that special prior training in traffic direction and control is necessary.) *(p. 1104)*
7. A child may have been involved. (This clue should prompt you to ask questions and complete a thorough search of the area.) *(p. 1106)*
8. **c.** A vehicle is stable when it can no longer move, rock, or bounce. *(p. 1106)*
9. **d.** Simply turns off the ignition *(p. 1106)*
10. Before disconnecting the power to the vehicle, you should try to move the seat backward, lower power windows, and unlock power door locks. This will give you greatest access to the patient. *(p. 1106)*
11. **a.** Remove the negative battery cable first. *(p. 1106)*
12. **b.** Complex access requires tools and specialized equipment. Simple access does not require tools. *(p. 1106)*
13. **a.** Breaking a window *(p. 1107)*
14. **c.** From the front (Approach facing the patient to keep him from moving his head.) *(p. 1107)*
15. **d.** Start your request by saying, "Without moving your head or neck." (If you wait until the end of your sentence to say this, the patient may move before you can finish.) *(p. 1107)*
16. **c.** Against the lower corner of the window *(p. 1108)*
17. **b.** Patient care always precedes removal from the vehicle *except* when delay would endanger the patient or rescue personnel. *(p. 1108)*
18. **d.** Use blankets, a tarp, or a spine board. *(p. 1109)*
19. **b.** Explain the activities, noises, and movements. *(p. 1110)*
20. **d.** The only exception to the rule that the spine must be stabilized and, if possible, immobilized before removing a patient from a vehicle is when there is an immediate threat to your patient's life or your own or when another patient blocks access to a critically injured patient. *(p. 1110)*

CASE STUDY

1. **a.** Secure an area that is more than 80 feet in all directions. Yell instructions to the patient to stay in the vehicle. Do not approach the car because power can be automatically restored. Trust only the power company or specialized teams trained in electrical hazards to tell you when it is safe.
2. **c.** Tell the patient to focus and keep his attention on an object directly in front of him.
3. Make the patient aware of how long the process may take, explain the activities and movements around him, explain the noises that will be present, ask the patient if he is ready to have the door opened, stay with the patient at all times, and reassure him constantly.

ENRICHMENT

1. **b.** The first step to properly stabilizing an upright vehicle is to immobilize the suspension. This is most often accomplished by positioning step chocks under the vehicle parallel to each wheel. *(p. 1110)*
2. **d.** The first step to securing a vehicle that is positioned on its side is to place a strong pulling device or chain from the undercarriage of the car to another vehicle or strong immovable object. *(p. 1111)*
3. **c.** Opening or removing doors during patient extrication will reduce the strength of the post and may cause the roof to collapse. *(p. 1112)*
4. **b.** Prying the latch site on the "B" posts most easily opens the front doors of a vehicle. The "A" posts are the front posts supporting the car roof (hinge side). The "C" posts are at the rear and the "B" posts are in the middle. *(p. 1112)*
5. **d.** If the vehicle is on its side, access is best gained through the rear window. Opening the trunk or rear hatch may cause the vehicle to become unstable, and the trunk will not allow access. Lifting the door on the top of the car is difficult and dangerous because of its weight. Removing the roof will likely make the vehicle unstable. *(p. 1112)*

Chapter 40: Hazardous Materials Emergencies

TERMS AN CONCEPTS

1. **a.** 3 **b.** 2 **c.** 4 **d.** 1 *(p. 1138)*

CONTENT REVIEW

1. **b.** Rescuer, public, and patient safety is always the primary concern at any hazardous material emergency. *(p. 1120)*
2. **c.** The four factors that determine a patient's response to hazardous material exposure are the dose, the concentration, route of exposure, and the time exposed to the material. *(p. 1120)*
3. **c.** A four-sided diamond shape. The placard contains a four-digit UN identification num-

ber and a legend that indicates whether the material is flammable, radioactive, explosive, or poisonous. *(p. 1124)*

4. **a.** A health hazard. The NFPA 704 system, for use in marking hazardous materials located at fixed facilities, identifies potential dangers with the use of background colors and numbers ranging from 0 to 4. Blue identifies a health hazard, red a fire hazard, yellow a reactivity hazard; the higher the number the greater the hazard. *(p. 1124)*

5. **a.** The Chemical Transportation Emergency Center, or CHEMTREC, may be reached at 1-800-424-9300 around the clock for advice on how to handle any emergency involving hazardous materials. *(p. 1126)*

6. **c.** Hazardous materials should not be detected by relying on your senses, are not always easily detectable, may create colored vapor clouds, and all spills should be treated as dangerous until proven otherwise. *(p. 1125)*

7. **b.** The principal dangers hazardous materials present are toxicity, flammability, and reactivity. *(p. 1120)*

8. **b.** *Emergency Response Guidebook* *(p. 1126)*

9. **b.** First Responder Awareness, First Responder Operations, Hazardous Materials Technician, and Hazardous Materials Specialist are the four levels of training that OSHA and EPA have identified. *(p. 1128)*

10. **c.** Threatens the immediate safety of victims and rescuers and threatens their long-term health. By carrying toxins and particles of hazardous materials through the air, smoke from a hazardous-materials fire not only threatens the immediate safety of victims and rescuers, it also may threaten long-term health, in some cases causing cancer and chronic poisoning affecting the brain, liver, lungs, and kidneys. *(p. 1130–1131)*

11. **c.** Before a hazardous material emergency occurs, one command officer should be appointed who will make all decisions, and a clear chain-of-command system must be developed. An established system of communications used throughout the emergency should be developed. The system should be one all rescuers are informed about, know how to use, and have access to. Predesignate the hospital receiving facilities that will be utilized, and train and prepare for the worst possible scenario that may occur in a local community. *(p. 1129)*

12. (1) Protect the safety of all rescuers and victims. (2) Provide patient care. (3) Decontaminate clothing, equipment, and the vehicle. *(p. 1129)*

13. **d.** Correct activities or actions in the hot zone include not allowing anyone (other than trained rescuers) in the hot zone; smoking, eating, and drinking are prohibited; establish one entry point. Only rescue, initial decontamination, and treatment of life threats are performed in the hot zone. *(p. 1132)*

14. **b.** Decontaminate the patient fully (A contaminated patient in a closed, tight space could affect the breathing or vision of the air transport team.) *(p. 1132)*

15. **c.** Keep uphill, upwind, upstream, and away from the danger. *(p. 1129)*

16. **b.** Failure to properly decontaminate equipment and the interior of the vehicle can result in chronic chemical exposure. *(p. 1134)*

CASE STUDY 1

1. **d.** Quickly call for additional assistance.
2. **c.** Keep uphill, upwind, and protect yourself and the patient. (Prevent others from approaching the accident site until specialized help arrives.)

CASE STUDY 2

1. **c.** Under the arms and in the groin (Contamination occurs most easily in areas of your body where the skin is thin or moist.)
2. **a.** Wash with mild detergent or green soap and plenty of running water. Irrigate exposed skin for at least 20 minutes.
3. **b.** Take precautions to protect your equipment and vehicle during transport, since there may still be some contamination on the patient. Cover exposed areas of the vehicle with plastic sheeting.

CASE STUDY 3

1. **a.** Remove the bystander, evacuate the area, contact dispatch. (Do not attempt or allow other untrained persons to attempt to put out the fire. Do not remain near the building. Because toxic fertilizers may be burning at this fire, evacuate to a safe area until specialized help arrives.)

ENRICHMENT

1. **c.** In a radiation accident the patient may suffer from both exposure to and contamination by radiation. Exposure occurs when the patient is in the presence of radioactive material without any of the radioactive material actually touching his clothing or body. The exposure he receives may be harmful to him, but the patient himself does not become radioactive and does not pose any major threat to rescue personnel. Contamination occurs when the patient has come into direct contact with the source of radioactivity or with radioactive gases, liquids, or particles. *(p. 1134)*
2. **d.** Alpha rays can be stopped by clothing. *(p. 1135)*
3. **a.** Radiation sickness is caused by exposure to large amounts of radiation. It starts the day after the exposure and can last from a few days to 7–8 weeks. *(p. 1136)*
4. **d.** The Federal Nuclear Regulatory Commission recommends that an individual in an emergency situation not be exposed to more than a one-time whole-body dose of 25 roentgens. *(p. 1136)*

5. d. This occurs when the patient has been exposed to a dangerous amount of internal radiation. It results in a host of diseases, including cancer and anemia. It is called radiation poisoning. *(p. 1136)*

DOCUMENTATION EXERCISE

1. b. Command for this situation should be assumed by one command officer.

2. a. The receiving facility to which the patient is being transported should be predesignated during preincident planning.

3. c. Tyrone auscultated Jill's chest for the presence of pulmonary edema that may be associated with inhalation of ammonia.

4. a. Tyrone and Colleen are most likely trained to the level of First Responder Awareness.

5. a. The area where contamination is present is called the hot zone.

Chapter 41: Multiple-Casualty Incidents

TERMS AND CONCEPTS

1. a. 8 **b.** 5 **c.** 2 **d.** 12 **e.** 4 **f.** 1 **g.** 9 **h.** 6 **i.** 3 **j.** 11 **k.** 7 **l.** 10 *(p. 1159)*

CONTENT REVIEW

1. b. The National Incident Management System (NIMS) provides a consistent approach to managing disasters by all responders. *(p. 1142)*

2. a. The incident commander is located or stationed in the mobile command unit. *(p. 1144)*

3. a. If the child is unresponsive to all stimuli or responds to pain with incomprehensible sounds or inappropriate movement (does not localize pain or has no purposeful flexion or extension), tag the child "red" and move on to the next patient. *(p. 1149, Fig. 41-8)*

4. c. Any patient who is able to walk at the scene of a multiple-casualty incident is initially tagged as a "green" or low-priority patient. *(pp. 1146–1147)*

5. b. Primary triage is conducted at the actual site of the incident if it is safe—example: inside the bus before the patients are moved. *(pp. 1145–1146)*

6. a. Triage is a system used to sort patients according to criticality. *(p. 1145)*

7. d. Secondary triage is performed when the patient is moved to the triage unit. It is designed to reevaluate the initial patient categorization, during which the patient may be upgraded, downgraded, or kept the same. *(p. 1146)*

8. d. Check ability to walk, respirations, perfusion, and mental status (ARPM) *(p. 1146)*

9. b. This patient is deceased. Tag the patient as "black" and move on to the next patient. *(p. 1147)*

10. a. Priority 1 patients are transported first, followed by Priority 2, then Priority 3 patients. Priority 4 patients are deceased. *(p. 1146)*

11. a. A patient with respirations greater than 30 per minute is assigned to Priority 1 (red). *(p. 1147)*

12. a. Red indicates high priority. (Tagging helps arriving EMTs quickly and efficiently identify treatment and transport priorities.) *(p. 1150)*

13. d. Triage or priority level (Color flags or ribbons should be erected at the ends of each row to designate the respective treatment areas. Place the patient in the appropriate row according to the color or level triaged.) *(p. 1151)*

14. c. Provide plenty of nourishing food and drinks. Rest every 1–2 hours; rapidly remove any rescue worker who becomes hysterical and transport to the hospital; encourage rescuers to talk among themselves. *(p. 1154)*

15. d. The JumpSTART pediatric triage system was specifically designed by Dr. Lou Romig for children between the ages of 1 and 8. However, Dr. Romig now recommends that JumpSTART be used on any patient that appears to be a child and START be used on any patient who appears to be a young adult or older. *(p. 1148)*

CASE STUDY

1. b. Request additional help and assistance *early* in the MCI. It's better to call too many rescuers than too few.

2. b. If the child is alert, responds to voice, or responds to pain by localizing it, withdrawing from it, or trying to push it away, the patient is tagged "yellow."

3. b. The transport unit leader is responsible for notification of the hospital; the unit should be located close to where the ambulances stage or arrive; it should be clearly marked; and if necessary, more than one treatment unit may be required.

4. a. Green **b.** Red **c.** Yellow **d.** Red **e.** Black

ENRICHMENT

1. b. Safe routes to take out of the area, the nature of the disaster and its estimated time of impact, a description of the expected severity, and appropriate destinations for those who evacuate are all appropriate. *(pp. 1155–1156)*

2. d. Preadolescents and adolescents are most likely to experience extreme aggression and stress that is severe enough to disrupt their lives. *(p. 1156)*

3. b. Always tell the truth. Giving false assurances to patients does not help them deal with the reality of the event. Encourage patients to talk about the disaster and its potential long-term effects. Reuniting of families should occur as soon as possible to lessen the emotional stress. Encouraging patients to do necessary chores will help them return to normal. *(pp. 1156–1157)*

Chapter 42: EMS Response to Weapons of Mass Destruction

TERMS AND CONCEPTS

1. a. 2 b. 3 c. 4 d. 1 e. 5 f. 6 *(p. 1176–1177)*

CONTENT REVIEW

1. a. Coordinated community preplanning for a WMD attack is necessary, and a single EMS agency is unlikely to have enough equipment to handle a WMD attack. Local, regional, and state disaster agencies should develop weapons-of-mass-destruction disaster plans, and the general approach is similar to that for any disaster involving multiple casualties, with some additional considerations. *(p. 1163)*
2. d. Explosive and incendiary agents are the most widely used weapons of mass destruction used by terrorists. *(p. 1165)*
3. c. Incendiary devices produce a different injury pattern from conventional explosives. They are easy to improvise and manufacture and include napalm, thermite, and magnesium. Incendiary-device burns are assessed in the same manner as thermal burns. *(p. 1166)*
4. a. The mnemonic SLUDGE (for salivation, lacrimation, urination, defecation, and gastric emptying) stands for the signs and symptoms associated with nerve agent exposure. *(p. 1168)*
5. b. Two drugs used to counteract the effects of nerve agents are atropine and pralidoxime (Protopam). *(p. 1168)*
6. c. Vesicants cause blistering, burning, and tissue damage on contact. *(p. 1168)*
7. b. Cyanide disrupts the ability of the cell to use oxygen and leads to cellular hypoxia and eventually death. The pulse oximeter may provide a false sense of reassurance, since the blood is being oxygenated well, yet the cell cannot use the oxygen. *(p. 1169)*
8. d. Phosgene, halogen compounds, and nitrogen–oxygen compounds are examples of pulmonary agents. *(p. 1169)*
9. b. The management for exposure to riot-control agents should focus first on removing the patient from the environment. Activated charcoal, amyl nitrite, and sodium nitrite are not administered for this purpose. The eyes should be irrigated. *(p. 1170)*
10. a. Biological agents are categorized into four groups: pneumonia-like agents, encephalitis-like agents, biological toxins, and other agents. *(p. 1171)*
11. a. The two common encephalitis-like agents are smallpox and Venezuelan equine encephalitis. *(p. 1171)*
12. b. The three primary mechanisms of death or injury associated with nuclear detonation are radiation, blast, and thermal burns. *(p. 1173)*
13. a. Gamma radiation is the most penetrating type of radiation and can travel long distances. *(p. 1173)*
14. b. There are two types of radiation exposure associated with a nuclear explosion. After primary exposure, fallout is the second form of radiation exposure, containing radioactive dust and particles. *(p. 1173)*
15. a. A conventional explosive attached to radioactive materials is referred to as a radiological dispersal device (RDD) or a "dirty bomb." *(p. 1174)*

CASE STUDY

1. a. The mechanism that causes most deaths and injury associated with nuclear detonation is the blast wave and thermal burns.
2. d. The nuclear ignition produces an explosively expanding gas cloud and the shock-wave injuries from nuclear detonation are similar to shock-wave injuries produced by conventional weapons. The intensity of shockwave injuries is greater the closer the victim is to ground zero, and the windblast is strong enough to cause structural collapse, crush injuries, and entrapment.
3. b. It's true that personnel with hazardous materials (HAZMAT) training are prepared to act as an initial response crew in a nuclear event because similar principles apply.

Chapter 43: Advanced Airway Management

MEDICAL TERMINOLOGY

1. b. Inflammation
2. a. Condition of
3. d. Narrowing
4. c. Mouth
5. c. Viewing, examining

TERMS AND CONCEPTS

1. a. 7 b. 10 c. 9 d. 1 e. 5 f. 6 g. 3 h. 2 i. 4 j. 11 k. 8 *(p. 1224)*

CONTENT REVIEW

1. A. Vallecula B. Epiglottis C. Tongue D. Glossoepiglottic ligament *(p. 1183)*
2. A. Epiglottis B. False vocal cords C. Aryepiglottic fold D. True vocal cords E. Glottis F. Cuneiform cartilage G. Corniculate cartilage *(p. 1183)*
3. d. The right mainstem bronchus is almost in line with the trachea. (Choices a and b refer to the bronchioles, which branch from the bronchi, not the trachea.) *(p. 1184)*
4. a. Place a small, folded towel under the child's shoulders; this will help place the patient in a more natural position due to the proportionately larger head. *(p. 1185)*
5. c. Snoring (or sonorous) airway sounds indicate that the tongue is occluding the upper airway. This is the most common mechanism of

airway obstruction in the unresponsive adult. *(p. 1182)*

6. **d.** Gurgling indicates fluid that needs to be removed prior to using advanced airway techniques. *(p. 1186)*

7. **c.** Permits better ventilation and oxygen delivery (the bag-valve device can be connected directly to the tracheal tube). Other advantages of tracheal intubation include the following: (a) provides complete control of the airway (a direct route for ventilation and oxygenation; (b) prevents the tongue from blocking the airway so manual maneuvers such as a head-tilt/chin-lift are not necessary); (c) isolates the trachea, lessening the risk of aspiration; (d) allows for deeper suctioning through the tracheal tube. *(p. 1192)*

8. **d.** After inserting an OPA and ventilating the patient, you determine the patient cannot protect her own airway. Indications for tracheal intubation include (a) inability to ventilate the apneic patient effectively with standard methods; (b) inability of the patient to protect her own airway (is unresponsive to any type of stimulus; has no gag reflex). *(p. 1192)*

9. **d.** The end-tidal CO_2 and esophageal detectors are applied as secondary placement confirmation. Direct visualization assures correct passage of the tracheal tube through the glottic opening and vocal cords. Primary confirmation of placement is obtained through auscultation of the epigastrium and chest. *(pp. 1191, 1196)*

10. **b.** You are able to insert an oropharyngeal airway without the patient's gagging. (Don't insert your fingers; the patient may bite you.) *(p. 1199)*

11. **d.** A nonporous gown may be used but is not a required body substance isolation device when performing tracheal intubation. Remember, your face will be very close to the patient's mouth; your eyes, nose, and mouth should all be protected, in addition to your wearing gloves. *(p. 1211)*

12. **a.** The best position for cricoid pressure follows the mnemonic BURP, which stands for backward, upward, rightward pressure. *(p. 1195)*

13. **d.** Hold the tongue out of the way *(p. 1188)*

14. **b.** Pressing on the glossoepiglottic ligament to lift the epiglottis indirectly (The curved blade is inserted into the vallecula, which presses on the glossoepiglottic ligament.) *(p. 1188)*

15. Check whether the blade is securely locked, whether the bulb is tightly screwed into the socket, and whether the bulb or the batteries need to be changed. *(p. 1188)*

16. **b.** 7.5 mm i.d. *(p. 1189)*

17. **A.** 15 mm adapter **B.** Centimeter marker **C.** Pilot balloon **D.** Inflation port **E.** Cuff **F.** Bevel **G.** Murphy eye *(p. 1190)*

18. **a.** Permits airflow if the tube is obstructed *(p. 1190)*

19. **b.** Distal tip of tube should be in the trachea, midway between the carina and the vocal cords. *(p. 1190)*

20. **c.** Never extend the stylet past the end of the tube; it may cause severe trauma to the patient's airway. *(p. 1190)*

21. **b.** Inflate the cuff with 10 cc of air. *(p. 1191)*

22. **d.** The purpose of the cuff is to seal the trachea (not to secure the tube in place). The cuff prevents regurgitation of stomach contents by sealing the trachea, not the esophagus. *(p. 1191)*

23. **a.** Place the index finger and thumb of one hand on the anterior aspect of the throat just lateral to the midline of the cricoid cartilage; then apply pressure backward to close off the esophagus. (Cricoid pressure decreases the chance of vomitus coming up the esophagus and into the airway; it also pushes the glottic structures into the visual field during intubation.) *(p. 1192)*

24. **b.** Most laryngoscope blades are designed to be held in the left hand and to sweep the tongue to the left. *(pp. 1188, 1195)*

25. **d.** Oval sphincterous passageway (The three landmarks that identify the glottic opening are (a) the cartilaginous structures surround the glottic opening; (b) the glottic opening is round, not oval like the esophageal opening; and (c) the glottic opening contains the vocal cords through which the tube will pass.) *(p. 1183)*

26. To verify correct tracheal-tube placement (in addition to watching the tube pass through the vocal cords), primary techniques of confirmation are the following: (a) Auscultate over the epigastrium. (Gurgling or breath sounds over the stomach indicate improper tube placement in the esophagus—deflate and remove the tube at once.) (b) Watch for chest rise and fall during ventilations (assures tube placement in the trachea). (c) Auscultate breath sounds at the apex and base of the right and left lungs. (Presence of equal sounds in both lungs assures that the tube has not advanced into the right mainstem bronchus, depriving the left lung of air.) In addition, as secondary techniques of confirmation, you should use an end-tidal carbon dioxide detector to measure the concentration of exhaled carbon dioxide, an esophageal intubation detection device, or a pulse oximeter to measure the blood-oxygen level. Also observe the patient for signs of deterioration, combativeness, or cyanosis. *(p. 1196)*

27. **d.** 1, 2, 3, 4, and 5. All may occur in the adult patient who has been intubated. (The most common complications in an adult are hypertension, tachycardia, and dysrhythmias. Bradycardia and hypotension are more commonly seen in infants and children but may be experienced by some adults. Additional potential complications of intubation are hypoxia and trauma to the lips, tongue, gums, teeth, and airway structures.) *(p. 1198)*

28. **b.** The patient must be unresponsive and in severe respiratory distress. *(p. 1199)*
29. **d.** The straight blade lifts the epiglottis directly. The curved blade is placed into the vallecula to lift the epiglottis indirectly. *(p. 1200)*
30. **a.** Refer to a sizing chart or resuscitation tape. Other methods include matching the outside diameter of the tube to the child's little finger or using this formula: For the patient between the ages of 1 and 10 years, when using the uncuffed tracheal tube: uncuffed tube size = 4 + (age in years ÷ 4). *(p. 1201)*
31. **a.** The presence of gurgling during airway maintenance is indicative of fluid in the airway. *(p. 1186)*
32. **a.** Two indications for nasogastric intubation in infants and children are (1) you are unable to provide positive-pressure ventilation due to gastric distension, or (2) the patient is unresponsive and at risk of vomiting or developing gastric distention. *(p. 1204)*
33. Contraindications for nasogastric intubation in infants and children (situations in which the NG tube should not be inserted) are (a) the patient has suffered major facial, head, or spinal trauma (the tube could exacerbate the trauma or be pushed through a basilar skull fracture into the brain; do not insert an NG tube in such patients without consulting medical direction); or (b) airway disease such as epiglottitis or croup is suspected (the NG tube can cause spasms or exacerbate swelling to the point of occluding the airway). *(p. 1204)*
34. **b.** The esophageal detector may provide inaccurate results in a patient who is extremely obese, is in late pregnancy, is suffering from status asthmaticus, or has large amounts of secretions. *(p. 1197)*
35. **b.** Measure the NG tube from the tip of the nose around the ear, extending downward until the distal end is past the xiphoid process. (Don't forget to mark the length with tape; when inserting the tube, you will stop when the tape is at the nostrils.) *(p. 1205)*
36. Possible complications of orotracheal suctioning are (1) hypoxia caused by removing residual air and interrupting ventilations; (2) cardiac dysrhythmias, possibly lethal; (3) coughing, which can dangerously increase pressure within the skull and decrease blood flow to the brain; (4) trauma to the mucosa; and (5) bronchospasms if the catheter is inserted past the carina. *(p. 1208)*
37. **b.** DOPE is the mnemonic used to help determine causes of deterioration in the patient's oxygenation or ventilation status. DOPE stands for displacement, obstruction, pneumothorax, equipment. *(p. 1203)*
38. **d.** The esophageal detector should immediately reinflate and not remain collapsed. *(p. 1191)*
39. **b.** A suction unit with an adjustable regulator should be adjusted to provide negative pressure between 80 and 120 mmHg. A suction

device should also be readily available during the pediatric intubation procedure. *(p. 1200)*
40. **a.** When intubating a child patient with a cuffed tracheal tube per your medical direction, you should use the formula: tube size = 3 + (age in years ÷ 4). *(p. 1201)*

CASE STUDY

1. **b.** Always provide basic airway management before attempting intubation: Perform a jaw thrust, insert an oropharyngeal airway, and hyperoxygenate.
2. Yes. This patient should be intubated because the patient is unresponsive and cannot protect his own airway.
3. **c.** Suction the patient before performing any advanced airway techniques.
4. **a.** Ten to 12 breaths per minute for at least 1 minute (This will help saturate the blood with oxygen, which is necessary because there will be no ventilations while the tracheal tube is being inserted.)
5. Because this patient has a suspected spinal injury, you must maintain in-line stabilization. Have Jill stabilize the head and neck from below while you secure the head with your thighs. Jill should apply Sellick's maneuver to help push the glottic structures into the visual field.
6. **b.** 30 seconds (Intubation attempts longer than 30 seconds can cause hypoxia.)
7. **a.** One-half inch to 1 inch past the vocal cords (This will place the tip approximately halfway between the carina and vocal cords.)
8. **b.** The tube is past the carina and in the right mainstem bronchus. Deflate the cuff and pull back enough to restore lung sounds on the left. When equal lung sounds are confirmed, reinflate the cuff.

ENRICHMENT

1. **c.** During digital intubation, the EMT lifts the epiglottis directly by inserting his fingers into the patient's hypopharynx. Digital intubation is a blind procedure and may not be performed on the alert patient, who may have a gag reflex. The head and neck do not have to be manipulated during digital intubation. *(p. 1211)*
2. **a.** Since this technique requires seeing light of the stylet through the tissues of the neck, it can be difficult to see in bright ambient light. This technique can be effective in the trauma patient. A bright light appearing lateral to the upper aspect of the thyroid cartilage indicates placement in the right or left pyriform fossa. A light at the front of the neck that is diffuse, dim, or hard to see indicates that placement is in the esophagus. *(p. 1213)*
3. **d.** The 17-year-old unresponsive patient suffering from smoke inhalation would be an appropriate candidate for the PtL®. Contraindications for the PtL® include patients younger than 16 years, patients less than 5 feet tall, responsive patients, patients who have a gag reflex, patients who have

swallowed a caustic substance, or the presence of esophageal disease. *(p. 1214)*

4. b. If the patient regains responsiveness or develops a gag reflex, you should immediately remove the ETC and prepare to suction the patient. *(p. 1217)*

5. a. When inserting the LMA, you should advance the airway until resistance is met. *(p. 1219)*

6. c. Capnometry is the process of monitoring the exhaled carbon dioxide in the body. *(p. 1209)*

7. c. The normal physiological range for $ETCO_2$ is about 38–42 mmHg. End-tidal CO_2 ($ETCO_2$) represents the measurement of the CO_2 concentration at the end of expiration, which correlates with the maximum CO_2 content in the exhaled gas. *(p. 1209)*

8. a. The Bougie (Eschmann) tracheal-tube introducer is advanced during laryngoscopy so that the bent tip is inserted past the epiglottis and vocal cords into the trachea. After you feel the "bumps" of the tracheal rings and confirming the device is in the trachea, you should pass the tracheal tube over the end and into the trachea. Then the Bougie is removed; confirm ET placement. *(pp. 1210–1211)*

ANSWERS TO COURSE REVIEW SELF-TEST

The numbers following each answer refer to the textbook page(s) where the answer can be found or supported.

CH 1 1. d. *(p. 4)*

CH 8 2. b. *(p. 221)*   3. a. *(p. 224)*
4. d. *(p. 225)*

CH 9 5. b. *(p. 245)* 6. c. *(p. 346)* 7. b. *(p. 253)*
8. a. *(p. 259)* 9. b. *(p. 266)* 10. a. *(p. 286)*
11. c. *(p. 296)* 12. d. *(p. 302)* 13. b. *(p. 311)*
14. b. *(p. 318)* 15. c. *(pp. 310, 321)*

CH 14 16. d. *(p. 424)* 17. b. *(p. 427)*

CH 6 18. b. *(p. 127)* 19. a. *(p. 129)*

CH 39 20. d. *(p. 1110)*

CH 6 21. d. *(p. 139)*

CH 25 22. a. *(p. 694)* 23. a. *(p. 690)*
24. b. *(p. 691)* 25. d. *(p. 689)* 26. d. *(p. 690)*
27. b. *(p. 702)* 28. c. *(p. 711)*

CH 36 29. c. *(p. 992)* 30. b. *(p. 1008)*

CH 7 31. d. *(p. 171)* 32. c. *(p. 172)*
33. b. *(p. 173)* 34. a. *(p. 180)* 35. b. *(p. 197)*
36. d. *(p. 190)* 37. c. *(p. 195)* 38. d. *(p. 201)*
39. b. *(p. 203)* 40. c. *(p. 205)*

CH 15 41. b. *(p. 471)* 42. b. *(p. 475)*

CH 5 43. c. *(p. 107)* 44. a. *(p. 120)*
45. c. *(p. 104)*

CH 2 46. a. *(p. 25)* 47. c. *(p. 27)* 48. b. *(p. 28)*

CH 27 49. b. *(p. 749)* 50. c. *(p. 751)*
51. b. *(p. 761)*

CH 36 52. c. *(p. 989)* 53. a. *(pp. 996)*
54. b. *(p. 998)* 55. d. *(p. 999)* 56. a. *(p. 1001)*
57. d. *(p. 1024)* 58. c. *(p. 1026)* 59. b. *(p. 1037)*

CH 41 60. b. *(p. 1148)* 61. b. *(p. 1150)*

CH 13 62. b. *(p. 380)* 63. b. *(p. 386)*
64. c. *(p. 381)* 65. a. *(pp. 382, 385)*
66. c. *(p. 382)* 67. a. *(p. 388)*

CH 28 68. c. *(p. 777)* 69. a. *(p. 783)*
70. c. *(p. 783)*

CH 16 71. d. *(pp. 492–494)*
72. d. *(p. 501)*

CH 3 73. a. *(p. 45)* 74. d. *(p. 49)*

CH 14 75. c. *(p. 416)* 76. b. *(pp. 441, 446)*
77. c. *(p. 427)* 78. a. *(p. 446)* 79. b. *(p. 446)*

CH 29 80. b. *(p. 803)* 81. b. *(p. 810)*

CH 24 82. d. *(p. 674)* 83. b. *(p. 678)*

CH 11 84. c. *(p. 351)* 85. c. *(p. 350)*

CH 40 86. d. *(p. 1124)* 87. b. *(p. 1131)*
88. d. *(p. 1129)*

CH 32 89. b. *(p. 869)* 90. d. *(p. 871)*
91. c. *(p. 811)* 92. c. *(p. 893)* 93. a. *(p. 877)*

CH 19 94. a. *(pp. 551, 552)* 95. b. *(p. 557)*
96. d. *(p. 559)*

CH 35 97. b. *(p. 976)* 98. d. *(p. 979)*

CH 4 99. b. *(p. 62)* 100. a. *(p. 62)*
101. c. *(pp. 98, 59)* 102. a. *(p. 79)*
103. b. *(p. 88)* 104. d. *(p. 98)*

CH 22 105. b. *(p. 618)* 106. b. *(p. 619)*
107. d. *(p. 619)* 108. b. *(p. 637)*
109. d. *(p. 642)*

CH 31 110. c. *(p. 859)* 111. b. *(pp. 866, 854)*

CH 21 112. c. *(pp. 610–611)* 113. a. *(p. 603)*

CH 37 114. d. *(p. 1057)* 115. d. *(p. 1058)*
116. d. *(p. 1063)*

CH 39 117. c. *(p. 1107)* 118. a. *(p. 1108)*

CH 26 119. d. *(p. 730)* 120. b. *(p. 734)*
121. d. *(p. 739)* 122. c. *(p. 740)*
123. a. *(p. 740)* 124. d. *(p. 741)*

CH 30 125. d. *(p. 831)* 126. c. *(p. 831)*
127. a. *(p. 836)*

CH 10 128. b. *(p. 336)* 129. a. *(p. 339)*

CH 23 130. b. *(p. 655)* 131. c. *(p. 658)*

CH 38 132. b. *(p. 1078)* 133. d. *(pp. 1079–1080)* 134. c. *(p. 1082)* 135. d. *(p. 1093)* 136. c. *(p. 1094)*

CH 17 137. d. *(p. 511)* 138. b. *(p. 513)*

CH 20 139. a. *(p. 577)* 140. a. *(p. 583)*

CH 33 141. c. *(p. 922)* 142. a. *(p. 923)* 143. a. *(p. 925)* 144. a. *(p. 928)* 145. c. *(p. 936)*

CH 18 146. c. *(p. 538)* 147. c. *(pp. 532–533)*

CH 34 148. d. *(p. 950)* 149. a. *(p. 951)* 150. b. *(p. 959)*

CH 42 151. a. *(p. 1161)* 152. b. *(p. 1175)*

CH 43 (OPTIONAL: ADVANCED AIRWAY)
153. c. *(p. 1186)* 154. b. *(p. 1186)* 155. a. *(p. 1186)* 156. d. *(p. 1188)* 157. c. *(p. 1191)* 158. a. *(p. 1201)* 159. d. *(p. 1204)* 160. b. *(p. 1206)*

Answers to Course Review Self-Test   **487**

In addition to oxygen, there are six medications the EMT can administer or assist the patient in administering, with on-line or off-line approval from medical direction. They are activated charcoal, aspirin, epinephrine by auto-injector, metered dose inhaler, nitroglycerin, and oral glucose. Detailed information on each of these medications (as listed in the U.S. Department of Transportation's 1994 *Emergency Medical Technician-Basic: National Standard Curriculum*) is provided on the next pages in a format that you may cut from the book and carry with you for reference.

ACTIVATED CHARCOAL

Medication Name: Activated charcoal, SuperChar, InstaChar, Actidose, LiquiChar

Indications: Patients who have ingested poisons by mouth; administer after receiving orders from medical direction or the poison control center.

Contraindications: (1) Altered mental status (not fully conscious) (2) Swallowed acids or alkalis (3) Unable to swallow

Medication Form: 12.5 grams premixed in water; powder form should be avoided.

Dosage: 1 gram of activated charcoal per kilogram of body weight; usual adult dose 25 to 50 grams, infants and children 12.5 to 25 grams.

(see over)

ASPIRIN

Medication Name: ASA, Bayer, Ecotrin, St. Joseph's, Bufferin

Indications: Chest discomfort that is suggestive of a heart attack and approval from medical direction.

Contraindications: Patient with a known allergy to the drug. Relative contraindication: May trigger wheezing in patients with asthma.

Medication Form: Tablet

Dosage: 160–325 mg; recommended that 160 mg of baby aspirin be chewed and a second 160 mg aspirin be swallowed.

(see over)

Activated Charcoal (continued)

Administration: Consult medical direction; shake container; encourage patient to drink through a straw from a covered container; record time and response; if patient vomits, notify medical direction for repeat dose.

Actions: Binds with poisons in the stomach and prevents their absorption into the body

Side Effects: Blackening of the stools, possible vomiting

Reassessment: (1) Check for abdominal pain or distress upon administration. (2) Watch for vomiting; position the patient and be prepared to suction.

Aspirin (continued)

Administration: Determine the patient is suffering from an acute syndrome suggestive of a heart attack; obtain approval to administer the medication; ensure the aspirin is 160 mg or 325 mg and it is not expired; ensure the patient is alert and oriented; if baby aspirin, have patient chew a 160-mg tablet followed by swallowing a second 160-mg tablet; reassess the patient and record the vital signs.

Actions: Decreases the ability of platelets to clump together; this reduces the formation of additional clots at the site of the coronary artery blockage.

Side Effects: Generally few side effects; patients may report stomach irritation or heartburn, nausea, or vomiting.

Reassessment: Perform a reassessment after administration and perform an ongoing reassessment. The aspirin is not being used as a pain reliever but to prevent platelets from continuing to clump together and occlude the coronary artery. Record any changes in the patient's condition.

EPINEPHRINE AUTO-INJECTOR

Medication Name: Epinephrine, Adrenalin, EpiPen®, EpiPen® Jr.

Indications: (1) Signs and symptoms of a severe allergic reaction (anaphylaxis). (2) Medication is prescribed to the patient. (3) EMT has received an order from medical direction.

Contraindications: None, when used in the life-threatening allergic reaction

Medication Form: Liquid drug contained within an auto-injector

Dosage: Auto-injectors deliver a single dose; adult dose 0.3 mg, infant and child 0.15 mg

Administration: Push the uncapped tip of the auto-injector firmly against the lateral aspect of the thigh until the needle is deployed and the medication delivered.

(see over)

METERED DOSE INHALER

Medication Name: Albuterol, Metaproterenol, Isoetharine, Proventil®, Ventolin®, Metaprel®, Alupent®, Bronkosol®, Bronkometer®

Indications: (1) Exhibits signs and symptoms of breathing difficulty. (2) Patient has a physician-prescribed MDI. (3) EMT has received medical direction approval.

Contraindications: (1) Patient is not responsive enough to use the MDI. (2) MDI is not prescribed for the patient. (3) Maximum dose allowed is reached prior to your arrival. (4) Permission denied by medical direction.

Medication Form: Aerosolized medication in a metered dose inhaler

Dosage: Each depression of the MDI delivers a precise dose. The number of times the medication can be delivered is determined by medical direction.

(see over)

NITROGLYCERIN

Medication Name: Nitroglycerin, Nitrostat®, Nitrobid®, Nitrolingual® Spray

Indications: (1) Patient exhibits signs and symptoms of chest pain. (2) Patient has physician-prescribed nitroglycerin. (3) EMT has approval from medical direction.

Contraindications: (1) Baseline blood pressure below 100 mmHg systolic. (2) Suspected head injury. (3) Patient is a child or infant. (4) Three doses have already been taken.

Medication Form: Tablet or sublingual spray

Dosage: One tablet or one spray under the tongue; may be repeated in 3 to 5 minutes if (1) Patient experiences no relief. (2) Blood pressure remains above 100 mmHg systolic. (3) Medical direction gives approval.

(see over)

Epinephrine Auto-Injector (continued)

Actions: Mimics the response of the sympathetic nervous system:
(1) Constricts blood vessels to improve the blood pressure. (2) Relaxes smooth muscles in the lungs to improve breathing. (3) Stimulates the heartbeat. (4) Reverses swelling and hives.

Side Effects: Increased heart rate, pale skin (pallor), dizziness, chest pain, headache, nausea and vomiting, excitability and anxiousness

Reassessment: (1) Reassess for decreasing mental status, decreasing blood pressure, increased breathing difficulties. (2) If condition worsens you may have to call medical direction for second dose, treat for hypoperfusion, may need CPR and use of the AED.

Metered Dose Inhaler (continued)

Administration: (1) Ensure the medication is the patient's and the patient is alert; determine number of doses administered prior to your arrival. (2) Obtain order from medical direction. (3) Assure the MDI is at room temperature, shake for 30 seconds. (4) Administer while the patient is inhaling; encourage him to hold breath.

Actions: Beta agonist, relaxes the bronchiole smooth muscles, dilates the lower airway

Side Effects: Tachycardia, tremors, shakiness, nervousness, dry mouth

Reassessment: Perform an ongoing assessment, reassess vital signs, question patient about effect, focused history and physical exam, monitor airway, record and document.

Nitroglycerin (continued)

Administration: (1) Assure medication is the patient's, blood pressure greater than 100 mmHg systolic, approval from medical direction. (2) Assure patient is alert; check expiration date; ask patient when he took his last dose. (3) Place or spray medication under the tongue; keep mouth closed. (4) Reassess the blood pressure in 2 minutes; record your actions.

Actions: Relaxes blood vessels, decreases workload of the heart

Side Effects: Vessel dilation may cause headache, drop in blood pressure, pulse rate changes.

Reassessment: (1) Monitor blood pressure. (2) Question patient about effect. (3) Obtain approval from medical direction before re-administering. (4) Record and document all findings and reassessment.

ORAL GLUCOSE

Medication Name: Oral glucose, Glutose®, Insta-Glucose®

Indication: (1) Altered mental status with (2) history of diabetes controlled by medication and (3) ability to swallow the medication

Contraindications: (1) Unconscious (2) Unable to swallow the medication

Medication Form: Gel, in a toothpaste-type tube

Dosage: Typical dose is one tube.

Administration: Oral, squeeze or place a portion between the cheek and gum.

Action: Increases blood- and brain-sugar levels

(see over)

Oral Glucose (continued)

Side Effects: May cause an airway obstruction in the patient without a gag reflex

Reassessment: Reassess the mental status to determine if the drug has had an effect.